Seventh Edition

Skin Diseases and

Sexually Transmitted Infections

Text with Multiple Choice Questions

Seventh Edition

Skin Diseases and Sexually Transmitted Infections

Text with Multiple Choice Questions

Uday Khopkar
Professor and Head
Department of Dermatology
KEM Hospital and Seth GS Medical College
Parel, Mumbai, Maharashtra

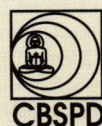

CBS Publishers & Distributors Pvt Ltd

New Delhi • Bengaluru • Chennai • Kochi • Kolkata • Lucknow • Mumbai
Hyderabad • Jharkhand • Nagpur • Patna • Pune • Uttarakhand

Seventh Edition

Skin
Diseases and
Sexually Transmitted
Infections

with Multiple Choice Questions

ISBN: 978-93-88108-45-4

Copyright © Author and Publisher

Seventh Edition 2019
  Reprint 2023, 2024
First Edition 1996
Second Edition 1997
Third Edition 1999
Fourth Edition 2001
  Reprint 2002, 2003
Fifth Edition 2004
  Reprint 2005, 2006
Sixth Edition 2009
  Revised Reprint 2011
  Reprint 2013, 2018

Published by Satish Kumar Jain and produced by Varun Jain for

CBS Publishers & Distributors Pvt Ltd
4819/XI Prahlad Street, 24 Ansari Road, Daryaganj, New Delhi 110 002, India
Ph: 011-23289259, 23266838

Website: www.cbspd.com
e-mail: delhi@cbspd.com

Corporate Office: 204 FIE, Industrial Area, Patparganj, Delhi 110 092, India
Ph: 0114934 4934   Fax: 011-4934 4935   e-mail: publishing@cbspd.com; publicity@cbspd.com

Branches

- **Bengaluru:** Seema House 2975, 17th Cross, K.R. Road, Banasankari 2nd Stage, Bengaluru 560 070, Karnataka, India
  Ph: +91-80-26771678/79   Fax: +91-80-26771680   e-mail: bangalore@cbspd.com
- **Chennai:** 7, Subbaraya Street, Shenoy Nagar, Chennai 600 030, Tamil Nadu, India
  Ph: +91-44-26680620, 26681266   Fax: +91-44-42032115   e-mail: chennai@cbspd.com
- **Kochi:** 42/1325, 1326, Power House Road, Opp KSEB, Power House, Ernakulam, Kochi, 682 018, Kerala, India
  Ph: +91-484-4059061-65,67   Fax: +91-484-4059065   e-mail: kochi@cbspd.com
- **Kolkata:** 147, Hind Ceramics Compound, 1st Floor, Nilgunj Road, Belghoria, Kolkata 700 056, West Bengal, India
  Ph: +91-33-25633055/56   e-mail: kolkata@cbspd.com
- **Lucknow:** Basement, Khushnuma Complex, 7-Meerabai Marg (behind Jawahar Bhawan), Lucknow 226 001, UP, India
  Ph: +91-522-4000032   e-mail: tiwari.lucknow@cbspd.com
- **Mumbai:** PWD Shed, Gala no. 25/26, Ramchandra Bhatt Marg, Next to JJ Hospital Gate no. 2,
  Opp. Union Bank of India, Noorbaug, Mumbai 400 009, Maharashtra, India
  Ph: +91-22-66661880/89   e-mail: mumbai@cbspd.com

Representatives

• **Hyderabad**	0-9885175004	• **Jharkhand**	0-9811541605	• **Nagpur**	0-8692091830
• **Patna**	0-9334159340	• **Pune**	0-9664372571	• **Uttarakhand**	0-9716462459

Printed at: Goyal Offset Works Pvt. Ltd, Kundli, Sonipat, Haryana

to

my parents
who, even now, toil
ceaselessly & silently
for me

Foreword

I have great pleasure in writing the Foreword to this handbook meant for undergraduate students. My pleasure in writing this foreword is multiplied by the fact that the author, Dr Uday Khopkar is my closet colleague. Since more than a decade, Dr Uday Khopkar has been taking keen interest in the conduct and teaching of undergraduate and postgraduate students and hence, has been able to gauge the pulse of our students as also their needs and requirements.

In this era of information explosion, a student has to study more and more materials and with this in mind, any attempt to ease the burden of studying for examinations is welcome. At the present moment, there is hardly any book authored by an Indian and meant for undergraduates. This book will serve to fill up this lacuna in undergraduate teaching material.

The book has also discussed many subjects with a clinical orientation. Important clinical points are highlighted in each section and are supported by an array of depictive illustration. In keeping with their public health importance, the subjects of leprosy and STDs, including HIV infection, have been dealt within detail. This would make the book useful from the viewpoint of general practitioners as well.

I wish all the success to this utility oriented book which will prove to be a boon for students and practitioners.

Dr SL Wadhwa
Ex. Professor and Head
Department of Dermatology
TN Medical College and Nair Hospital,
Mumbai 400 008

Preface to the Seventh Edition

I have tried to keep the book student-friendly like before and hope that the students continue to benefit from it. Some new chapters or topics have been added while, keeping with times, some others have been abridged.

I thank all those who have contributed to this effort. Especially noteworthy has been the contribution of Dr Akansha Chadha who has helped me not just embellishing the text but also ridding the book of errors. I thank all my postgraduates and colleagues for helping me with fresh clinical photographs as many of the old photos had to be replaced.

I thank CBS Publishers and Distributors and their team for bringing it out in an improved printing format and Mr Rajesh Bhalani for all the coordination efforts. I also appreciate the carefully redrawn diagrams by Mr Dattaram Wadekar. I also thank Mr Ramesh Krishnamachari for his meticulous and painstaking editing job.

Wishing all my dear students easy reading!

Uday Khopkar

Preface to the First Edition

As is true for attainment of knowledge in any field of science, there are three basic levels of attainment in the discipline of dermatology. First is survival, i.e. it allows a person to pass a certain standard set forth by the society. Second is skill, i.e. it makes a person an expert clinician who can diagnose common as well as the rare disorders with equal ease. Third and final is understanding, i.e. it enlightens a person about the intricate pathomechanisms of different diseases and various factors contributing to their occurrence. It is only when this last level of attainment of knowledge is reached can the training be said to near completion. Although it is desirable to attain this ideal this book obviously concerns itself with the first knowledge level necessary for success at undergraduate examinations!

No attempt has been made to make this a comprehensive text on the subject. Topics important from examination and practical standpoint are dealt within piecemeal fashion. Sections on Leprosy, STDs and HIV infection are more detailed due to their importance. Readers are requested to bring to the author's notice any errors of omission or commission, so that they may be corrected in future. However, broad generalisations and purposeful oversimplifications have been made, at times, even at the risk of minor inaccuracies.

Several individuals have contributed in bringing out this handbook. Dr Rajiv Joshi helped in ridding the book of serious errors and in taking and selecting photographs. Dr Rajeshree Chavan drew the sketches. Dr Aparna Santhanam helped in reading proofs. Dr SL Wadhwa, apart from providing encouragement and material in this venture, has been my teacher in clinical dermatology and venereology and it is my pleasure and good fortune to put some of his teachings in print through this small venture. Bhalani Publishers and, Mr Rajesh Bhalani and Mr Suketu Deliwala in particular, took great efforts to see that the publication came out in time and shape. My sincere thanks to all these individuals without whom it would have been impossible to bring out this handbook. I am especially greatful to our hospital Dean. Dr (Mrs) KD Nihalani who not only permitted me the use of our hospital patient's photographs for this publication but has also served as a source of constant encouragement and inspiration in our efforts to develop our department. I am also thankful to Dr RG Valia who kindly consented to review this manuscript and to Dr SL Wadhawa for acceding to all the demands that I made including a request to pen the forward.

With hope that this venture proves useful to those for whom it is meant.

Uday Khopkar

Contents

Section 1: BASIC CONSIDERATIONS

Section 2: SKIN DISEASES

Section 3: SEXUALLY TRANSMITTED INFECTIONS INCLUDING HIV INFECTION

Section 4: DERMATOTHERAPEUTICS

SECTION 1

Basic Considerations

Structure and Functions of Skin

STRUCTURE OF SKIN

Epidermis is the keratinising stratified squamous epithelium that covers the body. Under it lies the dermis and the subcutaneous fat (hypodermis). Within the dermis are present epidermal appendages viz. hair follicles, eccrine and apocrine sweat units and nail units. Structure of skin is shown in Fig. 1.1.

Epidermis

Epidermis provides a tough, dry and semipermeable covering for the body (Fig. 1.2). It does this by producing a protein called keratin. Hence, epidermal cells are known as keratinocytes. The epidermal basal layer is the germinative layer of the epidermis and is thus continuously multiplying. Ordinarily, epidermal layer is 10–15 cells thick.

As the basal columnar epidermal cells multiply, mature and produce more and more keratin, they move up towards the surface and assume polygonal shapes. These polygonal cells are connected to each other by desmosomal bridges that are seen as spines under the ordinary microscope. Hence,

this layer, which forms the substance of the epidermis, is known as the spinous layer (stratum spinosum).

Further maturation and upward movement of keratinocytes is accompanied by appearance of keratohyaline granules within the cells, which now become flattened (elongated on cross section). This layer is called granular layer (stratum granulosum). Keratohyaline granules provide the matrix for the fibrous protein, keratin.

Stratum corneum or the cornified layer is the topmost layer of epidermis. Its fully matured red cells contain keratin in its final form. As keratinocytes mature they lose their nuclei and cellular organelles and hence the stratum corneum cells are dead cells without nuclei. After some days, these cornified cells are gradually shed as individual squames and their place is taken by newly formed cells.

Epidermis is thus in a state of dynamic balance between multiplication of basal cells and shedding of cornified cells.

Melanin, the pigment responsible for skin colour, is made by melanocytes. Melanocytes are situated in the basal layer of the skin and distribute

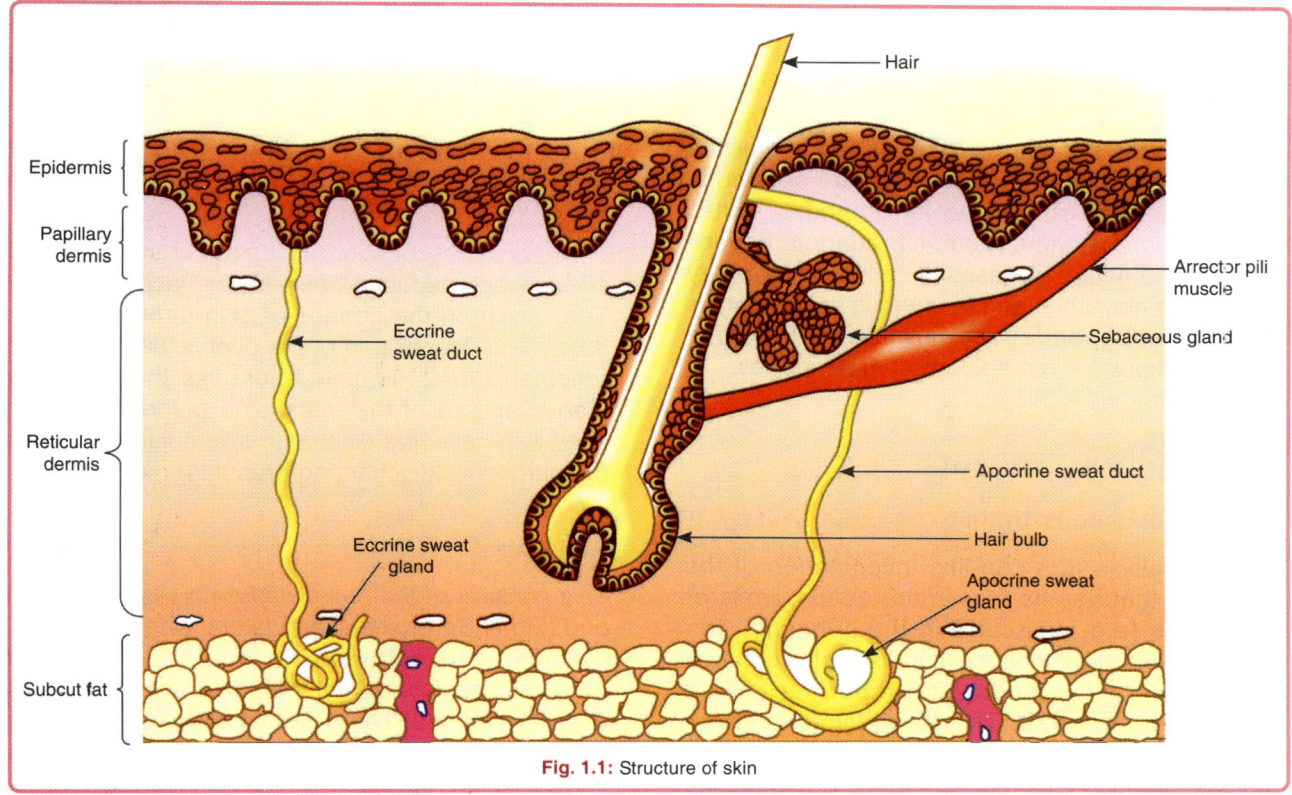

Epidermis
Papillary dermis
Reticular dermis
Subcut fat

Hair
Arrector pili muscle
Sebaceous gland
Apocrine sweat duct
Hair bulb
Apocrine sweat gland
Eccrine sweat duct
Eccrine sweat gland

Fig. 1.1: Structure of skin

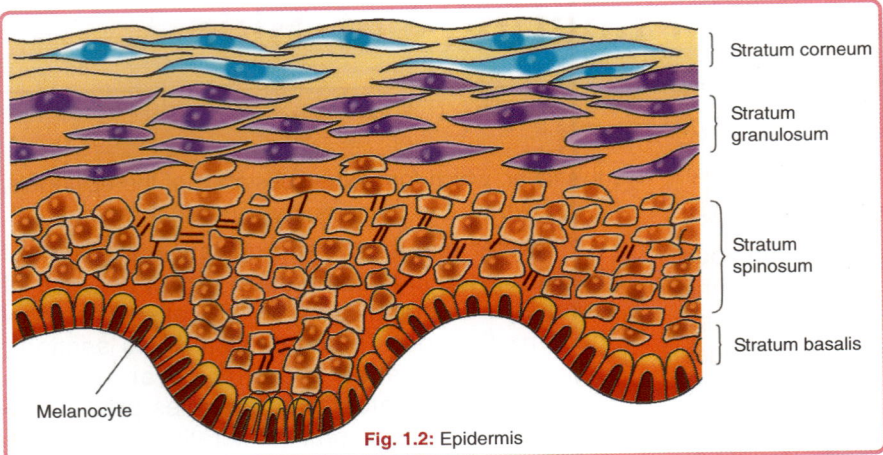
Fig. 1.2: Epidermis

their pigments by means of dendrites to the surrounding keratinocytes.

> **Dermoepidermal junction :** The epidermal-dermal interface is not a straight line but an undulating one. The alternating thicker parts of the epidermis are known as the rete pegs as they fit like pegs into complementary valleys in the papillary dermis. The corresponding alternating projecting parts of the papillary dermis are called dermal papillae. The dermoepidermal junction is also known as the basement membrane zone (BMZ). It consists of a lamina lucida, lamina densa and anchoring filaments.

Dermis

The dermis is made up of reticular dermis, which forms the substance of the skin, and the adventitial dermis. Reticular dermis provides strength and resilience to the skin through the collagen and elastic fibres that constitute it. These fibres are situated in a 'watery' matrix of mucopolysaccharides, called the ground substance. Adventitial dermis houses vascular and neural plexuses. It comprises papillary dermis that nourishes and innervates the epidermis and the periappendageal dermis that does the same functions for the epidermal appendages.

CUTANEOUS APPENDAGES

Folliculosebaceous Units

The hair follicle is a cup-like invagination of the epidermis that has its root in the deep dermis or sometimes (e.g. on scalp) in the subcutis. The germinative and matrical cells in its root produce a different keratin product that emerges on the surface as hair shaft. The hair follicle is continuously passing through the growth phase (anagen), degeneration phase (catagen) and resting phase (telogen). (Please *see* chapter on alopecia for details). Hair follicles are present all over the body, except the palms/soles and mucocutaneous junctions. However, in some regions, e.g. over face, hair shafts are very thin and short (vellus hair), so that the hair are hardly visible.

The sebaceous glands are lobulated structures that produce sebum. Sebum is produced as a holocrine secretion by discharging the whole of the mature fat laden sebocytes into sebaceous ducts that open into the follicular canal. Arrector pili muscles attach to the deeper portion of follicles and straighten them under the influence of the autonomic nerves (resulting in goose pimples). The point of attachment of arrector pilorum muscle is thicker than the rest of the follicle and is called the 'bulge' of the follicle. The follicular stem cells reside in the bulge area of the follicle. During early anagen, a new follicle develops from these cells.

Apocrine Sweat Units

These are present only in the axillae, groins, areola, perianal and perigenital regions. They may open into follicles or on the surface of skin through apocrine ducts. The apocrine gland is a coiled structure that lies at the junction of the dermis and subcutis, and is lined by secretory cells that make the apocrine sweat by discharging their terminal portions into the lumen by a process of 'pinching off'.

Eccrine Sweat Units

These are present over most parts of the body and are concentrated over palms/soles, face and scalp. They open on the surface of skin through eccrine ducts. The deeper part of the duct, situated in deep reticular dermis, is coiled, just like the secretory glandular part of the units. The glandular part is lined with cells that discharge sweat into the lumen by merocrine (discharging granules) method.

Nail Unit

This consists of the nail plate which sits on the nail bed (Fig. 1.3). Proximal and lateral sides of the nail plate fit into cutaneous invaginations called proximal and lateral nail folds that are continuous with the nail bed. The potential space between the nail plate and the proximal and lateral nail folds is sealed by the cuticle which is an extension of the

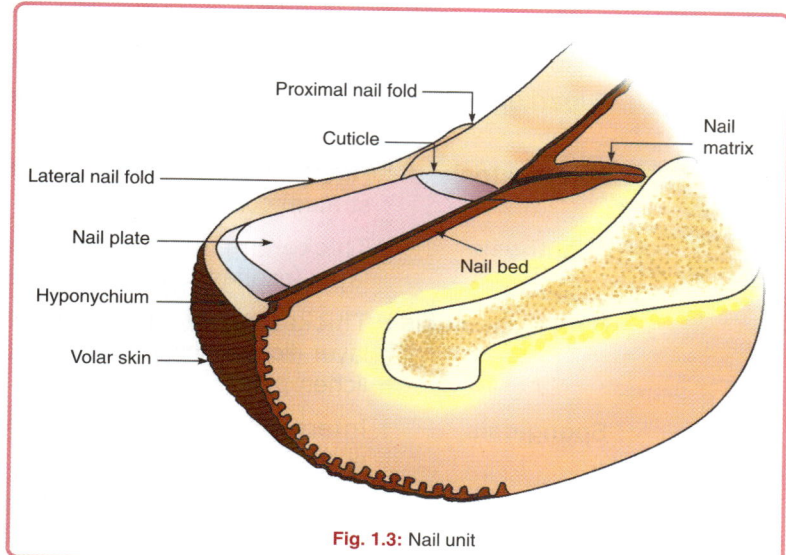

Fig. 1.3: Nail unit

stratum corneum of nail folds onto the nail plate. The proximal nail fold contains the nail matrix, the keratinocytes of which mature (keratinize) and form the nail plate.

Hypodermis (Subcutaneous Fat)

This is arranged as fat lobules that contain individual fat cells (adipocytes) amid a rich vascular plexus. The lobules are separated by fibrous septa that house larger vessels and nerves.

Organelles for Sensations

Special organelles are present in the skin for sensing various physical stimuli. Pain, temperature, crude touch and itch sensations are detected by free nerve endings. Meissner's corpuscles mediate the sensation of fine touch and are present mainly over the palms and soles. Pacinian corpuscles sense pressure and are also found over palms and soles. Sensation of cold is perceived by end bulb of Krause while end organ of Ruffini detects the sensation of heat.

Summary : Skin consists of the epidermis, dermis and hypodermis. Epidermal cells (keratinocytes) are continually multiplying and maturing (keratinising) to provide the protective stratum corneum. The epidermal layers from base to the top are stratum basalis, stratum spinosum, stratum granulosum and stratum corneum. Melanocytes within the epidermis produce melanin. Dermis consists of connective tissue, blood vessels and nerves situated in a matrix of 'ground substance'. Folliculosebaceous units, eccrine and apocrine sweat units and nail units are the cutaneous appendages.

FUNCTIONS OF SKIN

Skin is the largest organ of the body, both in terms of volume and weight. Its functions are as follows.

Protective Interface

The keratinised epidermis acts as an effective barrier against a variety of insults. These may be:

- **Chemical** (because it is impermeable to harmful water soluble substances).
- **Mechanical** (because the skin is tough and the subcutaneous fat provides a cushioning effect against blunt trauma).
- **Biological** (dryness, acidic pH and protective normal flora ward off infections).
- **Radiational** (melanin, the protective skin pigment, absorbs a wide range of harmful rays and hence minimises the risk of skin cancers).

Sensitive Interface

The sensations of touch, pain, temperature, etc., are essential for **protection** against danger. The sensation of touch is also used, between individuals, to express **emotions.** Facial skin reacts to emotions very fast.

Maintaining Balances

Skin maintains **water and electrolyte** balance by avoiding undue evaporation of body water or absorption of it. It has the capacity to concentrate or dilute sodium in sweat.

It maintains **thermal balance** by:
- Increased sweating causes cooling due to evaporation of sweat.
- Subcutaneous fat protects against excessive cold.
- The amount of blood flowing through the skin can be varied by peripheral vasodilation and opening up of arteriovenous shunts. This can suitably adjust the core temperature.

By peripheral vasodilation or constriction skin helps in maintaining normal **blood volume.**

Other Metabolic Functions

In the presence of sunlight, skin **manufactures vitamin D** from cholesterol. Subcutaneous fat acts

Chapter 1

Structure and Functions of Skin

as a storehouse of energy in the form of fat. Fat cells actively participate in the dynamic lipid metabolism.

Aesthetic Function

Smooth, soft glowing skin is aesthetically valued. Feminine 'curves' and masculine 'cuts' are largely on account of the difference in the distribution of subcutaneous fat between women and men.

> **Summary :** Skin not only serves the function of a protective and sensitive interface between the internal milieu of the body and the external environment, but also participates in regulating body temperature, water and electrolyte balance.

Pathology of the Skin

A skin biopsy is frequently needed to make or confirm a diagnosis in patients who pose diagnostic difficulty or do not respond adequately to therapy. Compared to biopsies of other organs, it is relatively non-invasive, can be carried out in a dermatologist's office under local anaesthesia and usually causes only an insignificant scar. Various terms are used to describe the skin pathology under the microscope. Some of those terms are :

Hyperkeratosis	: Thickening of stratum corneum (lichen simplex chronicus)
Parakeratosis	: Retention of nuclei by cells in stratum corneum (psoriasis)
Acanthosis	: Thickening of the spinous layer (psoriasis, lichen planus)
Hypergranulosis	: Thickening of the granular layer (lichen simplex chronicus, lichen planus)
Spongiosis	: Intercellular oedema of the spinous layer (eczemas)
Ballooning	: Intracellular oedema of keratinocytes (herpes infection)
Acantholysis	: Separation of keratinocytes due to loss of intercellular bridges (pemphigus)
Dyskeratosis	: Collection of abnormal keratin within keratinocytes (squamous cell carcinoma, inherited disorders of keratinisation like Darier's disease)

MCQs

1. **The most superficial layer of epidermis is:**
   a. Stratum germinativum
   b. Stratum corneum
   c. Stratum lucidum
   d. Stratum granulosum

2. **The lowermost layer of epidermis is:**
   a. Stratum germinativum
   b. Stratum corneum
   c. Stratum lucidum
   d. Stratum granulosum

3. **The germinative layer of epidermis is called:**
   a. Stratum basalis
   b. Stratum corneum
   c. Stratum lucidum
   d. Stratum granulosum

4. **The non-nucleated layer of epidermis is called:**
   a. Stratum basalis
   b. Stratum corneum
   c. Stratum malpighi
   d. Stratum granulosum

5. **The nucleated epidermis is called:**
   a. Stratum basalis
   b. Stratum corneum
   c. Stratum malpighi
   d. Stratum granulosum

6. **The term 'spines' in the epidermis refers to:**
   a. Keratohyaline granules
   b. Odland bodies
   c. Hemidesmosomes
   d. Desmosomes

7. **Cells of this layer of epidermis are columnar:**
   a. Stratum basalis
   b. Stratum spinosum
   c. Stratum malpighi
   d. Stratum granulosum

8. **Cells of this layer of epidermis are polygonal:**
   a. Stratum basalis
   b. Stratum spinosum
   c. Stratum germinativum
   d. Stratum granulosum

9. **The main protein in the epidermis is called:**
   a. Desmin
   b. Collagen
   c. Elastin
   d. Keratin

10. **The cells of epidermis are held together by:**
    a. Keratohyaline granules
    b. Odland bodies
    c. Hemidesmosomes
    d. Desmosomes

11. **The barrier of the epidermis lies within the:**
    a. Stratum basalis
    b. Stratum spinosum
    c. Basement membrane
    d. Stratum corneum

12. **Which of the following is a function of the skin?**
    a. Protect against mechanical, chemical or biological attack
    b. Maintain water and electrolyte balance
    c. Maintain body temperature
    d. All of the above

13. **The term hypodermis refers to:**
    a. Epidermis
    b. Lower part of dermis
    c. Reticular dermis
    d. Subcutaneous fat

14. **The cell organelles that help in maintaining the barrier function of the skin are:**
    a. Keratohyaline granules
    b. Odland bodies
    c. Hemidesmosomes
    d. Desmosomes

15. **The layer of epidermis which is usually seen only on the palms and soles is:**
    a. Stratum basalis
    b. Stratum spinosum
    c. Stratum lucidum
    d. Stratum granulosum

16. **Apocrine glands are present at all the following sites *except*:**
    a. Palms and soles
    b. Areola
    c. Perineum
    d. Axillae

17. **The apocrine duct opens into:**
    a. Acrosyringium
    b. Infundibulum
    c. Sebaceous duct
    d. None of these

Chapter

1

Structure and Functions of Skin

18. **The process of secretion of apocrine sweat is called:**
    a. Pinching off
    b. Apocopation
    c. Merocrine
    d. Holocrine

19. **The process of secretion of eccrine sweat is called:**
    a. Apocopation
    b. Holocrine
    c. Merocrine
    d. Pinching off

20. **Maximum density of eccrine glands is found on:**
    a. Palms and soles
    b. Areola
    c. Perineum
    d. Axillae

21. **The spiral part of the eccrine duct within the epidermis is called:**
    a. Apocrine duct
    b. Eccrine pore
    c. Acrosyringium
    d. Infundibulum

22. **Which of the following skin glands has a lobulated structure?**
    a. Apocrine
    b. Sebaceous
    c. Eccrine
    d. Merocrine

23. **Sebaceous glands are a type of:**
    a. Eccrine glands
    b. Apocrine glands
    c. Holocrine glands
    d. Merocrine glands

24. **Glands involved in the pathogenesis of acne are:**
    a. Eccrine glands
    b. Apocrine glands
    c. Sebaceous glands
    d. Thyroid glands

25. **Receptors responsible for fine touch sensation are:**
    a. End bulb of Krause
    b. Pacinian corpuscle
    c. End organ of Ruffini
    d. Meissner's corpuscle

26. **Receptors responsible for pressure sensation are:**
    a. Free nerve endings
    b. Pacinian corpuscle
    c. End organ of Ruffini
    d. Meissner's corpuscle

27. **Receptors responsible for pain sensation are:**
    a. End bulb of Krause
    b. Merkel cells
    c. Free nerve endings
    d. Meissner's corpuscle

28. **Which of the following is not a dendritic cell in the epidermis?**
    a. Langerhans cell
    b. Merkel cell
    c. Melanocyte
    d. Dermal dendrocyte

29. **The part of the hair follicle to which the arrector pilorum muscle is attached is called:**
    a. Infundibulum
    b. Isthmus
    c. Bulge
    d. Bulb

30. **The part of the hair follicle in which the follicular stem cells reside is:**
    a. Matrix
    b. Germinative layer
    c. Bulge
    d. Bulb

31. **The germinative cells of the hair follicle reside in:**
    a. Infundibulum
    b. Isthmus
    c. Bulge
    d. Bulb

32. **The part of the hair follicle which is lined by layers resembling the epidermis is:**
    a. Infundibulum
    b. Stem
    c. Isthmus
    d. Bulb

33. **The growth phase of the hair follicle cycle is called:**
    a. Anagen
    b. Catagen
    c. Telogen
    d. Nanogen

34. **The number of scalp hair follicles at birth is approximately:**
    a. 10,000
    b. 100,000
    c. 10,00,000
    d. 10,000,000

35. **The resting phase of the hair follicle cycle is called:**
    a. Anagen
    b. Catagen
    c. Telogen
    d. Nanogen

36. **In healthy scalp at any given time the proportion of telogen follicles is about:**
    a. 1–2%
    b. 5%
    c. 10%
    d. 25%

37. **The nail plate is mainly produced by matrix cells located in the:**
    a. Nail bed
    b. Proximal nail fold
    c. Distal nail fold
    d. Lateral nail fold

38. **The nail plate is made of:**
    a. Hard collagen
    b. Calcium and phosphorus
    c. Keratin
    d. Elastin

Chapter
1

Structure and Functions of Skin

39. The rate of growth of nail is related to:
- a. Length of finger
- b. Age of person
- c. Physiological state
- d. All of the above

40. Which of the following cells is derived from the neural crest?
- a. Langerhans cells
- b. Keratinocyte
- c. Melanocytes
- d. Adipocytes

41. The basement membrane zone consists of all of the following *except*:
- a. Lamina lucida
- b. Desmosomes
- c. Anchoring filaments
- d. Lamina densa

42. Thickening of the spinous layer is called:
- a. Parakeratosis
- b. Acanthosis
- c. Spongiosis
- d. Dyskeratosis

43. The pigment responsible for absorbing harmful radiation is:
- a. Haeme
- b. Melanin
- c. Rhodopsin
- d. Carotene

44. The majority of the vellus hair is on:
- a. Axilla
- b. Scalp
- c. Face
- d. Perineum

45. The longest phase of the hair cycle is:
- a. Anagen
- b. Telogen
- c. Catagen
- d. Nanogen

Chapter 1

Structure and Functions of Skin

ANSWERS

1-b,	2-a,	3-a,	4-b,	5-c,	6-d,	7-a,	8-b,	9-d,	10-d,
11-d,	12-d,	13-d,	14-b,	15-c,	16-a,	17-b,	18-a,	19-c,	20-a,
21-c,	22-b,	23-c,	24-c,	25-d,	26-b,	27-c,	28-b,	29-c,	30-c,
31-d,	32-a,	33-a,	34-b,	35-c,	36-c,	37-b,	38-c,	39-d,	40-c,
41-b,	42-b,	43-b,	44-c,	45-a					

Section A: Basic Lesions: The Building Blocks of Dermatologic Description
Section B: Principles of Diagnosis

SECTION – A

Basic Lesions: Building Blocks of Dermatologic Description

Communication is the vital link in any scientific exchange. Communication in dermatology, which is a science based largely on visual information, needs exact description of the skin affection. Without intelligible description a bedside scientific dialogue could sound like:

- What is that?
- Psoriasis.
- How do you know?
- Because it looks like psoriasis.
- What does psoriasis look like?
- It looks like that!

Since English language did not have suitable terms for classifying skin lesions based on their morphology, new terms had to be invented. These terms are called basic lesions because they form the building blocks of accurate description of skin lesions. In order that the dermatologic terms used, are understood by both parties, it is necessary to ensure uniformity of meaning of these various terms.

Basic lesions in dermatology may either appear de novo (primary lesions) or may develop by a change in a preexisting lesion (secondary lesions). Traditionally, primary lesions include macule, patch, papule, plaque, nodule, vesicle, pustule and bulla. Secondary lesions like scale, crust, erosion, ulcer, etc. pertain to changes occurring in a primary lesion.

Parameters to be Noted in Detailed Description of Basic Lesions

- **Number :** Whether single, few, multiple, numerous or innumerable.
- **Size (in cm or inches) :** Whether much variation in size or of uniform size.
- **Shape :** Circular, oval, or polygonal.
- **Surface :** Smooth, rough, dry or oily.
- **Contour :** Rounded, conical/acuminate, dome shaped, or papillated.
- **Colour :** Hyperpigmented (brown, black, or bluish), hypopigmented, depigmented, red (bright red, dull red, etc.) or yellowish. Red colour of skin lesions is caused by either:
  - ❑ *Erythema,* temporary dilation of blood vessels (with resultant increase in blood flow) or
  - ❑ *Purpura,* extravasation of red blood cells (RBCs). Red colour due to purpura can't be blanched whereas that due to erythema can be blanched by light pressure.
  - ❑ *Telangiectasia* are due to permanent dilation of small blood vessels. They may be either linear, macular, papular, mat like or spider like.

Hence, a detailed morphologic description of the papular lesions of molluscum contagiosum would be 'multiple, 2–5 mm, round, smooth, dome shaped, pearly white papules'.

PRIMARY LESIONS

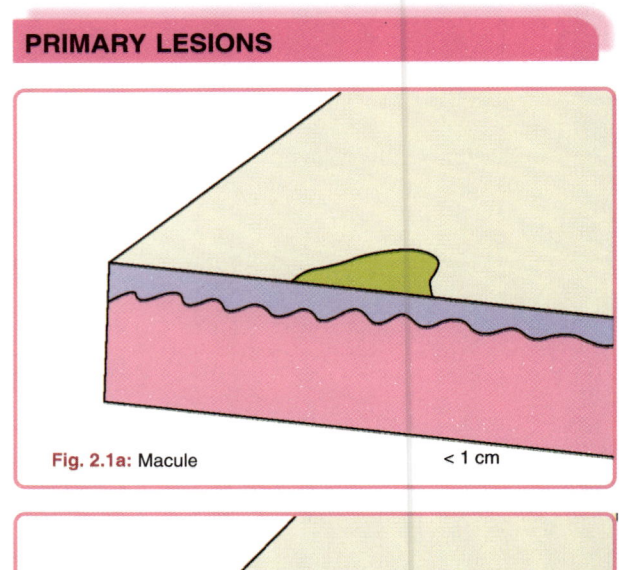

Fig. 2.1a: Macule   < 1 cm

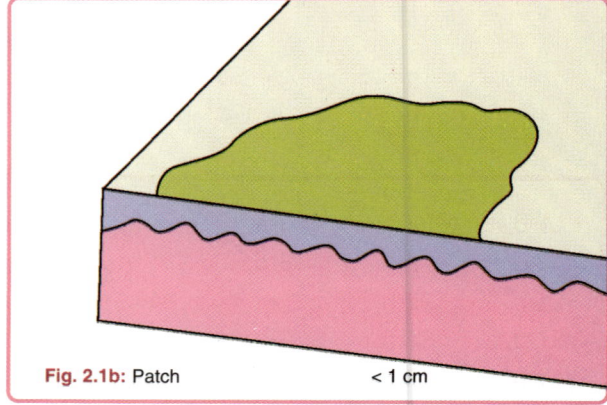

Fig. 2.1b: Patch   < 1 cm

TABLE 2.1 : Primary lesions of the skin		
Primary lesion	**Morphological subtype**	**Examples**
Macule: Circumscribed skin discoloration, less than 1 cm in diameter without any elevation or depression (Fig. 2.1a)	Hyperpigmented Hypopigmented Depigmented Dyspigmented Erythematous Purpuric	Freckles, lentigines, tattoo Pityriasis versicolor Vitiligo Morphea Rubella Thrombocytopenic purpura
Patch: Circumscribed skin discoloration, more than 1 cm in diameter, without any elevation or depression (Fig. 2.1b)	Hyperpigmented Hypopigmented Depigmented Erythematous Telangiectatic Purpuric	Café au lait spots, fixed drug eruption Leprosy, pityriasis alba, pityriasis versicolor Vitiligo Sunburn, fixed drug eruption Port wine stain Senile purpura
Papule: Circumscribed solid, elevated skin lesion less than 1 cm in diameter (Fig. 2.1c)	Erythematous Violaceus Skin coloured Yellow Rounded Conical Flat topped Dome shaped	Allergic contact dermatitis Lichen planus Phrynoderma, closed comedones Molluscum contagiosum Measles Phrynoderma Lichen planus Molluscum contagiosum
Nodule: Circumscribed solid elevated skin lesion more than 1 cm in diameter, the vertical dimensions, (height + depth) of which equal or exceed the horizontal dimensions (diameter) (Fig. 2.1d)	Skin coloured Erythematous Hyperpigmented Soft Firm Hard	Neurofibroma, lipoma Furuncle, erythema nodosum Prurigo nodularis Neurofibroma Fibroma Calcinosis cutis
Plaque: Circumscribed solid elevated skin lesion more than 1 cm in diameter, the horizontal dimensions of which exceed the vertical dimension (Fig. 2.1e)	Erythematous Violaceous Skin coloured Hyperpigmented Hypopigmented	Psoriasis Lichen planus Sclerema, mucinosis, sarcoidosis Lichen simplex chronicus Morphea
Vesicle: Circumscribed elevated skin lesion of less than 1 cm in diameter containing free fluid other than pus (Fig. 2.1f)	Clear Haemorrhagic Cloudy vesicle/vesicopustule	Chickenpox, herpes zoster Haemorrhagic chickenpox or zoster Impetigo

Pustule: Circumscribed elevated skin lesion of less than 1 cm in diameter containing pus (Fig. 2.1g)	Follicular pustule
	Non-follicular pustule :
	    Superficial
	    Deep
		Folliculitis
		Impetigo, candidiasis
		Pustular psoriasis, impetigo
		Ecthyma

Bulla: Circumscribed elevated lesion of more than 1 cm in diameter containing free fluid (Fig. 2.1h)	Tense Flaccid Clear fluid filled Pus filled Haemorrhagic fluid	Bullous pemphigoid Pemphigus Bullous pemphigoid Bullous impetigo Stevens Johnson syndrome

Chapter
2

Section A: Basic Lesions: The Building Blocks of Dermatologic Description
Section B: Principles of Diagnosis

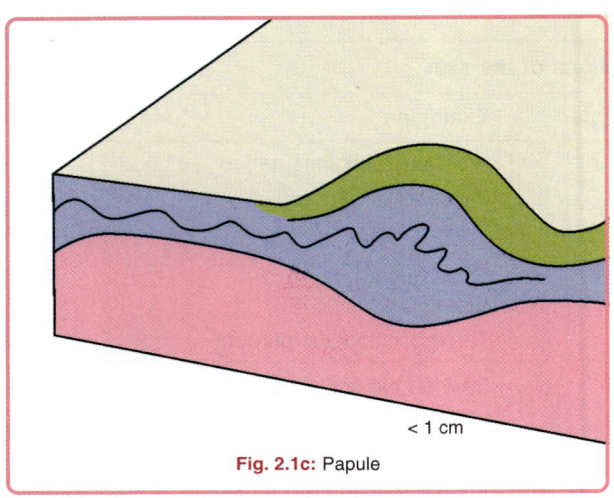

Fig. 2.1c: Papule

< 1 cm

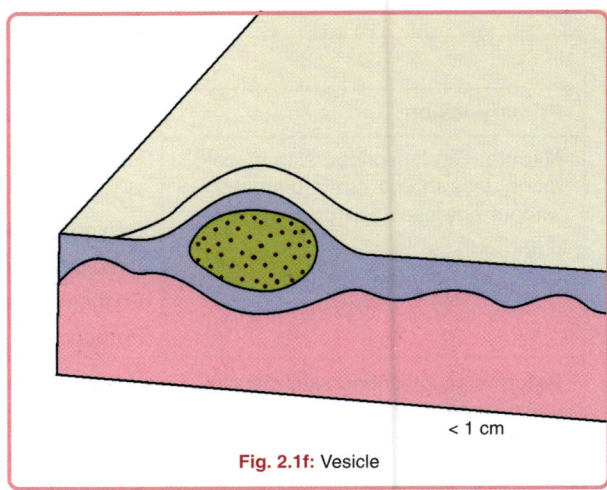

Fig. 2.1f: Vesicle

< 1 cm

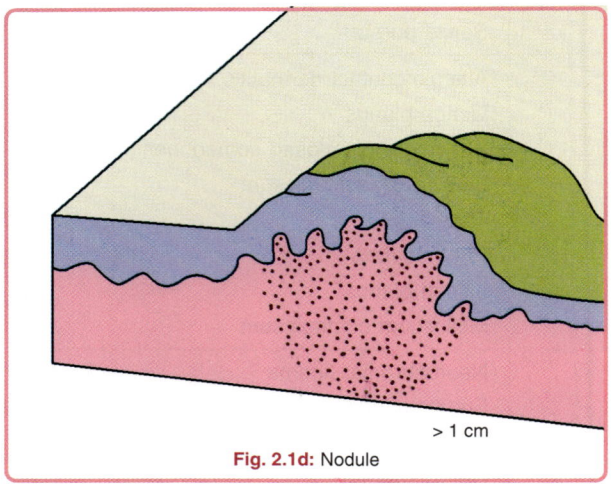

Fig. 2.1d: Nodule

> 1 cm

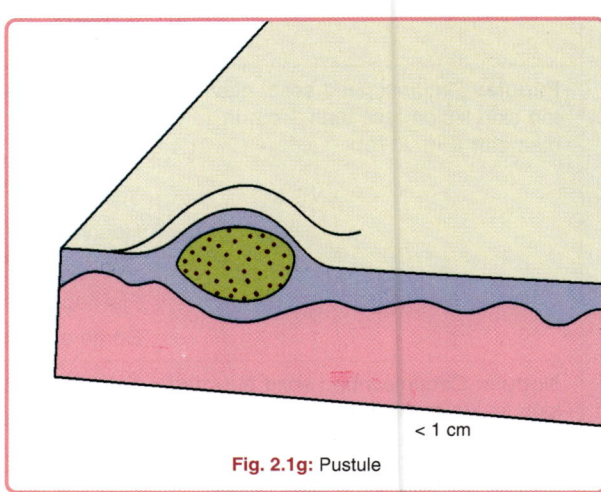

Fig. 2.1g: Pustule

< 1 cm

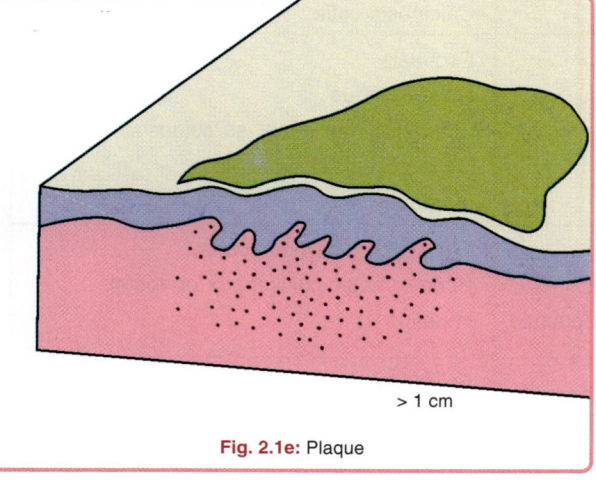

Fig. 2.1e: Plaque

> 1 cm

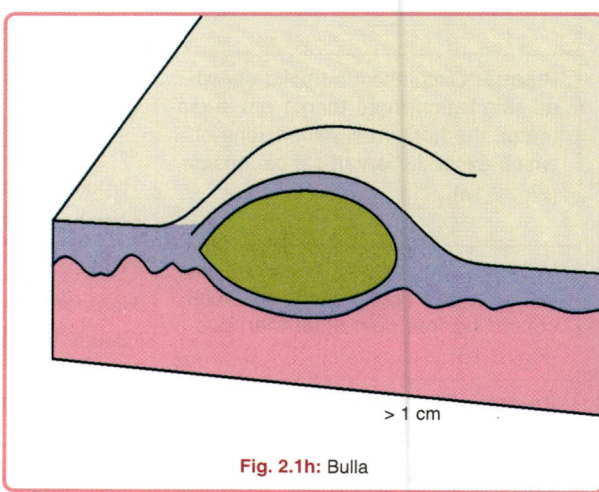

Fig. 2.1h: Bulla

> 1 cm

Occasionally, when doubt exists as to whether a particular skin lesion is a papule or a vesicle, puncture with a sterile needle may be done to elicit fluid from a vesicle. Papulovesicle is a vesicle that sits atop a papule, e.g. in an insect bite reaction (prurigo simplex). Vesicles may be:

- clear (clear fluid—chickenpox, herpes simplex) (Fig. 2.14)

- haemorrhagic (haemorrhagic chickenpox or zoster)

- cloudy (vesicopustule in impetigo)

SECONDARY LESIONS

Secondary lesion	Morphologic subtype	Examples
Erosion: It is breach on skin continuity due to loss of part or whole of epidermis and without any dermal damage (Fig. 2.2a)	Superficial	Impetigo, staphylococcal scalded skin syndrome
	Deep	Pemphigus, bullous pemphigoid and Stevens Johnson syndrome
Ulcer: It is breach in skin continuity due to loss of epidermis and at least a part of dermis (Fig. 2.2b)	Superficial	Arterial ulcers, dermatitis artefacta
	Deep	Venous ulcers, neuropathic ulcers and ecthyma
Scale: It is a visible exfoliation of the skin (Fig. 2.2c)	Thin	Dermatophytosis
	Thick	Psoriasis
	Adherent	Discoid lupus erythematosus
	Easily removable	Psoriasis
	Silvery white	Psoriasis
	Yellowish greasy	Seborrheic dermatitis
	Branny	Pityriasis versicolor
	Collarette like scale	Pityriasis rosea
	Fish like scales	Ichthyosis
Crust : It is dried up exudate consisting of serous fluid, blood, dead inflammatory cells as well as epidermal and/or dermal elements (Fig. 2.2d)	Purulent	Bacterial eczema
	Seropurulent	Impetigo
	Haemorrhagic	Stevens Johnson Syndrome, ecthyma
	Serosanguinous	Excoriations

TABLE 2.2 : Secondary lesions of the skin

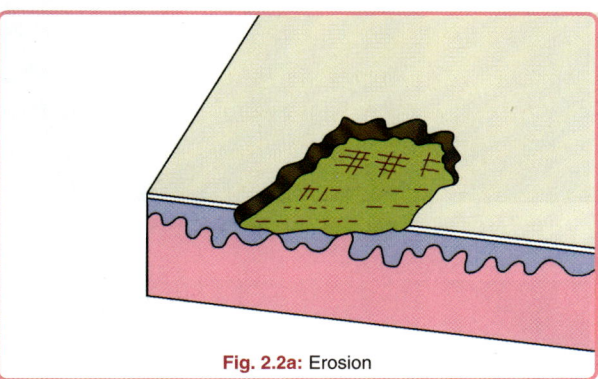

Fig. 2.2a: Erosion

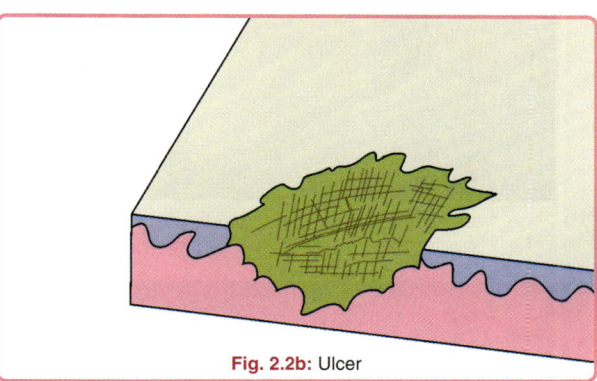

Fig. 2.2b: Ulcer

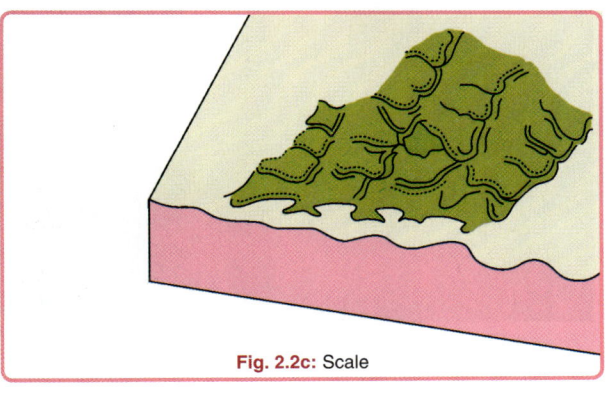

Fig. 2.2c: Scale

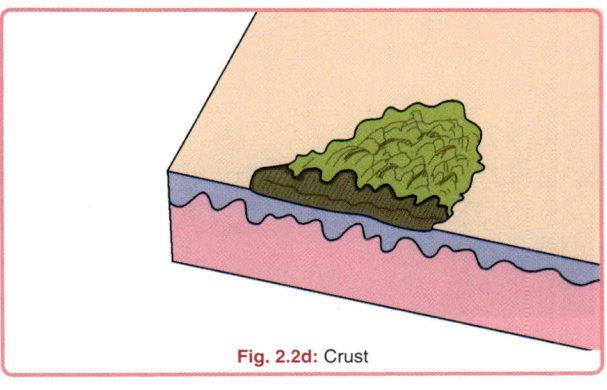

Fig. 2.2d: Crust

Chapter
2

Section A: Basic Lesions: The Building Blocks of Dermatologic Description
Section B: Principles of Diagnosis

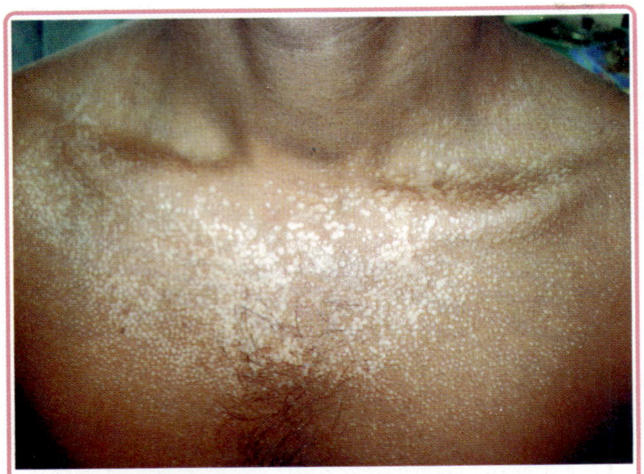

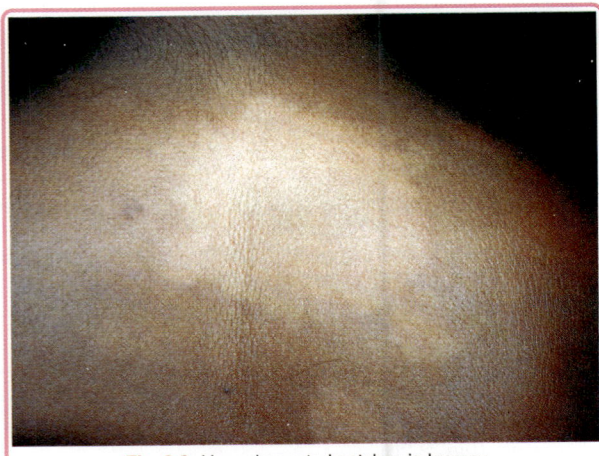

Fig. 2.3: Hypopigmented macules and patches in pityriasis versicolor

Fig. 2.6: Hypopigmented patches in leprosy

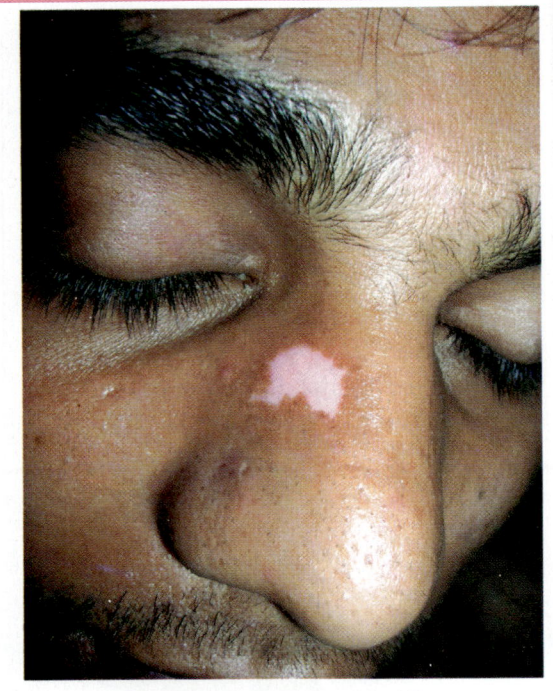

Fig. 2.4: Depigmented patch in vitiligo

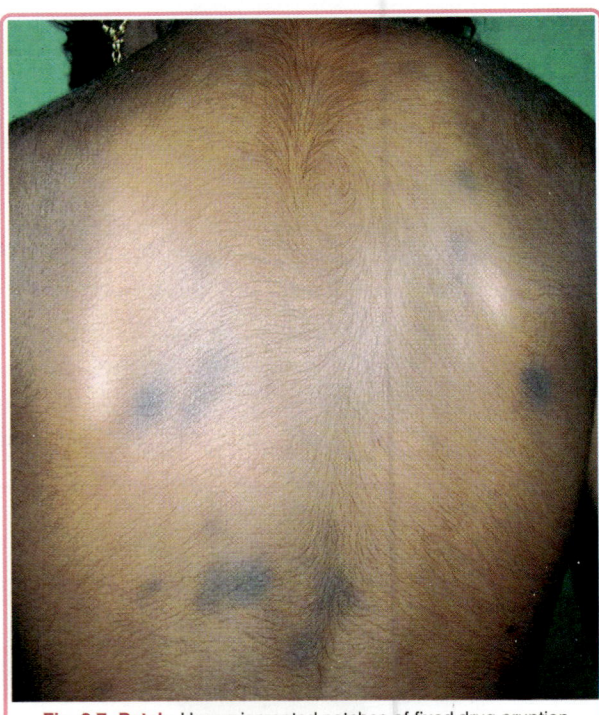

Fig. 2.7: Patch: Hyperpigmented patches of fixed drug eruption

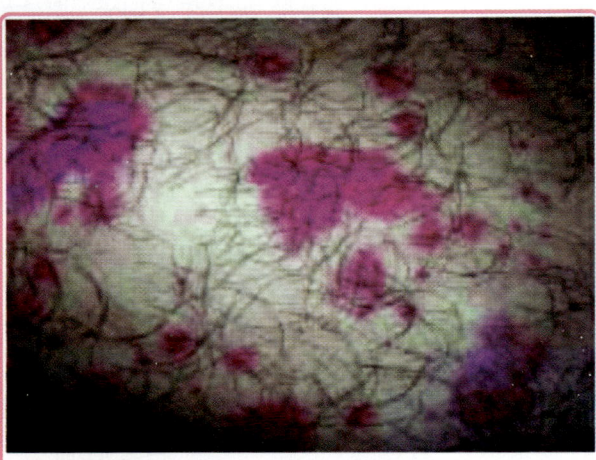

Fig. 2.5: Palpable purpura : Nonblanchable red coloured papules and plaques

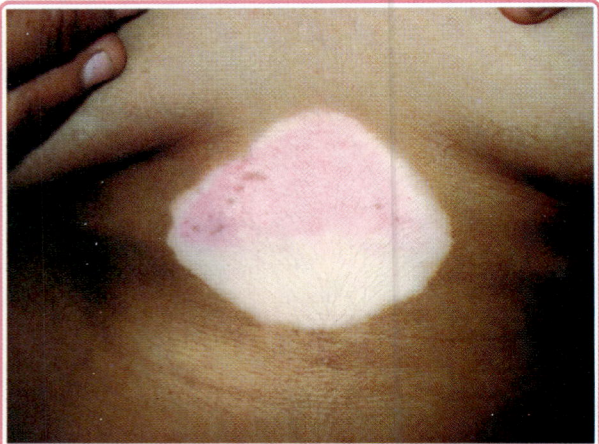

Fig. 2.8: Depigmented patch of vitiligo with hyperpigmented macules within it

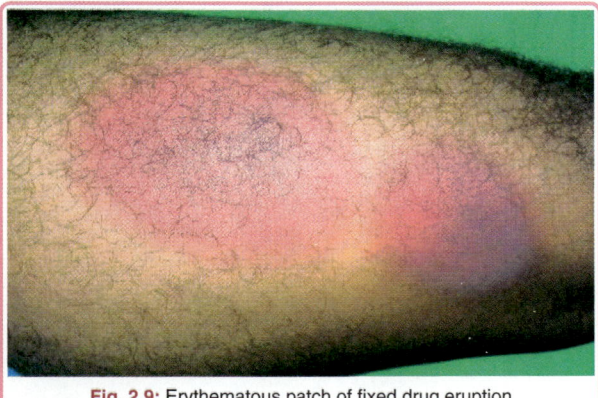

Fig. 2.9: Erythematous patch of fixed drug eruption

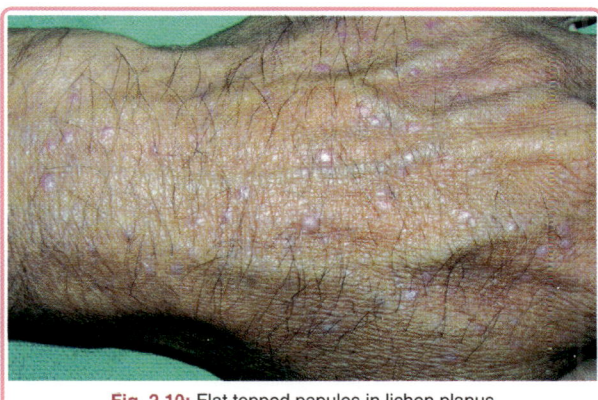

Fig. 2.10: Flat topped papules in lichen planus

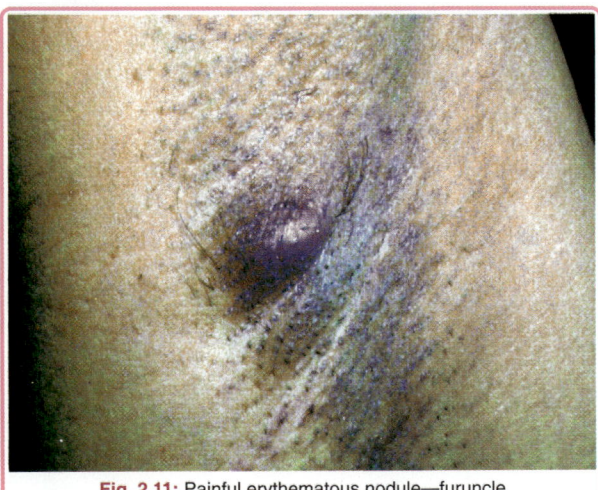

Fig. 2.11: Painful erythematous nodule—furuncle

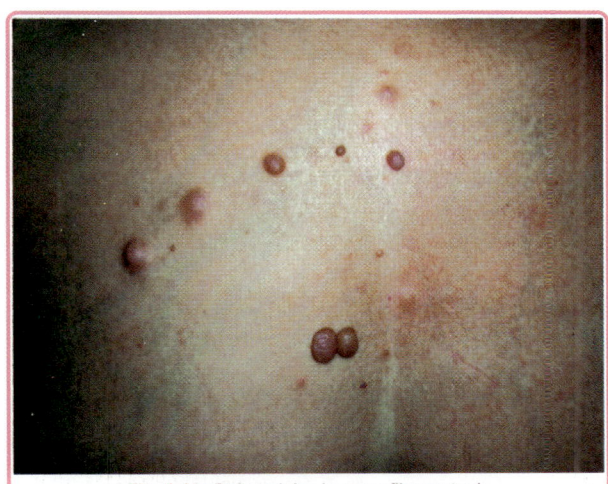

Fig. 2.12: Soft nodules in neurofibromatosis

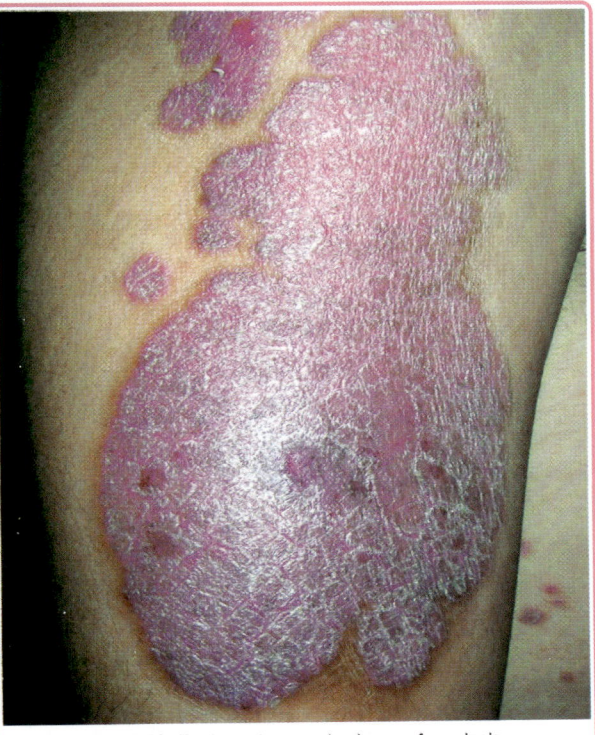

Fig. 2.13: Erythematous scaly plaque of psoriasis

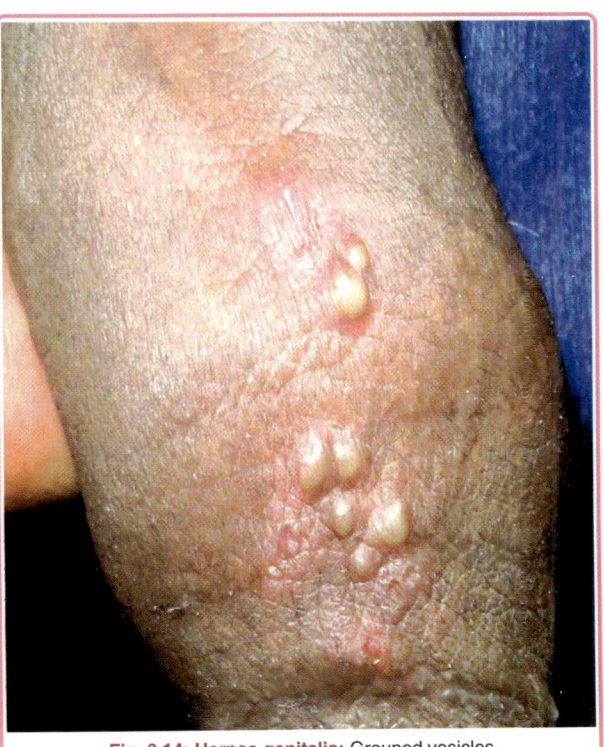

Fig. 2.14: Herpes genitalis: Grouped vesicles

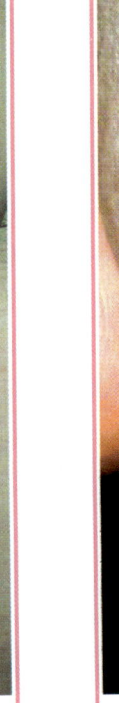

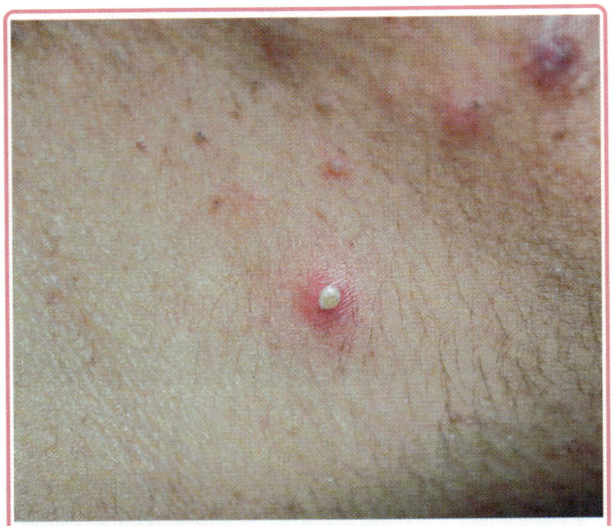

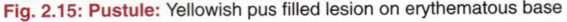

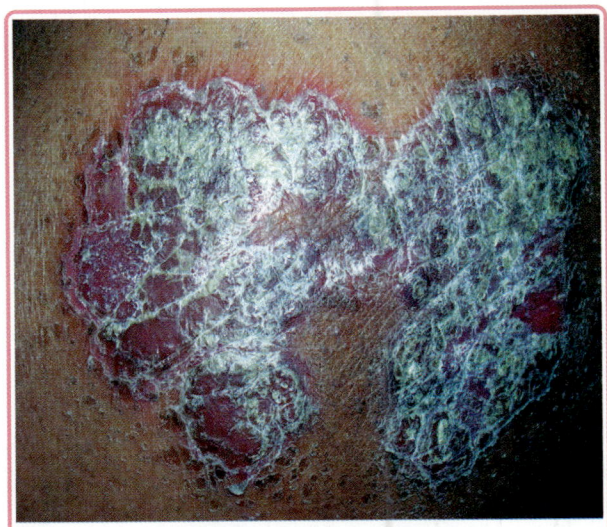

Fig. 2.15: Pustule: Yellowish pus filled lesion on erythematous base

Fig. 2.18: Thick silvery white scales in psoriasis

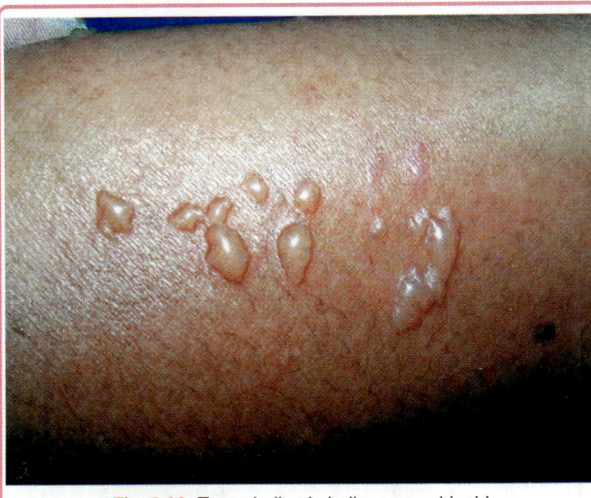

Fig. 2.16: Tense bullae in bullous pemphigoid

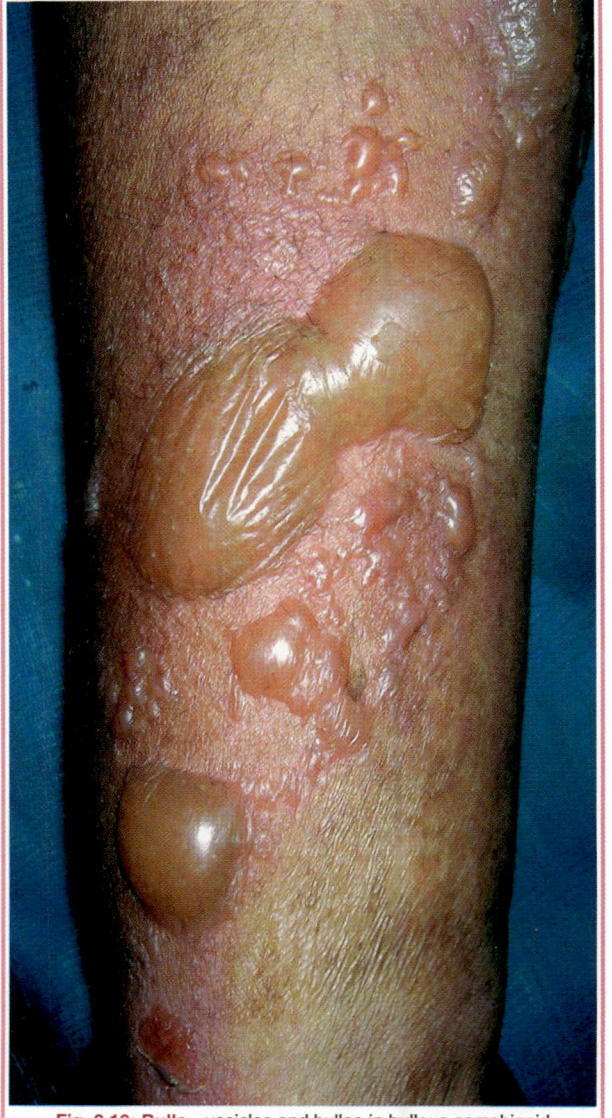

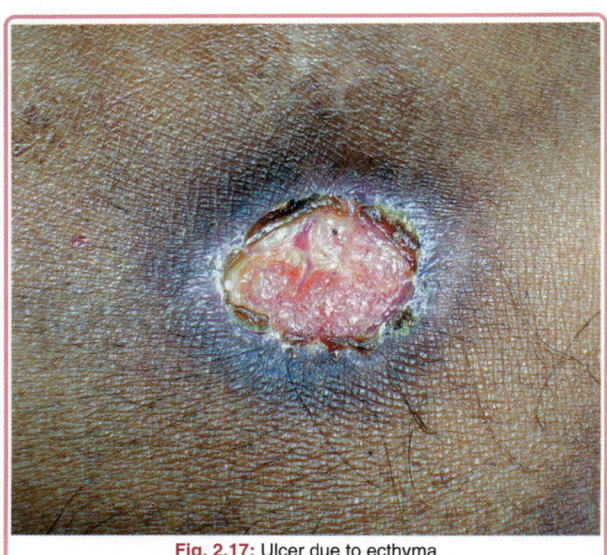

Fig. 2.17: Ulcer due to ecthyma

Fig. 2.19: Bulla—vesicles and bullae in bullous pemphigoid

SPECIAL TERMS

Comedone or Comedo (Plural—Comedones or Comedoes)

It is the result of impaction of the opening of a pilosebaceous unit with a plug of cornified cells. Clinically, a conical papule that has either a white spot at the top (whitehead or closed comedone) or a black coloured plug within a dilated follicular opening at its summit (blackhead or open comedone) is seen. These lesions are typical of acne vulgaris.

Burrow

This is a tortuous tunnel dug by the scabies mite beneath the stratum corneum. It is seen as a greyish brown wavy line about 5–10 mm in length.

Scar

It is a reparative fibrosing inflammation that results in replacement of the original normal tissues with fibrous tissue. Scars may be atrophic, hypertrophic, pock like (resembling small pox) or bridge like. They may follow trauma, infections or inflammations.

Atrophy

Loss of or reduction in structural components (epidermis, collagen, elastin, hair, sebaceous or sweat glands) of the skin is termed as atrophy. It implies a preceding process that has destroyed these structural components. Clinically, atrophy is seen as loss of the normal crisscross skin markings, excessive wrinkling, thinning, loss of hair, dryness (due to loss of sweat and sebaceous activity), hypopigmentation and telangiectasia.

Hypertrophic

Used only as an adjective to indicate skin lesions that are more elevated or thicker than is usually expected.

Induration

Induration is said to be present when the skin feels thicker and firmer than normal. It is seen as a result of chronic granulomatous and fibrosing inflammation (tuberculosis, syphilis, keloid and scleroderma) or due to oedema (erysipelas) or deposition of extracellular material like mucin (myxoedema) or infiltration with malignant cells (squamous cell carcinoma).

Lichenification

Lichenification is a combination of accentuation of the normal, crisscross, diamond shaped skin markings, thickening of the skin and hyperpigmentation. It results primarily from a thickening of the epidermis and papillary dermis and is a response to persistent rubbing or scratching.

SECTION – B

Principles of Diagnosis

METHOD OF DESCRIPTION OF SKIN LESIONS

There are three components of description of skin lesions : morphology, distribution and configuration.

- **Morphology**

   Basic lesions are terms used for classifying skin lesions based on their morphology alone. Hence, a lesion of psoriasis would be described as 'plaque covered with scales' wherein plaque is the primary lesion and scale is the secondary lesion. Taking help of common adjectives to describe the shape, size, colour, etc., of the lesion, a complete description would be 'a 5 cm diameter, well defined circular erythematous plaque covered with thick silvery scales'.

- **Distribution**

   The sites of involvement in a particular patient provide important clues to diagnosis. This is because certain sites are commonly affected in certain diseases. For example, psoriasis typically affects elbows, knees, extensor aspects of extremities, scalp, lower back, palms and soles.

Certain other patterns of distribution include:

- *Sun-exposed sites:* In photosensitive dermatoses like pellagra, polymorphous light eruption and lupus erythematosus

- *Exposed sites:* In prurigo simplex (hypersensitivity to insect bites)

- *Seborrhoeic distribution:* In seborrhoeic dermatitis

- *Flexural:* Intertrigo, candidiasis, dermatophytosis and inverse psoriasis

- *Segmental (restricted to a nerve segment):* Herpes zoster and segmental vitiligo

□ *Acral (hands and feet):* Palmoplantar psoriasis and pompholyx

□ *Sites of trauma (bony prominences and acral):* Epidermolysis bullosa

- **Configuration**

The pattern of arrangement of multiple skin lesions and their relationship to each other is termed as configuration. The various configuration include:

□ *Grouped (agminate):* That is closely clustered as in herpes simplex

□ *Scattered:* Chickenpox

□ *Annular:* Tinea corporis, some cases of secondary syphilis, lichen planus and psoriasis

□ *Linear:* Some cases of psoriasis, lichen simplex and lichen planus.

CASE STUDY IN DERMATOLOGY AND STDs

In order to focus on a patient's problem, it is necessary to perform an initial examination of patient's skin lesions before detailed history taking can progress. Hence, after the initial question 'What's your problem?' examination of skin lesions and history taking usually go hand-in-hand and it is frequent for a dermatologist to continue taking relevant history while examination is in progress.

In addition to finding out about the origin, duration and progress of the skin lesions, certain points that a dermatologist commonly elicits and that may prove helpful, are:

- other sites of affection
- history of pruritus, severity, relation with time or activity
- family history of similar lesions
- history of fever
- history of drug ingestion drug allergies
- history of exposure to STD for genital lesions and non-pruritic rash in an adult
- occupational history especially for hand lesions
- history of local trauma/insect bites
- past history of skin disease

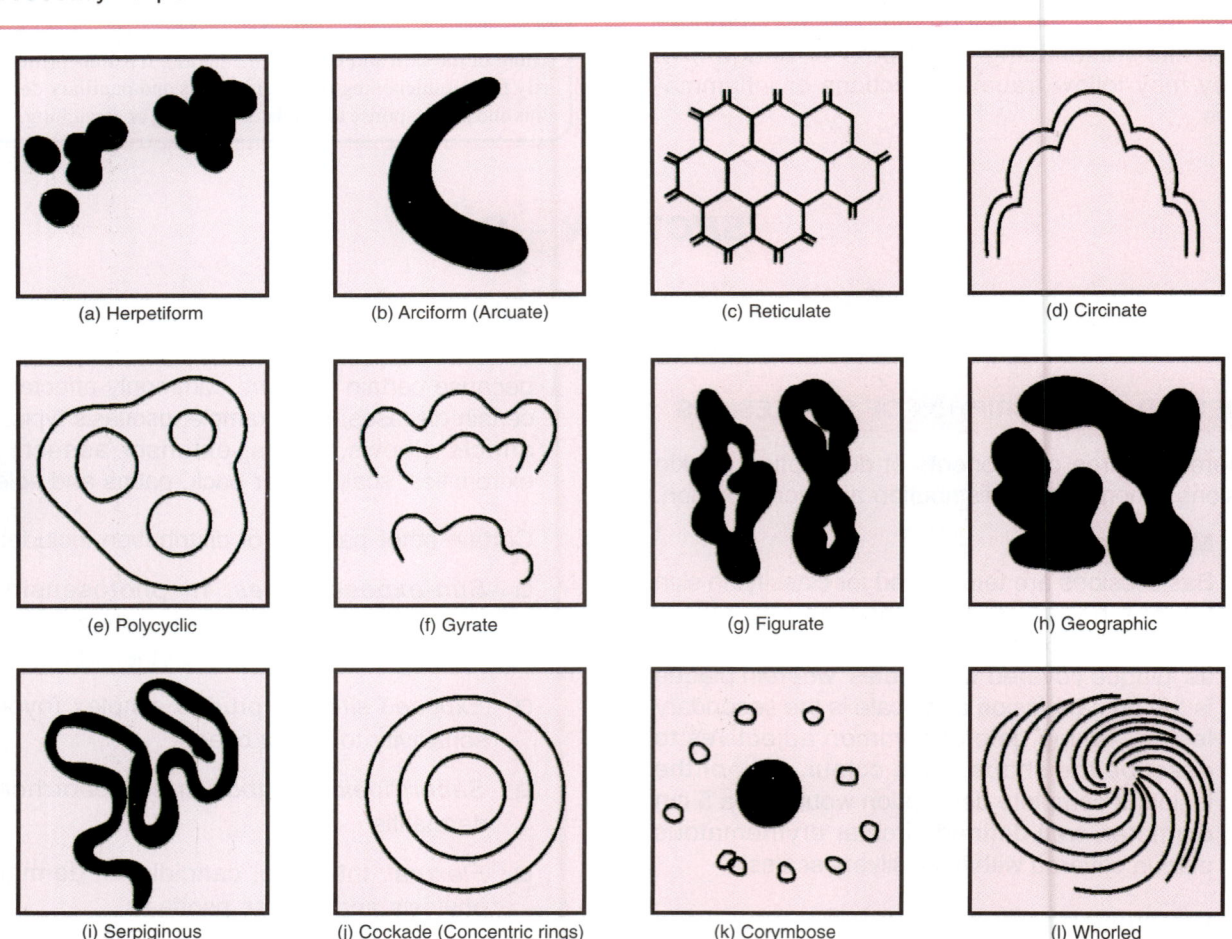

(a) Herpetiform (b) Arciform (Arcuate) (c) Reticulate (d) Circinate

(e) Polycyclic (f) Gyrate (g) Figurate (h) Geographic

(i) Serpiginous (j) Cockade (Concentric rings) (k) Corymbose (l) Whorled

Fig. 2.20: Uncommon configurations

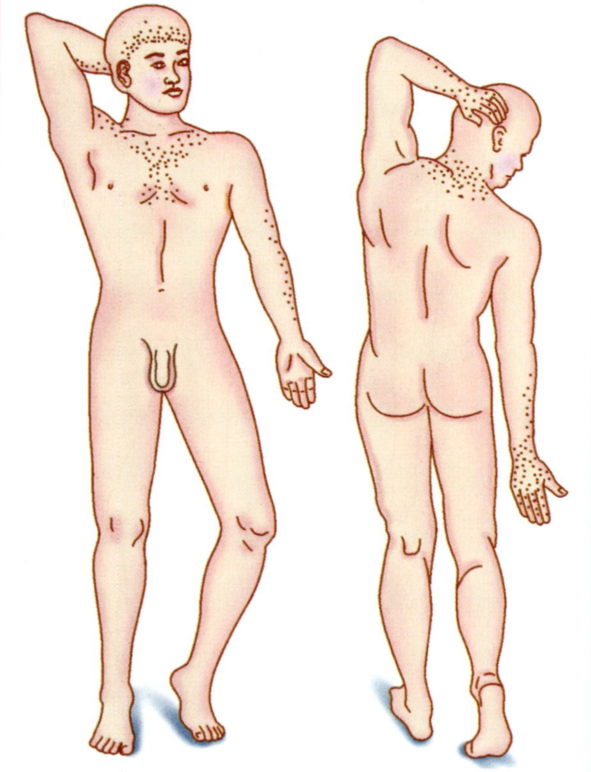

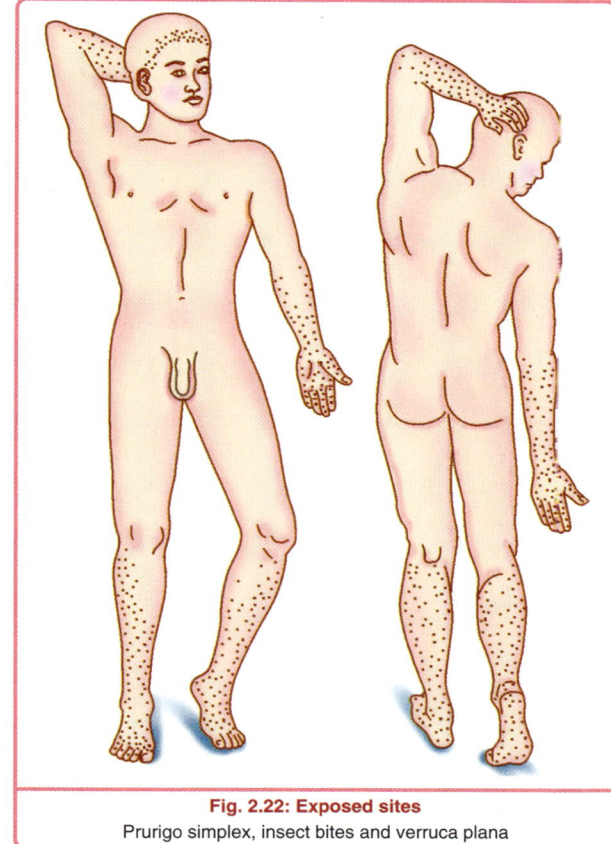

Fig. 2.21: Sun-exposed sites
Photoallergic dermatitis, polymorphous light eruption, pallagra and discoid lupus

Fig. 2.22: Exposed sites
Prurigo simplex, insect bites and verruca plana

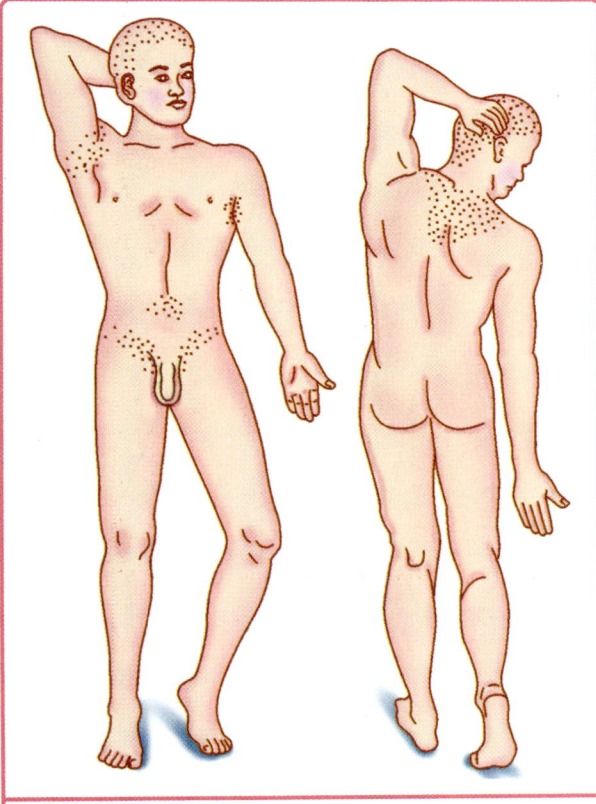

Fig. 2.23: Seborrhoeic pattern
Seborrhoeic dermatitis, pemphigus foliaceus and pityriasis versicolor

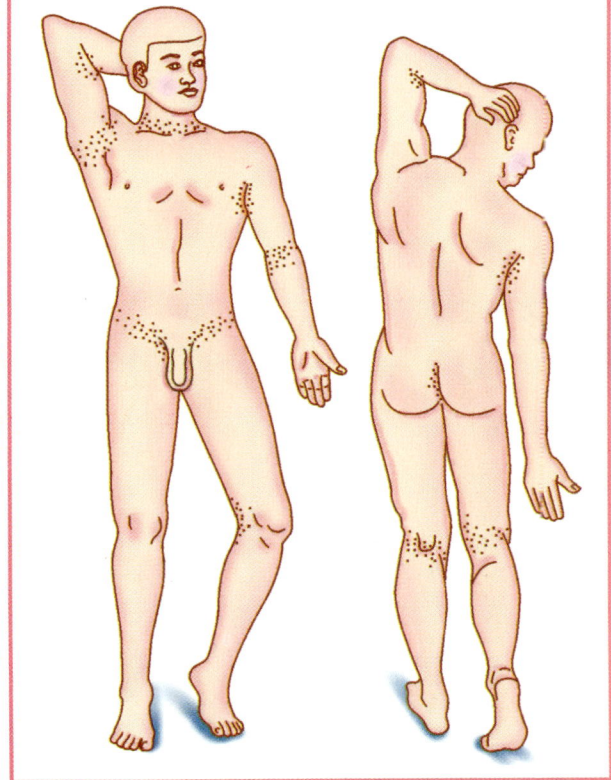

Fig. 2.24: Flexural pattern
Atopic dermatitis, candidiasis, intertrigo, condyloma lata and erythrasma

Chapter
2

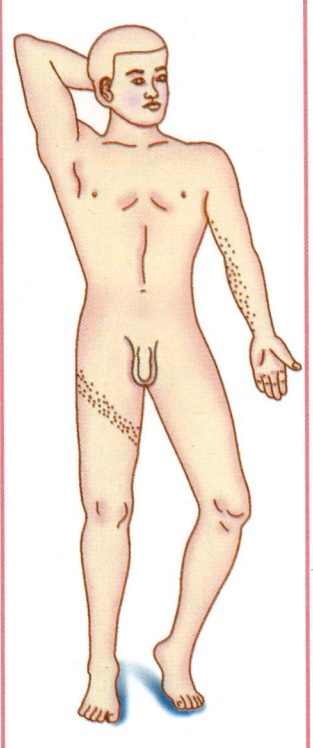

Fig. 2.25: Segmental pattern
Epidermal nevus, linear lichen planus and herpes zoster

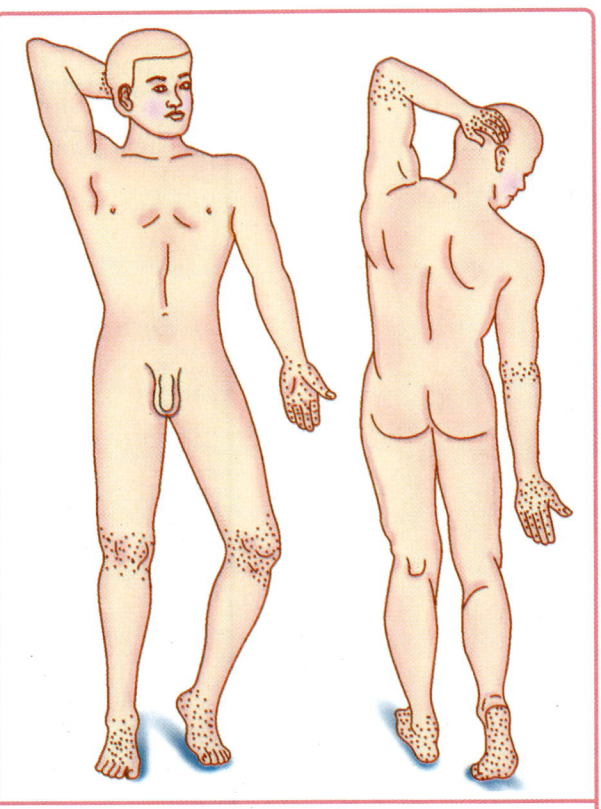

Fig. 2.26: Sites of trauma
Psoriasis, eczema, tuberculosis verrucosa cutis and epidermolysis bullosa

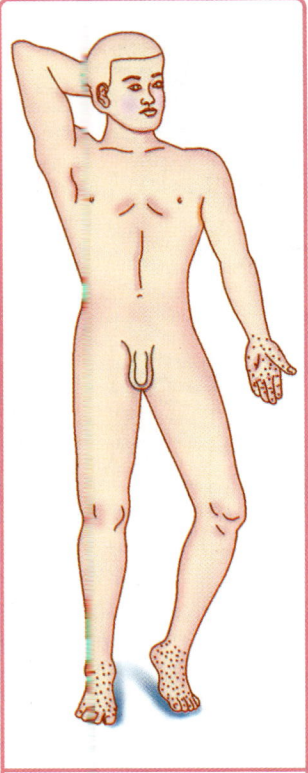

Fig. 2.27: Acral pattern
Psoriasis, pompholyx, vitiligo and keratoderma

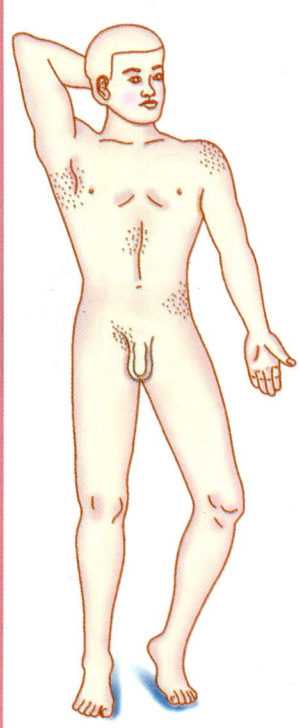

Fig. 2.28: Grouped lesions
Herpes simplex, herpes zoster, dermatitis herpetiformis and insect bites

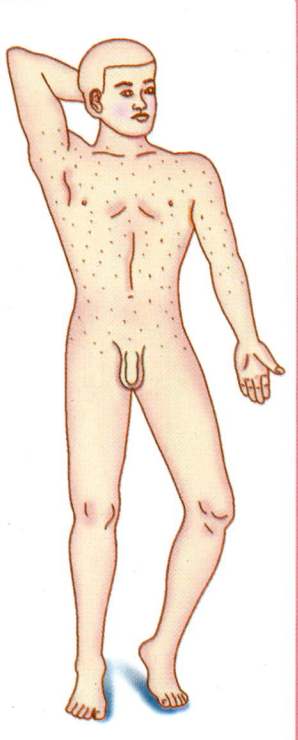

Fig. 2.29: Scattered lesions
Chicken pox, secondary syphilis, and pityriasis lichenoides

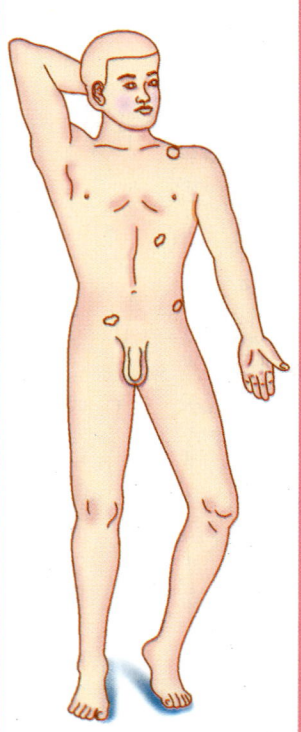

Fig. 2.30: Annular lesions
Pityriasis rosea, tinea corporis, annular syphilid, psoriasis and lichen planus

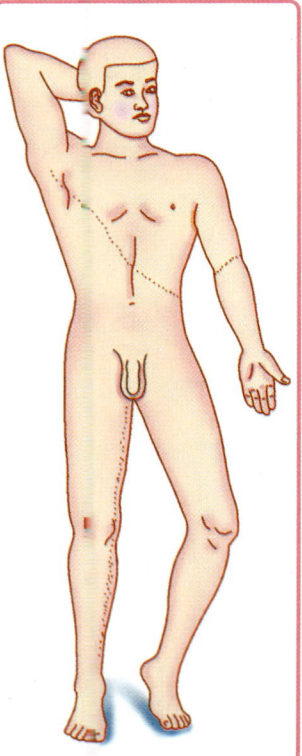

Fig. 2.31: Linear lesions
Whiplash injury, acute dermatitis due to plant contact and bed-bug bites

Chapter 2

Section A: Basic Lesions: The Building Blocks of Dermatologic Description
Section B: Principles of Diagnosis

- history of recent change of job, place of residence or lifestyle or food habits, history of recent stressful event
- past history of drug allergy/treatment taken

Examination findings should be categorised under the heads of morphology, distribution and configuration. Once adequate history has been elicited, it should be integrated with these observations to reach a diagnosis or a differential diagnosis.

BEDSIDE INVESTIGATIONS IN DERMATOLOGY AND STDs

Several bedside investigations help confirm a diagnosis or differentiate between a list of possible diagnoses. These include:

- **Magnifying glass examination:** To look for signs that are difficult to appreciate with the naked eye, e.g. Wickham's striae in lichen planus, exclamation mark hair in alopecia areata, Auspitz sign in psoriasis.
- **Diascopy:** Viewing the skin by applying pressure with a transparent firm object like a glass slide is termed as diascopy. This is used for differentiation between erythema and purpura.
- **Wood's lamp examination:** Wood's lamp, an ultraviolet light with a wavelength of 365 nm, is used for demonstrating fluorescence in lesions of tinea capitis, pityriasis versicolor and erythrasma.

- **Scraping and KOH mount:** For fungal infections like dermatophytosis, candidiasis.
- **Tzanck smear:** Giemsa stain or Wright's stain to demonstrate acantholytic cells in pemphigus and multinucleated epithelial giant cells in herpes infections.
- **Smear of discharge for organisms:** Gram's stain—staphylococci (impetigo), gonococci (gonorrhoea), meningococci (meningococcaemia), *Haemophilus ducreyi* (chancroid), candida (candidiasis)

Ziehl Nielsen stain—*Mycobacterium tuberculosis* (tuberculosis), *M. leprae* (leprosy).

TIPS FOR DIAGNOSIS IN DERMATOLOGY AND STDs

- Examine in good light. If you can't see skin lesions, you can't diagnose them.
- Subtle elevation of some skin lesions, can be better appreciated under tangential and reduced illumination.
- Use a magnifying lens when required.
- Examine all the affected body regions, even if the patient thinks it is unrelated. Otherwise, you may miss a skin lesion that may be the most important for diagnosis.
- Diagnose common conditions commonly.
- As far as possible, try to fit all the symptoms and signs in a single diagnosis.

MCQs — SECTION - A

1. **Papule is:**
   a. A flat lesion
   b. A fluid filled lesion
   c. An elevated lesion
   d. More than one centimeter in diameter

2. **A nodule is:**
   a. More in depth than in height
   b. More in diameter than its height
   c. Less than 1 cm in height
   d. More in its vertical dimensions than its horizontal dimensions

3. **Plaques are seen in:**
   a. Lichen simplex chronicus
   b. Impetigo
   c. Pemphigus
   d. Vitiligo

4. **Bullae are seen in all *except*:**
   a. Impetigo
   b. Psoriasis
   c. Pemphigus
   d. Eczema

5. **Wheals are characteristic of:**
   a. Scabies
   b. Erythema multiforme
   c. Urticaria
   d. Prurigo simplex

6. **Burrow is a typical lesion of:**
   a. Pediculosis pubis
   b. Larva migrans
   c. Scabies
   d. Loa loa

7. **Which of the following is not a type of scale?**
   a. Collarette
   b. Silvery
   c. Haemorrhagic
   d. Adherent

8. **Nodules are a primary lesion seen in all of the following *except*:**
   a. Erythema multiforme
   b. Erythema nodosum
   c. Erythema induratum
   d. Type II lepra reaction

9. **Which of the following is a secondary lesion?**
   a. Papule
   b. Vesicle
   c. Pustule
   d. Scale

10. **Which of the following is not a type of crust?**
    a. Haemorrhagic
    b. Serous
    c. Greasy
    d. Purulent

11. **Which of the following is a primary lesion of the skin?**
    a. Scale
    b. Burrow
    c. Erosion
    d. Bulla

12. **Which of the following is a secondary lesion of the skin?**
    a. Nodule
    b. Ulcer
    c. Vesicle
    d. Pustule

13. **Which of the following is a lesion less than 1 cm in diameter?**
    a. Plaque
    b. Bulla
    c. Patch
    d. Pustule

14. **Hypopigmented macules are seen in all, *except*:**
    a. Vitiligo
    b. Pityriasis versicolor
    c. Neurofibromatosis
    d. Pityriasis alba

15. **Hyperpigmented macules are seen in all, *except*:**
    a. Pityriasis versicolor
    b. Melasma
    c. Portwine stain
    d. Lichen planus

16. **Diascopy involves use of:**
    a. Magnifying lens
    b. Measuring tape
    c. Wood's lamp
    d. Glass slide

17. **All of the following are types of papules, *except*:**
    a. Conical
    b. Flaccid
    c. Dome shaped
    d. Keratotic

18. **All of the following are types of plaques *except*:**
    a. Erythematous
    b. Indurated
    c. Cystic
    d. Scaly

19. **Macules may be all *except*:**
    a. Erythematous
    b. Purpuric
    c. Depigmented
    d. Urticarial

20. **A plaque is:**
    a. A flat lesion
    b. An elevated lesion
    c. A fluid filled lesion
    d. Less than one centimeter in diameter

21. **A magnifying glass is used for observing all *except*:**
    a. Telangiectasia
    b. Auspitz sign
    c. Koebner phenomenon
    d. Burrow

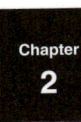

Chapter 2

Section A: Basic Lesions: The Building Blocks of Dermatologic Description
Section B: Principles of Diagnosis

22. All of the following are types of scales except:
a. Powdery
b. Fish-like
c. Stuck-on
d. Wafer-like

23. A bulla may contain within it:
a. Clear fluid
b. Pus
c. Haemorrhagic fluid
d. Any of these

24. All of the following are types of telangiectasia except:
a. Cherry angioma
b. Spider angioma
c. Linear
d. Mat-like

25. All of the following are types of scars except:
a. Bridge-like
b. Keratotic
c. Varioliform
d. Hypertrophic

26. All of the following are configurations of skin lesions except:
a. Linear
b. Dome shaped
c. Grouped
d. Annular

27. Which of the following sites are spared in dermatoses affecting exposed areas?
a. Face
b. Hands
c. Hairy scalp
d. Ankles

28. Which of the following sites is affected in photodermatoses?
a. Legs
b. Retroauricular region
c. Lower lip
d. Upper lip

29. Which of the following sites is not affected in photodermatoses?
a. Retroauricular region
b. Bald scalp
c. Hands
d. V area of chest

30. Which of the following sites is affected in seborrhoeic distribution of lesions?
a. Upper central back
b. Forearms
c. Legs
d. Palms and soles

31. Grouped configurations of lesions is seen in all except:
a. Lichen planus
b. Chickenpox
c. Insect bite
d. Phrynoderma

32. Annular configuration of lesions is seen in all except:
a. Psoriasis
b. Lichen planus
c. Secondary syphilis
d. Prurigo simplex

33. Acral pattern of distribution of lesions is seen in:
a. Vitiligo
b. Prurigo simplex
c. Lichen planus
d. Psoriasis

34. Flexural pattern of distribution of lesions is seen in all of the following except:
a. Atopic dermatitis in adults
b. Candidiasis
c. Lichen planus
d. Inverse psoriasis

35. Tzanck smear is useful for diagnosis of all, except:
a. Pemphigus
b. Impetigo
c. Chickenpox
d. Herpes zoster

36. All of the following skin lesions show induration except:
a. Lupus vulgaris
b. Neurofibroma
c. Erysipelas
d. Scleroderma

37. All the following may appear in segmental distribution except:
a. Vitiligo
b. Herpes zoster
c. Plexiform neurofibroma
d. Measles

38. Loss of epidermis and part of dermis is called:
a. Erosion
b. Ulcer
c. Excoriation
d. Crust

39. Scale is defined as:
a. Exfoliation of skin
b. Visible exfoliation of skin
c. Dry skin
d. None of the above

40. Typical lesion of acne is a:
a. Pustule
b. Nodule
c. Papule
d. Comedone

41. Atrophy consists of all of the following except:
a. Excessive wrinkling
b. Dry skin
c. Loss of hair
d. Thickening

Chapter 2

Section A: Basic Lesions: The Building Blocks of Dermatologic Description
Section B: Principles of Diagnosis

ANSWERS

1-c,	2-d,	3-a,	4-b,	5-c,	6-c,	7-c,	8-a,	9-d,	10-c,
11-d,	12-b,	13-d,	14-c,	15-c,	16-d,	17-b,	18-c,	19-d,	20-b,
21-c,	22-c,	23-d,	24-a,	25-b,	26-b,	27-a,	28-c,	29-a,	30-a,
31-b,	32-d,	33-a,	34-c,	35-b,	36-b,	37-d,	38-b,	39-b,	40-d,
41-d									

MCQs — SECTION – B

1. **Wood's lamp is not useful in the diagnosis of:**
   a. Tinea capitis
   b. Eerythrasma
   c. Pityriasis rosea
   d. Pityriasis versicolor
   e. Porphyrias

2. **Diascopy is useful for:**
   a. Differentiation of vitiligo from leprosy
   b. Testing for capillary fragility
   c. Testing for contact allergy
   d. Differentiating erythema from purpura
   e. Differentiating vitiligo from fungal infection

3. **The skin disease that is not pruritic is:**
   a. Lichen planus
   b. Atopic dermatitis
   c. Dermatophytosis
   d. Scleroderma
   e. Dermatitis herpetiformis

4. **Which of the following lesions is not palpable?**
   a. Papule
   b. Macule
   c. Vesicle
   d. Pustule
   e. Plaque

5. **Sezary cells in skin are found in:**
   a. Sezary syndrome
   b. Sezary syndrome and mycosis fungoides
   c. All types of cutaneous T cell lymphomas
   d. All T cell lymphomas and leukaemias
   e. All of the above and many benign dermatoses

6. **All of the following are primary skin lesions except:**
   a. Papule
   b. Macule
   c. Plaque
   d. Scale
   e. Vesicle

7. **All of the following are secondary skin lesions except:**
   a. Vesicle
   b. Scale
   c. Crust
   d. Erosion
   e. Ulcer

8. **All of the following are primary skin lesions except:**
   a. Papule
   b. Macule
   c. Plaque
   d. Wheal
   e. Vesicle

9. **Indurated plaques are seen in all of the following except:**
   a. Lupus vulgaris
   b. Keloid
   c. Erythema multiforme
   d. Morphea
   e. Squamous cell carcinoma

10. **Colloid bodies are found in:**
    a. Psoriasis
    b. Pityriasis rosea
    c. Contact allergic dermatitis
    d. Polymorphous light eruption
    e. Lichen planus

11. **Which of the following hypersensitivity reaction is IgE mediated?**
    a. Type I
    b. Type II
    c. Type III
    d. Type IV
    e. None of the above

12. **Which of the following hypersensitivity reactions is immune complex mediated?**
    a. Type I
    b. Type II
    c. Type III
    d. Type IV
    e. None of the above

13. **Angioneurotic oedema is:**
    a. A type of subcutaneous oedema
    b. Seen in neurotic individuals
    c. A vascular malformation
    d. Severely pruritic
    e. Unrelated to urticaria

14. **Angiooedema is an example of which type of hypersensitivity reaction?**
    a. Type I
    b. Type II
    c. Type III
    d. Type IV
    e. None of the above

15. **Allergic contact dermatitis is an example of which type of hypersensitivity reaction?**
    a. Type I
    b. Type II
    c. Type III
    d. Type IV
    e. None of the above

16. **Grattage is useful for:**
    a. Differentiating vitiligo from fungal infection
    b. Testing for capillary fragility
    c. Testing for contact allergy
    d. Differentiating erythema from purpura
    e. Differentiation of vitiligo from leprosy

17. **Toxic epidermal necrolysis is an example of which type of hypersensitivity reaction?**
    a. Type I
    b. Type II
    c. Type III
    d. Type IV
    e. None of the above

18. **Which of the following hypersensitivity reactions is of the delayed type?**
    a. Type I
    b. Type II
    c. Type III
    d. Type IV
    e. None of the above

19. **Which of the following hypersensitivity reactions is of the cytotoxic type?**
    a. Type I
    b. Type II
    c. Type III
    d. Type IV
    e. None of the above

20. **Which is an example of immune complex mediated hypersensitivity?**
    a. Allergic contact dermatitis
    b. Erythema nodosum leprosum
    c. Erythema nodosum
    d. Urticaria
    e. Irritant contact dermatitis

21. **Irritant dermatitis is an example of which type of hypersensitivity reaction?**
    a. Type I
    b. Type II
    c. Type III
    d. Type IV
    e. None of the above

22. **Basal cell degeneration is a predominant feature of:**
    a. Pityriasis rosea
    b. Lichen planus
    c. Psoriasis
    d. Contact dermatitis
    e. Nummular eczema

23. **The test that confirms diagnosis of contact dermatitis is:**
    a. Patch test
    b. Scratch test
    c. Prick test
    d. Conjunctival test
    e. Intradermal injection of allergens

24. **Which of the following do not leave behind a scar?**
    a. Lupus vulgaris
    b. Carbuncle
    c. Ecthyma
    d. Impetigo
    e. Discoid lupus erythematosus

25. **Tzanck cell is seen in:**
    a. All spongiotic dermatitides
    b. Pemphigus
    c. Bullous pemphigoid
    d. Dermatitis herpetiformis
    e. Cicatricial pemphigoid

26. **Tzanck cells are:**
    a. Macrophages
    b. Multinucleated giant cells in donovanosis
    c. Multinucleated giant cells in chickenpox
    d. Acantholytic cells in pemphigus
    e. Acanthotic epidermal cells

27. **Urticaria is an example of which type of hypersensitivity reaction?**
    a. Type I
    b. Type II
    c. Type III
    d. Type IV
    e. None of the above

28. **Hypertrophic scars commonly follow all of the following *except*:**
    a. Acne vulgaris
    b. Traumatic wounds
    c. Lupus vulgaris
    d. Lichen planus
    e. Scrofuloderma

29. **Ultraviolet A light spectrum is:**
    a. 200–250 nm
    b. 200–280 nm
    c. 280–320 nm
    d. 320–400 nm
    e. 400–560 nm

30. **Immediate hypersensitivity skin tests are assessed by presence of:**
    a. Erythema/Oedema
    b. Vesiculation
    c. Induration
    d. Ulceration
    e. All of the above

31. **Delayed hypersensitivity skin tests are assessed by presence of:**
    a. Erythema/Oedema
    b. Vesiculation
    c. Induration
    d. Ulceration
    e. All of the above

32. **All of the following dermatoses are extremely pruritic *except*:**
    a. Lichen planus
    b. Psoriasis
    c. Lichenified eczema
    d. Pediculosis corporis
    e. Dermatitis herpetiformis

33. **Virchow cells are bacilli containing giant cells in**
    a. Tuberculosis
    b. Leprosy
    c. Rhinoscleroma
    d. Bacterial vaginosis
    e. Donovanosis

34. **Tzanck cell is actually a:**
    a. Lymphocyte
    b. Plasma cell
    c. Histiocyte
    d. Keratinocyte
    e. Langerhans cell

35. **Occurrence of a wheal upon stroking the skin is called:**
    a. Nikolsky's sign
    b. Darier's sign
    c. Crowe's sign
    d. Auspitz sign
    e. Bulla spread sign

Chapter
2

Section A: Basic Lesions: The Building Blocks of Dermatologic Description
Section B: Principles of Diagnosis

36. All of the following present as keratotic papules *except*:

a. Keratosis pilaris
b. Phrynoderma
c. Follicular lichen planus
d. Verruca vulgaris
e. Molluscum contagiosum

37. Rhinophyma refers to:

a. Cutaneous horn
b. Thickened and curved nails
c. Enlargement of nose
d. Lymphoedema of genitals
e. Type of fungal infection of nose

38. Herpes iris lesions are characteristic of:

a. Erythema multiforme
b. Dermatitis herpetiformis
c. Urticaria
d. Herpes simplex
e. Herpes zoster

39. Testing sensations is useful for:

a. Differentiating vitiligo from fungal infection
b. Testing for capillary fragility
c. Testing for contact allergy
d. Differentiating erythema from purpura
e. Differentiation of vitiligo from leprosy

40. Patch testing is useful for:

a. Differentiating vitiligo from fungal infection
b. Testing for capillary fragility
c. Testing for contact allergy
d. Differentiating erythema from purpura
e. Differentiation of vitiligo from leprosy

41. Kerion is a scalp infection by:

a. Bacteria
b. Candida
c. Anaerobes
d. Dermatophytes
e. Larvae of flies

42. Favus is a type of:

a. Alopecia areata
b. Tinea capitis
c. Cicatrising alopecia
d. Pityriasis capitis
e. Yellow fluorescence

ANSWERS

1-c,	2-d,	3-d,	4-b,	5-e,	6-d,	7-a,	8-d,	9-c,	10-e,
11-a,	12-c,	13-a,	14-a,	15-d,	16-a,	17-b,	18-d,	19-b,	20-b,
21-e,	22-b,	23-a,	24-d,	25-b,	26-d,	27-a,	28-d,	29-d,	30-a,
31-c,	32-b,	33-b,	34-d,	35-b,	36-e,	37-c,	38-a,	39-e,	40-c,
41-d,	42-b								

CHAPTER 3

Physiological Variations in Skin and Age Related Diseases

The normal skin shows tremendous variation in its morphological features and even physiologic functioning at different ages. Moreover, age related changes in the skin makes it vulnerable to certain diseases depending on these variations. This chapter tries to trace the changes and introduce the reader to such age related diseases.

PHYSIOLOGIC VARIATIONS IN INFANCY

The skin in infants (except in premature babies) is fully mature with respect to the barrier function. The water content and vascularity is high which makes it appear red and soft. Vascular thermal adapta-tion is not fully developed (especially in hypothyroid) in young infants leading to cutis marmorata (marbled skin) over limbs. Systemic absorption of topical medications is a distinct possibility due to the high body surface to weight ratio and the occlusive environment that the infant is kept in.

SKIN DISEASES IN INFANCY

Both infectious and non-infectious diseases can occur during infancy.

Pustular Eruptions in Infancy

Pustular Eruptions in Infancy
• Toxic erythema of newborn
• Transient neonatal pustular melanosis
• Miliaria pustulosa
• Impetigo
• Candidiasis

Toxic erythema of newborn

This benign, self-limiting condition occurs in term infants as variably sized macules or patches of erythema topped with pustules and less commonly vesicles. Lesions appear on first or second day after birth. Lesions commonly affect the trunk. Smear from the pustule shows eosinophils. No treatment is required as lesions heal within a week.

Transient neonatal pustular melanosis

This transient condition is commoner in the dark skinned. Tiny pustular lesions occur on erythema-tous background which subside with hyperpigmen-tation. Smear from the pustule shows neutrophils. The condition is self-limiting and heals within 1–2 weeks.

Miliaria rubra and miliaria pustulosa

They occur as multiple tiny papulopustules over the sites of occlusion and trunk (Fig. 3.1). Covered areas of the body are commonly involved. The condition is more common in hot and humid climates and affects neonates and infants due to occlusive or tight baby wraps.

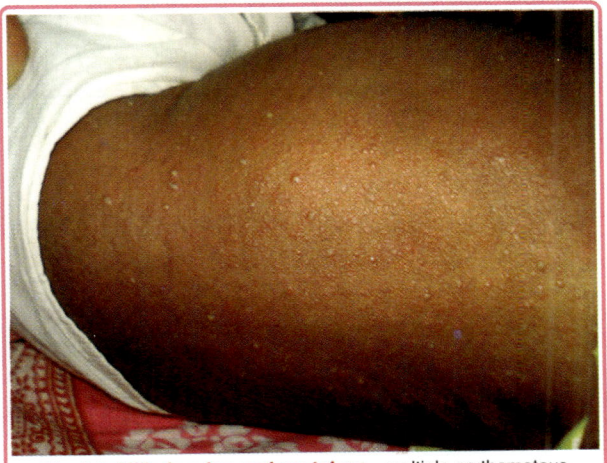

Fig. 3.1: Miliaria rubra and pustulosa—multiple erythematous papules and pustules

Candidiasis

Premature babies are more prone to develop can-didiasis due to low immunity. Curdy white patches with surrounding erythema are seen over the tongue and buccal mucosa (thrush). Skin lesions appear as 2–4 mm pustules in flexors along with maceration and erythema in the skin folds. Lesions subside with formation of collarette of scale.

Vesiculobullous Eruptions in Infancy and Childhood

Impetigo and staphylococcal scalded skin syndrome

Impetigo is the commonest bacterial infection affecting infants. Lesions tend to form large clear bullae as against small pustules or crusted erosions in children. For more details *see* page 45.

Herpes virus infection

Active herpes simplex virus infection in mothers during labour, may lead to widespread herpes infection in neonates that may at times involve the lungs or the brain and may be fatal. Scattered clear vesicles with central umbilication and surrounding erythema are the characteristics.

Epidermolysis bullosa

Bullae and erosions develop on the trauma prone sites like hands, feet, knees, elbows and even the mouth. For more information please refer to page 248.

Hand, foot and mouth diseases

Papules and vesicles appear suddenly in toddlers and older children over limbs, buttocks, face and in the mouth. This enteroviral infection is self-limiting to a few weeks and only requires supportive treatment (Fig. 3.2).

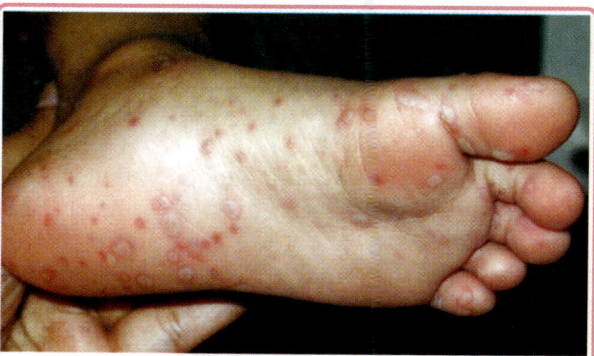

Fig. 3.2: Hand, foot and mouth disease—papulovesicles over foot in a 4-year-old child

---

Vesiculobullous Eruptions in Childhood

- Impetigo
- Bullous impetigo
- Staphylococcal scalded skin syndrome (SSSS)
- Chickenpox
- Hand foot and mouth disease
- Pompholyx
- Insect bite reaction
- Scabies
- Prurigo simplex
- Atopic dermatitis
- Epidermolysis bullosa

Pigmentary Conditions in Infancy

Mongolian spots

These are blue gray macules or patches over lumbosacral region and that are noticed at birth or in the first few months of life (Fig. 3.3). The lesions resolve by the age of 5 years.

Pigmented Lesions in Childhood and Adolescence

- Mongolian spots
- Café au lait spots (coffee with milk spots)
- Congenital melanocytic nevus
- Lentigines
- Freckles
- Junctional nevi
- Epidermal nevi

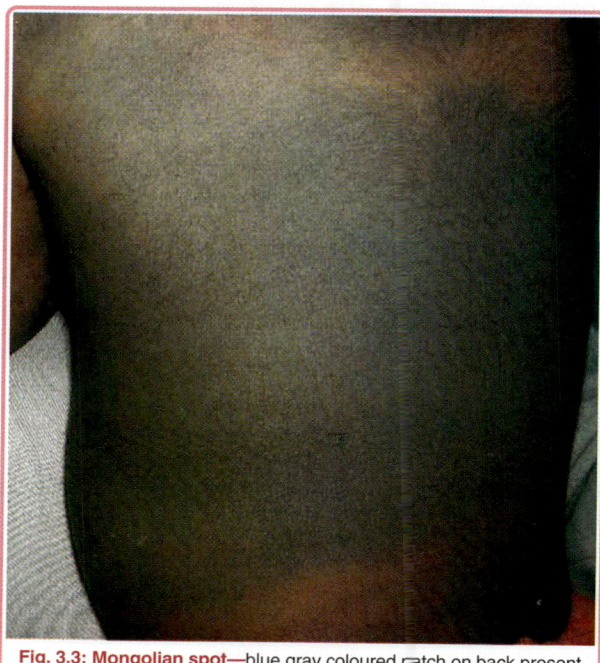

Fig. 3.3: Mongolian spot—blue gray coloured patch on back present since birth

Café au lait (coffee with milk) spots

These are well defined light brown or coffee coloured macules or patches. They can occur in up to 5% of normal persons or may be a cutaneous manifestation of neurofibromatosis. The spots persist unchanged though they may grow in size with the growth of the baby. Presence of more than 6 spots of more than 0.5 cm diameter at birth, are suggestive of the diagnosis of neurofibromatosis (Fig. 3.4)

Vascular Neoplasms and Malformations

Strawberry haemangioma

This is seen as bright red, circular or oval, compressible plaque or nodule, noticed at or soon after birth and that grows rapidly during the first 6 months. Most lesions regress completely by the age of 5 years. For more details *see* page 237.

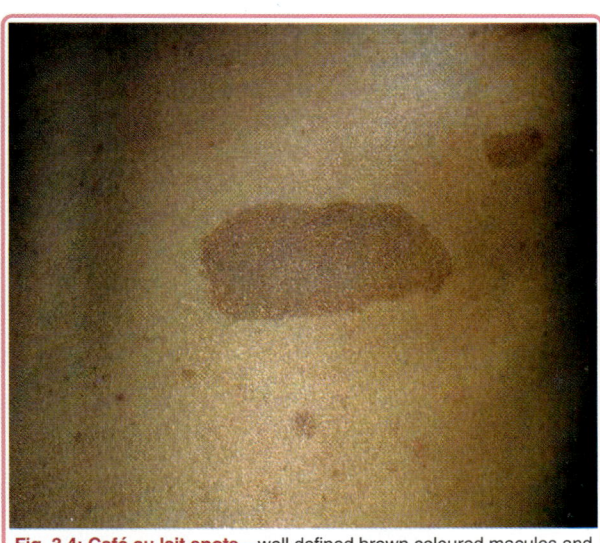

Fig. 3.4: Café au lait spots—well defined brown coloured macules and patches

Salmon patch (angel's kiss/nevus flammeus)

This capillary malformation is seen at birth as a pink to red, blanchable flat lesion on the nape of the neck. It usually subsides in a few months without any treatment.

Vascular and Lymphatic Malformations
- Strawberry haemangioma
- Salmon patch (angel's kiss/nevus flammeus)
- Port wine stain
- Lymphangioma circumscriptum
- Cystic hygroma
- Lymphoedema

Port wine stain

These are flat capillary malformations that occur as sharply defined, irregular, bright or dark red, patches that are difficult to blanch and remain largely unchanged since birth. Please *see* page 204 for further details.

Lymphangioma circumscriptum

This focal malformation of lymphatics affects the shoulder girdle or the pelvic girdle or the flanks. Lesions are seen as clustered, clear and umbilicated vesicles that ooze clear fluid on trauma. Treatment is ablative but recurrences are common. Due to its slow progress, the lesions are noticed in later childhood.

Cystic hygroma

This is usually seen as a single, large soft, cystic and translucent mass present since birth in the neck. If large it can compress airway and oesophagus making breathing or feeding difficult.

PHYSIOLOGIC VARIATIONS IN CHILDHOOD

Skin is soft due to higher water content but is not oily. It is thinner with a higher number of vellus follicles and hence has more vellus hair. Although fully mature, the skin in children is more prone to steroid induced atrophy. Due to the higher body surface to weight ratio chances of systemic absorption of topically applied medications is higher. Prolonged and generalised application of a potent topical steroid may lead to iatrogenic Cushing's syndrome.

SKIN DISEASES IN CHILDREN

Developmental and genetic diseases are common in children. However, in day-to-day practice, the types of skin diseases seen commonly in children are either infective or allergic in origin. Impetigo, scabies, molluscum contagiosum or viral warts are common in children. Atopic dermatitis typically affects children of almost all ages and may differ in its presentation according to the age-group affected.

PHYSIOLOGIC VARIATIONS IN ADOLESCENCE

Hormonal changes (increased sex hormones) are the initiating event for skin changes in adolescence. The skin develops a glow during the adolescence probably due to the stimulated action of the sebaceous glands. Development of secondary sexual characteristics including conversion of vellus hair to terminal hair in axillae and pubic area occurs during adolescence. In males, hair over beard and moustache regions convert to terminal type while those over anterior temple and forehead convert to vellus type (pubertal recession).

SKIN DISEASES IN ADOLESCENT

Commonest skin condition seen in adolescents is acne vulgaris. Highly active sebaceous glands initiate development of acne in many otherwise normal adolescents. They also promote occurrence of pityriasis versicolor over the seborrhoeic areas of the trunk and face. Seborrhoeic dermatitis and androgenetic alopecia also begin during adolescence.

BECKER'S NEVUS

A large patch of coffee brown pigmentation is seen with or without hypertrichosis over it. The lesion appears over shoulder, chest, arm or buttocks; the lesion appears after puberty and remains static thereafter.

PHYSIOLOGIC VARIATIONS IN OLD AGE (SKIN AGING)

Aging of skin occurs due to two factors sunlight (photoaging) and true aging. Sun-exposed areas of the body are more severely affected and show changes of solar elastosis. Solar elastosis is seen as slightly thickened, leathery, yellowish coloured skin with prominence of the crisscross skin markings. Aged skin looks dry, thin and wrinkled (Fig. 3.5). Deep wrinkles lead to the crow lines at the outer canthus and the deepened and fixed lines of expression lead to the forehead furrows. Over a period of time, telangiectasia, solar lentigo, seborrhoeic keratoses and dyspigmentation appear. Solar keratoses are uncommon in the brown skinned Indians but may be seen in the habitually sun-exposed fair coloured individuals.

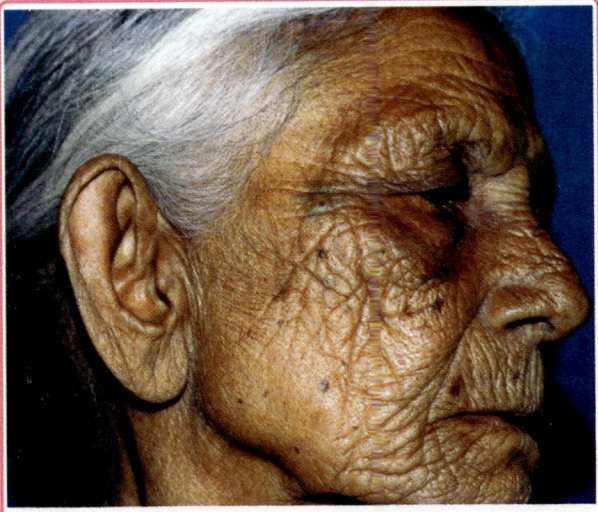

Fig. 3.5: Aging—wrinkled, yellowish leathery skin due to solar damage

---

Signs of Skin Aging

Photoaging signs (solar elastosis)

- Thickened, leathery skin
- Deep coarse wrinkles
- Yellowish colour (elastosis)
- Crisscross skin markings
- Solar lentigo
- Seborrhoeic keratoses
- Dyspigmentation
- Solar keratosis (actinic keratosis)

True aging

- Dry skin
- Thin and wrinkled
- Deep fine wrinkles
- Forehead furrows
- Telangiectasia

SKIN DISEASES IN ELDERLY

Pruritus

Due to reduced sweating and sebaceous gland activity, the elderly are prone to develop xerosis of the skin. Besides, aging is associated with reduced water content of the skin, itching and dry skin with or without mild scaling occur. Exacerbation in winter is common. Progression to xerotic eczema (winter eczema) may occur if dry skin is not taken care of. Even without the dry skin, pruritus is a common skin complaint in elderly. Renal failure, hepatic disorders, haematological malignancies like lymphoma, leukaemias and even drugs may cause pruritus. Lichen simplex chronicus may occur due to persistent rubbing and scratching.

Stasis Dermatitis

Impaired venous return in the legs reduces capacity to withstand long periods of standing and leads to haemosiderin induced hyper-pigmentation, itching and eczematisation around the ankles. Progression may lead to stasis ulcers around the medial or lateral malleoli and these are resistant to healing.

Infections

Decreased immunity with aging leads to susceptibility to bacterial, fungal and viral infections. Associated diseases like diabetes and compromised circulation make them vulnerable to infections like carbuncle, erysipelas, cellulitis or lymphangiitis. Oral candidiasis is common and herpes zoster is commoner and more severe.

Benign and Malignant Neoplasms

Both benign and malignant neoplasms are much more common in the elderly. Common benign neoplasms include, seborrhoeic keratoses and melanocytic nevi while common malignant neoplasms include, basal cell carcinoma, squamous cell carcinoma and Bowen's disease. For their detailed descriptions refer page 230.

Autoimmune Bullous Diseases

Some of the autoimmune bullous diseases like bullous pemphigoid, mucosal pemphigoid are commoner in the elderly. They need to be managed with special care due to the numerous co-morbidities and drug interactions likely to occur in the elderly.

PHYSIOLOGIC CHANGES IN PREGNANCY

The skin in pregnancy is more vascular, soft and smooth. Vascular spiders are occasionally seen. The skin also becomes more pigmented especially over nipples, areola and mucocutaneous junctions. A pigmentary line may develop in the midline of the trunk (linea nigra). Pre-existing nevi and scars may darken. Late pregnancy is associated with vulval oedema and varicosities. Stretch marks (striae) commonly occur during pregnancy. Striae appear over the abdomen, breasts and thighs as linear pinkish or hypopigmented marks. They may improve in appearance after pregnancy but usually persist.

SKIN DISEASES IN PREGNANCY

Pregnancy Mask (Melasma, Chloasma)

This is seen as symmetrical, light brown, blotchy pigmentation over the butterfly area of the face and forehead. The pigmentation commonly appears during pregnancy but persists indefinitely thereafter (Please *see* under 'Melasma' page 161 for details).

Pruritus Gravidarum

This is also called intrahepatic cholestasis of pregnancy and is common in the third trimester of pregnancy. It starts as generalised itching without any skin lesions. Excoriations on the skin may be seen due to vigorous scratching. Icterus and yellowish discolouration of skin can occur in severe cases. Condition remits within a few weeks after delivery but may recur in subsequent pregnancies. Management is symptomatic which includes topical application of soothing and antipruritic agents and if needed, oral antihistaminics.

Prurigo of Pregnancy

This is an extremely pruritic, excoriated papular eruption over trunk and extremities that occurs during the third trimester. The condition responds poorly to treatment but resolves after pregnancy.

Pruritic Urticarial Papules and Plaques of Pregnancy

It is seen as itchy erythematous papules and plaques in third trimester of pregnancy. Lesions characteristically begin over the striae. Treatment is symptomatic; however, drug usage should be minimized in pregnancy. Severe cases may need to be treated with antihistaminics and topical steroids.

Herpes Gestationis (Bullous Pemphigoid of Pregnancy)

This is a rare autoimmune bullous disease resembling bullous pemphigoid that presents during the third trimester or in the post-partum period. Without intervention with systemic steroids the condition may adversely affect the prognosis of the baby.

MCQs

1. **All of the following are self-resolving except:**
   a. Mongolian spot   b. Nevus flammeus
   c. Capillary haemangioma d. Port wine stain

2. **Eosinophils in smear are seen in:**
   a. Toxic erythema of newborn
   b. Transient neonatal pustulosis
   c. Miliaria pustulosa
   d. None of the above

3. **Most common organism causing bullous impetigo is:**
   a. *Staphylococcus aureus*
   b. *Streptococcus pyogenes*
   c. *Micrococcus sedentarius*
   d. *Corynebacterium minutissisum*

4. **All of the following are associated with pruritus in the elderly except:**
   a. Liver disorder   b. Kidney disorder
   c. Peripheral neuropathy d. None of these

5. **Adolescence is associated with:**
   a. Becker's nevus   b. Onset of acne
   c. Oily skin   d. All of these

6. **Which of the following is associated with adverse foetal outcome?**
   a. Prurigo of pregnancy
   b. Pruritic urticarial papules and plaques of pregnancy
   c. Herpes gestationis
   d. None of the above

7. **An 18-year-old male came with a new onset hairy patch on his left shoulder. He denied any family history of similar lesions. The diagnosis is:**
   a. Cafe au lait spot   b. Dermal melasma
   c. Becker's nevus   d. Mongolian spot

8. **All of the following are signs of aging except:**
   a. Dry wrinkled skin
   b. Seborrhoeic keratoses
   c. Thickened skin
   d. Telangiectasias

9. **Which of the following is true for infants?**
   a. Systemic absorption of topical medications is high
   b. The skin is immature even in full term babies
   c. Hand foot and mouth disease is common n infants
   d. Miliaria rubra is common in uncovered areas of the body

10. **A 3-month-old baby is having thick yellow greasy scales on scalp. Diagnosis is:**
    a. Occlusion miliaria
    b. Seborrhoeic dermatitis
    c. Candidiasis
    d. Atopic dermatitis

11. **A common disease seen in children:**
    a. Molluscum contagiosum
    b. Acne
    c. Seborrhoeic dermatitis
    d. Erythrodermic psoriasis

12. **Common site of stasis ulcer is:**
    a. Medial malleolus   b. Lateral malleolus
    c. Dorsa of foot   d. Calf

13. **Trigger factor for the development of melasma is:**
    a. Adolescence   b. Obesity
    c. Pregnancy   d. Chronic infections

14. **A 70-year-old male came with history of fluid filled lesions over the left side of the back along with severe burning pain. Diagnosis is:**
    a. Candidiasis   b. Herpes zoster
    c. Carbuncle   d. Folliculitis

15. **Which of the following bullous disease is particularly common in the elderly?**
    a. Pemphigus vulgaris
    b. Dermatitis herpetiformis
    c. Bullous pemphigoid
    d. Pemphigus foliaceus

--- ANSWERS ---

1-d,	2-a,	3-a,	4-d,	5-d,	6-c,	7-c,	8-c,	9-a,	10-b,
11-a,	12-a,	13-c,	14-b,	15-c					

SECTION 2

Skin Diseases

Cutaneous Infections—Scabies and Pediculosis

SCABIES

This is a common ectoparasitic infestation caused by the mite *Sarcoptes scabiei* (Figs 4.1 and 4.2) that is transmitted by close skin to skin contact.

Patient Profile

Affects children, more frequently than young adults. Overcrowding facilitates transmission.

Incubation Period

Incubation period of about 1 month passes before pruritus (itching) begins due to development of hypersensitivity to mite antigens.

> **Clinical implication:** Since pruritus is due to hypersensitivity to mite products, it may persist for a few weeks even after adequate and successful therapy with a miticidal agent.

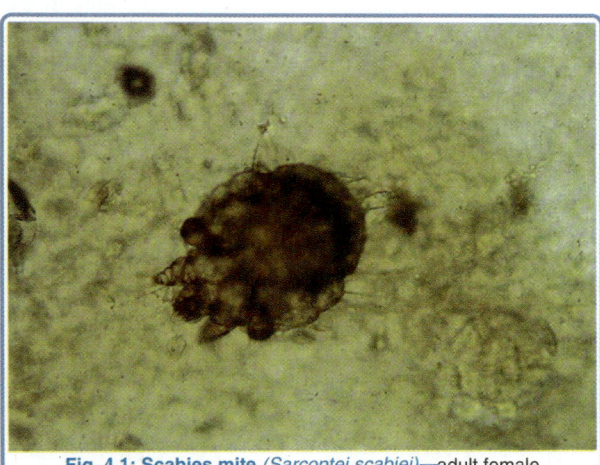

Fig. 4.1: Scabies mite *(Sarcoptei scabiei)*—adult female

Life Cycle

Transfer of a fertilised female mite (size about 300 microns) is necessary for transmission of infection. It lays eggs in a burrow. Passing through larval and nymphal stages, they than turn into adults in 10–14 days.

> **Clinical implication:** Since most antiscabietics are not ovicidal a second application after 10 days is needed to kill larvae and nymphs which are, newly formed unaffected ova.

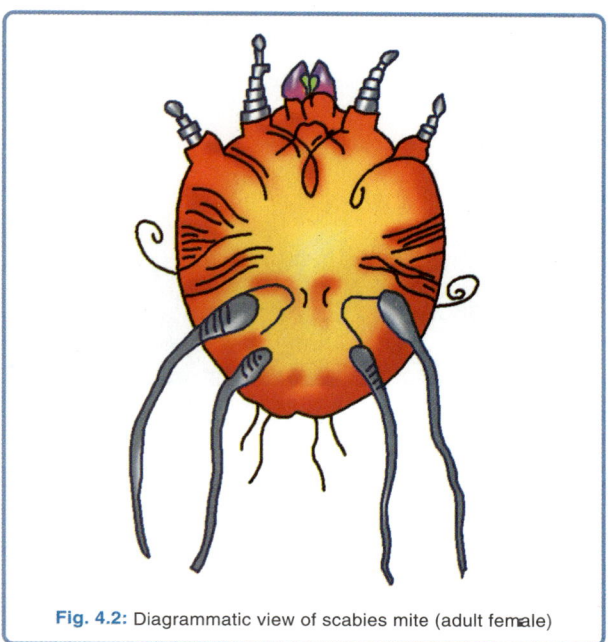

Fig. 4.2: Diagrammatic view of scabies mite (adult female)

Clinical Features

History

Severe **pruritus,** that gets worse at night, is a rule. More than one family member is usually affected. Commonly scabies is transmitted from one family to another family through young children. Occasionally, in adults, it is transmitted through sexual contact.

Examination

The mite of scabies resides in the superficial epidermis between the cornified and the granular layer. It digs a tunnel at this level which is visible clinically as an irregular gray-brown line **(burrow)** about 5 mm long over the wrists, finger webs, genitalia and in young children, over palms/soles. Presence of a burrow is diagnostic of scabies.

Other skin lesions have uncharacteristic morphology but **characteristic distribution.** Tiny erythematous papules, excoriated papules and papulo-vesicles are located in the web spaces, wrists (Fig. 4.3), ulnar border of forearm and arm, anterior axillary fold, nipple and areola in women, periumbilical region, and especially in the male, over genitalia, anterior thighs, buttocks and natal cleft. Face, scalp, back, palms and soles are spared in adults, but are commonly involved in infants and young children. Erythematous follicular papules over anterior thighs are common in adults (Fig. 4.4).

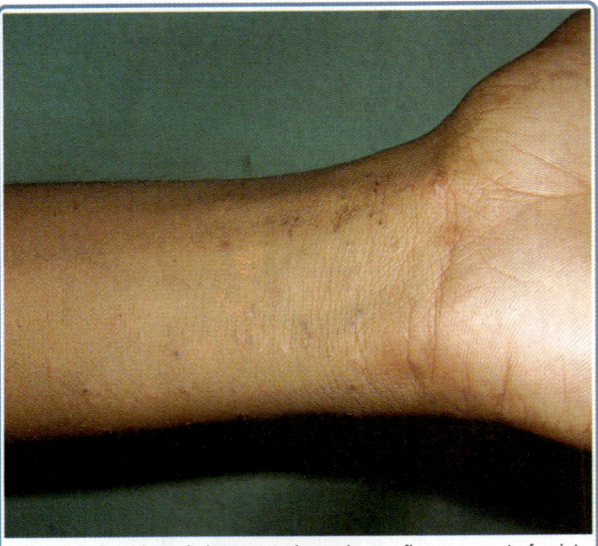

Fig. 4.3: Scabies—itchy, crusted papules on flexor aspect of wrist

Variations

Genital scabies occurs in sexually active adult males and presents as reddish excoriated papules on the glans and shaft of penis, scrotum and inner thighs.

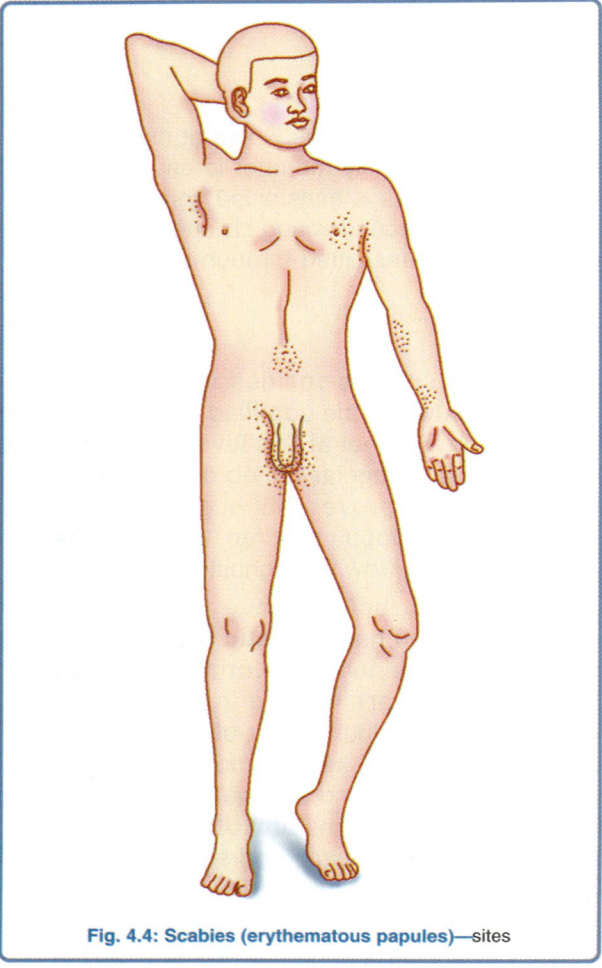

Fig. 4.4: Scabies (erythematous papules)—sites

Scabies in the 'clean' is seen in individuals with better personal hygiene. These patients have fewer lesions, some of which are at atypical sites, but severe pruritus.

Clinical implication: Without a high index of suspicion, this diagnosis may be missed. Prescription of topical or systemic steroids at this stage may induce 'scabies' incognito'.

Clinical Features of Scabies

1. Classical scabies
2. Eczematised scabies
3. Infected scabies
4. Genital scabies
5. Scabies in the 'clean'
6. Nodular scabies
7. Keratotic scabies

Nodular scabies

This is a hypersensitive response to the mite antigens and commonly follows an episode of typical scabies. Erythematous or Skin coloured papulonodules occur over genitalia, especially in the male, or axillae. Lesions are extremely pruritic. Mite or Mite products can't be demonstrated from these skin lesions. Typical lesions of scabies are frequently absent (Fig. 4.5).

Keratotic scabies

Develops in the special categories of patients mentioned later (*see* page 38).

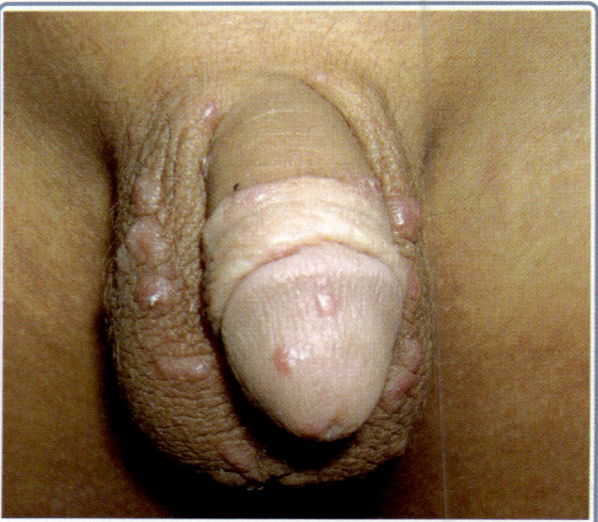

Fig. 4.5 : Nodular scabies—intensely itchy, erythematous papules and nodules

Complications

Bacterial infection (infected scabies)

If left untreated, a case of classical scabies develops secondary bacterial infection with streptococci or staphylococci.

Pre-existing lesions of scabies turn into pustules and at times bullae filled with pus. As these lesions burst, they get covered with purulent (yellowish) crusts. Due to scratching, erosions results. Uninfected lesions of scabies are also present.

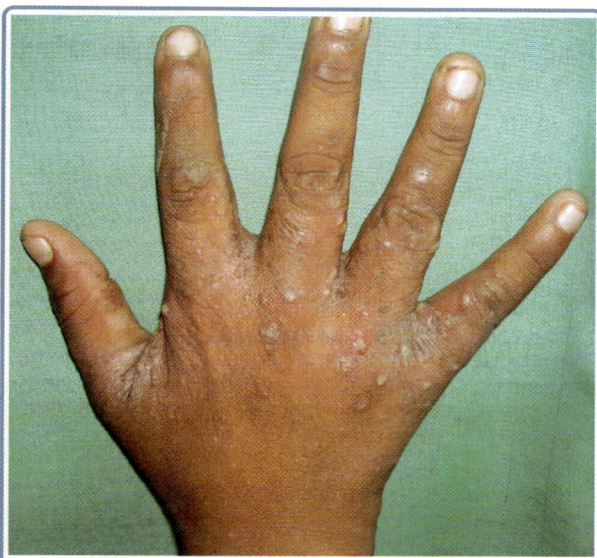

Fig. 4.6: Scabies with secondary infection—pustules and papules in web spaces and dorsum of hand

Eczematisation (eczematised scabies)

Infants and young children frequently develop this complication. Affected areas of trunk and extremities display erythema, oedema, vesiculation, oozing and sanguinous crusting. Face is commonly involved in infants. Typical lesions of scabies are present in

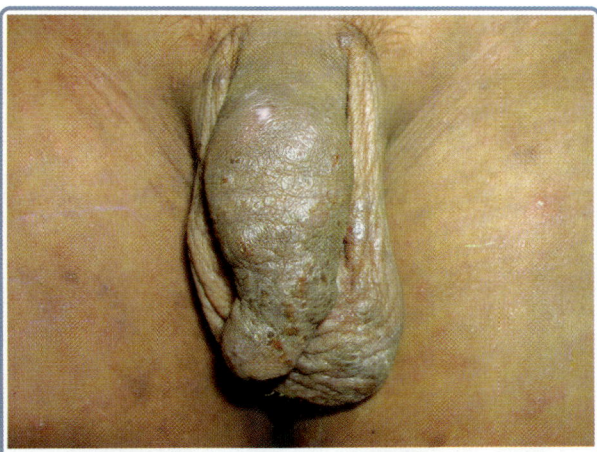

Fig. 4.7: Eczematised scabies on genitals—crusted papules on penis and scrotum

characteristic locations in addition to the eczematous patches (Fig. 4.7).

Paraphimosis

Inability to take forward the retracted oedematous preputial skin is a complication of scabies peculiar to children.

Immunologic sequelae

Due to associated streptococcal infection, glomerulonephritis and rheumatic fever are potential complications in children.

Diagnosis

In India, a country that is endemic for scabies, the diagnosis is based on personal or family history or pruritus and examination findings typical for scabies. Mites can be demonstrated by scraping the skin lesions or by extracting a mite from a burrow. However, this is not always easy except in cases of keratotic scabies.

Treatment

All **family members,** at least all the children in the family and the spouse of the affected person, must be treated simultaneously (Table 4.1).

Therapy consists of overnight application of a scabicide from neck to toe, carefully covering all parts, after a scrub bath. Application must be repeated after 10 days if the agent is not ovicidal. **Gamma benzene hexachloride** (1%, one application), permethrin (5%, one application, miticidal and ovicidal agent) benzyl benzoate (25%, 3 applications) are popular effective remedies, but benzyl benzoate should be avoided because of its irritant potential. Crotamiton and precipitated sulphur are only moderately effective.

Antihistaminics like hydroxyzine hydrochloride help relieve pruritus. Non-sedative antihistaminics like desloratidine or levocetirizine or fexofenadine may be used if sedation is to be avoided. Oral ivermectin in a single dose of 0.2 mg/kg is moderately effective but its safety in children and pregnant women is yet to be proved. Permethrin is the drug of choice in these cases.

Ordinarily, it takes 1–2 weeks for relief of pruritus. Therapeutic failure is usually due to non-compliance with the instructions regarding application of anti-scabietic agent or due to reinfestation from a family member or, very rarely due to resistance to a scabicide. Combination therapy of topical permethrin

	GBH	Permethrin	Benzyl benzoate	Sulphur	Crotamiton
TABLE 4.1 : Topical therapy of scabies					
Concentration [%]	1	5	25	5	10
No. of applications	1	1	3	3	3
Irritation	No	No	Yes	Yes	No
Relative contraindications	Infants, pregnancy	Nil	Children, infected or eczematised scabies	Infected or eczematised scabies	Nil
Efficacy	Good	Good	Good	Moderate	Moderate
Repeat after 10 days	Yes	Not needed	Yes	Yes	Yes
Advantage	Effective and inexpensive	Ovicidal and effective as one application	Inexpensive	Inexpensive	Additional antipruritic action
Disadvantage	Neurotoxicity in infants if over-used	Safe in pregnancy and infants (> 2 months of age)	Causes severe burning	Stains, stinks and sticks	Safe but less efficacious

N.B. : GBH = Gamma Benzene Hexachloride

and oral ivermectin is needed for severe or unresponsive cases or in communities or families where the chain of transmission is difficult to break.

Treatment of Complications

Complication like bacterial infection, eczematisation and paraphimosis need to be treated before antiscabietic applications.

Bacterial infections are easily controlled with oral erythromycin or cefadroxyl, or roxithromycin, or cloxacillin. Topical antibiotics like neomycin (1%) and framycetin [1%] are useful adjuncts. Improving personal hygiene helps hasten recovery.

Eczematisation should be treated, in the acute oozing phase, with cold soaks or compresses using Condy's solution. Topical steroids may then be added. Topical or oral antibiotics are commonly added to control accompanying secondary bacterial infection. The fact that the original underlying condition is scabies that needs separate treatment at a later date should be explained to the patient. Administering topical or systemic steroids to a patient with scabies will result into **'scabies incognito'**. In this condition, which may be missed if the history of steroid administration is not elicited, pruritus is mild or absent and skin lesions occur at atypical sites and appear less inflamed.

Nodular scabies responds to topical or intralesional steroids.

Keratotic scabies (Norwegian scabies) is a rare variant of scabies that affects immunosuppressed persons [lymphoma, human immunodeficiency virus (HIV) infection and immunosuppressive therapy] or those who have lost the sensation of pruritus (leprosy) or are unable to take care of themselves (mental retardation, Down's syndrome). Keratotic and scaly erythematous plaques over trunk, extremities, scalp and face characterise this condition (Fig. 4.8). Sometimes, this condition presents as generalised erythroderma. This type of scabies is likely to be missed unless a high index of suspicion is maintained. Such delays in instituting correct treatment may result in epidemics of scabies in the community because these patients are highly infectious. Norwegian scabies responds to ivermectin combined with a topical keratolytic, like 3% salicylic acid, and repeated applications of an antiscabietic.

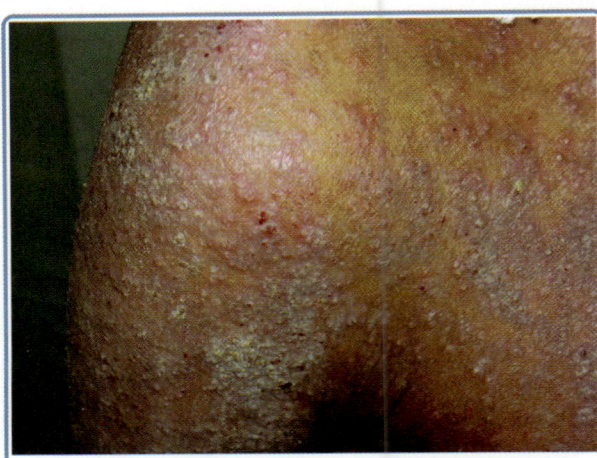

Fig. 4.8: Crusted scabies—keratotic and erythematous papules

Summary: Scabies is caused by the mite, *Sarcoptes scabiei*. Diagnosis is based on nocturnal pruritus, family history of pruritus and the presence of excoriated papules in finger web spaces, wrists, axillae, genitals, thighs and buttocks. Burrows, though diagnostic, are difficult to find. Treat the family and the patient with topical 1% gamma benzene hexachloride lotion from neck to toe and repeat it after 10 days. Permethrin is effective as a single application. Oral ivermectin is moderately effective.

PEDICULOSIS

These ectoparasitic infestations are caused by the lice *Pediculus capitis*, *Pediculus corporis* and *Phthirius pubis* that cause pediculosis capitis, pediculosis corporis and pediculosis pubis respectively. Lice live on host blood and cannot survive for long without a host.

Body lice are responsible for transmission of louse borne relapsing fever, louse borne typhus and viral encephalitis.

Pediculosis Capitis (Head Louse Infestation)

This is the commonest of the lice infestations that is transmitted by close contact, e.g. sharing a bed or when children are playing (Figs 4.9 and 4.10).

Patient profile

Children and women are typically affected. Overcrowded communities provide an ideal setting. Infrequent combing and washing predispose to this infestation.

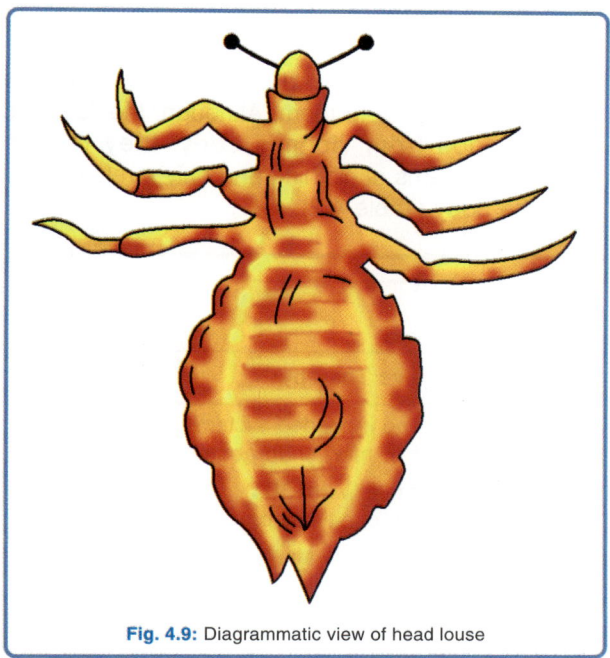

Fig. 4.9: Diagrammatic view of head louse

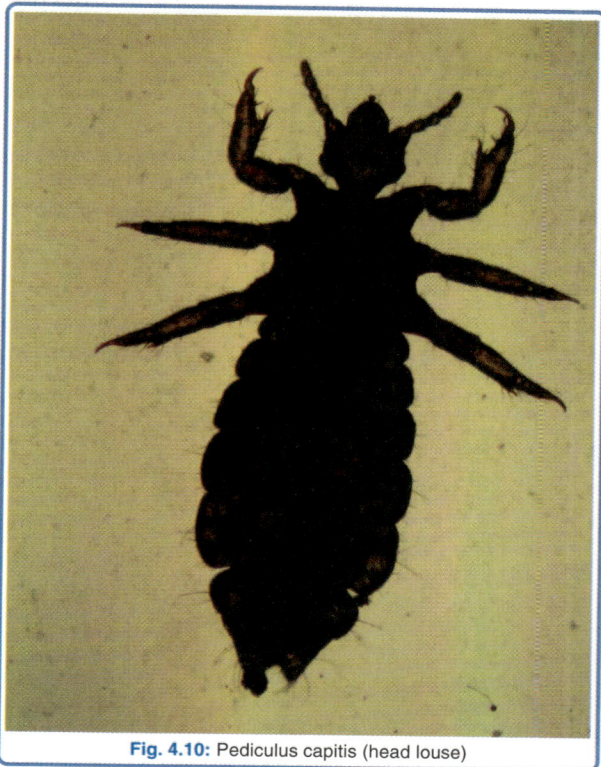

Fig. 4.10: Pediculus capitis (head louse)

History

Early infestations present with scalp pruritus. Advanced cases complain of pruritus and 'boils' in the scalp or glands in the neck. Most patients are aware of lice or nits in the scalp.

Morphology

Nits (egg), (Figs 4.11–4.13) are always detectable even when lice are not seen. Lice are difficult to find except in the heavily infested. Nits are differentiated from scales of 'dandruff' by their firm adherence to hair (dandruff can be flicked off hair). Under the microscope nits are seen as smooth surfaced oval structures attached to the hair at an angle of about 30 degrees. The free end of a nit point away from the hair root and is usually closed by an operculum (lid) if the nit is alive (Fig. 4.13).

Complications that arise due to persistent scratching include excoriated papules, which develop secondary streptococcal infection. Pustules, crusts and matting of scalp hair characterise this stage. Posterior cervical lymphadenopathy is a common presentation of pediculosis capitis.

Distribution

Hair of the postauricular and occipital regions of the scalp typically bear the nits. Nits survive in these areas probably because these regions are least attended to during hair grooming.

Chapter
4

Cutaneous Infections—Scabies and Pediculosis

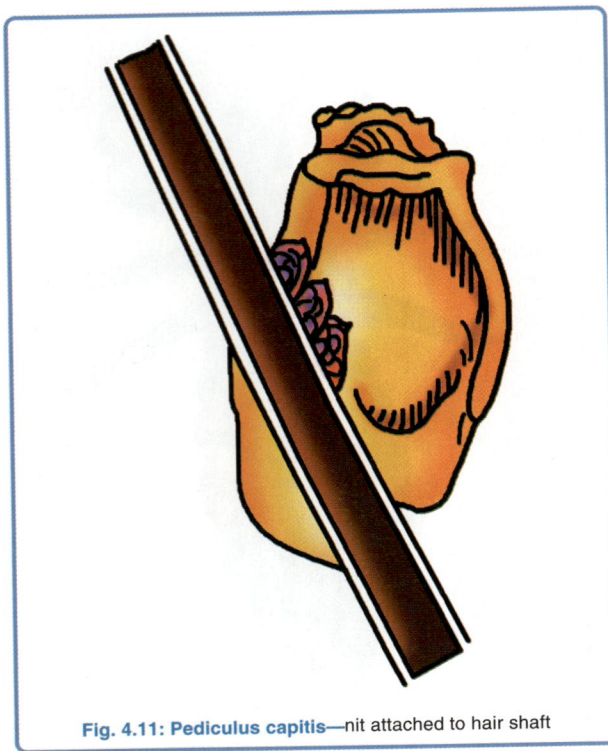

Fig. 4.11: Pediculus capitis—nit attached to hair shaft

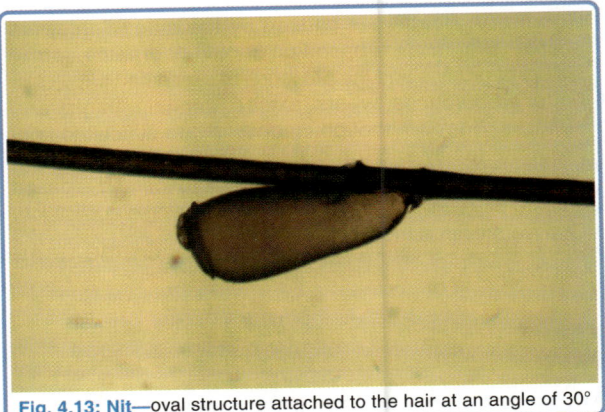

Fig. 4.13: Nit—oval structure attached to the hair at an angle of 30°

Single application of **gamma benzene hexachloride (1%), malathion (0.5%),** or permethrin (2%) is very effective. It is safer to repeat the application once after 10 days. Nits can be killed by applying kerosene **(5%)** or removed by combing the hair with a fine toothed comb following application of vinegar (dilute acetic acid) that loosens them.

Supportive therapy includes the use of a **shampoo** to cleanse the scalp, an **antihistaminic** to relieve pruritus and oral and topical **antibacterial agents** for the therapy of bacterial infection and/or cervical lymphadenopathy.

Summary: Pediculosis capitis is caused by the head louse. Women and children are affected because of close contact. Diagnosis is based on finding nits (eggs) with or without scalp pruritus, pustules, crusts and cervical lymphadenopathy. Scalp applications of 1% gamma benzene hexachloride or 1% permethrin are curative.

Pediculosis Corporis (Vagabond's Disease, Body Louse Infestation)

Skin lesions are produced due to the feeding by lice and hypersensitivity to them. Although, the lice feed on the blood from victim's body, they remain attached to seams of clothing and only rarely venture on to the body (Table 4.2).

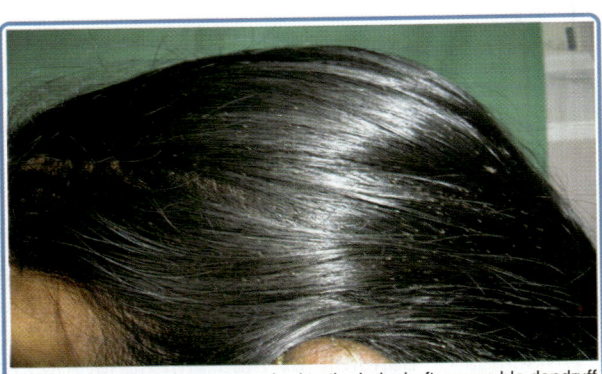

Fig. 4.12: Numerous nits, attached to the hair shafts resemble dandruff

Treatment

All predisposed family members especially those sharing beds with the patient should be treated.

TABLE 4.2 : Therapy of pediculosis		
Type	**Main Therapy**	**Supportive Therapy**
Capitis	Gamma-benzene hexachloride (GBH) 1% or Permethrin 2% or Malathion 0.5% apply overnight to scalp	Topical and if needed systemic antibacterials, removal of nits, shampooing
Corporis	Wash clothes in boiling water and press with hot iron	Treat clothes with DDT or GBH. Treat ped. capitis, if present.
Pubis	Apply 1% GBH or 2% permethrin to pubis, perineum, genitals, perianal region, thighs, lower abdomen and other involved hairy parts.	Shave hair from affected sites.

Patient profile

Affected adults are usually male, who, unfortunately, are unable to wash their clothes regularly. Most of these persons lack a home and hence the name, vagabond's disease.

Morphology

Numerous petechial and erythematous macules, papules with haemorrhagic puncta, some in linear array, and excoriations typify this disease.

Distribution

Upper back over the scapulae, shoulders, infra-axillary region and waistline are commonly affected. Examination of clothing seams that touch these regions reveals lice and nits. The latter can be detected with a lens.

Diagnosis

Severe pruritus over the trunk, especially the back that is out of proportion for existing skin lesions arouses suspicion. History of infrequent laundering of clothes is helpful. Lice and nits can be demonstrated in the clothing and confirmed under the microscope.

Treatment

Immersing all clothes in boiling water, thorough washing and hot ironing with special attention to the seams is curative. Powdering clothes and bedding with a disinfectant like DDT (10%), gamma benzene hexachloride (1%), pyrethrin or malathion is an alternative. Improving personal hygiene and regular washing of clothes is crucial for preventing a recurrence.

Summary: Pediculosis corporis affects those unfortunate persons who are unable to wash their clothes with regularity. Severe pruritus over trunk demands a search for lice that cling to seams of underclothes. Treatment of clothes with boiling water followed by hot ironing or treating clothes with a pediculicide is curative.

Pediculosis Pubis

This sexually transmitted condition is caused by infestation with the pubic louse (also called crab louse because of its resemblance to a crab) (Figs 4.14 and 4.15). Affected young adults complain of intense pruritus of the pubis, inner thighs, perineum and other hairy parts. With a hand lens, lice can be seen burying their heads into follicular orifices and nits are attached to hair shafts. Excoriations and occasional bluish macules (maculae cerulae) are the only skin lesions. Treatment consists of single application of 1% gamma benzene hexachloride or 2% permethrin to the affected parts. Sexual partner needs to be treated. Shaving off hair in the affected parts is helpful. In unresponsive cases, the application may be repeated after 10 days.

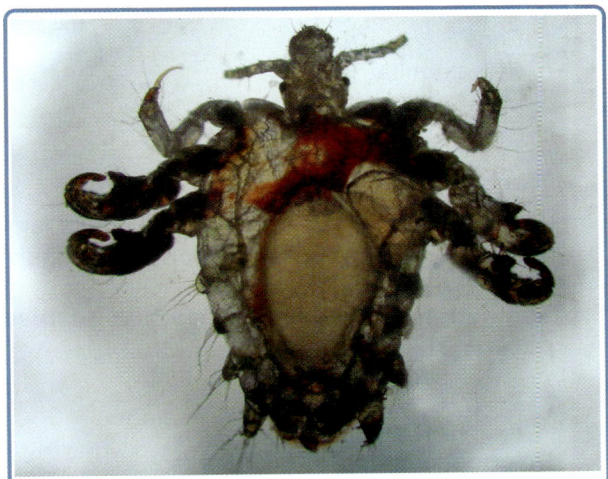

Fig. 4.14: Phthirus pubis (crab louse)

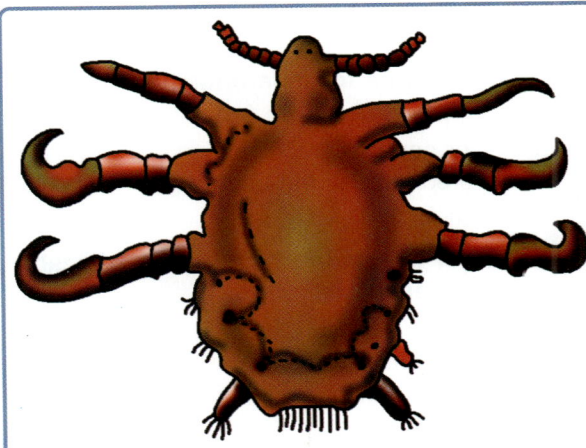

Fig. 4.15: Diagrammatic view of pubic louse (crab louse)

Chapter
4

Cutaneous Infections—Scabies and Pediculosis

MCQs

1. **The pruritus in scabies is worse:**
   a. After bath
   b. At night
   c. After hand washing
   d. Early in the morning

2. **Scabies spreads by:**
   a. Skin to skin contact
   b. Through fomites
   c. By droplet infection
   d. By sharing food

3. **Scabies is usually transmitted by transfer of:**
   a. Eggs
   b. Female mite
   c. Male and female mites
   d. Fertilised female mite

4. **The scabies mite has:**
   a. Two pairs of legs
   b. Three pairs of legs
   c. Four pairs of legs
   d. Six pairs of legs

5. **The average number of mites in a scabies patient is:**
   a. 1–2
   b. 2–4
   c. 10–12
   d. Hundreds

6. **Diagnostic lesion of scabies is:**
   a. Papule
   b. Vesicle
   c. Burrow
   d. Crusts containing mite

7. **Scabies tends to preferentially affect:**
   a. Acral regions
   b. Flexor aspects of the body
   c. Covered parts of the body
   d. Genitals

8. **The layer of skin in which burrow of scabies mite is present, is:**
   a. Dermis
   b. Basal layer of epidermis
   c. Granular layer of epidermis
   d. Spinous layer of epidermis

9. **The incubation period of scabies is:**
   a. 1–2 days
   b. 1 week
   c. 2 weeks
   d. 1 month

10. **The circle of Hebra in scabies does not include:**
    a. Hand
    b. Axilla
    c. Nipple
    d. Neck

11. **All of the following types of lesions occur in scabies *except*:**
    a. Pustule
    b. Plaque
    c. Papule
    d. Vesicle

12. **Scabies usually spreads within:**
    a. Families
    b. Communities
    c. Schools
    d. All of these

13. **Antiscabietic application must be made:**
    a. To the whole body
    b. To the whole body below neck
    c. To affected areas only
    d. Over the skin lesions only

14. **The antiscabietic that is safe in infants is all *except*:**
    a. Gamma benzene hexachloride
    b. Permethrin
    c. Precipitated sulphur
    d. Benzyle benzoate

15. **The percentage of permethrin cream used in scabies is:**
    a. 0.5%
    b. 1%
    c. 2%
    d. 5%

16. **The percentage of gamma benzene hexachloride used for scabies is:**
    a. 0.5%
    b. 1%
    c. 2%
    d. 5%

17. **The percentage of sulphur ointment used for treatment of scabies is:**
    a. 1%
    b. 2%
    c. 5%
    d. 10%

18. **The percentage of crotamiton used for treatment of scabies is:**
    a. 1%
    b. 2%
    c. 5%
    d. 10%

19. **A 2-year-old boy is brought to you with genital pruritus and on examination you find burrows on his hands. He has 3 siblings aged 4, 7 and 12 years who do not have any itching or skin lesions. Whom will you treat?**
    a. The whole family
    b. All the four siblings
    c. The three siblings less than 12 years
    d. The patient alone

20. **The drug of choice for treatment of scabies in pregnant women is:**
    a. Permethrin
    b. Gamma benzene hexachloride
    c. Precipitated sulphur
    d. Crotamiton

21. **A drug which is useful for oral treatment of scabies is:**
    a. Permethrin
    b. Precipitated sulphur
    c. Ivemectin
    d. Crotamiton

22. **The dose of ivermectin in scabies is:**
    a. 50 mcg/kg body weight
    b. 200 mcg/kg body weight
    c. 2 mg/kg body weight
    d. 5 mg/kg body weight

23. **A drug which acts on eggs of scabies mite is:**
    a. Permethrin
    b. Gamma benzene hexachloride
    c. Precipitated sulphur
    d. Crotamiton

24. **The preferred contact time for antiscabietic applications is:**
    a. 2 minutes
    b. 5 minutes
    c. 2 hours
    d. 8 hours

25. **Nodular scabies affects:**
    a. Genitals
    b. Axillae
    c. Elbows
    d. All of these

26. **Treatment of nodular scabies is:**
    a. Antiscabietic application to the lesions
    b. Antiscabietic application to the region
    c. Antiscabietic application to the whole body below neck
    d. Topical steroids

27. **Pediculosis capitis is:**
    a. Head louse infestation
    b. Another name for dandruff
    c. Side effect of pedicure
    d. Inflammatory condition of the foot

28. **Pediculosis capitis spreads by:**
    a. Skin to skin contact
    b. Sharing of combs
    c. Sharing of bed
    d. All of the above

29. **Pediculus capitis has:**
    a. Two pairs of legs
    b. Three pairs of legs
    c. Four pairs of legs
    d. Six pairs of legs

30. **Easily demonstrable sign of pediculosis capitis is:**
    a. Presence of lice
    b. Presence of nits
    c. Presence of hair casts
    d. All of the above

31. **The most common complaint of pediculosis capitis is:**
    a. Pruritus
    b. Pain
    c. Boils in scalp
    d. All of these

32. **A complication of pediculosis capitis is:**
    a. Bacterial infection in the scalp
    b. Lymphadenopathy
    c. Matting of hair
    d. All of the above

33. **Nits are:**
    a. Small lice
    b. Larvae of lice
    c. Eggs of lice
    d. Excreta of lice

34. **Nits of lice are:**
    a. Present on the scalp skin
    b. Lie freely on hair surface
    c. Firmly attached to hair
    d. All of the above

35. **Nits are usually found on the scalp in the:**
    a. Occipital region
    b. Frontal region
    c. Temporal region
    d. Vertical region

36. **Nits are differentiated from dandruff by:**
    a. Flicking
    b. Feeling
    c. Use of a magnifying lens
    d. All of the above

37. **Nits of lice are attached to hair:**
    a. At right angles
    b. At an angle of 60°
    c. At an angle of 30°
    d. Parallel to the hair shaft

38. **Treatment of choice for pediculosis capitis is application of:**
    a. Gamma benzene hexachloride
    b. Permethrin
    c. Vinegar
    d. Kerosene

Chapter 4

Cutaneous Infections—Scabies and Pediculosis

39. **Which of the following treatment does not work against nits in pediculosis?**
    a. Gamma benzene hexachloride
    b. Permethrin
    c. Vinegar
    d. Kerosene

40. **Percentage of permethrin used for treatment of pediculosis capitis is:**
    a. 0.1%   b. 1%
    c. 2%   d. 5%

41. **Lice in pediculosis corporis are present over:**
    a. The skin of trunk
    b. The seams of clothing
    c. The hair on the body
    d. All of the above

42. **Treatment of pediculosis corporis must include:**
    a. Oral pediculicide
    b. Pediculicide application to the whole body
    c. Pediculicide application to the affected parts
    d. Pediculicide treatment of clothes

43. **Which of the following pediculosis is sexually transmitted?**
    a. Pediculosis pubis
    b. Pediculosis capitis
    c. Pediculosis corporis
    d. All of the above

44. **A young adult with multiple sex partners complained of severe itching in the pubic region. No skin lesions were seen. What is the likely diagnosis?**
    a. Scabies
    b. Pediculosis corporis
    c. Vagabond's disease
    d. Pediculosis pubis

45. **A 10-year-old boy is brought with severe generalised pruritus that is disturbing his sleep since 1 month. He was seen 15 days back by a doctor who prescribed him oral antihistamines and topical steroids. Examination shows no skin lesions. The most probable diagnosis is:**
    a. Pediculosis pubis
    b. Pediculosis corporis
    c. Scabies incognito
    d. Scabies in the clean

46. **All of the following are complications of scabies in young children except:**
    a. Paraphimosis
    b. Eczematisation
    c. Secondary infection
    d. Keratotic lesions

47. **Single application for scabies is recommended for:**
    a. Sulphur   b. Crotamiton
    c. Permethrin   d. Lindane

48. **Body lice are responsible for:**
    a. Relapsing fever
    b. Chagaes disease
    c. Rickettsial pox
    d. Pediculosis pubis

49. **In the case of pediculosis corporis all are true except:**
    a. It is also known as vagabond's disease
    b. Disinfection of clothes is a must
    c. Recommended overnight application of GBH all over body
    d. Regular washing of clothes is crucial to prevent recurrence

50. **Size of the fertile female mite causing scabies is:**
    a. 200 microns   b. 300 microns
    c. 400 microns   d. 500 microns

--- **ANSWERS** ---

1-b,	2-a,	3-d,	4-c,	5-c,	6-c,	7-b,	8-c,	9-d,	10-d,
11-b,	12-d,	13-b,	14-a,	15-d,	16-b,	17-c,	18-d,	19-a,	20-a,
21-c,	22-b,	23-a,	24-d,	25-d,	26-d,	27-a,	28-d,	29-b,	30-b,
31-a,	32-d,	33-c,	34-c,	35-a,	36-d,	37-c,	38-b,	39-a,	40-b,
41-b,	42-d,	43-a,	44-d,	45-c,	46-d,	47-c,	48-a,	49-c,	50-b

Cutaneous Infections with Pyogenic Bacteria

Primary bacterial **infections** of the skin arise de novo, have a characteristic lesional morphology and a predictable course. **Secondary infections** develop over an underlying skin disease, lack characteristic morphology and have a variable course.

TABLE 5.1: Primary vs secondary bacterial infections	
Primary	**Secondary**
Arise de novo	Arise over a pre-existing dermatoses
Have a characteristic morphology	Do not have a characteristic morphology
Course predictable	Course variable
Good response to appropriate antibacterial therapy	Response incomplete

Clinical implication: If a pyogenic bacterial infection cannot be neatly fitted into one of the primary types, then there must be an underlying skin disorder that needs to be treated after secondary bacterial infection clears with antibacterial therapy.

TABLE 5.2: Classification of pyogenic infections		
Primary pyodermas	Superficial	Impetigo
		Superficial folliculitis
	Deep	Deep folliculitis
		Furuncle
		Carbuncle
		Ecthyma
		Paronychia
		Periporitis
		Erysipelas
		Cellulitis
Secondary pyodermas may be superficial or deep and may follow eczema, scabies, fungal infection, burns or ulcers due to other causes (Fig. 5.1).		

Defenses Against Bacterial Infections

The several levels of skin's defense system against bacterial infections include:

- *Tough and intact stratum corneum:* Breached by mechanical (or chemical or thermal) trauma.
- *Dryness:* Simple desiccation kills most bacteria. This incredibly simple and effective defense is lost by occlusion and sweating especially in the flexures like axillae and groins.
- *pH:* Normal skin surface is slightly acidic (pH 5.4). Infection prone intertriginous regions have neutral pH.
- Normal bacterial flora of micrococci and corynebacteria provide a defense mechanism by producing enzymes and fatty acids that retard growth of pathogens.

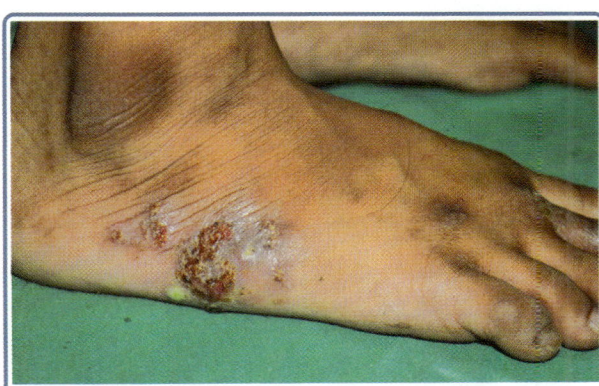
Fig. 5.1: Eczema with secondary pyoderma. Note pustules and seropurulent discharge

IMPETIGO (IMPETIGO CONTAGIOSA)

This is a superficial bacterial infection caused by staphylococci or streptococci.

Patient Profile

Young children (2–5 years) are typically affected. Infants, especially neonates, are susceptible to the serious bullous variant of this disease. Epidemics among neonates in nurseries are known. Lesions are asymptomatic.

Morphology

Each lesion begins as a red macule that evolves within 24 hours into a vesicle and then a pustule. These then burst leading to yellow-brown crusts with 'stuck-on' appearance and under which are superficial erosions (Fig. 5.2). Purulent fluid tends to gravitate to the bottom of large vesicopustules (hypopyon sign) (Figs 5.3–5.5).

Clinical Implication: Since individual lesions evolve rapidly, at the time of presentation, most lesions are erosions covered with honey colored (brownish yellow) crusts that have a 'stuck-on' appearance. Vesicles or Pustules are difficult to find.

Distribution

Face, especially perinasal and perioral areas, is the commonest site affected (Figs 5.2 and 5.7). Uncommonly axillae, trunk, scalp, and extremities are involved.

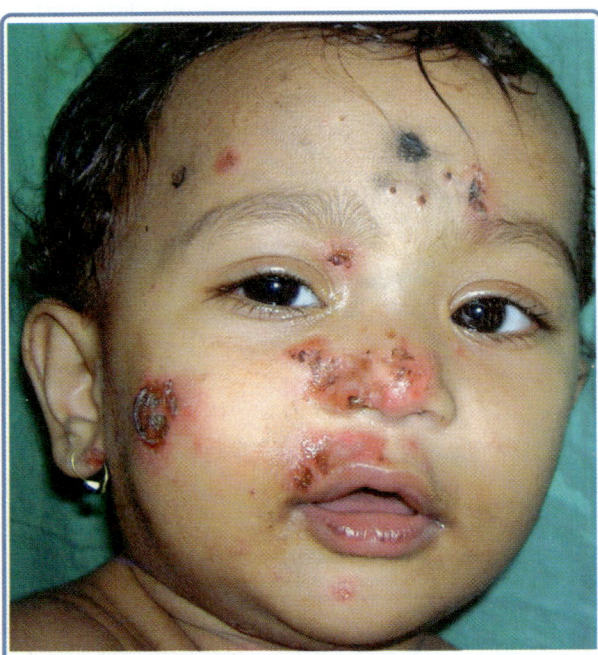

Fig. 5.2: Impetigo—erosions covered with seropurulent (honey coloured) crusts

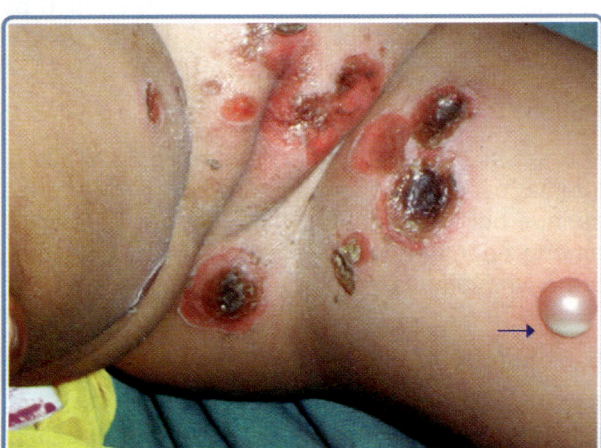

Fig. 5.3: Bullous impetigo—erosions covered with honey coloured crusts and a bulla with hypopyon sign (arrow)

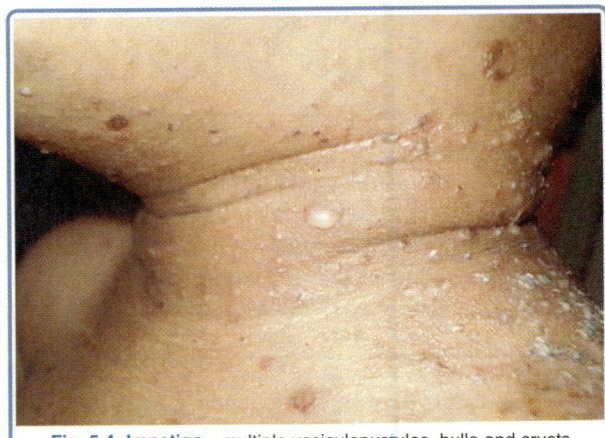

Fig. 5.4: Impetigo—multiple vesiculopustules, bulla and crusts

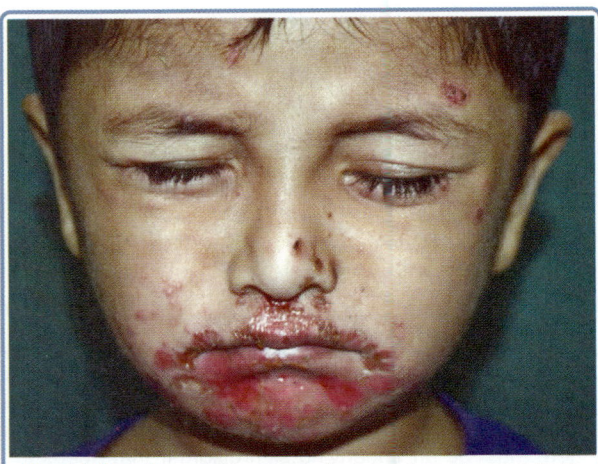

Fig. 5.5: Impetigo—erosions around nose and mouth covered with thin crusts

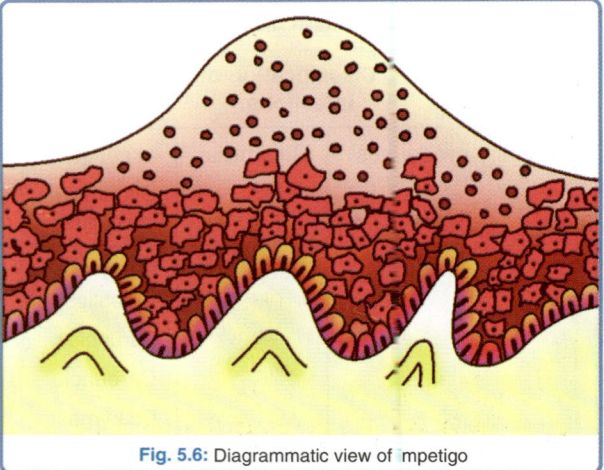

Fig. 5.6: Diagrammatic view of impetigo

Variations

Bullous impetigo is caused by staphylococci and shows intact vesicles, pustules and bullae predominating over erosions and crusts. Hypopyon sign is usually present (Fig. 5.3). Disseminated lesions are common and rapid institution of systemic antibiotics is essential.

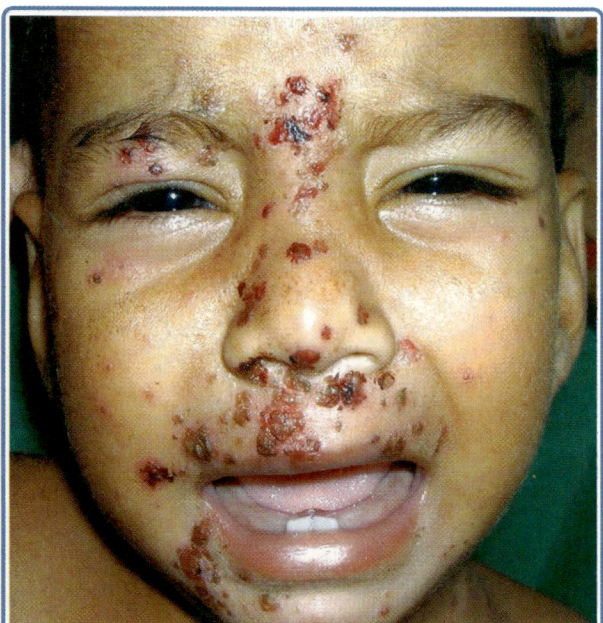

Fig. 5.7: Impetigo—erosions covered with seropurulent (honey coloured) crusts. Note absence of vesicles and pustules

Diagnosis

Classical morphology and distribution in the susceptible population is enough to initiate therapy. Demonstration of staphylococci or streptococci within neutrophils by Gram's stain of discharge or crust is diagnostic. Culture and antibiotic sensitivity to prevent test are useful recurrences. Bullous lesions grow staphylococci while crusted lesions commonly grow streptococci.

Treatment

See treatment of bacterial infection (page 53).

> **Staphylococcal scalded skin syndrome (SSSS)** is induced by an exotoxin (epidermolytin) produced by a focus of staphylococcal infection (cutaneous or otherwise). Infants and adults with renal compromise are the usual victims. Widespread, coalescing, thin roofed, flaccid bullae and shedding of the superficial epidermal layers with resultant erosions characterise the disease. If untreated, extensive denudation of the skin and resultant disturbances of water, electrolyte and temperature balance may occasionally lead to death. The condition responds well to cloxacillin.

Summary: Impetigo is a superficial staphylococcal or streptococcal skin infection that presents in young children as erosions covered with thin honey coloured crusts on face. Lesions begin as vesicles/pustules. Oral azithromycin or cefadroxyl (or cloxacillin) is frequently necessary in addition to a topical antibiotic.

ECTHYMA

This deep bacterial infection, caused by streptococci, involves the dermis (Fig. 5.8).

> **Clinical implication:** As against impetigo, which is superficial, ecthyma lesions heal with scarring due to dermal damage.

Patient Profile

Young adults, adolescents and older children with poor personal hygiene are typically affected drug abusers, alcoholics and debilitated patients are also involved. Most patients are males. Trauma or Insect bites may play a role in initiation of lesions.

Morphology

Although, the earliest lesion is a macule, at the time of presentation, pustules and/or **ulcers covered with thick crusts** are present. Ecthyma pustules are non-follicular, have an erythematous, oedematous base and are tender. Within 1 or 2 days they rupture resulting in rounded ulcers that tend to get covered with thick, heaped up, purulent or haemorrhagic (yellow-brown to black) crusts (Fig. 2.17). Removal of the crust reveals a pool of pus that covers the ulcer floor.

> Patients under therapy or those with improved hygiene may lack the typical crust and consequently have only rounded ulcers with purulent or sero-sanguinous discharge.

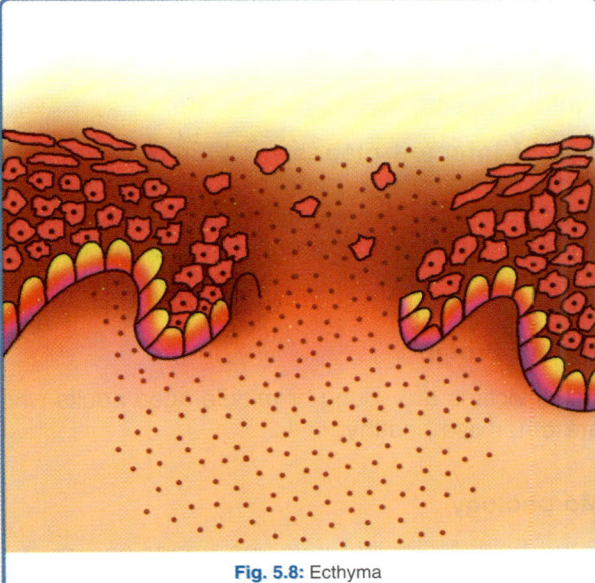

Fig. 5.8: Ecthyma

Chapter
5

Cutaneous Infections with Pyogenic Bacteria

Distribution

Extremities, especially lower legs, are the pre-disposed sites.

Diagnosis

Clinical diagnosis is based on morphology, distribution and patient profile. Beta haemolytic streptococci can be grown on blood agar from pus or crusts.

Treatment

See treatment of bacterial infections (page 53).

> **Ecthyma gangrenosum** has nothing to do with ecthyma. It is a skin manifestation of pseudomonas septicaemia. Haemorrhagic pustules, that turn into ulcers, occurring in seriously ill patients suggest the diagnosis. Prognosis is grim.

Summary: Ecthyma is a deep streptococcal skin infection seen in older children or adolescents with poor hygiene as rounded ulcers covered with thick crusts over lower legs. Lesions heal with scarring after local cold compresses, topical antibiotics and oral azithromycin or cefadroxil or cloxacillin.

FOLLICULITIS

Although literally this term means inflammation of the hair follicle. It is commonly used to denote follicular infection with pyogenic organisms. The most common causative agent is staphylococcus but occasionally streptococci and gram negative rods (*Escherichia coli*, Klebsiella, Proteus and Pseudomonas) are implicated.

Pathogenesis

Use of infected blades for hair removal is a common initiating event for sycosis barbae (folliculitis of beard region). The traditional practice in North India of application of oil to the body is implicated in folliculitis of legs.

Patient Profile

Usual victims are young or middle aged adults who are otherwise healthy.

Morphology

Superficial folliculitis involves upper part of the follicle (infundibulum) with acute (neutrophilic)

inflammation and pustule formation (Figs 5.11 and 5.12) that heals without follicular scarring

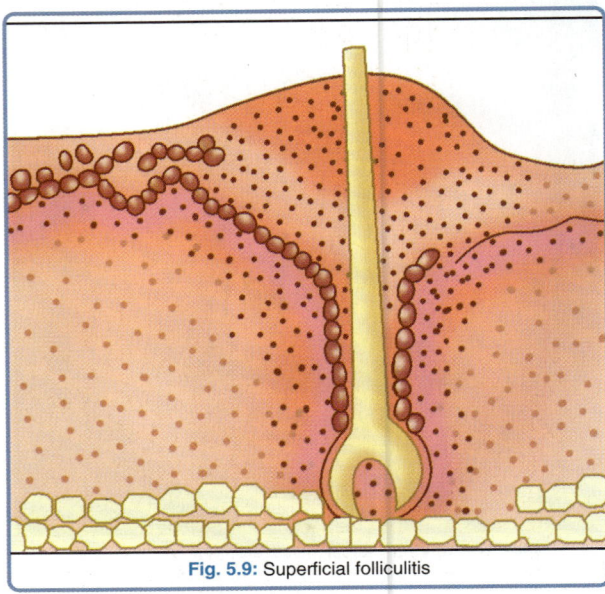

Fig. 5.9: Superficial folliculitis

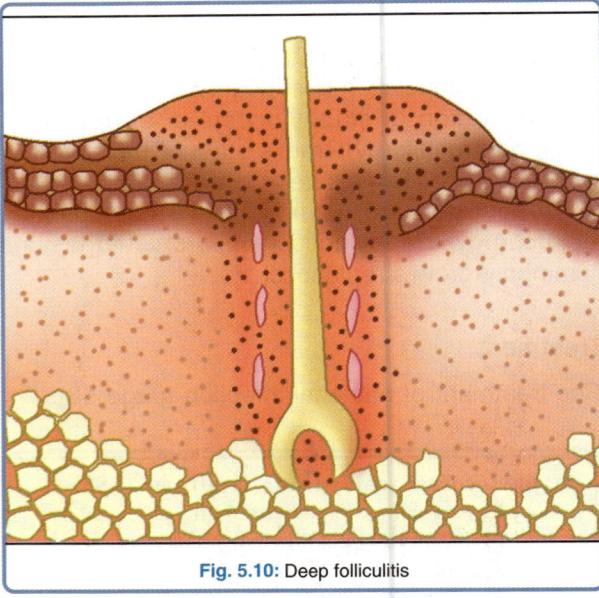

Fig. 5.10: Deep folliculitis

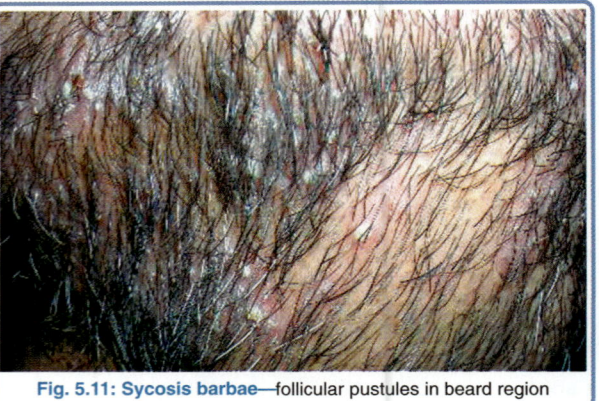

Fig. 5.11: Sycosis barbae—follicular pustules in beard region

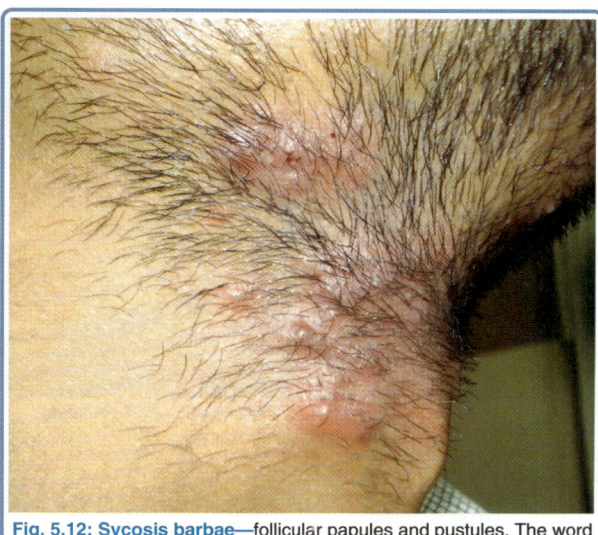

Fig. 5.12: Sycosis barbae—follicular papules and pustules. The word sycosis refers to resemblance to a cut fig

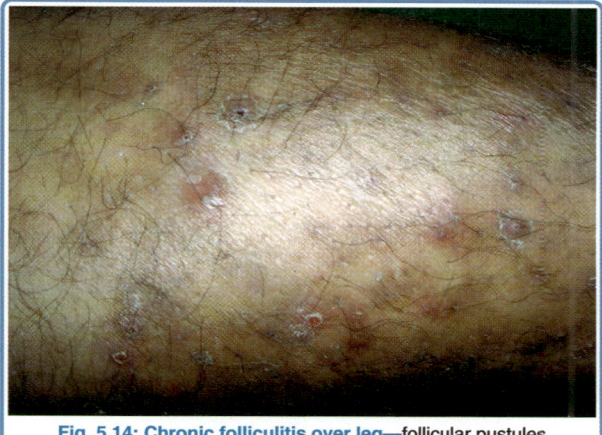

Fig. 5.14: Chronic folliculitis over leg—follicular pustules and scaling with erythema and atrophy

(permanent loss of involved hair). Clinically, grouped tiny follicular pustules with a narrow rim of erythema are observed.

Deep folliculitis involves the whole length of the follicle up to the level of deep dermis and heals with follicular scarring (Figs 5.13 and 5.14). Erythematous follicular papules, 2–3 mm in diameter, topped by tiny pustules characterise the condition. Hair shaft of the involved follicle can be pulled out with a light tug.

Distribution

Common sites of affection are the beard and must-ache areas and anterior legs in males (Figs 5.11–5.15). Axillae, pubic region, scalp or other body sites with terminal (thick) hair may also be affected.

Treatment

See page 53 for therapy of bacterial infections.

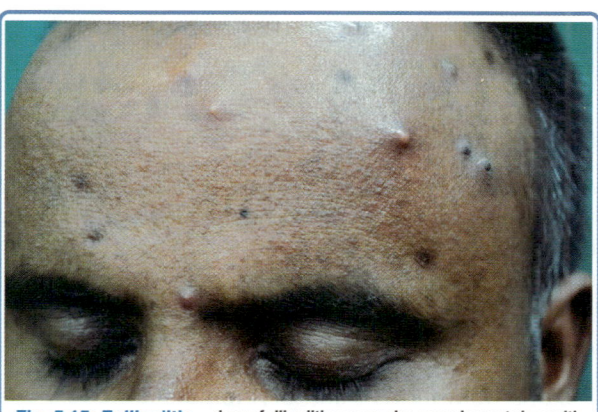

Fig. 5.15: Folliculitis—deep folliculitis on scalp; papulopustules with surrounding erythema

Summary: Folliculitis is a staphylococcal infection of the hair follicle that affects adult males. Follicular pustules or papulopustules over beard region or anterior legs characterise the condition. Extended application of a topical antibiotic is usually needed in addition to a short course of oral azithromycin or cefadroxyl or cloxacillin.

FURUNCLE AND CARBUNCLE

These two conditions, though clinically distinct, are essential forms of deep folliculitis that involve, deep dermis and subcutaneous fat. Terminal (thick) hair follicles that extend to the subcutaneous fat are preferentially affected. Staphylococcus is the usual offender. Whereas furuncle involves a single hair follicle, carbuncle affects a group of contiguous follicles.

Furuncle (Common Boil)

It is the commonest pyogenic skin infection.

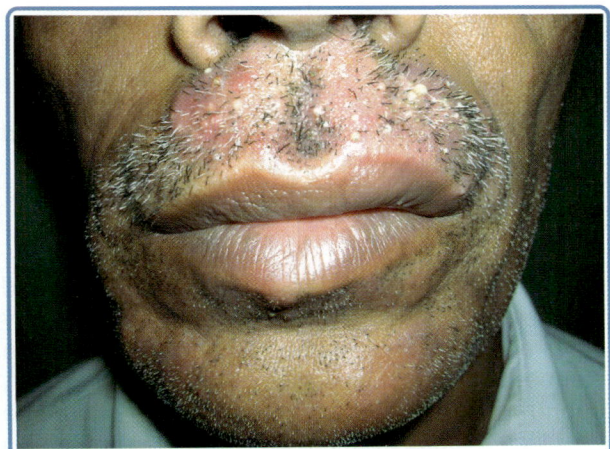

Fig. 5.13: Chronic folliculitis—multiple pustules and broken stubs of hair

Chapter
5

Cutaneous Infections with Pyogenic Bacteria

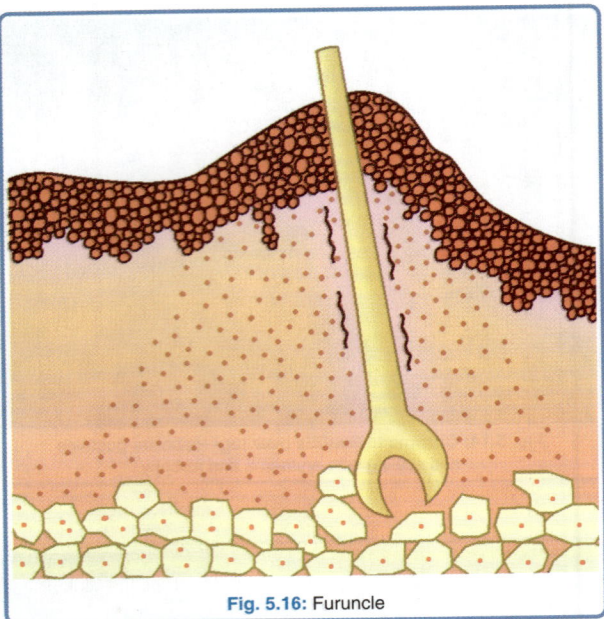

Fig. 5.16: Furuncle

Patient profile

Anyone (usually adults) may be affected. Excessive sweating, occlusive clothing, poor hygiene, and diabetes mellitus predispose to multiple and recurrent lesions.

Morphology

It starts as a tender, firm erythematous nodule that is better felt than seen. Within a few days the barely elevated nodule enlarges and develops central pointing (Fig. 5.17). A tiny pustule commonly forms at the central point through which emerges a hair. After a few more days, the nodule softens in the centre and bursts, discharging inspissated matter and then pus (Fig. 5.18). Pain and tenderness subsides after a lesion bursts. Healing without a visible scar (but with follicular loss), takes a few more days.

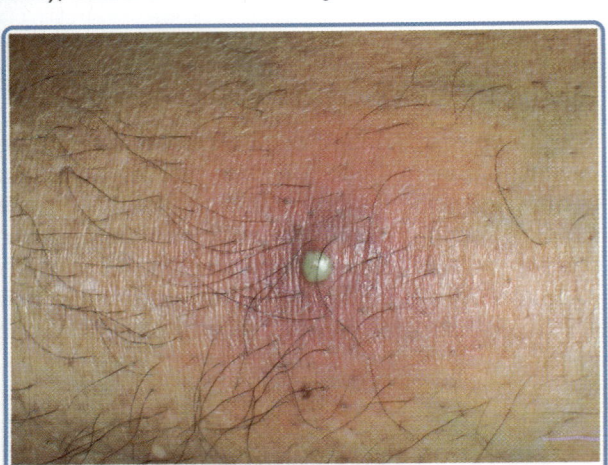

Fig. 5.17: Furuncle—tender erythematous nodule topped with a pustule

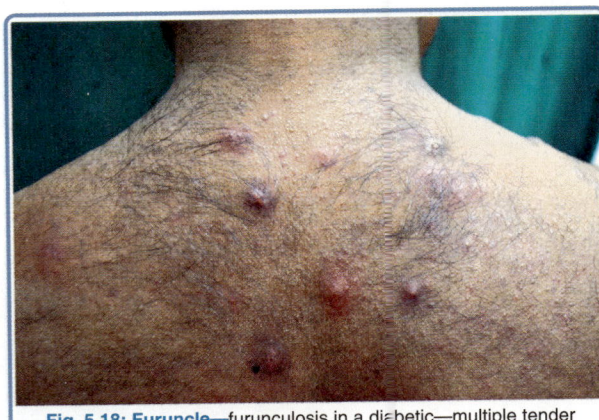

Fig. 5.18: Furuncle—furunculosis in a diabetic—multiple tender nodules with pus pointing

Distribution

Axillae, buttocks, perianal region, thighs and face are common sites. Other parts of extremities and trunk may be affected.

Diagnosis

Morphology is characteristic to permit clinical diagnosis. Culture and antibiotic sensitivity testing are useful from therapeutic viewpoint, particularly in patients with recurrent or multiple lesions.

Treatment

See therapy of bacterial infections (page 53).

> **Summary:** Furuncle is a deep staphylococcal infection of a terminal (thick) follicle that reaches up to the fat. A painful, tender, erythematous nodule with central pointing is seen over either the axillae, buttocks of face. Abscess forms in a few days, bursts or needs drainage. Topical antibiotics are useful for a single lesion but oral cloxacillin or azithromycin or cefadroxil are needed for multiple or recurrent lesions.

Carbuncle

Patient profile

Most patients are adults with poorly controlled diabetes. Children are spared.

Morphology

An extremely tender erythematous indurated plaque, that has considerable depth but is barely elevated, is the initial lesion. After a few days, the plaque develops multiple points of softening that, upon pressure, discharge pus through sieve-like openings (Figs 5.19 and 5.20). The intervening skin becomes necrotic and forms a dark, thick eschar.

At a later stage, the whole surface of the plaque sloughs off leading to a large, deep ulcer (Fig. 5.21). Healing with scarring takes weeks or even months.

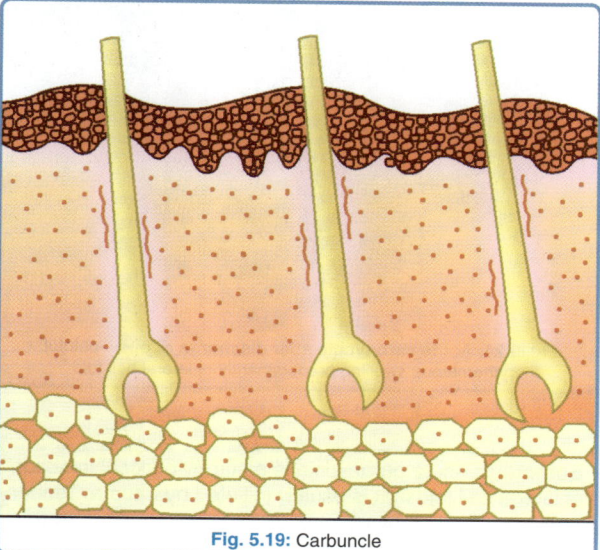

Fig. 5.19: Carbuncle

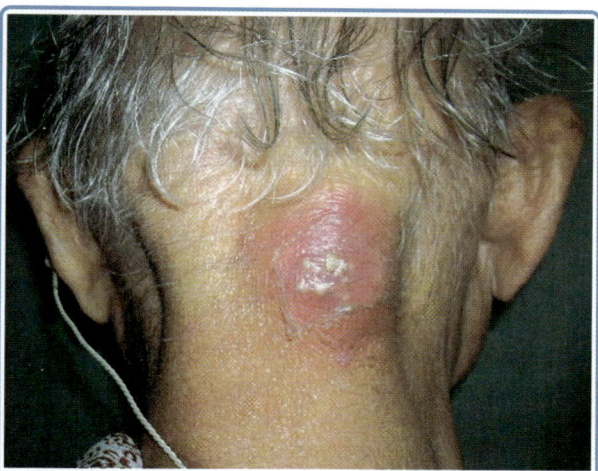

Fig. 5.20: Carbuncle—Erythematous tender nodule with multiple pus pointings

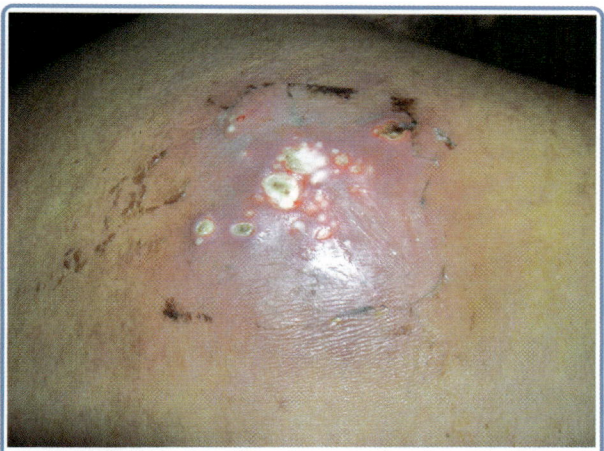

Fig. 5.21: Carbuncle after rupture—indurated plaque discharging pus through multiple openings. The centre commonly turns necrotic

Distribution

Nape of the neck is the classic site. Trunk and proximal extremities are affected less commonly.

Diagnosis

Classic morphology and typical site are diagnostic. Culture and antibiotic sensitivity testing are important to decide upon the choice of antibiotic. Diabetes mellitus must be ruled out by doing blood sugars.

Treatment

In addition to systemic antibiotics, (please *see* treatment of bacterial infections) oral nonsteroidal antiinflammatory drugs (NSAIDs) in the initial stages, and later, once the skin overlying the plaque is necrotic, surgical desloughing necessary. The resultant ulcer has to be treated with regular dressings with antiseptics and granulation promoting agents. Skin grafting may be done once the ulcer floor has healthy granulation tissue.

Summary: Carbuncle is a deep staphylococcal infection affecting a group of contiguous follicles that reach up to the subcutaneous fat. It typically affects diabetics. An extremely tender indurated erythematous plaque that, upon pressure, discharges pus through its sieve like openings and later forms a deep ulcer over the nape of neck is the characteristic. Desloughing, and later, grafting may be needed in addition to oral cloxacillin or clavulanate potentiated amoxycillin.

ACUTE PARONYCHIA

Paronychia is inflammation of the nail fold. Acute paronychia is caused by bacteria, mainly staphylococci whereas chronic paronychia is usually initiated and perpetuated by candida albicans (Fig. 5.22).

Clinical Features

Young adults of both sexes are affected. Trauma is a common initiating event. Pain is the predominant symptom. The condition begins as tender erythema and oedema involving the lateral nail fold and progresses to form an abscess of the lateral nail fold (Fig. 5.23). Within a few days, the abscess develops and is seen as a yellowish spot of pointing. Excruciating pain and tenderness characterise this stage. If left untreated, the abscess bursts after a couple of days and this relieves the pain (Fig. 5.24).

Chapter 5

Cutaneous Infections with Pyogenic Bacteria

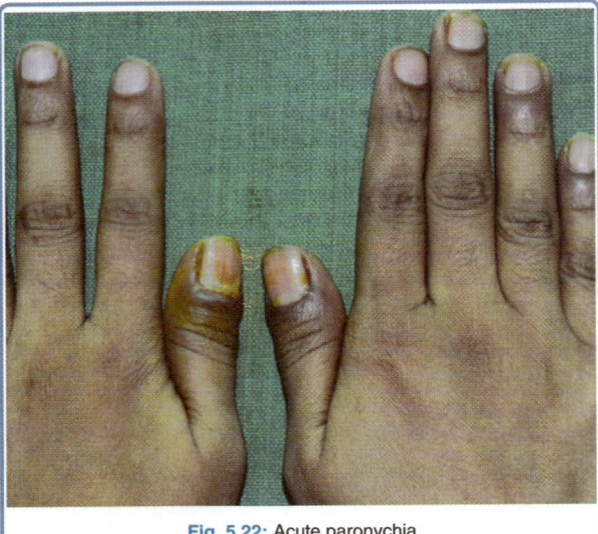

Fig. 5.22: Acute paronychia

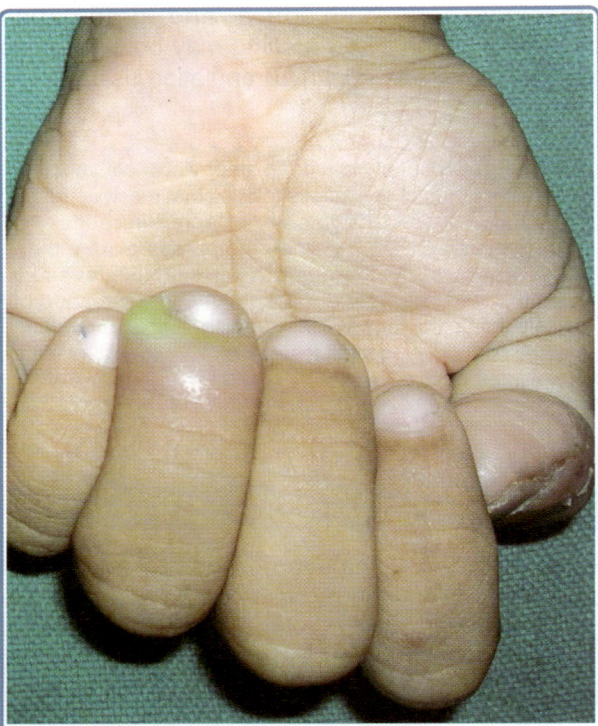

Fig. 5.23: Acute paronychia—extremely painful swelling with pus collection involving lateral nail

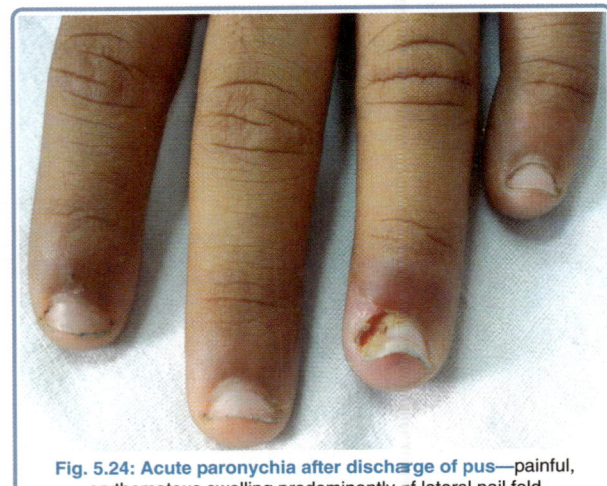

Fig. 5.24: Acute paronychia after discharge of pus—painful, erythematous swelling predominantly of lateral nail fold

Summary: Acute paronychia is a staphylococcal infection of lateral nail fold that is usually initiated by trauma. Tender erythema and swelling evolves into an abscess that is extremely painful. Oral cloxacillin and NSAIDs are needed in addition to incision and drainage for relief of pain.

PERIPORITIS (MULTIPLE SWEAT GLAND ABSCESSES)

It is a common staphylococcal infection of children in the summer; malnutrition and poor hygiene are the risk factors for it (Fig. 5.25).

Clinical Features

Lesions begin as multiple erythematous papules and nodules over forehead, face (Fig. 5.26), scalp and upper trunk. Over several days, they progress

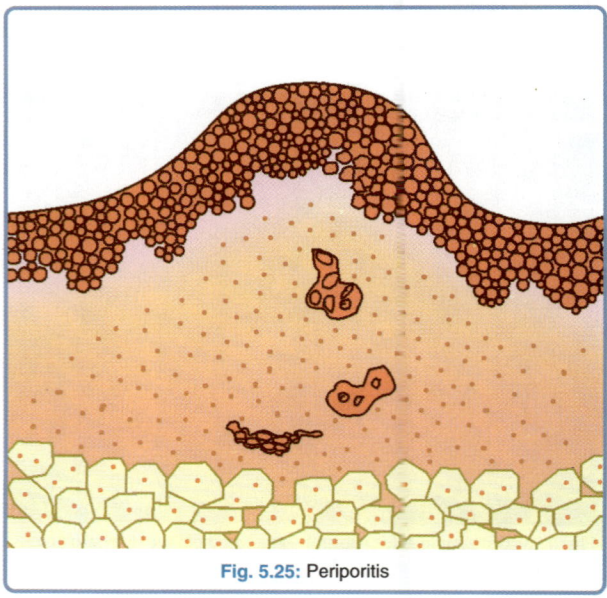

Fig. 5.25: Periporitis

Management

Culture and antibiotic sensitivity test may be done for establishing the diagnosis. However, most of the times the pain is too pressing to wait for lab results. Hence, therapy is initiated with cloxacillin 250 mg qds along with an anti-inflammatory agent like ibuprofen 400 mg tid. Once the abscess has developed, pain is best relieved by incising the abscess at the site of pointing. This is followed up with antibiotic therapy.

Chapter 5

Cutaneous Infections with Pyogenic Bacteria

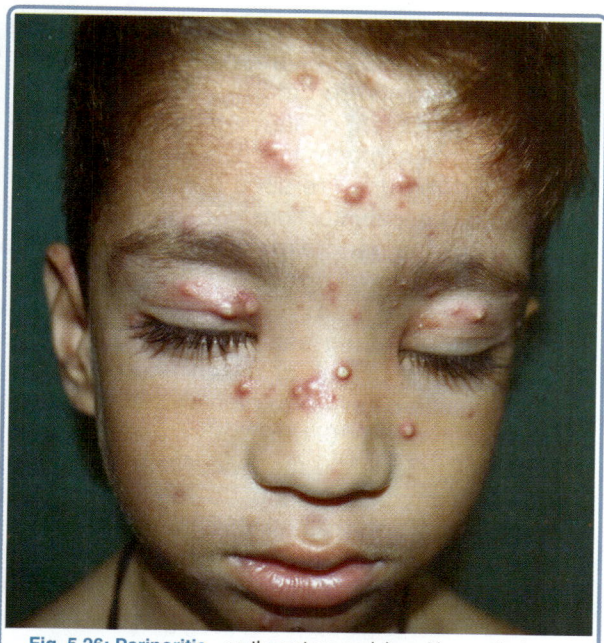

Fig. 5.26: Periporitis—erythematous nodules with pus discharge

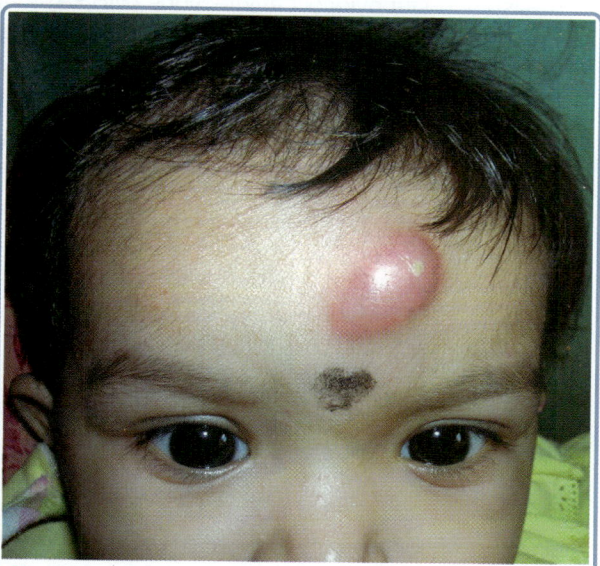

Fig. 5.27: Periporitis (sweat gland abscess)—large dome shaped, nontender erythematous fluctuant nodule

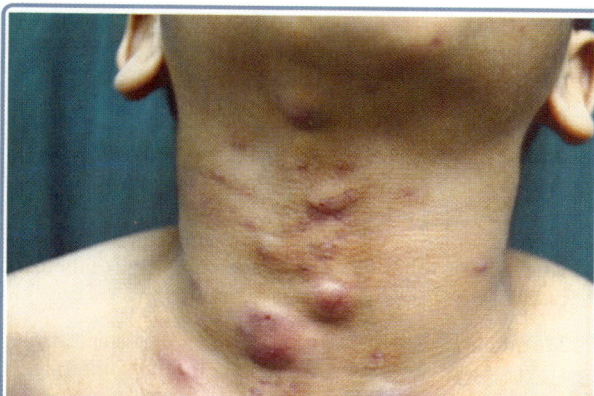

Fig. 5.28: Periporitis—multiple sweat gland abscesses, nodules that lack tenderness

to form non-tender fluctuant thin walled abscess of 0.5–3 cm diameter (Figs 5.27 and 5.28). Differentiation from furunculosis is based on absence of pain and tenderness as well as the lack of central follicular pointing.

Treatment

See below for treatment of bacterial infections.

> **Summary:** Periporitis is a staphylococcal infection of facial skin of malnourished children. Lesions are non-tender, erythematous, rounded papulonodules that may evolve into abscesses. Oral azithromycin or cloxacillin, improving hygiene and nutrition and drainage of large abscesses is needed.

TREATMENT OF BACTERIAL INFECTIONS

Principles of the therapy are:

- **Removal of crusts**

    Crusts, not only provide a moist and nourishing milieu for bacteria, but also prevent antibiotics from reaching the bacteria. Hence, their removal hastens healing. Thin crusts, as in impetigo, may be removed by repeated gentle washing with water and soap. Thicker crusts, as in ecthyma, can be softened before removal by the action of wet compresses with potassium permanganate. Scalp lesions need shampooing.

- **Attention to predisposing factors**

    Poor personal hygiene, malnutrition, uncontrolled diabetes mellitus, hot and humid environment, tendency to excessive sweating, obesity, and occlusive clothing are some partially or fully correctable predisposing factors. If an underlying primary dermatosis like scabies, pediculosis, prurigo simplex, etc., is not attended to, persistence of bacterial infection is to be expected. An underlying immunodeficiency disorder (commonest of which is diabetes mellitus) may be suspected in pyogenic bacterial infections that are recurrent, persistent or unusually severe.

- **Topical antibiotics**

    Since these are easily administered, lack systemic side effects when applied over limited body regions and provide good concentration of the antibacterial in the skin, they are used in almost all pyogenic bacterial infections. Their

Chapter 5

Cutaneous Infections with Pyogenic Bacteria

only side effect, contact allergic dermatitis, is uncommon. It is preferable to use antibacterials that are not commonly used systemically since topical use promotes development of resistant strains in a community.

TABLE 5.3: Topical antibacterials	
Antibacterials	Activity spectrum
Neomycin 1%	Gram-negative bacteria
Fusidic acid 2%	Gram-positive bacteria
Bacitracin	Gram-positive cocci
Polymyxin B	Pseudomonas
Mupirocin 2% and retapamulin	Resistant superficial infections
Povidone iodine (solution 10%)	Broad antimicrobial activity used as an antiseptic to treat wounds
Silver sulphadiazine 1%	Broad antimicrobial activity for prevention and treatment of infections in burn wounds
Framycetin sulphate	Broad spectrum

Neomycin 1%, fusidic acid 2%, framycetin 1%, chlorhexidine 1%, and mupirocin 1% are some of the commonly employed preparations. A combination of neomycin (for gram-negative bacteria), bacitracin (for gram-positive cocci) and polymyxin B (for Pseudomonas) is also available. Topical mupirocin and retapamulin are effective for resistant superficial bacterial infections. Application to the skin lesions and perilesional skin 2–3 times a day gives good results. Topical antibiotics should preferably be continued for a week after all the lesions have healed, as this prevents reinfections and allows gradual regrowth of protective normal bacterial flora. Topical antibacterials have the potential to get absorbed and cause systemic side effects when applied over large eroded areas particularly in infants.

- **Systemic antibiotics**

Indications for systemic treatment include extensive infections or infections that recur or persist after adequate topical therapy. Associated regional lymphadenopathy and fever are other indications. Poor compliance for topical therapy, as in young children, is another situation for systemic therapy. In ordinary infections, 1–2 weeks of systemic therapy is sufficient. For recurrent infections, longer duration of therapy may be necessary.

Antibiotic sensitivity test should ideally be utilised for choosing the right agent. However, such testing is commonly reserved for recurrent, persistent or life threatening infections. Cloxacillin, erythromycin, cephalexin in doses of 250–500 mg qds are used for staphylococcal or streptococcal infections. Cephalosporins like cefadroxyl or macrolide antibiotics are also effective. Broad spectrum antibiotics like ampicillin or amoxycillin with or without cloxacillin (250 mg each) are popular agents but are most useful for mixed and secondary bacterial infections. Alternatively, one may use azithromycin 500 mg daily for 3 days or cefadroxyl 250–500 mg twice daily for 5 days or clindamycin 300 mg tid for 5 days. For unresponsive infections, a combination of amoxycillin (500 mg) with clavulanic acid (125 mg) 2–3 times daily is recommended for a duration of 5–7 days depending on the extent and severity of infections. For methicilium resistance staphylococcal infections (MRSA) that are usually resistant to multiple antibacterials linezolid 600 mg twice daily or cotrimoxazole two tablets twice daily are effective.

TABLE 5.4: Systemic antibacterials	
Antibacterial group	Infection
Penicillins (cloxacillin) cephalosporins (cephalexin, cefadroxyl) and macrolides (erythromycin, azithromycin)	Gram positive cocci
Clindamycin, amoxycillin-clavulanate, cotrimoxazole, tetracyclins	Mixed infections
Linezolid, vancomycin, cotrimoxazole	MRSA

Erysipelas and Cellulitis

These infections of the skin and the subcutis, respectively, are caused usually by streptococci and occasionally by staphylococci. They are dermatologic emergencies and should be treated urgently (Figs 5.29 and 5.30).

Patient Profile: Middle aged males are the most frequent victims. Trauma, infected ulcers and primary bacterial infections may act as initiating events. Compromise of immune function either locally (lymphoedema due to filariasis or other causes) or systemically (diabetes mellitus) may underlie these infections.

Morphology: Erysipelas is seen as a sharply demarcated, single, large, bright red erythematous and sometimes purpuric, indurated plaque that is warm to touch and

(Contd.)

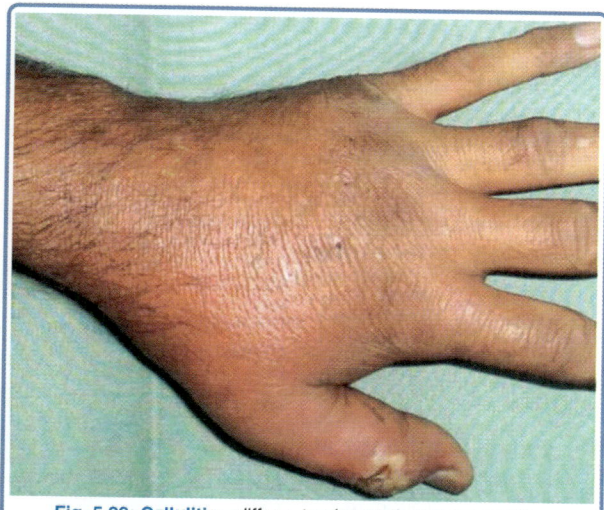

Fig. 5.29: **Cellulitis**—diffuse, tender, erythematous swelling

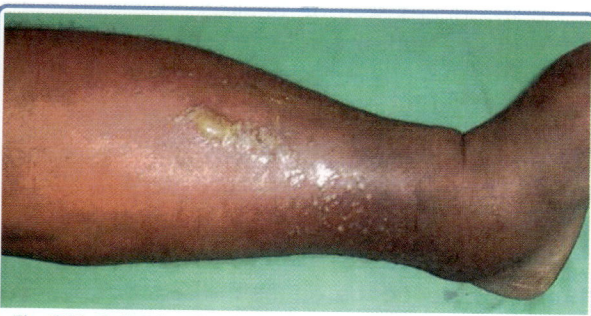

Fig. 5.30: **Cellulitis**—ill defined, erythematous, tender, warm plaque with vesicles, pustules and bullae

(Contd.)

Morphology: As suggested by the name, lesions consist of sharply circumscribed, small (1–2 mm) to broad (several centimetres) rounded areas of keratolysis (loss of the thick keratin layer of palms or soles) seen as pits or craters (Figs 5.31–5.33).

Distribution: Palms and soles are almost exclusively affected.

Therapy: Success of therapy depends heavily on the ability of the patient to keep hands or feet dry. Careful drying and even powdering of hands and feet is a must after wet work is finished. Topical and oral antibacterials as well as topical salicylic acid hasten improvement.

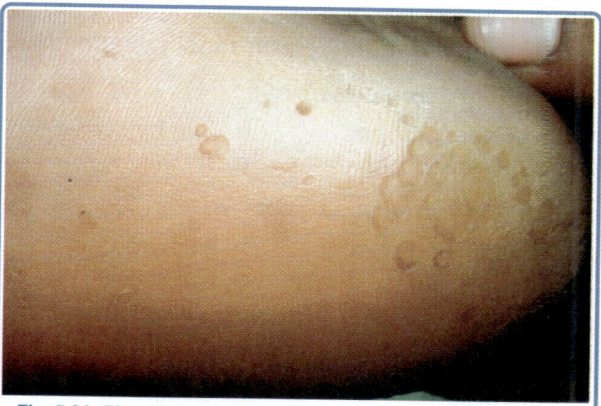

Fig. 5.31: **Pitted keratolysis**—multiple small and large, coalescing, superficial circular craters

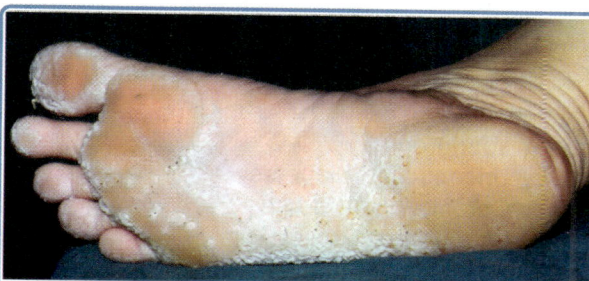

Fig. 5.32: **Pitted keratolysis**—multiple pits and sodden skin in a house maid

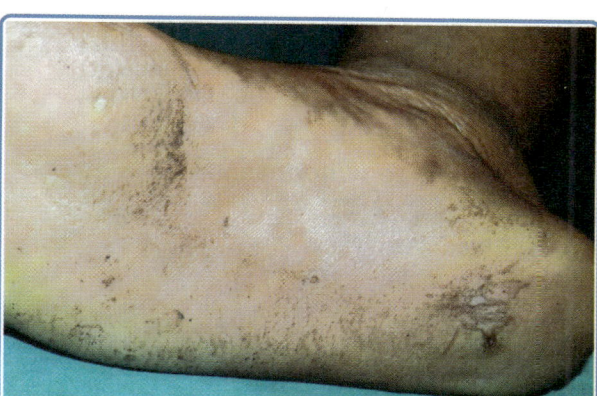

Fig. 5.33: **Pitted keratolysis**—multiple pits over sole in a male with hyperhidrosis

tender. Fever is a common accompaniment and blisters may superimpose over the plaque. Cellulitis differs by being a diffuse swelling that is not as indurated. Constitutional symptoms like fever, body ache and toxicity may vary from mild to severe.

Distribution: A lower extremity, especially the leg, is most commonly affected. Upper limb and face may be occasionally involved.

Treatment: Urgent institution of effective antibiotics is crucial. Orally, cloxacillin 500 mg QDS or clavulanated amoxycillin 1000 mg bid are effective, if begun early. Later, intravenous crystalline penicillin 10 lac IU 4 hourly or, for hospital infections and in immunocompromised patients, intravenous ceftriaxone 500 mg 8 hourly is advisable. For serious and disseminated infections intravenous piperacillin, tazobactum or/and linezolid/vancomycin can be used.

Pitted Keratolysis

Overgrowth of an opportunistic corynebacterium, Dermatophilus congolensis, occurs in persons involved in wet work. Hence, domestic servants, dishwashers, hotel boys, sharbat vendors, seamen and occasionally housewives are affected. At times, underlying hyperhidrosis may be responsible.

Chapter 5

Cutaneous Infections with Pyogenic Bacteria

MCQs

1. **The following features of skin protect against bacterial infection *except*:**
   a. Acidic pH
   b. Sweating
   c. Normal flora of the skin
   d. Dryness

2. **Staphylococcal scalded skin syndrome occurs in:**
   a. Elderly
   b. Pregnant women
   c. Chronic liver disease
   d. Infants and those with renal compromise

3. **Ecthyma is caused by:**
   a. Pseudomonas
   b. Staphylococci
   c. Streptococci
   d. *E.coli*

4. **Hypopyon sign is seen in:**
   a. Bullous impetigo
   b. Ecthyma
   c. Cellulitis
   d. Folliculitis

5. **Most common site of impetigo is:**
   a. Hands
   b. Face
   c. Axilla
   d. Scalp

6. **'Sycosis' literally means:**
   a. Fig
   b. Tamarind
   c. Berry
   d. Plum

7. **Predisposing factors for development of carbuncle:**
   a. Young age
   b. Uncontrolled diabetes
   c. Chronic NSAIDs use
   d. Skin graft sites

8. **Scarring after resolution is seen in:**
   a. Ecthyma
   b. Folliculitis
   c. Periporitis
   d. Impetigo

9. **Drug of choice for infection with MRSA is:**
   a. Azithromycin
   b. Linezolid
   c. Teicoplanin
   d. Amikacin

10. **Pus pointing is not seen in:**
    a. Folliculitis
    b. Pitted keratolysis
    c. Carbuncle
    d. Furuncle

11. **Factors promoting the growth of bacteria include:**
    a. Crusts
    b. Healthy granulation tissue
    c. Dry skin
    d. None of the above

12. **Following are the indications of systemic antibacterial therapy:**
    a. Fever
    b. Regional lymphadenopathy
    c. Inadequate response to therapy
    d. All of the above

13. **False statement about impetigo is:**
    a. Mostly caused by staphylococcus or streptococcus or both
    b. It predisposes to glomerulonephritis
    c. Produces scar on healing
    d. It is a contagious lesion

14. **Impetigo is:**
    a. common on face
    b. viral infection
    c. Characterised by thick crust
    d. Common in adults

15. **Staphylococcus causes all *except*:**
    a. Scarlet fever
    b. Toxic shock syndrome
    c. Carbuncle
    d. Sycosis barbae

16. **Staphylococcus causes all diseases *except*:**
    a. Carbuncle
    b. Impetigo herpetiformis
    c. Furuncle
    d. Folliculitis

17. **Impetigo contangiosa is most commonly due to:**
    a. Group B streptococcus
    b. Streptococus viridans
    c. Moniliasis
    d. Staphylococcus

18. **A 3-month-old infant developed otitis media for which he was given a course of cotrimoxazole. A few days later he developed extensive peeling of skin, there were no mucosal lesions and the baby was not toxic. The most likely diagnosis is:**
    a. Toxic epidermal necrolysis
    b. Staphylococcal scalded skin syndrome
    c. Stevens Johnson syndrome
    d. Infantile pemphigus

19. **Which of the following is a bacterial infection?**
    a. Pyoderma gangrenosum
    b. Impetigo herpetiformis
    c. Pitted keratolysis
    d. Mycosis fungoides

20. **Erythrasma is caused by:**
    a. Corynebacterium
    b. Staphylococcus
    c. Streptococcus
    d. Coronavirus

21. *Corynebacterium minutissimum* **causes:**
    a. Erysipelas
    b. Erythrasma
    c. Ecthyma
    d. Trichomycosis axillaris

22. **The dominant symptom of pyoderma is:**
    a. Pain
    b. Pruritus
    c. Watering
    d. Bleeding

23. **Pyogenic infection of skin spreads by:**
    a. Skin to skin contact
    b. Through fomites
    c. Keeping poor hygiene
    d. All of these

24. **Crusted lesions of impetigo usually grow:**
    a. Staphylococci
    b. Streptococci
    c. Pseudomonas
    d. All of these

25. **Bullous impetigo is caused by:**
    a. Staphylococci
    b. Streptococci
    c. Corynebacterium
    d. Pseudomonas

26. **Characteristic lesion of impetigo is:**
    a. Thin scale with thin roof
    b. Vesicle
    c. Crust containing blood
    d. Stuck-on honey coloured crust

27. **Impetigo tends to preferentially affect:**
    a. Acral regions
    b. Flexor aspects of the body
    c. Face
    d. Genitals

28. **Bacterial infection in impetigo is develop in this layer of skin:**
    a. Papillary dermis
    b. Basal epidermis
    c. Granular layer of epidermis
    d. Spinous layer of epidermis

29. **The organism causing furuncle is:**
    a. Staphylococcus
    b. Streptococcus
    c. Corynebacterium
    d. Pseudomonas

30. **One of the commonest sites of affection in furuncle is:**
    a. Hand
    b. Axilla
    c. Nipple
    d. Neck

31. **The organism responsible for carbuncle is:**
    a. Staphylococcus
    b. Streptococcus
    c. Proteus
    d. Pseudomonas

32. **Pyodermas usually spreads within:**
    a. Families
    b. Schools
    c. Communities
    d. All of these

33. **Topical antibacterial application must be made:**
    a. To the whole body
    b. On body folds
    c. Over the skin lesions only
    d. On and around the skin lesions

34. **Secondary pyoderma may superimpose upon:**
    a. Scabies
    b. Eczema
    c. Dermatophytoses
    d. All of these

35. **Percentage of fusidic acid cream used in pyoderma:**
    a. 0.5%
    b. 1%
    c. 2%
    d. 5%

36. **Percentage of mupirocin cream used for pyoderma:**
    a. 0.5%
    b. 1%
    c. 2%
    d. 5%

37. **Organism causing common bacterial folliculitis:**
    a. Staphylococcus
    b. Streptococcus
    c. Proteus
    d. Corynebacterium

38. **Common predisposing factor for recurrent furunculosis:**
    a. Sweating
    b. Poor hygiene
    c. Diabetes mellitus
    d. All of these

39. **The commonest site of affection for carbuncle is:**
    a. Axilla
    b. Scalp
    c. Neck
    d. Foot

40. **Periporitis is associated with:**
    a. Hot and humid climate
    b. Malnutrition
    c. Miliaria
    d. All of the above

Chapter 5

Cutaneous Infections with Pyogenic Bacteria

41. Periporitis typically affects:

 a. Forehead
 b. Forearm
 c. Forefoot
 d. All of the above

42. The type of crust in ecthyma is:

 a. Thin honey coloured
 b. Thin papery
 c. Thick heaped up
 d. Serosanguinous

43. A furuncle is also known as:

 a. Blind boil   b. Common boil
 c. Infected cyst   d. All of these

44. Bacterial infection which heals with permanent hair loss is:

 a. Impetigo
 b. Impetigo bockhart
 c. Deep folliculitis
 d. Periporitis

45. Ecthyma gangrenosum is caused by septicaemia due to:

 a. Staphylococcus
 a. Staphylococci
 b. Streptococci
 c. Pseudomonas
 d. Corynebacterium

ANSWERS

1-b,	2-d,	3-c,	4-a,	5-b,	6-a,	7-b,	8-a,	9-b,	10-b,
11-a,	12-d,	13-c,	14-a,	15-a,	16-b,	17-d,	18-b,	19-c,	20-a,
21-b,	22-a,	23-d,	24-b,	25-a,	26-d,	27-c,	28-c,	29-a,	30-b,
31-a,	32-d,	33-d,	34-d,	35-c,	36-c,	37-a,	38-d,	39-c,	40-d,
41-a,	42-c,	43-b,	44-c,	45-c					

Cutaneous Tuberculosis

Based upon the manner in which the skin is invaded by the tubercle bacilli, tuberculosis of the skin is divided into:

1. Primary inoculation tuberculosis (tuberculous chancre)

This is rare since the usual site of primary infection is the lung.

It is seen in young children, not previously exposed to tuberculosis, it presents as a non-healing ulcer on an extremity with or without regional matted lymphadenopathy. Ulceration following bacillus Calmette-Guérin (BCG) vaccination may take long time to heal in the immunocompromised and this may resemble primary tuberculous chancre.

2. Reinoculation tuberculosis

This is seen in persons who were exposed to tuberculosis in the past, have developed immunity to it and are being reinoculated with tubercle bacilli, through penetrating cutaneous trauma. These commonest forms of skin tuberculosis include:

- **lupus vulgaris** (refer to section on next page)
- **tuberculosis verrucosa cutis** (refer to section on page 61)

3. Contiguous spread tuberculosis

Skin involvement through spread from underlying organs **(scrofuloderma)**. This commonly occurs following lymph node affection (especially cervical) but even follows chest, abdomen, joint or bone tuberculosis. (*see* section on scrofuloderma)

4. Haematogenous spread to the skin (miliary tuberculosis)

5. Auto-inoculation tuberculosis (periorificial tuberculosis) which is due to reinoculation of tubercle bacilli into draining orifices in cases of uncontrolled tuberculosis of internal organs (e.g. in and around the mouth in pulmonary tuberculosis or periurethral in renal tuberculosis).

Clinical implication: Categories 1 and 2 have good prognosis due to lower bacterial load and good immunity whereas 3, 4 and 5 have internal organ involvement, higher bacterial load and poorer immunity.

Diagnosis

A high index of suspicion, based on the clinical features, is necessary because tuberculosis has many widely differing presentations. Demonstration of *Mycobacterium tuberculosis* in **smear of discharge**, is usually possible from cases with ulcerated lesions (especially tuberculous chancre, scrofuloderma, periorificial tuberculosis). Fine needle aspiration cytology (FNAC) of lymph nodes may demonstrate bacilli or granulomatous cytology.

Mantoux test is positive in patients with good immunity, e.g. lupus vulgaris and may be negative in those with poor immunity, e.g. miliary tuberculosis. Tuberculoid granuloma is seen in **skin biopsy**. Other routine investigations to rule out an internal focus of tuberculosis include a **chest X-ray,** white blood cells (WBC) count and **ESR** or Creative protein or Adenosine deaminase level. Recent tests include interferon gamma and tuberculosis polymerase chain reaction (TB PCR). When suspicion of a particular organ involvement exists, additional investigations may be done.

Treatment

Antituberculous therapy as for pulmonary tuberculosis is recommended. A common short duration regimen for an adult includes:

- **Ethambutol**   800 mg/day
- **Pyrazinamide**   1500 mg/day
- **INH**   300 mg/day
- **Rifampicin**   450 mg/day

All for 2 months, and followed by the latter two drugs for a further period of 4 months. Alternatively one may follow the directly observed treatment short-course (DOTS) regimens.

Summary: Cutaneous tuberculosis may occur as a result of primary inoculation (tuberculous chancre), reinoculation lupus vulgaris, tuberculosis verrucosa cutis, contiguous spread (scrofuloderma) or uncommonly as autoinoculation (periorificial tuberculosis) or through haematogenous spread (miliary tuberculosis). Prognosis is poor in the latter two. Diagnosis can be established by demonstration of bacilli and/or a granuloma on biopsy. A four drug regimen for two months followed by two drugs for 4 months is effective.

LUPUS VULGARIS

This is a common form of localised cutaneous tuberculosis. It occurs due to inoculation, with tubercle bacilli, of persons who have been previously exposed to the infection (reinoculation tuberculosis). A common mode of inoculation is through contamination of traumatic ulcers.

Patient Profile

Older children, adolescents and young adults are affected, probably because of increased chances of trauma. Males are more prone. Most of these patients are otherwise healthy and do not have another active tuberculous focus.

History

A slowly progressive (over several months or years), asymptomatic lesion that follows trauma is the usual presentation.

Morphology

A well defined reddish brown plaque that has a beaded (papulonodular) border is characteristic. Diascopy (pressure with a transparent firm object like a glass slide) elicits the light brown (apple jelly) coloured nodules considered typical of the condition. Long standing lesions (over 6 months) may display self healing in the centre or on one side and extension on the other side (Figs 6.1–6.4). Healing occurs with an atrophic scar.

Distribution

Elbows, knees, buttocks, extensor aspects of extremities are common sites. Face is involved less commonly than reported in the Western literature.

> **Variations:** In addition to the classic plaque type, other variants include:
> - Verrucous—surface of the plaque is keratotic (Fig. 6.4).
> - Papulo-nodular—coalescence into plaque is absent.
> - Atrophic/Cicatrising—scarring is prominent.
> - Ulcerative.
>
> Tumid—indurated oedematous tumorous plaque.

Diagnosis

Skin biopsy is diagnostic. It shows a tuberculoid granuloma made of epitheloid cells and Langhan's giant cells surrounded by lymphocytes and plasma cells. Mantoux test is usually positive. Organisms are difficult to demonstrate from biopsy or smears.

Treatment

Antituberculous therapy leads to prompt resolution. Please refer page 59 for further details.

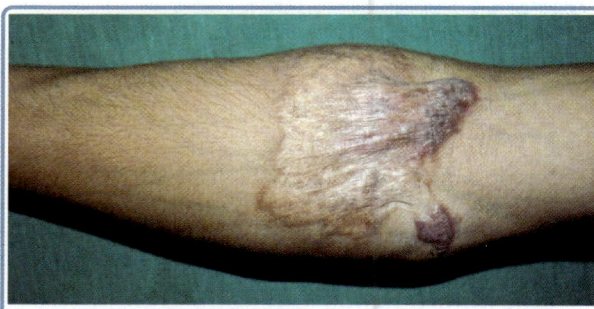

Fig. 6.1: Lupus vulgaris—erythematous plaque progressing towards right and healing with hypertrophic scarring towards the left

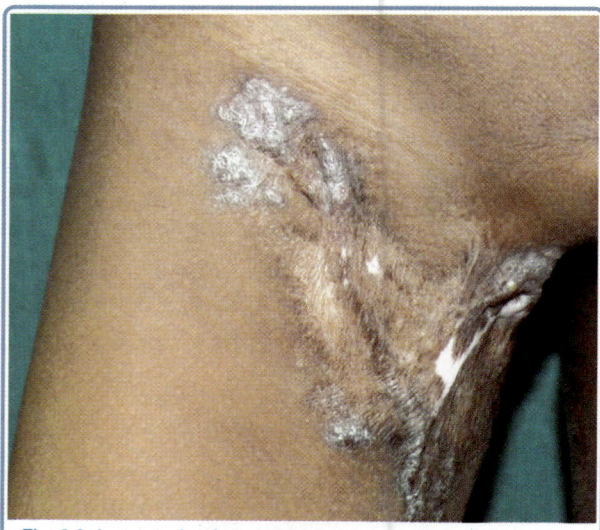

Fig. 6.2: Lupus vulgaris—around puckered scars of scrofuloderma following tuberculous lymphadenitis

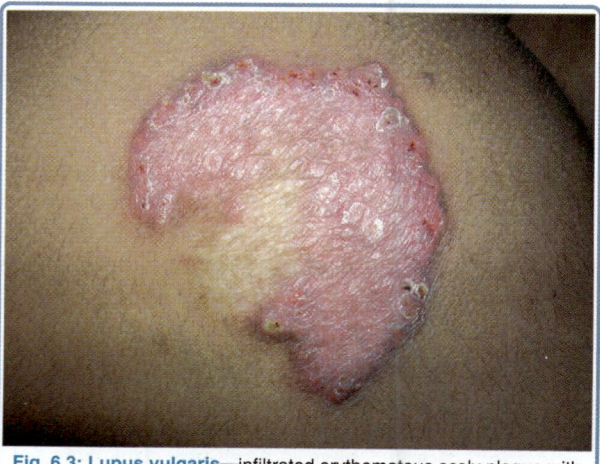

Fig. 6.3: Lupus vulgaris—infiltrated erythematous scaly plaque with focal atrophy

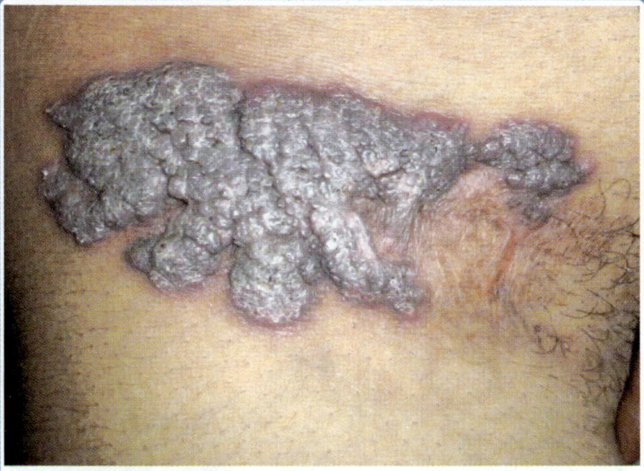

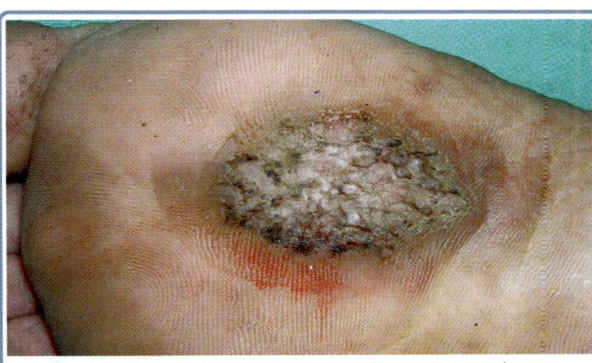

Fig. 6.4: Verrucous lupus vulgaris—keratotic erythematous indurated plaque with healing at one end

Summary: Lupus vulgaris occurs due to reinoculation with *M. tuberculosis* in persons with good immunity to it. A slowly evolving asymptomatic reddish brown plaque that shows apple jelly colour on diascopy, over extensors of extremities in young individuals is the typical presentation. Healing occurs with scarring. Biopsy shows a tuberculoid granuloma. Antituberculous therapy leads to prompt resolution.

TUBERCULOSIS VERRUCOSA CUTIS (ANATOMIST'S WART) (PROSECTOR'S WART)

This is another common localised form of reinoculation tuberculosis.

Patient Profile

Adults who have a chance of getting exposed to the tubercle bacillus, while performing their duties, e.g. prosectors, anatomists, butchers are characteristically affected. However, in India, it is seen more commonly in young adults who walk barefoot. Probably due to higher chances of trauma, males are more commonly affected. Patients are otherwise healthy.

History

A slowly progressive, asymptomatic lesion that follows penetrating trauma is the usual presentation.

Morphology

A well defined verrucous (rough surfaced, grayish) plaque (Fig. 6.5), that has a tendency to heal at one end and progress at the other is characteristic. Healing occurs with an atrophic scar. Superimposed pustules and purulent crusts are common.

Distribution

Palms, soles, especially fingers and toes are involved in most cases (Figs 6.5 and 6.6). Elbows, knees and extensor aspects of extremities are other less common sites.

Diagnosis

Skin biopsy is diagnostic. The epidermis shows pseudocarcinomatous hyperplasia while the dermis shows papillomatosis. A tuberculoid granulomatous infiltrate is seen in addition to neutrophilic infiltrate. Mantoux test is usually positive. Organisms are difficult to demonstrate in biopsy or smears.

Treatment

Please refer to section on cutaneous tuberculosis on page 59.

Summary: Tuberculosis verrucosa cutis is a reinoculation tuberculosis that follows penetrating injuries to hands and feet. An indolent asymptomatic verrucous plaque that is covered with purulent crust is typical. Lesion tends to heal at one end, with scarring. Biopsy shows hyperplastic epidermis and a tuberculoid granuloma in the dermis. Antituberculous therapy leads to prompt clearing.

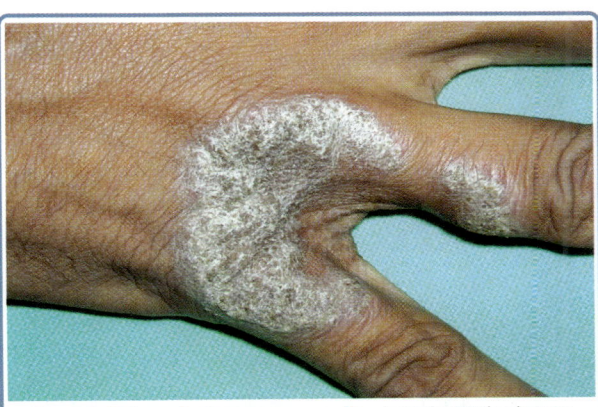

Fig. 6.5: Tuberculosis verrucosa cutis—verrucous plaque resembling plantar wart

Fig. 6.6: Tuberculosis verrucosa cutis—hyperkeratotic plaques interrupted by areas of atrophy

Chapter 6

Cutaneous Tuberculosis

SCROFULODERMA

Scrofuloderma represents involvement of skin by extension from an internal organ like lymph node or joint. As compared to reinoculation tuberculosis (lupus vulgaris), body's immunity against tuberculosis is poorer. This may manifest as higher bacillary count in lesional discharge and a weakly positive Mantoux test.

Patient Profile

As opposed to reinoculation tuberculosis these patients always have an underlying tuberculous focus and may be ill from its systemic effects.

Morphology

Multiple discharging sinuses that are connected to underlying non-tender swellings is the general pattern of presentation. Most commonly, the swellings consist of few or many, matted, soft to firm, non-tender lymph nodes (tuberculous lymphadenitis). However, tuberculosis of joints, bones, chest (empyema), abdomen (ileocaecal) or any other organ may underlie these sinuses. Sinuses discharge purulent and later serosanguinous material and are marked by undermined edges.

Distribution

Cervical lymphadenitis is the most common site of affection (Fig. 6.7). Axillary (Fig. 6.8) and inguinal lymphadenitis are next common. Joints, bones, chest and abdomen are less commonly involved.

Diagnosis

Biopsy of sinus mouth shows suppurative foci surrounded by a tuberculoid granulomatous infiltrate. Tubercle bacilli are demonstrable in biopsy tissue. Bacilli are demonstrable in smears and can be cultured.

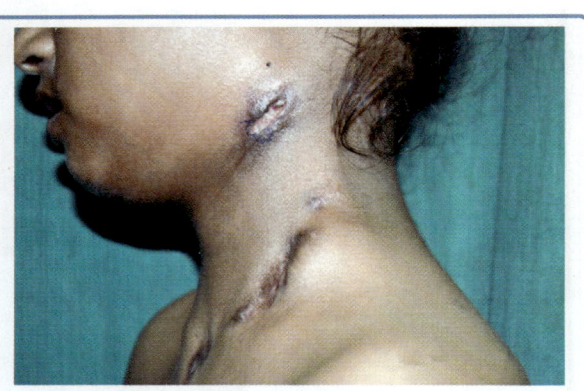

Fig. 6.7: Scrofuloderma—multiple discharging sinuses over matted lymphadenopathy. Neck is the commonest site of affection

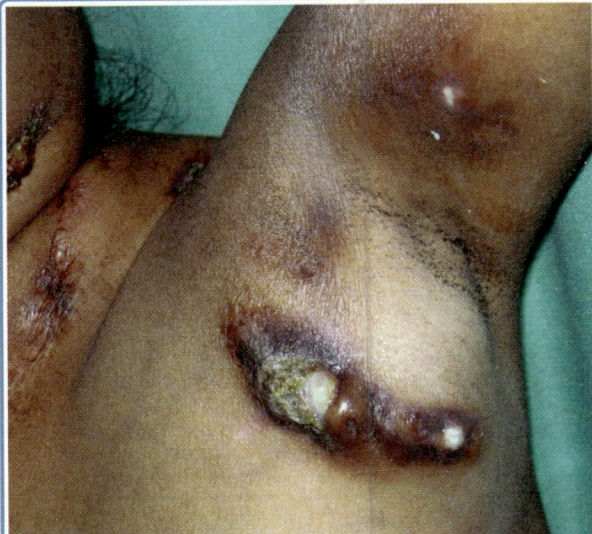

Fig. 6.8: Scrofuloderma—pus discharging sinuses and nodules with underlying matted lymph nodes in axilla and neck

Treatment

Please *see* section on cutaneous tuberculosis on page 59. Underlying tuberculous focus needs to be treated appropriately.

Summary: Being a progressive form of tuberculosis, prognosis in scrofuloderma is related to the underlying organ affected. Multiple discharging sinuses, that have undermined edges, and which overlie matted lymph nodes is the standard presentation. Lymph nodes in the neck, axillae or groins may be affected. Occasionally sinuses may be related to joint, bone, chest or abdominal tuberculosis. Bacilli can be seen and cultured from the serosanguinous discharge. Therapy is that of underlying organ tuberculosis.

Tuberculids

Tuberculids are a group of skin rashes caused by hypersensitivity of the skin to circulating tuberculous antigens. Tuberculous antigens are pushed into circulation by an active tuberculous focus in another organ or occasionally in the skin. Their general characteristics are:

- Mycobacteria cannot be demonstrated from the skin lesions of tuberculids.
- A tuberculoid granuloma is seen on skin biopsy.
- The Mantoux test is strongly positive.
- Tuberculids resolve after the active tuberculous focus elsewhere is treated with antitubercular therapy.

Tuberculids may occur as:

- Lichen scrofulosorum (Fig. 6.9)—an asymptomatic scaly grouped micropapular rash over trunk

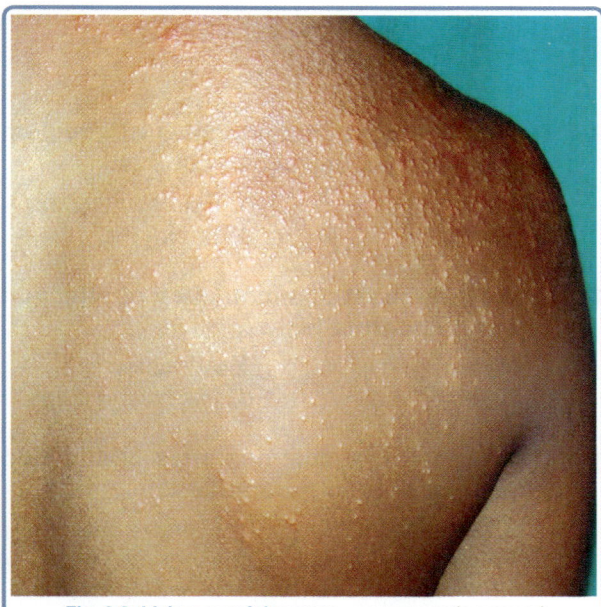

Fig. 6.9: Lichen scrofulosorum—asymptomatic grouped erythematous micropapules

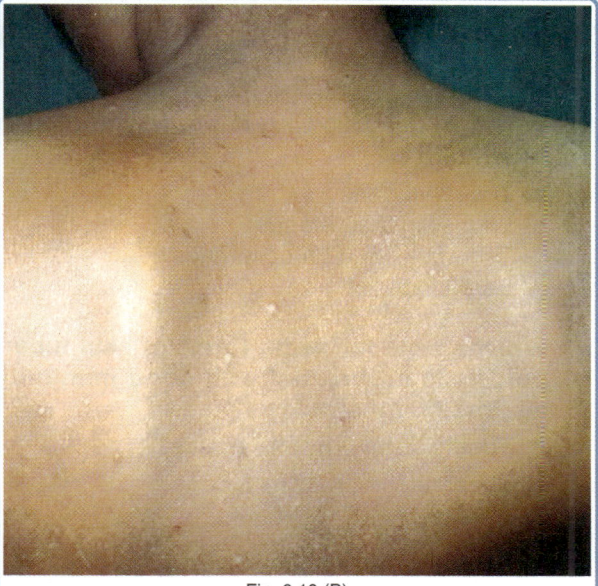

Fig. 6.10 (B)

Fig. 6.10A and B: Papulonecrotic tuberculid—symmetrically distributed papules with central necrosis resolving with scars

especially in young girls. The lesions heal without scarring following antitubercular therapy.

- *Papulonecrotic tuberculid*—asymptomatic, scattered papules topped by a pustule or a necrotic centre over extensors of extremities, elbows, knees, back, face, genitals and palms and soles in that order of frequency. Histopathology shows vasculitis in addition to a tuberculoid granuloma in the dermis. The lesions affect adults and heal with atrophic scars (Fig. 6.10A and B).

- Erythema induratum or Bazin's disease— painful nodules over the back or sides of legs of young women that may break down leading

to deep ulcers. Ulcers heal over several weeks to leave behind atrophic scars. Histopathology shows vasculitis and granulomatous panniculitis. The conditions responds slowly to antitubercular therapy (Fig. 6.11).

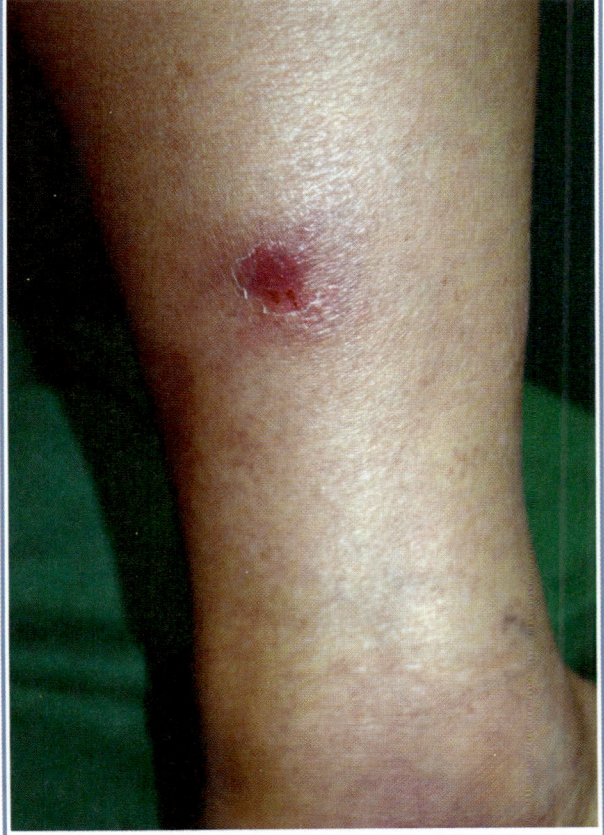

Fig. 6.11: Erythema induratum—erythematous indurated nodule with central softening on back of leg

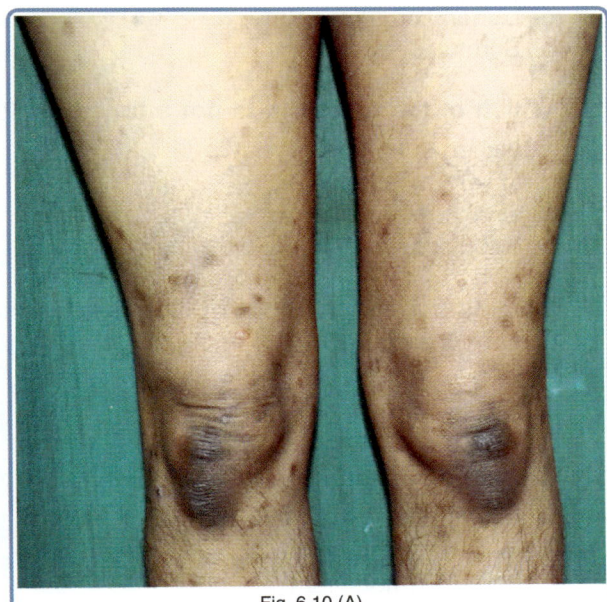

Fig. 6.10 (A)

Chapter 6

Cutaneous Tuberculosis

MCQs

1. **Which of the following is not a type of skin tuberculosis?**
   a. Lupus vulgaris
   b. Lupus erythematosus
   c. Tuberculosis verrucosa cutis
   d. Scrofuloderma

2. **Which of the following forms of skin tuberculosis is associated with good immunity against *M. tuberculosis*?**
   a. Tuberculosis verrucosa cutis
   b. Tuberculous chancre
   c. Miliary tuberculosis
   d. Scrofuloderma

3. **The sign of apple jelly nodules is seen in:**
   a. Discoid lupus erythematosus
   b. Lepromatous leprosy
   c. Lupus vulgaris
   d. Erythema nodosum

4. **The commonest morphology of lupus vulgaris is:**
   a. Papule   b. Plaque
   c. Nodule   d. Ulcer

5. **Anatomist's wart refers to:**
   a. Verruca vulgaris in an anatomist
   b. Tuberculosis verrucosa cutis
   c. Condyloma acuminata
   d. Condyloma lata

6. **Which of the following forms of tuberculosis is not associated with good immunity against *M. tuberculosis*?**
   a. Lupus vulgaris
   b. Tuberculosis verrucosa cutis
   c. Scrofuloderma
   d. Papulonecrotic tuberculid

7. **Penetrating injury usually precedes this form of tuberculosis:**
   a. Scrofuloderma
   b. Papulonecrotic tuberculid
   c. Tuberculosis verrucosa cutis
   d. Miliary tuberculosis

8. **One of the most common sites of affection of lupus vulgaris is:**
   a. Knees and elbows   b. Palms and soles
   c. Back   d. Fingers

9. **One of the most common sites of affection of tuberculosis verrucosa cutis is:**
   a. Neck   b. Palms and soles
   c. Face   d. Back

10. **One of the most common sites of affection of scrofuloderma is:**
    a. Neck   b. Abdomen
    c. Back   d. Palms and soles

11. **One of the most common sites of affection of papulonecrotic tuberculid is:**
    a. Knees and elbows   b. Palms and soles
    c. Face   d. Fingers

12. **Which of the following forms of cutaneous tuberculosis is not preceded by penetrating injury?**
    a. Tuberculous chancre
    b. Tuberculosis verrucosa cutis
    c. Papulonecrotic tuberculid
    d. Lupus vulgaris

13. **Which of the following forms of cutaneous tuberculosis is not associated with lymphadenopathy?**
    a. Lupus vulgaris   b. Scrofuloderma
    c. Tuberculous chancre   d. Cold abscess

14. **Which of the following is a tuberculid?**
    a. Lichen nitidus
    b. Lichen planus
    c. Lichen scrofulosorum
    d. Scrofuloderma

15. **Which of the following is not a tuberculid?**
    a. Lichen scrofulosorum
    b. Miliary tuberculosis
    c. Erythema induratum
    d. Papulonecrotic tuberculid

16. **What is the usual colour of skin lesions in lupus vulgaris?**
    a. Pink   b. Yellowish red
    c. Brown red   d. Red

17. **Bazin's disease refers to:**
    a. Papulonecrotic tuberculid
    b. Erythema induratum
    c. Erythema nodosum
    d. Recurrent oral aphthae and genital ulcers

18. **Bazin's disease occurs most commonly over:**
    a. Feet
    b. Calves
    c. Shins
    d. Thighs

19. **The commonest site of affection of scrofuloderma is:**
    a. Axilla
    b. Groin
    c. Neck
    d. Knee

20. **Commonest underlying organ affected in scrofuloderma is:**
    a. Joint
    b. Pleura
    c. Peritoneum
    d. Lymph node

21. **A scaly plaque of lupus vulgaris is differentiated from psoriasis by:**
    a. Modularity
    b. Apple jelly sign
    c. Atrophy
    d. All of these

22. **A characteristic of cutaneous tuberculids is:**
    a. Presence of acid fast bacilli
    b. Positive Mantoux test
    c. No response to antituberculous therapy
    d. Macrophage granuloma

23. **Tuberculous lymph nodes are described as:**
    a. Shotty
    b. Rubbery
    c. Knotted
    d. Matted

24. **An asymptomatic verrucous plaque with focal atrophy over foot is likely to be:**
    a. Mosaic wart
    b. Tuberculosis verrucous cutis
    c. verrucous psoriasis
    d. Viral wart

25. **The most common form of cutaneous tuberculosis in India:**
    a. Tuberculous verrucous chancre
    b. Miliary tuberculosis
    c. Scrofuloderma
    d. Lupus vulgaris

26. **Apple jelly nodules are typically described to occur in:**
    a. Granuloma faciale
    b. Lupus vulgaris
    c. Sarcoidosis
    d. Leprosy

27. **Mantoux test will be negative in:**
    a. Scrofuloderma
    b. Lichen scrofulosorum
    c. Lupus vulgaris
    d. Tuberculosis verrucosa cutis

28. **Cutaneous analogue of Ghon's focus in the lungs is:**
    a. Tuberculous chancre
    b. Scrofuloderma
    c. Erythema induratum
    d. Papulonecrotic tuberculid

29. **Butcher's wart is another name for:**
    a. Scrofuloderma
    b. Erythema induratum
    c. Lupus vulgaris
    d. Tuberculosis verrucosa cutis

Chapter
6

Cutaneous Tuberculosis

ANSWERS

1-b,	2-a,	3-c,	4-b	5-b,	6-c,	7-c,	8-a,	9-b,	10-a,
11-a,	12-c,	13-a,	14-c,	15-b,	16-c,	17-b,	18-b,	19-a,	20-d,
21-d,	22-b,	23-d,	24-b	25-d,	26-b,	27-a,	28-a,	29-d	

Cutaneous Fungal Infections

SUPERFICIAL FUNGAL INFECTIONS

Pityriasis Versicolor (Tinea Versicolor)

A common infection caused by overgrowth of the lipophilic fungus *Malassezia furfur* which is also a normal commensal. It has nothing to do with the other tinea (ringworm) infections that are caused by dermatophytes (Fig. 7.1).

> **Clinical implication:** The organisms, being lipophilic, inhabit the sebaceous duct and follicular infundibulum and cause lesions in 'seborrhoeic regions' of young adults whose sebaceous glands are most active. However, the face is usually spared.

Patient profile

Young adults and adolescents are typical patients; children are affected less frequently. It is more common in males. Oily skin and sweating predispose to this infection. Acne vulgaris and seborrhoeic dermatitis are common associations.

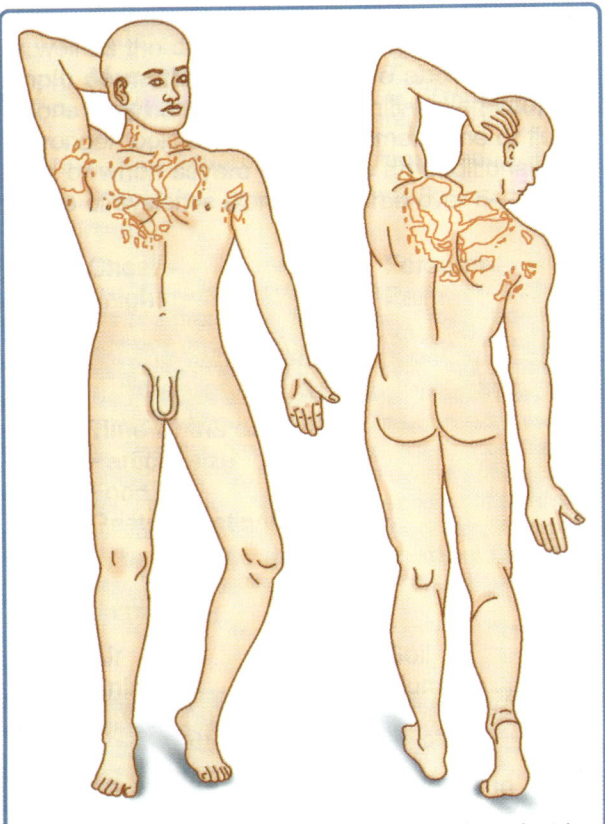

Fig. 7.1: Pityriasis versicolor—hypopigmented macules and patches

Morphology

Asymptomatic, variably sized, well defined hypo-pigmented (Figs 7.2 and 7.3) or hyperpigmented brownish macules and patches (Fig. 7.4) covered with barely visible, powdery, thin scales characterise this condition. Scales can be made more prominent by scraping lesions with a sharp object (scratch sign or Besnier's sign). Occasionally, lesions may be variously coloured as reddish brown, dark brown or black, hence the name, versicolor, i.e. variously coloured.

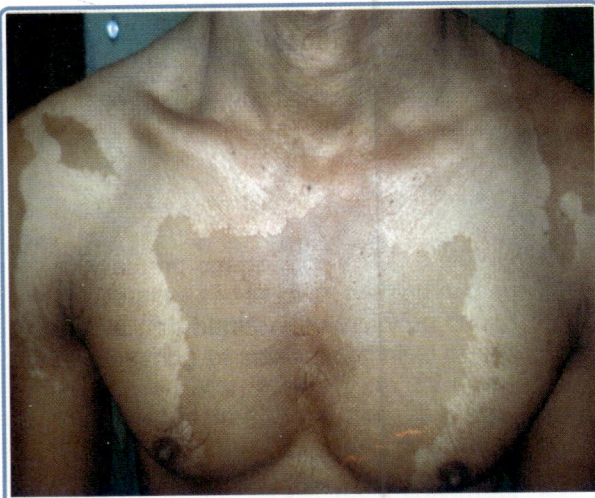

Fig. 7.2: Pityriasis versicolor—large, sharply defined, coalescing hypopigmented patches with powdery scales

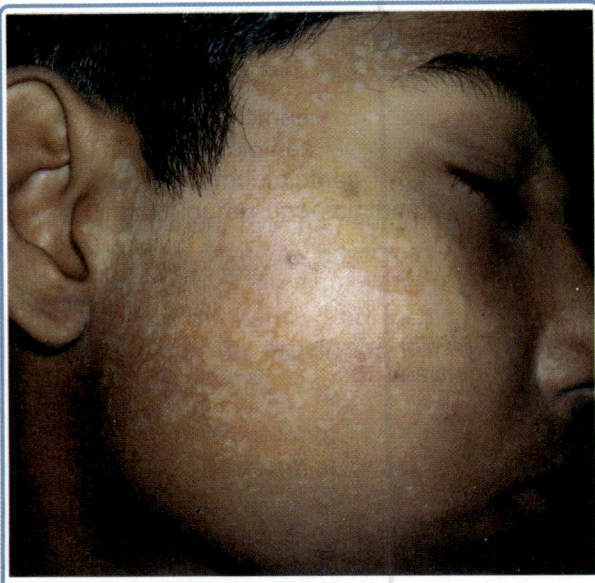

Fig. 7.3: Pityriasis versicolor—hypopigmented, well defined macules coalescing to form patches. Face is involved in children

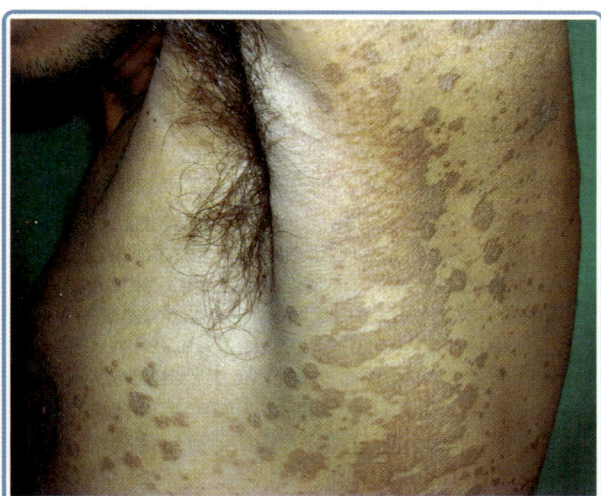

Fig. 7.4: Hyperpigmented pityriasis versicolor—well defined, brown coloured macules and patches with fine scaling

TABLE 7.1: Treatment modalities of pityriasis versicolor

Topicals	Systemic
Azoles like 1% clotrimazole, 2% ketoconazole, 2% miconazole	Single dose oral fluconazole 400 mg
Topical sulphur—40% sodium thiosulphate, 2% selenium sulphide	Itraconazole 100 mg bd for 10 days

Summary: Caused by the fungus, Malassezia, pityriasis versicolor affects young adults. Hypopigmented macules and patches covered with fine, powdery scales, that are accentuated with stroking, typify this condition. Upper trunk, neck and axillae are usually involved. KOH mount demonstrates fungal spores and hyphae. Once daily topical use of 1% clotrimazole or 2% selenium sulphice for two weeks is curative. Oral itraconazole or fluconazole are also effective.

Distribution

Central chest, upper central back, neck, axillae, other parts of trunk, groins, proximal extremities and occasionally, face and inframammary folds in females are affected.

Diagnosis

Clinical picture in a young adult is diagnostic. When examined with a Wood's lamp, scales fluoresce golden yellow. Scraping the lesions and mounting the scales in 10% KOH solution demonstrates short, broad septate hyphae and clusters of thick walled, refractile, round spores that resemble 'spaghetti and meatballs'. Diagnosis may be proved by culture or biopsy.

Treatment

Oral fluconazole in a single dose of 400 mg provides a convenient therapeutic option. Topical antifungal solutions like 1% clotrimazole, 2% miconazole, 1% tolnaftate, 2% ketoconazole are all effective. Alternatively, topical sulphur preparations like 40% sodium thiosulphite or 2% selenium sulphide can be used. Application to the lesions and surrounding normal skin is needed once a day for 2 weeks. Other oral antifungals like itraconazole 100 mg BD for 10 days are better reserved for persistence or recurrence. Pigmentary change takes 1–2 months to resolve after antifungal therapy is initiated.

Clinical implication: Patient needs to be assured that the skin colour will return to normal after a couple of months even though the fungal infection is controlled within 2 weeks.

CANDIDIASIS

This is an opportunistic yeast infection caused by *Candida albicans* and occasionally by other candida species. The yeast proliferates whenever a conducive (i.e. hot and humid) environment exists with or without lowered body resistance (Fig. 7.5).

Clinical Implication: Hot and humid environment is present at certain body sites (i.e. body folds and mucosae) which may be exacerbated by climatic conditions. Low immunity is encountered in young infants and elderly, diabetics, debilitating disorders, patients on steroids and immunosuppressives, haematologic malignancies and ecologic imbalances as with broad spectrum antibacterial therapy.

According to the site of affection, the different syndromes of candidiasis include the following:

Candidial Intertrigo

This inflammation of body folds is usually initiated by friction between apposing surfaces that allows candida to gain a foothold. Accompanying humidity and heat promotes proliferation of candida. Secondary bacterial proliferation is not uncommon.

Patient profile

Overweight adults and chubby infants are common victims. Diabetes mellitus is a common predisposing factor in adults. Affection of toe webs and

Chapter 7

Cutaneous Fungal Infections

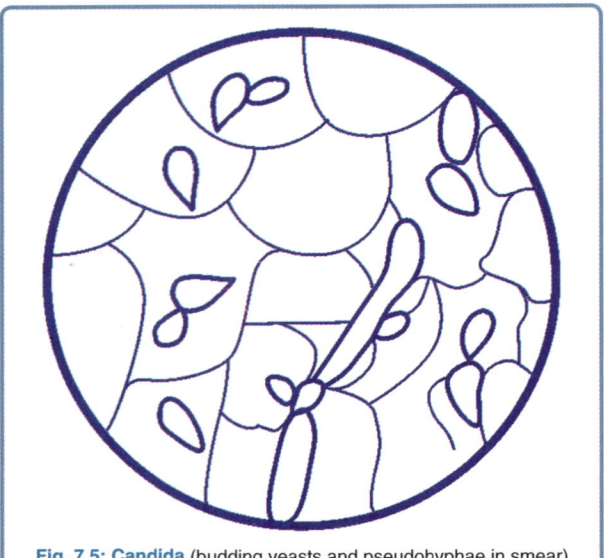

Fig. 7.5: Candida (budding yeasts and pseudohyphae in smear)

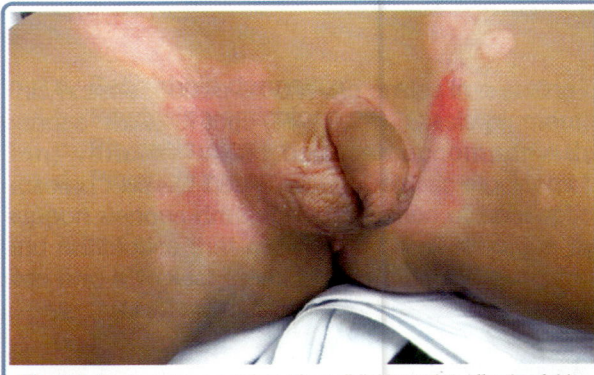

Fig. 7.7: Erythematous patches of candidial intertrigo affecting folds. Lesions frequently resolve with postinflammatory hypopigmentation

finger webs is common in occupations involving wet work, e.g. housemaids, dishwashers or washermen. A tendency to sweat excessively may be a contributory factor especially in those wearing closed footwear.

Morphology

Moist erythematous patches restricted to apposing surfaces of body folds characterize this disease (Figs 7.6–7.8). The periphery of relatively dryer patches may show a collarette of thin scale. Tiny superficial pustules are present beyond the periphery (Fig. 7.8). In advanced cases, the surface of these patches may be eroded or even ulcerated and may discharge serous or sero-purulent fluid.

Over regions covered with thick stratum corneum, i.e. toe webs or finger webs, the lesions appear as moist, white coloured plaques (Figs 7.9 and 7.10). This is due to the hydration of the thick stratum corneum that swells up and becomes white.

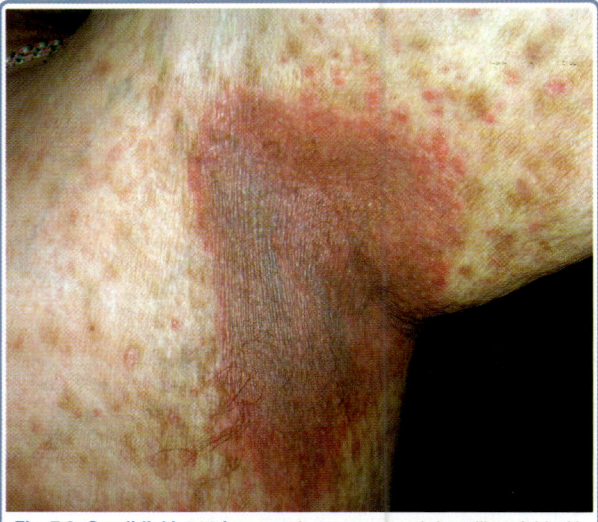

Fig. 7.8: Candidial intertrigo—erythematous patch in axillary fold with satellite lesions

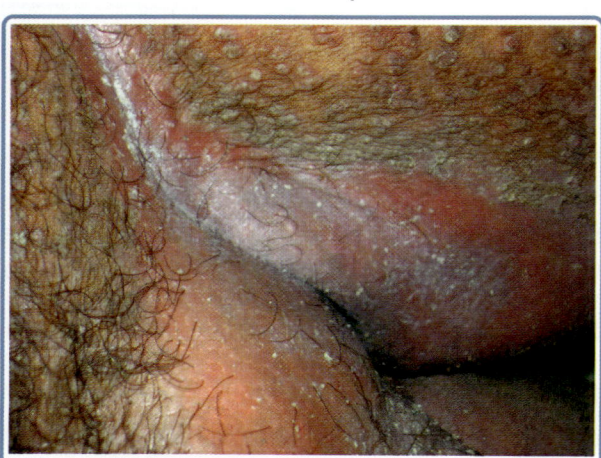

Fig. 7.6: Candidial intertrigo—shiny erythema in inguinal fold with satellite pustules

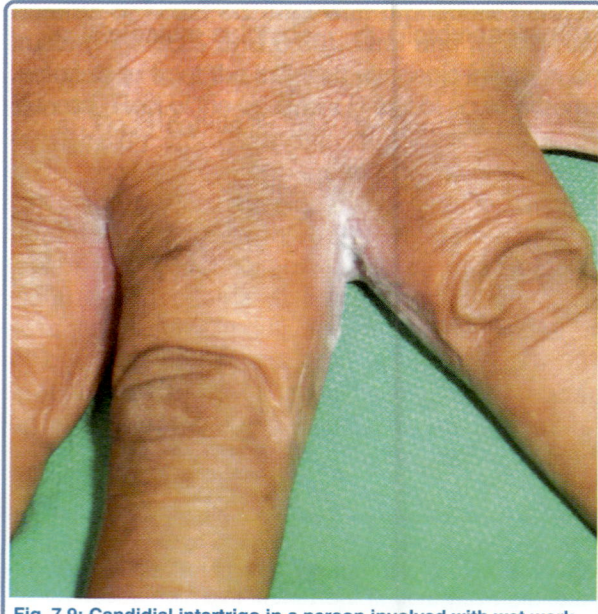

Fig. 7.9: Candidial intertrigo in a person involved with wet work—erythema, fissuring and scaling in the web spaces

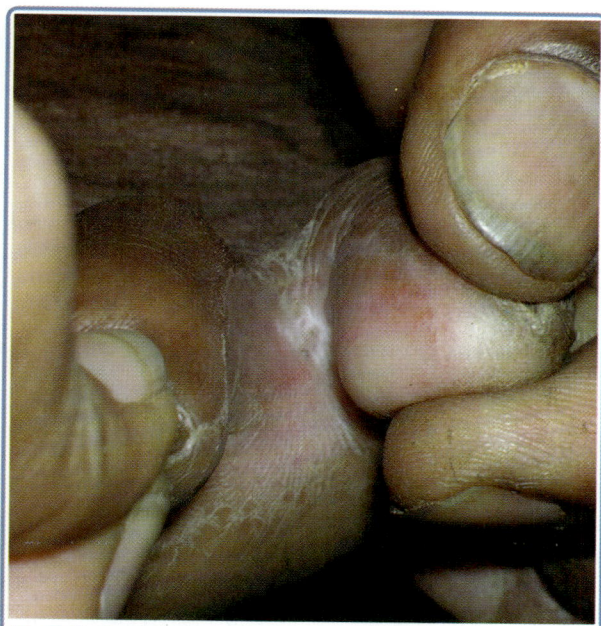

Fig. 7.10: Candidial Intertrigo—erythema and sodden white skin due to maceration

Summary: Candidial intertrigo affects closely apposing and rubbing body folds that provide hot and humid environment for candida to grow. Obese, diabetic adults and chubby infants are frequent victims. Oozing erythematous erosions with marginal scales and satellite pustules are typical. Groins, axillae, inframammary and interdigital folds are involved. Smear shows budding yeasts and pseudohyphae. Topical 1% clotrimazole and correction of predisposing factors is curative. Oral fluconazole is useful in persistent or recurrent cases.

Clinical Presentations of Candidiasis

- Candidial intertrigo
- Napkin candidiasis
- Candidial stomatitis (oral thrush, median rhomboid glossitis and perleche)
- Candidial vulvovaginitis and perianal candidiasis
- Candidial balanoposthitis
- Congenital cutaneous candidiasis
- Neonatal candidiasis
- Candidial paronychia
- Candidial granuloma

Distribution

Virtually any body fold may be affected. Groins, axillae, submammary folds (in females), toe webs and finger webs are common sites of affection. Neck fold and natal cleft are involved in chubby infants and obese adults.

Diagnosis

Smear of scraping from the surface (especially the periphery) of the lesions reveals budding candida spores and pseudohyphae. Candida can be cultured on Sabouraud's agar. Diabetes mellitus needs to be ruled out in an adult, particularly with difficult to control or recurrent infections.

Treatment

Application of clotrimazole 1% or miconazole 2% in cream or lotion form twice daily will clear lesions within a week. Recovery may be hastened by adding a topical antibacterial to control secondary infection, if this is present. Oral fluconazole 50 mg per day for 2 weeks is needed for persistent or relapsing cases.

Correction of the hot and humid environment is crucial in preventing relapse. This can be achieved by meticulously drying affected surfaces after bathing or washing, powdering the region with clotrimazole or miconazole powder and then wearing thin, loose, cotton clothing. For toe web affection, wearing chappals or sandals instead of shoes is helpful.

Candidial Paronychia (Chronic Paronychia)

In a normal nail unit, the potential space between proximal nail fold and the nail plate is sealed by an extension of stratum corneum from the nail fold to the nail plate [cuticle].

When the cuticle is damaged due to persistent action of water and chemicals [usually soaps and detergents] the opened space [Refer Diagram on page 3] provides ideal humid environment for the growth of candida. Superadded staphylococcal infection leads to periodic exacerbations.

Patient profile

Persons involved in work with water and soap, e.g. housemaids, housewives, cooks, etc., are at risk.

Morphology and distribution

Erythema, oedema and hyperpigmentation of proximal nail folds of involved finger and toe nails suggests the diagnosis (Figs 7.11 and 7.12). The cuticle is commonly lost or damaged over the proximal nail fold resulting in the separation of the nail fold from the nail plate. Finger nails are more frequently affected than toe nails. Affection of multiple nails is common (Fig. 7.11). Pressure upon the boggy swelling of the proximal nail fold is painful and may elicit a bead of pus from underneath the nail fold.

Chapter 7

Cutaneous Fungal Infections

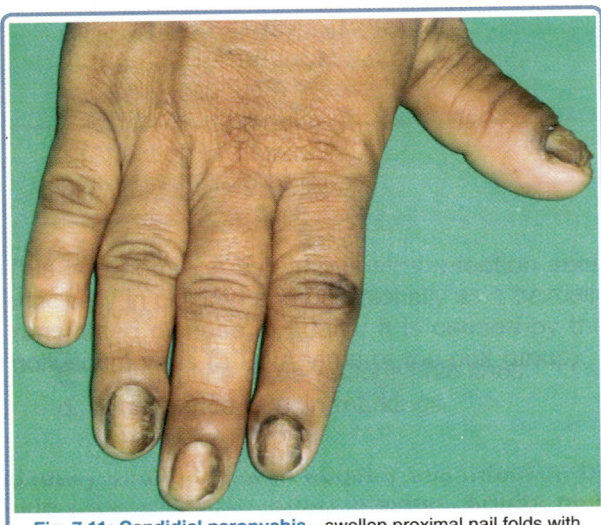

Fig. 7.11: Candidial paronychia—swollen proximal nail folds with involvement of nail plates

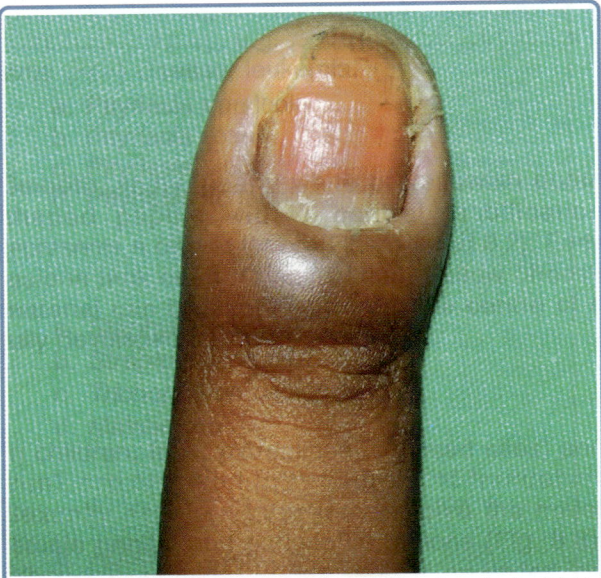

Fig. 7.12: Chronic paronychia—boggy swelling of proximal nail fold with loss of cuticle and nail dystrophy

Diagnosis

Candida can be demonstrated, in addition to staphylococci, by microbiological techniques from a smear of the discharge from the nail fold.

Treatment

A multi-pronged approach of correction of predisposing factors and the use of antifungal and antibacterial agents is needed to induce remission, which may take several weeks even with adequate therapy. Topical antifungals like clotrimazole 1% or miconazole 2% or ciclopirox olamine 1% in lotion forms need to be administered twice daily for 2-4 weeks, sometimes longer. Antibiotic and anti-inflammatory agents are used to control the symptoms of superadded bacterial infection.

Difficult to treat infections will be helped by oral fluconazole 50 mg od or ketoconazole 200 mg od for 2 weeks.

Summary: Candida thrives in the subcuticular space opened up due to damage to the cuticle by prolonged contact with soap and water. Pain, swelling, erythema and tenderness of proximal nail fold of fingers in housewives is the typical presentation. Avoiding soap and water and using topical clotrimazole solution promotes healing. Oral fluconazole helps resistant infections.

Candidial Stomatitis (Oral Thrush, Candidial Glossitis)

Neonates, infants, malnourished, debilitated, immunocompromised individuals [including human immunodeficiency virus (HIV) infected], patients on systemic steroids or antibiotics, diabetics, denture users, elderly or those overusing antiseptic lozenges develop this form of candidiasis. Presence of a curdy white pseudomembrane on the buccal, labial, tongue, gingival or palatal mucosa is characteristic (Figs 7.13 and 7.14). Dislodging the membrane-like white matter with a spatula reveals underlying erythema or erosions. Smear of the discharge proves the diagnosis. Identifying and correcting the predisposing factor is essential. Topical antifungal mouth paint (clotrimazole 1%) hastens healing. Oral fluconazole 50–100 mg daily for 5–7 days or 150 mg/week for 3 per week rapidly clears mucosal candidiasis and is especially needed for immunocompromised or debilitated persons.

Perlèche (Candidial Angular Stomatitis)

This peculiar form of candidiasis is seen as erythema and whitish discolouration of the lips at the angles of the mouth (Fig. 7.15). Excess moisture in this region resulting from overlapping of

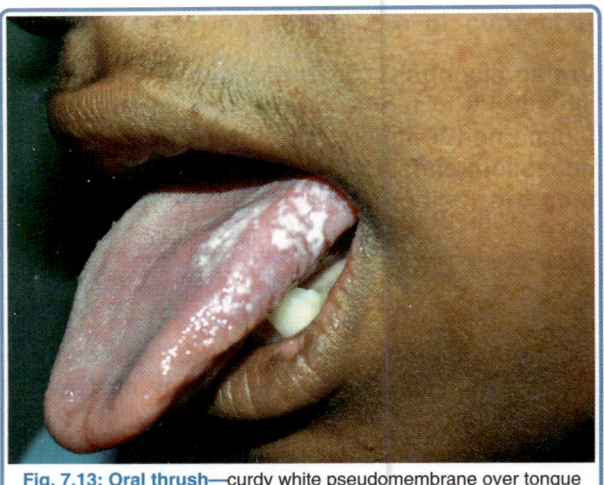

Fig. 7.13: Oral thrush—curdy white pseudomembrane over tongue in a child on antibiotics

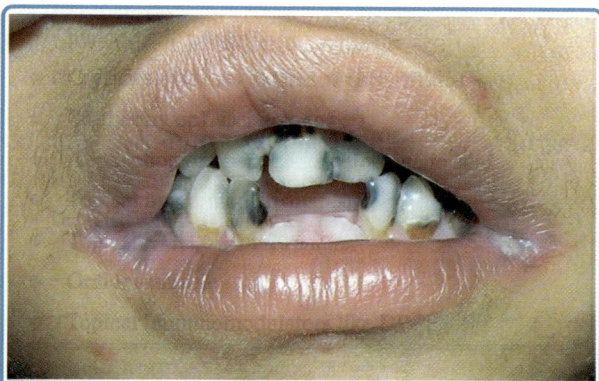

Fig. 7.14: Extensive oral candidiasis in a HIV seropositive— erythema with curdy white discharge

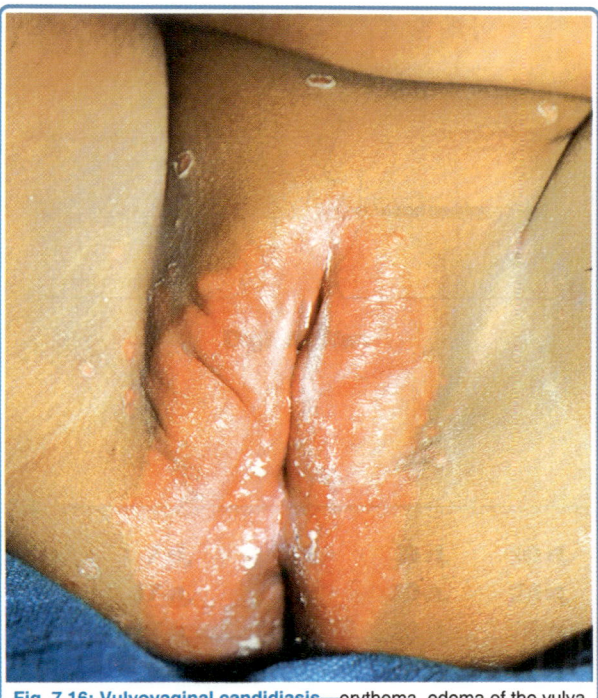

Fig. 7.15: Perieche—erythema, whitening and fissuring at the angles of mouth

lips due to loss of teeth in the elderly or from ill-fitting dentures is a common cause. Deficiency of B complex vitamins may initiate the process. Topical antifungals and correction of the predisposing factors are sufficient. Many a times, it accompanies oral thrush and then needs management on those lines.

Candidial Vaginitis

Normal acidic pH of the vagina prevents the growth of candida. Oral contraceptives, oral antibiotics, pregnancy, menstruation, altered pH predisposes to vaginal candidiasis. Complaints are pruritus, burning and whitish discharge per vaginum. Speculum examination reveals curdy white discharge, erythema and erosions of vaginal walls and introitus. Mounting the white discharge under the microscope demonstrates the budding yeasts. For treatment, the patient is instructed to insert an antifungal vaginal tablet at bed time (Clotrimazole 100 mg for 6 days or 200 mg for 3 days). Nystatin and miconazole can also be used instead. Oral fluconazole 150 mg once a week for 3 weeks is

usually curative. For recurrent or persistent infections, fluconazole 50 mg once or twice a day for 10–14 days is effective.

Candidial Vulvovaginitis

This is seen in young girls as pruritic erythema, oedema of the vulva with curdy whitish discharge from the vagina (Fig. 7.16). Topical clotrimazole lotion and, if required, oral fluconazole is used for therapy.

Perianal Candidiasis

Infants and young children develop this form commonly following an episode of diarrhoea. Erythema, erosions, whitish discharge and marginal pustules are seen over the perianal skin. Lesions that do not respond to topical clotrimazole cream may need oral nystatin for treating candidial superinfection of the bowels. Oral fluconazole is useful in persistent cases. The condition needs to be differentiated from napkin dermatitis that spares folds but affects the rounds of buttocks.

Candidial Balanoposthitis

A stereotypical case is an uncircumcised male with either an affected sex partner or underlying uncontrolled diabetes mellitus. Pruritic erythema, white discharge over the glans and prepuce and radial fissures along the inner aspect of prepuce characterise the disease. Persistent infection leads

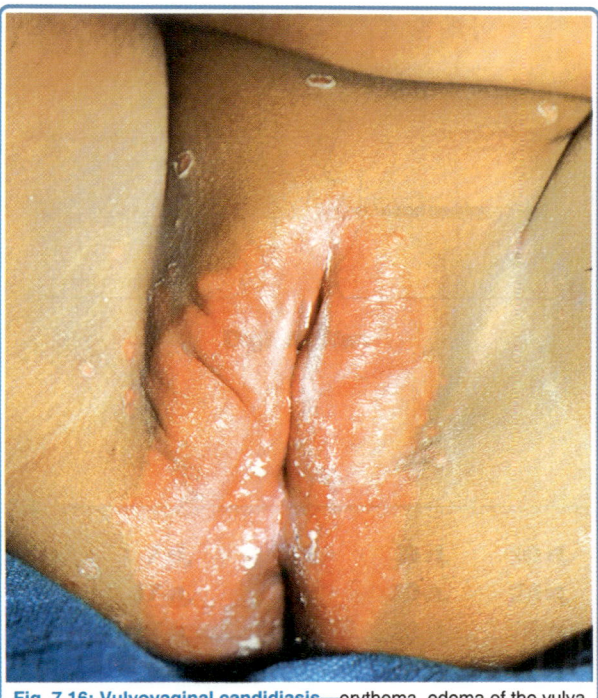

Fig. 7.16: Vulvovaginal candidiasis—erythema, edema of the vulva with curdy white discharge of satellite pustules in a child

Chapter
7

Cutaneous Fungal Infections

to oedema of the prepuce and phimosis. Treatment of the partner and management of diabetes, if any, is necessary. Topical clotrimazole or miconazole lotion is generally effective. Oral fluconazole is also effective.

> **Summary of candidiasis:** Candidiasis is an opportunistic, yeast infection caused by *Candida albicans* that thrives either in the warmth and moisture provided by body folds or when host immunity is compromised (diabetes mellitus, leukaemia, steroid or immunosuppressive therapy). Erythema, tiny superficial pustules, erosions and a curdy white discharge that overlies them typify the disease. Oral thrush, vulvovaginitis, intertrigo, paronychia are the common manifestations of candidiasis. Correction of predisposing factors and topical antifungals (clotrimazole, nystatin) are effective. Oral fluconazole or itraconazole are needed in unresponsive or immuno-compromised cases.

DERMATOPHYTOSIS (RINGWORM)

The commonest of all fungal infections, dermato-phytosis is caused by dermatophytes, a group of fungi that survive by living on keratin. These may spread from human to human (anthropophilic, by sharing of clothes and personal articles), animal to human (zoophilic, by close contact with pets) and soil to human (geophilic, contact with soil). Microbiologically, these fungi have been classified into three genera, trichophyton, microsporum and epidermophyton.

Dermatophytosis is extremely common in our country due to its tropical climate. According to the site of affection dermatophytosis is classified into tinea corporis, tinea barbae, tinea cruris, etc. Pruritus is common to all types of dermatophytoses except tinea incognito, tinea unguium and some cases of non-inflammatory tinea pedis and manuum.

Patient Profile

Adults, young and middle aged, are typically affected. Obesity, diabetes mellitus, sweating tendency, high temperatures at work place (e.g. kitchens, near boilers and furnaces), wearing damp or non-absorbent or thick clothing or closed footwear in a humid atmosphere, sharing personal articles like towels, all predispose to these infections. Sharing caps, combs and shaving blades may lead to tinea capitis and tinea barbae respectively.

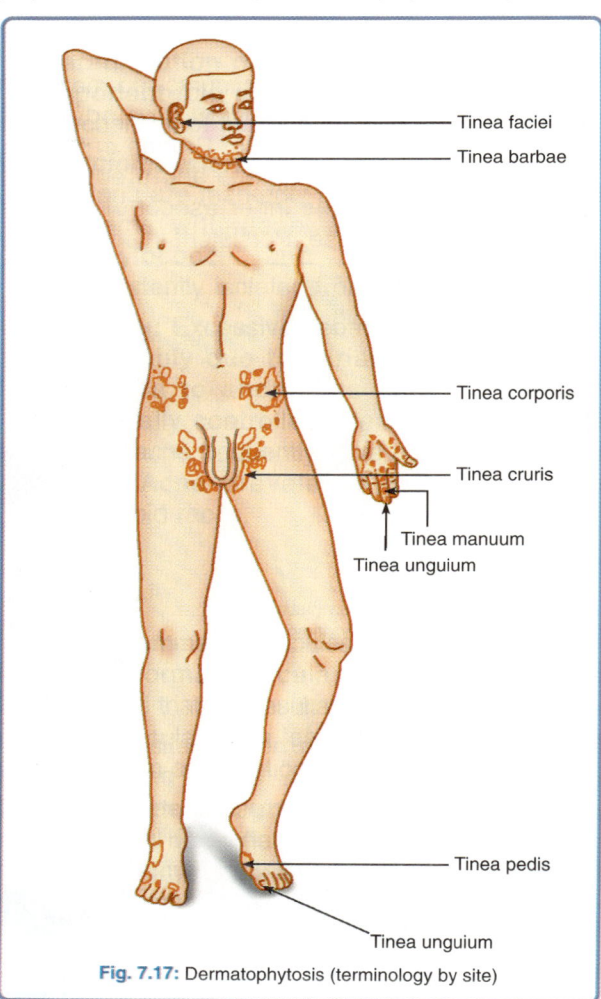

Fig. 7.17: Dermatophytosis (terminology by site)

TABLE 7.2: Types of dermatophytoses based on region of affection	
Types of dermatophytoses	**Region affected**
• Tinea capitis	• Scalp
• Tinea corporis	• Trunk and proximal limbs
• Tinea cruris	• Groin
• Tinea pedis	• Feet
• Tinea faciei	• Face
• Tinea manuum	• Hand
• Tinea barbae	• Beard
• Tinea unguium	• nails

TINEA CORPORIS AND CRURIS (RINGWORM)

Morphology

A typical case has erythematous papules, tiny vesicles and pustules at the margins of a scaly variably pigmented patch. Secondary changes in this 'active margin' may result in crusting, scaling and erosions. Initial lesions are grouped reddish papules with a thin scale. Lesions subside centrally and progress peripherally to produce a ring-like (annular) lesion, hence the name ringworm.

Distribution

The appellation tinea cruris is used to indicate involvement of upper inner thighs (Figs 7.18 and 7.22); the commonest site of dermatophytosis in males. Tinea corporis affects waistline, axillae, buttocks (Fig. 7.19), other parts of the trunk (Figs 7.20–7.23) and extremities excluding palms and soles.

TINEA BARBAE

Grouped erythematous papules and pustules, some of which are follicular, in the beard region are suggestive. Presence of scaling over an adjacent erythematous patch is typical. Lesions may heal with loss of hair.

TINEA CAPITIS

Common presentation (non-inflammatory type) includes a scaly patch of partial alopecia over scalp in a child aged 5–10 years. The condition is

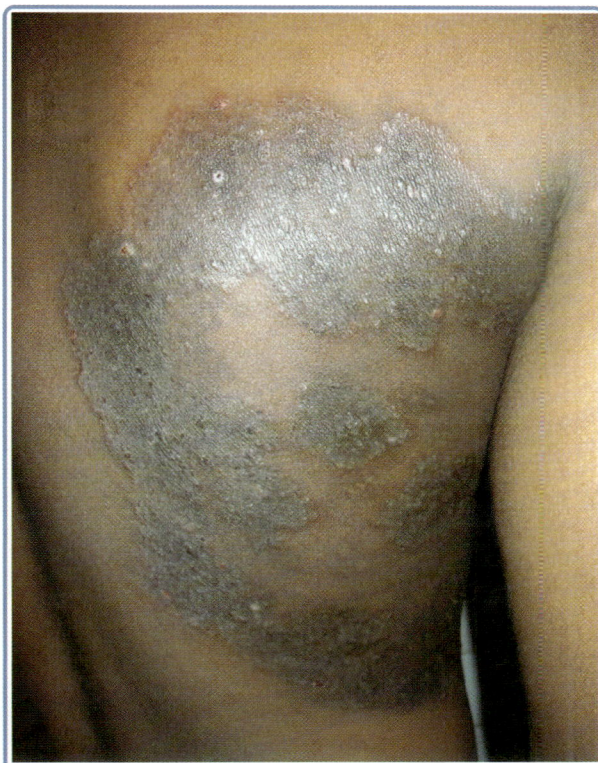

Fig. 7.20: Extensive tinea corporis—hyperpigmented coalescing scaly patches with active erythematous papular border

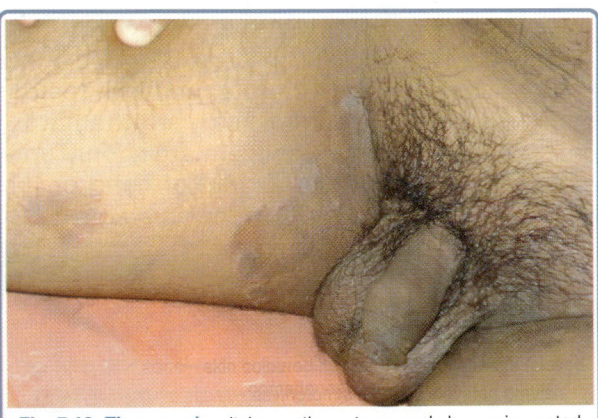

Fig. 7.18: Tinea cruris—itchy, erythematous, scaly hyperpigmented plaques in groin and on thigh

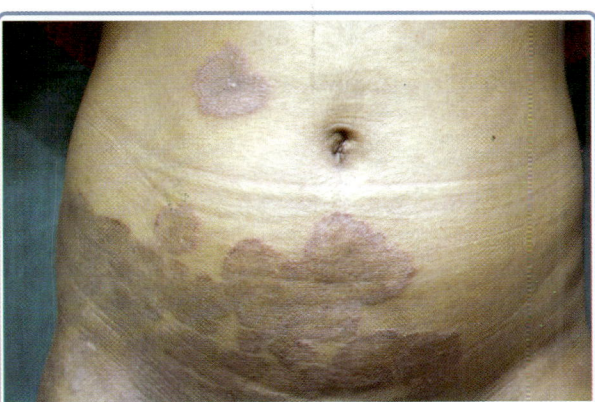

Fig. 7.21: Tinea corporis—involvement of lower trunk and waistline is frequent

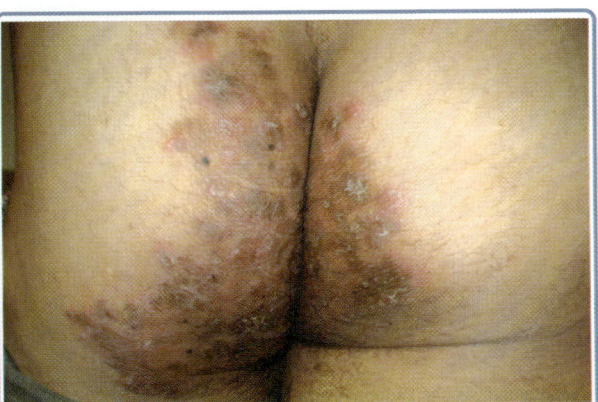

Fig. 7.19: Tinea cruris commonly extends to natal cleft and buttocks—itchy, erythematous scaly plaques with tiny crusts

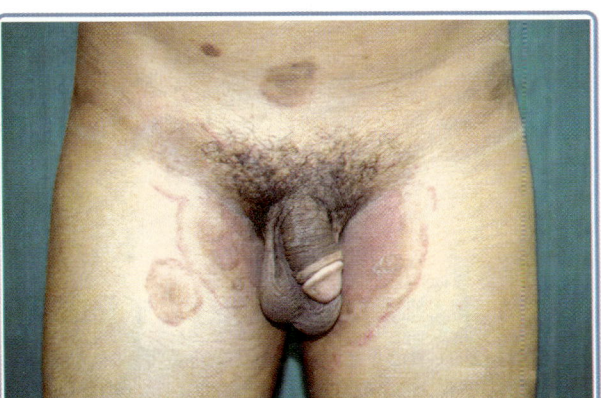

Fig. 7.22: Tinea cruris and corporis—itchy plaques with concentric erythematous rings

Chapter

7

Cutaneous Fungal Infections

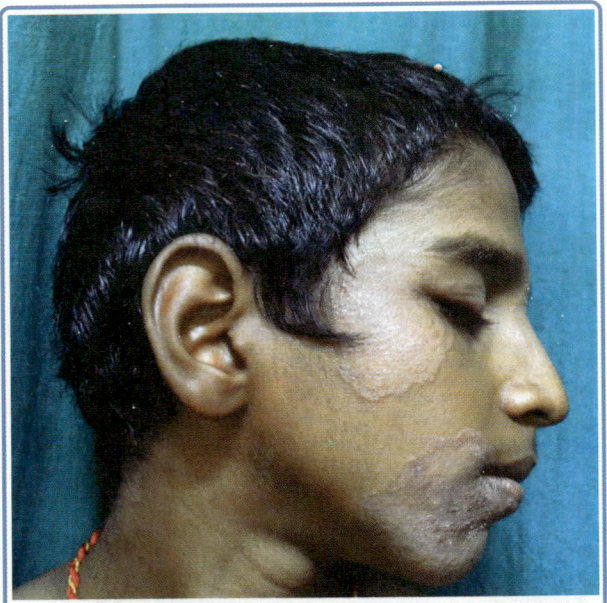

Fig. 7.23 : Tinea faciei—erythematous plaques with abundant fine scales. Active border seen in this case is not always present

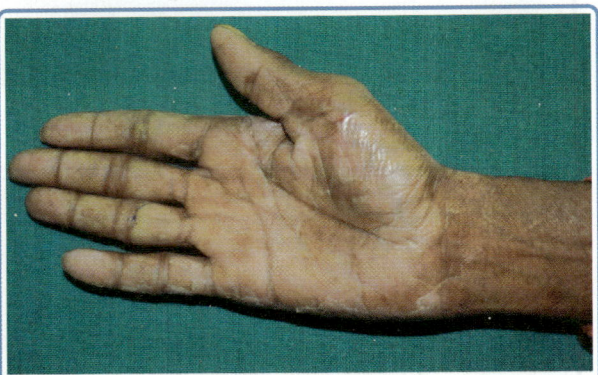

Fig. 7.24: Tinea manuum—ill-defined erythema and scaling of hand is a feature of non-inflammatory tinea manuum

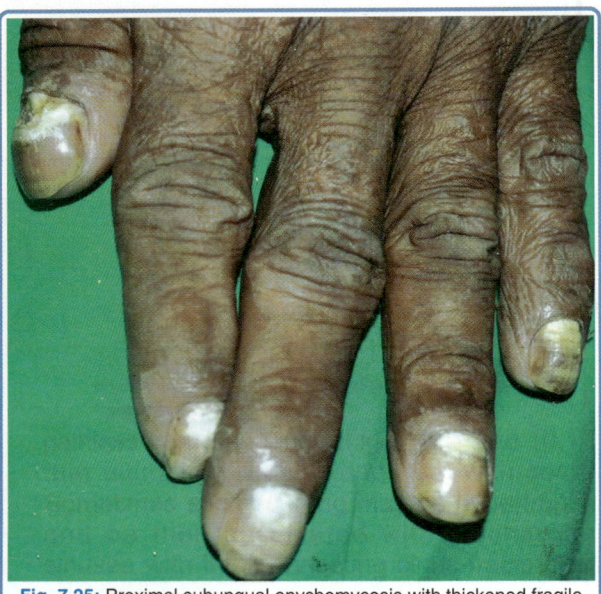

Fig. 7.25: Proximal subungual onychomycosis with thickened fragile nail plates in an immunocompromised patient

commonest in those using caps. Hair within the patch are fragile and lustreless. Uncommonly, a tender oedematous indurated plaque with super-added follicular pustules (inflammatory type, kerion) may be seen (Fig. 7.26). Another inflammatory variety (favus) shows large concave purulent crusts that fluoresce with Wood's light.

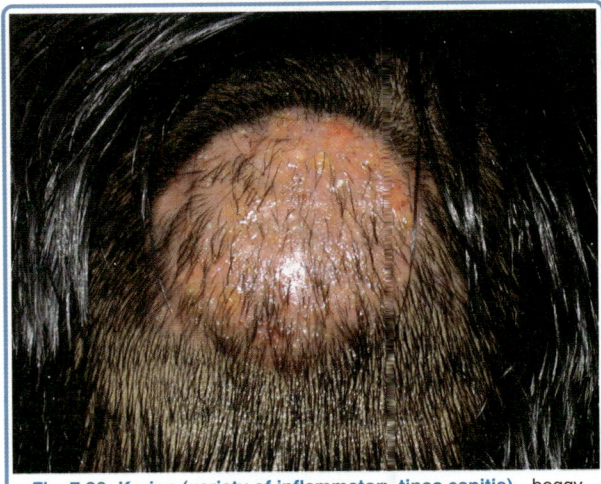

Fig. 7.26: Kerion (variety of inflammatory tinea capitis)—boggy inflammatory swelling studded with pustules and broken hair shafts

TINEA MANUUM AND TINEA PEDIS

Affection of hands (manuum) and feet (pedis) has many similarities. Non-inflammatory lesions comprise poorly defined scaly erythematous patches that show the 'active margin' only upon extension to the dorsal aspect of hand or foot (Figs 7.24, 7.27 and 7.28). Thin scaling is accentuated

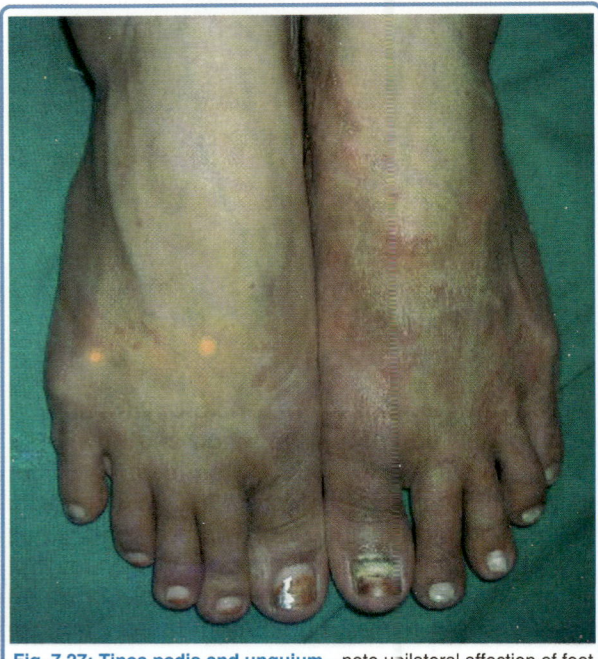

Fig. 7.27: Tinea pedis and unguium—note unilateral affection of foot and nails

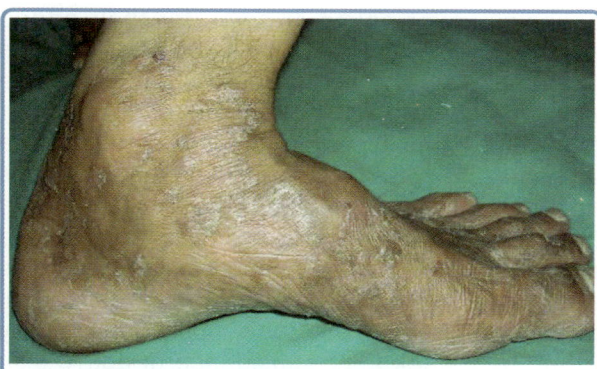

Fig. 7.28: Tinea pedis—erythematous, scaly patches and plaques

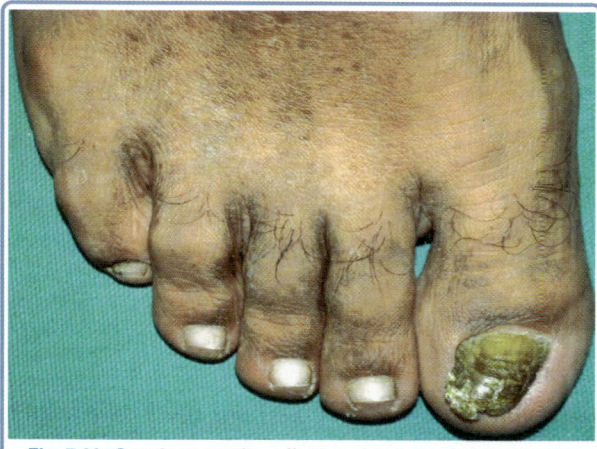

Fig. 7.29: Onychomycosis—affection of great toe nail-thickening, discolouration and dystrophy of the whole nail plate with subungual hyperkeratosis

in volar creases. (Fig. 7.30) inflammatory types are characterised by grouped vesicles based on erythema and oedema. These can progress to tender bullae, erosions with foul smelling discharge due to superadded bacterial and anaerobic infection especially in the toe web spaces (athlete's foot).

TINEA UNGUIUM

Commonly accompanies tinea manuum and pedis with asymmetric nail involvement (Fig. 7.27). All the nails are rarely affected. Involved nails become thick, fragile, yellowish or grayish brown in colour and develop subungual hyperkeratosis (Fig. 7.29). They may separate from the nail bed (onycholysis) or may be distorted (dystrophy).

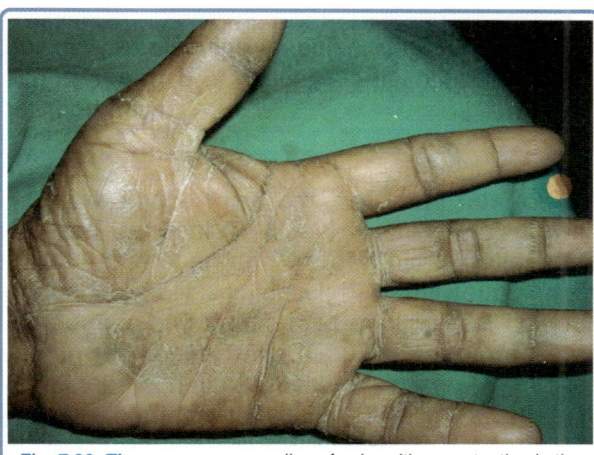

Fig. 7.30: Tinea manuum—scaling of palm with accentuation in the flexion creases

| TABLE 7.3: Types of tinea unguium ||
Type	Comments
Distal lateral subungual onychomycosis	Yellowish discolouration of distal and lateral nail plate with subungual hyperkeratosis, splinter hemorrhages
Proximal subungual onchymycosis	Whitish to brownish discolouration of proximal nail plate, seen in the HIV infected and peripheral vascular disease
White superficial onychomycosis	Powdery white patches away from the distal end of the nail, surface rough and friable
Endonyx	Milky white patches without subungual hyperkeratosis or onycholysis
Total nail dystrophy	Total nail destruction

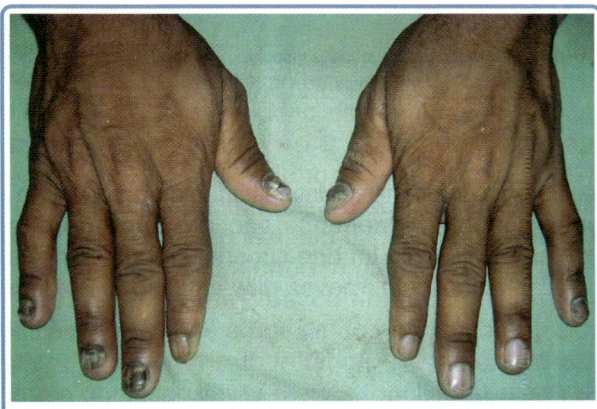

Fig. 7.31: Onychomycosis—dark and yellowish discolouration of the nail plates with thickening and sparing of some nails

Tinea Incognito (Not Recognisable)

Inadvertent treatment of dermatophytosis with topical steroids leads to loss of its typical clinical features like pruritus, ring like lesions, etc. (Fig. 7.32). Such an atypical clinical appearance of dermatophytosis is termed as tinea incognito. Such lesions are usually widespread, less itchy, less scaly, less erythematous and may lack active inflammatory border.

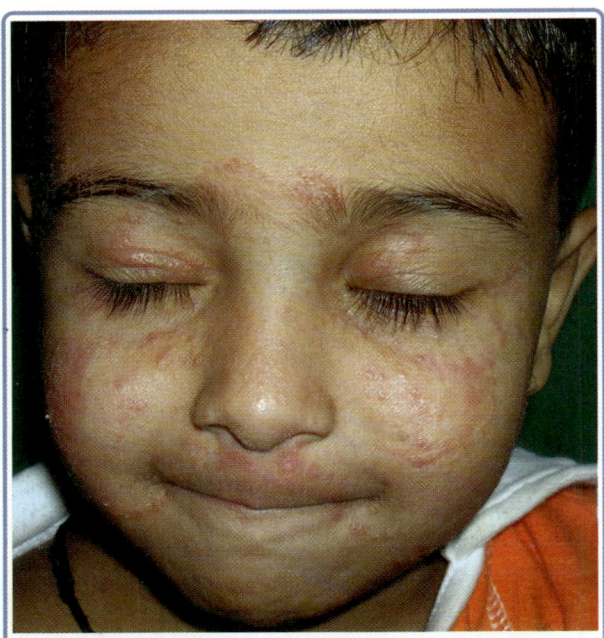

Fig. 7.32: Tinea incognito—multiple erythematous, ill-defined annular plaques

INVESTIGATIONS IN DERMATOPHYTE INFECTIONS

Tinea capitis caused by some dermatophytes fluoresces bluish green under Wood's lamp. Dermatophytes are seen (as hyphae and spores) when scales in tinea corporis, cruris, manuum, pedis, incognito and at times in tinea barbae and tinea capitis, are mounted in KOH (10–20% for 30 minutes). Nail and hair clippings require to be heated, after mounting in KOH, in order to dissolve the keratin and visualise hyphae and spores. Culture on Sabouraud's agar for identifying the organism or on dermatophyte test medium (DTM) for rapid result may be done. Biopsy is rarely needed for diagnosis.

THERAPY OF DERMATOPHYTE INFECTIONS

General Principles

In addition to the administration of antifungal agents, it is mandatory to look for and correct internal (diabetes mellitus, immunodeficiency) or external (hot, humid environment and occlusive clothing/footwear) contributory factors. Prevention of recurrences is more dependent on such corrective steps rather than a course of antifungal therapy.

Topical Antifungals

Older antifungal agents like Whitfield's ointment (salicylic acid 6% and benzoic acid 12%) are useful especially over palms or soles for their added keratolytic activity. Imidazole group of antifungals (clotrimazole 1%, miconazole 2%, ketoconazole 2%) are used widely in lotion, cream and powder forms. Topical oxiconazole, butenafine, terbinafine or bifonazole are also extremely effective. Lotions and powders are desirable for use in intertriginous areas like groins and toe webs as they cause drying. Lotions or Gels spread easily over groins and hairy areas like scalp and beard. Topical antifungals usually need to be applied twice daily for up to 1 week after subsidence of active skin lesions (i.e. erythema, papules or scaling).

Topical Antifungals

Whitfield's ointment (6% salicylic acid + 12% benzoic acid)

Imidazoles (clotrimazole 1%, miconazole 2%, ketoconazole 2%, eberconazole 1%, luliconazole 1%)

Terbinafine cream 1%

Amorolfine cream 0.25%

Ciclopirox olamine cream 0.77%

Systemic Antifungals

Indications for systemic therapy (Table 7.4) include:

- **Tinea unguium, tinea pedis, tinea manuum, tinea capitis since topical antifungals do not penetrate to** the desired depth in these conditions.
- **Widespread tinea** corporis or tinea corporis/cruris/faciei/barbae unresponsive to or **recurring** after adequate topical therapy.
- Underlying **contributory factor** that is difficult to correct, e.g. uncontrolled diabetes mellitus, immunodeficiency and obesity.

Griseofulvin (micronised form) 250 mg twice a day (10 mg/kg/day in children) for 3–4 weeks for tinea cruris/corporis/faciei, 6 weeks for tinea manuum and capitis, 8 weeks for tinea pedis, 6 months to 1 year for fingernails and 1–2 years for toe nails is the traditional choice of therapy. It is best taken after meals to facilitate absorption. Side effects, except for headache, are rarely encountered with griseofulvin. Treatment failures are common with nail infections.

Terbinafine 250 mg twice daily for 3–4 weeks for tinea corporis/cruris, for 4–6 weeks for tinea manuum/pedis and capitis provides an effective and safe option. For itraconazole doses refer Table 7.4. However, for nail infections itraconazole is preferred as it is effective against non-dermatophyte moulds.

TABLE 7.4 : Systemic antifungal agents

Drug	PV	Dermatophytosis	Candidiasis	Side Effects	Precautions	Comment
Griseofulvin	NA	**10 mg/kg x 4 weeks for corporis, x 6 weeks for manuum/capitis, x 8 weeks for pedis, 6 month to 1 year for finger nail, for toe nail-high failure rate.	NA	Uncommon headache, skin rashes	To be taken with food to improve absorption	Safe, inexpensive effective in dermatophytosis except nail infections
Ketoconazole	*200 mg OD 10 days	200 mg OD x 3–6 weeks for corp. x 6–8 weeks for cap/man/pedis x 6 months for finger nail and x 1 year for toe nail.	200–400 mg OD for 2 weeks	Hepatotoxicity	To monitor hepatic transaminases	Hepatitis seen in 1:1000
Fluconazole	*400 mg single dose	150 mg once daily for 4 weeks in combination with topicals is successful in corporis, manuum/pedis in a good proportion of cases	**150 mg once a week for 3 weeks or 50–100 mg OD for 3–7 days or 2 weeks in immuno-suppressed	Gastritis rarely, hepatitis	Take with food to avoid gastritis	Expensive but effective and safe in candidiasis
Itraconazole	*200 mg BD 5 days	*200 mg BD for 1 week per month x 2 months for finger nails and x 3 months for toe nails 200 mg BD x 1 week for tinea manuum/pedis/capitis 100 mg BD for 3–4 weeks for tinea corporis/cruris	200 mg OD for 3 days. Not for oropharyn-geal candidiasis	Rare, reversible hepatitis	—	Expensive but effective and safe Reduces treatment duration
Terbinafine	NA	*250 mg/day x 4 weeks for finger nail and x 8 weeks for toe nails; 250 mg/day x 3 weeks for tinea corporis 250 mg BD x 1 week per month for 2 months for finger nail infection and for 3 months for toe nail infection	NA	Rare, hepatitis	—	Expensive but effective in dermatophytosis. Reduces treatment duration

N.B. : NA = Not available due to lower activity.   **PV** = Pityriasis versicolor

** drug of choice

* effective

Pulse therapy is popularly practised for nail infections as itraconazole 200 mg bid or terbinafine 250 mg bid for 1 week every month for 2–3 months in tinea unguium. Itraconazole has a broader spectrum of action and is useful against deep as well as superficial fungal infections. Continuous therapy with terbinafine 250 mg/day or itraconazole 100 mg bid for 1–2 months is effective for fingernail and toe nail infections respectively. *See* Table 7.4 for details.

In recent years efficacy of oral antifungals has been dented though resistance to antifungals has not been demonstrated in laboratory. More attention should be paid to compliance and preventive measures and treatment of family members.

Summary: Dermatophytes are fungi that live on keratin. According to the site of affection, dermatophytosis is classified into tinea capitis (scalp hair), tinea faciei (face), tinea cruris (groins), tinea corporis (trunk), tinea manuum (hand), tinea pedis (foot) and tinea unguium (nail). Typical lesion is a ring shaped arrangement of erythematous papules, vesicles and pustules with central clearing. Hyphae and spores are seen when scraping is mounted in KOH. Localised lesions respond to topical antifungals (clotrimazole) whereas widespread and unresponsive cases need griseofulvin 10 mg/kg/day for 4–6 weeks (corporis, cruris, manuum and capitis), 8 weeks (pedis) and 6 months to 2 years (unguium). Itraconazole, fluconazole, and terbinafine are newer drugs.

DEEP FUNGAL INFECTIONS

Most of the common fungi affecting the skin restrict themselves to the stratum corneum of the epidermis. Any fungal infection that penetrates the skin beyond the epidermis is termed as a deep fungal infection. Based on the pathogenicity of causative fungi, such infections can be categorised into:

- **Subcutaneous fungal infections:** These are caused by fungi that can gain entry into the body only through a penetrating injury, e.g. by thorn prick or by infection of a pre-existing wound. These fungi cause localised subcutaneous fungal infections, e.g. eumycotic mycetoma, sporotrichosis or chromomycosis. They do not disseminate to other organs (do not threaten life) but cause chronic smouldering infections that may last for years or decades.

- **Systemic infections caused by pathogenic fungi:** These fungi are present in soil and cause a self healing primary pulmonary infection (as in tuberculosis) in immuno-competent hosts. Skin lesions occur after many years due to reinoculation or an immune

deficiency occurring in later life. Histoplasmosis and blastomycosis are examples of this group.

- **Systemic infections caused by opportunist fungi:** These fungi are present as normal human flora and only cause disease in immunocompromised hosts. Cryptococcosis and mucormycosis are examples of this group.

Subcutaneous Fungal Infections

As mentioned above eumycotic mycetoma, sporotrichosis and chromomycosis are the fungal infections in this category that are seen in India. Eumycotic mycetoma is discussed in more detail later in this chapter.

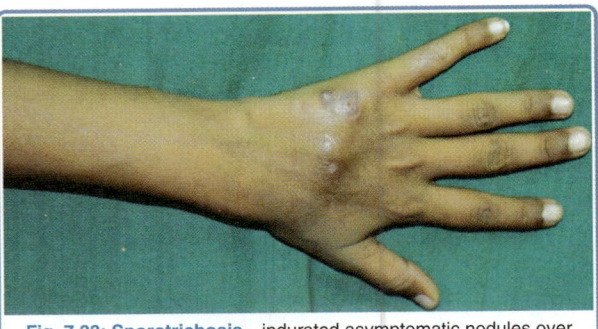

Fig. 7.33: Sporotrichosis—indurated asymptomatic nodules over hand, a common site of inoculation

Sporotrichosis usually presents as erythematous nodules arranged in linear pattern over an extremity. After a penetrating injury by a thorn a noduloulcerative lesion forms at the site. Infection spreads proximally along lymphatics and results in linear arrangement of nodules. Intervening lymphatics are thickened (pipestem lymphatics). Diagnosis can be confirmed by biopsy or culture of the fungus, *Sporothrix schenkii*. This infection responds well to oral potassium iodide or itraconazole.

Chromomycosis (chromoblastomycosis) is seen as sessile or pedunculated or cauliflower-like nodules or plaques with rough, verrucous surface over an extremity. The lesions may extend proximally and secondary infection and lympho-edema are common. The brown coloured fungus can be demonstrated in biopsy or culture. The condition responds to oral itraconazole (Fig. 7.34).

Rhinosporidiosis is a parasitic infection affecting nasal mucosa in those with a history of bathing in stagnant freshwater. Organisms can be demons-trated by biopsy in nasal papillomas.

Opportunistic Fungal Infections

Histoplasmosis is seen in previously ill HIV infected or debilitated patients as erythematous or ulcerated

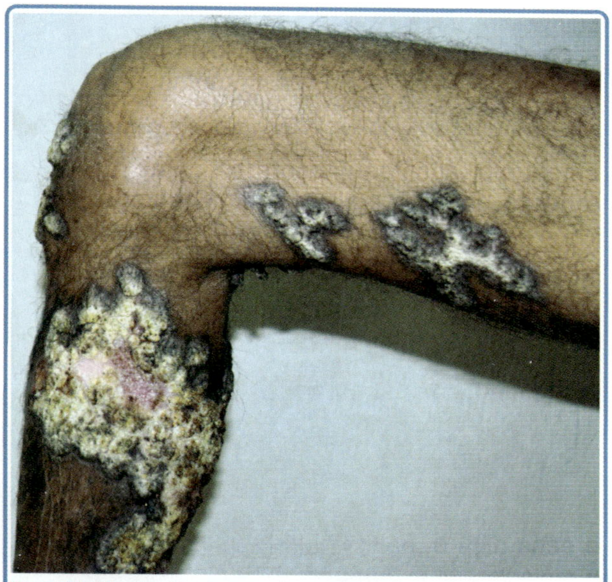

Fig. 7.34: Chromoblastomycosis—verrucous indurated and hyperpigmented plaques with central scarring resembling verrucous tuberculosis

nodules or plaques anywhere on the body. The lesions show a predilection for mucocutaneous junctions and mucosae where they show a tendency to ulceration. The fungus, *Histoplasma capsulatum* is easy to demonstrate on smear, culture or biopsy. The drug of choice remains amphotericin B though some patients may respond to itraconazole.

Cryptococcosis

This opportunistic infection is caused by *Cryptococcus neoformans* that is present in pigeon excreta. History of contact with pigeons is usually associated with fungaemia and affection of other systems like meningitis or pneumonia. It occurs in immunocompromised conditions like HIV infection, lymphomas, leukaemias or in patients on cytotoxic or systemic steroid therapy.

They may develop either cryptococcal meningitis without any skin lesions or they may develop chronic cryptococcaemia leading to scattered, smooth surfaced, skin coloured or slightly erythematous papules with or without slight central necrosis. Larger papules or nodules tend to resemble molluscum contagiosum due to the central depression (umbilication). The lesions affect the face, neck and extremities, but may be widespread. Large ulcerated lesions discharge gelatinous or mucinous material.

Organisms are easy to demonstrate on smear, culture or biopsy. Skin smear shows capsulated yeast forms especially with the India ink preparation. Biopsy shows a granuloma surrounding the organisms in the dermis. Treatment of cutaneous cryptococcosis is similar to systemic cryptococcosis. Courses of intravenous fluconazole or amphotericin B need to be followed up with long term oral high doses of fluconazole (400 mg once daily) to prevent relapse till the immunocompromised condition is corrected.

MYCETOMA (MADURA FOOT)

This is a recalcitrant subcutaneous infection with either filamentous bacteria (actinomycotic mycetoma) or fungi (eumycotic mycetoma) with a tendency to form large colonies in tissues. These

TABLE 7.5 : Treatment of mycetoma foot	
Eumycotic mycetoma	
Medical	Surgical (assist in wound healing)
Itraconazole, amphotericin B Voriconazole, posaconaole given long term for more than 2 years	Exploration and drainage of sinus tracts, debridement of diseased tissue, removal of bone cysts
Actinomycotic mycetoma	
Medical	
Streptomycin with cotrimoxazole	
Rifampicin, amikacin, amoxycillin-clavulanic acid, dapsone and potassium iodide	
Welsch regimen : Inj. amikacin 15 mg/kg/day divided into 2 doses for 21 days. Constitutes 1 cycle. 1–3 such cycle at the interval of 15 days along with tab. Trimethoprim-sulphamethoxazole (7 and 35 mg/kg/day resp.) for a period of 6 months.	
Modified Welsch regimen : Addition of rifampicin to the Welsch regimen	

Chapter

7

Cutaneous Fungal Infections

colonies are discharged as granular matter through sinuses and are called 'grains', which form a pathognomonic feature of mycetoma.

The thin filamentous gram positive bacteria that commonly cause actinomycotic mycetoma in Western and Southern India belong to the genera of Nocardia, Actinomadura and Streptomyces. In North India, eumycotic mycetoma, producing black coloured grains, caused by Madurella spp. is commoner. These causative organisms, which abound in the environment, are not pathogenic unless introduced into the body by a penetrating injury (Table 7.5).

Morphology

Initial lesions are clustered erythematous indurated nodules that have a tendency to soften in the centre and burst, discharging purulent fluid. Asymptomatic and indolent nature of the disease invariably leads to neglect in the initial stages. As the disease progresses over months, lesions evolve into deep seated, ill defined, indurated swellings punctuated with multiple points of softening and that eventually burst to form numerous discharging sinuses (Figs 7.35 and 7.36). Firm pressure may express pus as well as grains. Old sinuses may heal with scars although new nodules keep appearing.

Distribution

Foot being prone to trauma, is most frequently affected. Hand, buttock, arm and shoulder are uncommon sites.

Diagnosis

Indurated nodules, discharging sinuses and grains are enough to make a clinical diagnosis of mycetoma. Aetiologic diagnosis requires examination of grains under the microscope and culture of the organisms.

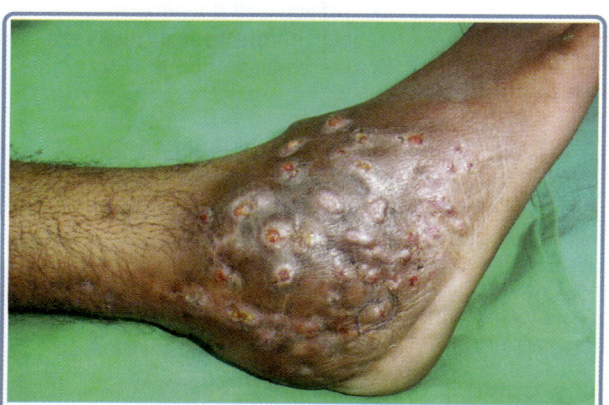

Fig. 7.35: Mycetoma—multiple discharging sinuses and nodules overlying diffuse swelling of foot

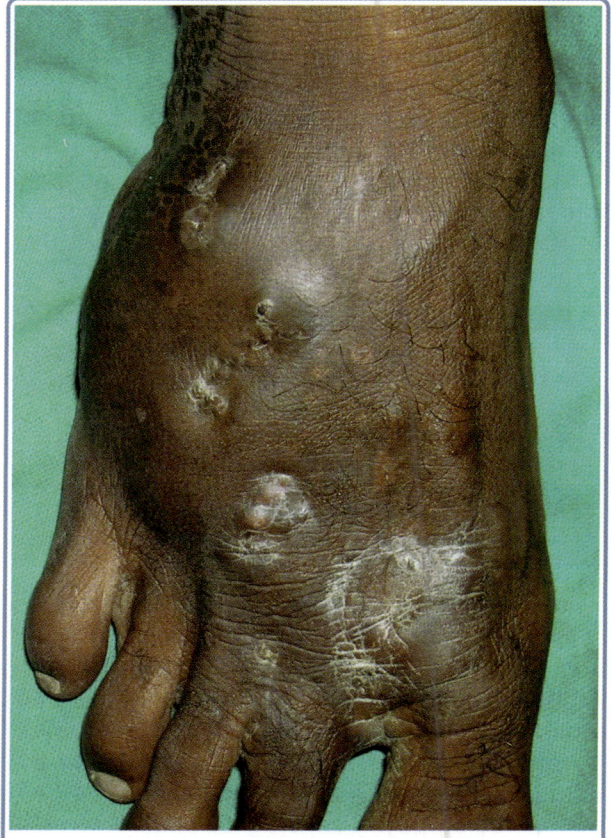

Fig. 7.36: Mycetoma—swelling and multiple sinuses

Biopsy is frequently helpful. Osteolytic areas in underlying bones are a sign of bony affection.

Therapy

Routine short course of antibiotics is inadequate as tissue levels of drugs are lower than in ordinary infections. Besides, highly effective drugs against these organisms, even *in vitro*, are unavailable. Hence, medical therapy is prolonged and relapses are common.

Actinomycotic mycetomas due to actinomadura respond to high doses of penicillin whereas those due to nocardia and streptomyces respond to prolonged therapy with streptomycin in combination with cotrimoxazole. Rifampicin, amikacin, amoxycillin + clavulinic acid, sulphadiazine, dapsone and potassium iodide are other useful agents. Eumycotic mycetomas respond to itraconazole 200 mg twice a day for 6–9 months. Monitoring of hepatic enzymes for hepatotoxicity is essential. Amphotericin B may be used (1–2 mg/kg/day) only in progressive and unresponsive cases (Fig. 7.37).

Other modalities of treatment used in mycetomas include thermal pads, regional perfusion of antibacterials and antifungals, surgical excision, debulking and, as an extreme measure, amputation.

Chapter 7

Cutaneous Fungal Infections

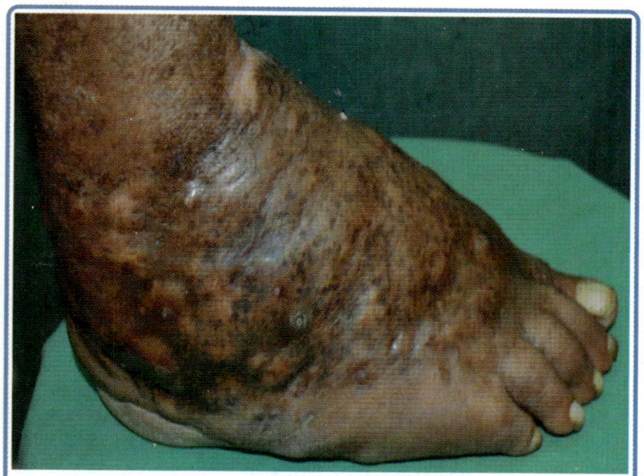

Fig. 7.37: **Mycetoma**—advanced condition. The bones are affected in later stages

Crystalline penicillin 10–20 MU daily as a drip for 1–2 months.

Streptomycin 1 g intramuscular (IM) OD for 2–3 months.

Cotrimoxazole 2–4 tablets twice a day for 6–9 months.

Summary: Mycetoma is an uncommon subcutaneous infection caused by either actinomycetes or true fungi that are introduced into the body by penetrating trauma. Multiple grouped nodules on foot that discharge pus and colonies of organisms (granules) are diagnostic. Causative organism can be identified and cultured in the laboratory. Systemic antibiotic or antifungal therapy extended over many months may be successful. Surgical solutions may be considered, if response to medical treatment is inadequate.

Chapter

7

Cutaneous Fungal Infections

MCQs

1. **The organism causing tinea versicolor is:**
   a. *Pityrosporum orbiculare*
   b. *Trichophyton violaceum*
   c. *Pityrosporum ovale*
   d. *Malassezia furfur*

2. **The commonest organism causing candidiasis is:**
   a. *Candida tropicalis*
   b. *Candida subtropicalis*
   c. *Candida albicans*
   d. *Candida krusei*

3. **The commonest organism causing favus is:**
   a. *Trichophyton violaceum*
   b. *Microsporum canis*
   c. *Trichophyton mentagrophytes*
   d. *Trichophyton schoenleinii*

4. **Tinea capitis due to which of the following does not fluoresce under the Wood's lamp?**
   a. *M. audouinii*   b. *M. canis*
   c. *M. ferrugenium*   d. *T. rubrum*

5. **The commonest cause of tinea capitis in India is:**
   a. *M. canis*   b. *T. tonsurans*
   c. *M. gypseum*   d. *T. violaceum*

6. **Infection of which of the following sites is not included under the appellation of tinea corporis?**
   a. Chest   b. Forearm
   c. Thigh   d. Palm

7. **Following factors affect the gastrointestinal absorption of oral griseofulvin *except*:**
   a. Time of the day
   b. Particle size
   c. Food
   d. Gastrointestinal diseases

8. **Dermatophytes do not spread by contact with infected:**
   a. Air   b. Soil
   c. Animals   d. Humans

9. **The active border of dermatophytosis has all of the following *except*:**
   a. Pustules   b. Papules
   c. Vesicles   d. Telangiectasia

10. **Fluconazole has been used for dermatophytosis in pulse format every:**
    a. Year   b. Week
    c. Fortnigh   d. Month

11. **For tinea unguium pulse therapy with itraconazole is advocated:**
    a. Once every day
    b. One day every week
    c. One week every fortnight
    d. One week every month

12. **The commonest side effect of griseofulvin is:**
    a. Peripheral neuropathy
    b. Headache
    c. Nephropathy
    d. Drug rash

13. **Which one of the following is a predisposing factor for tinea pedis?**
    a. Wearing chappals
    b. Wearing shoes
    c. Walking barefoot
    d. Fissuring of soles

14. **Which one of the following is not a predisposing factor for tinea pedis?**
    a. Wearing closed footwear
    b. Work involving standing in water
    c. Excessive sweating
    d. None of the above

15. **Which one of the following is not a predisposing factor for tinea cruris?**
    a. Tight underclothes
    b. Thick underclothes
    c. Synthetic underclothes
    d. Dark coloured underclothes

16. **Which of the following is not a morphologic feature of mycetoma?**
    a. Grains   b. Tumefaction
    c. Sinuses   d. Vesicles

17. **A dishwasher presented with pain, erythema and white sodden appearance of finger webs. The diagnosis is:**
    a. Tinea manuum
    b. Candidial paronychia
    c. Pitted keratolysis
    d. Candidial intertrigo

18. **The colour of fluorescence in pityriasis versicolor with Wood's lamp is:**
   a. Whitish
   b. Blue green
   c. Golden yellow
   d. Coral red

19. **The positive sign in pityriasis versicolor is:**
   a. Collarette scale
   b. Christmas tree pattern
   c. Apple jelly nodules
   d. Scratch sign

20. **The colour, pityriasis versicolor does not show in its skin lesions, is:**
   a. Hypopigmented
   b. Brown
   c. Black
   d. Bluish

21. **Microscopic examination of scales in fungal infections of skin is done with:**
   a. 5% NaOH (sodium hydroxide)
   b. 10% KOH (potassium hydroxide)
   c. 5% KOH (potassium hydroxide)
   d. 1% KOH (potassium hydroxide)

22. **Which of the following is not useful for treating pityriasis versicolor?**
   a. Sodium hyposulphite
   b. Itraconazole
   c. Nystatin
   d. Clotrimazole

23. **Which of the following is used orally in treating pityriasis versicolor ?**
   a. Clotrimazole
   b. Miconazole
   c. Econazole
   d. Fluconazole

24. **Intertrigo does not affect:**
   a. Toe webs
   b. Inframammary folds
   c. Axillae
   d. Palms and soles

25. **The systemic treatment of choice for candidiasis is:**
   a. Ketoconazole
   b. Griseofulvin
   c. Nystatin
   d. Fluconazole

26. **The most common site of affection of mycetoma is:**
   a. Foot
   b. Hand
   c. Buttocks
   d. Knees

27. **All of the following may show ring like lesions *except*:**
   a. Tinea cruris
   b. Psoriasis
   c. Secondary syphilis
   d. Pityriasis versicolor

28. **The method which is commonly used to establish diagnosis in dermatophytosis, is:**
   a. Clinical examination
   b. KOH mount
   c. Biopsy
   d. Wood's lamp examination

29. **Candidiasis affects all of the following *except*:**
   a. Oral mucosa
   b. Glans penis
   c. Scalp
   d. Finger webs

30. **Dermatophytes are fungi that are:**
   a. Aquaphilic
   b. Lipophilic
   c. Keratinophilic
   d. Aerophilic

31. **Following are the transmission groups of dermatophytes *except*:**
   a. Zoophilic
   b. Anthropophilic
   c. Aerophilic
   d. Geophilic

32. **Dermatophyte infection is most difficult to eradicate from:**
   a. Groins
   b. Foot
   c. Hair
   d. Nails

33. **Which of the following is not a genus of dermatophytes?**
   a. Trichophyton
   b. Epidermophyton
   c. Trichosporon
   d. Microsporum

34. **The most common presentation of dermatophytosis is:**
   a. Tinea capitis
   b. Tinea corporis
   c. Tinea cruris
   d. Tinea pedis

35. **The most common morphology of tinea corporis is:**
   a. Rounded plaque
   b. Erythematous plaque
   c. Annular scaly plaque
   d. Scaly patch without erythema

36. **Following are the signs of fungal infection of nails *except*:**
   a. Onycholysis
   b. Thickening of nail plate
   c. Nail pits
   d. Subungual hyperkeratosis

37. **Which of the following is not a differential diagnosis of tinea pedis?**
   a. Pompholyx
   b. Candidiasis
   c. Footwear dermatitis
   d. Tinea versicolor

Chapter 7

Cutaneous Fungal Infections

38. **The two types of organisms causing mycetoma are eumycetes and:**
    a. Dermatophytes
    b. Madurella mycetomi
    c. Mucor
    d. Actinomycetes

39. **Mycetoma is transmitted by:**
    a. Skin-to-skin contact
    b. Insect bite
    c. Droplet infection
    d. Penetrating injury

40. **Madura foot refers to:**
    a. Complicated tinea pedis
    b. Contact dermatitis to Madura textile
    c. Pompholyx of foot
    d. Mycetoma of foot

41. **The type of scales in pityriasis versicolor is:**
    a. Powdery
    b. Collarette
    c. Mica like
    d. Yellowish greasy

42. **The most common association of candidial balanoposthitis is:**
    a. HIV infection
    b. Diabetes mellitus
    c. Chancroid
    d. Syphilis

43. **Candidial vaginitis is associated with all of the following *except*:**
    a. Pregnancy
    b. Diabetes
    c. HIV infection
    d. Menopause

44. **Treatment of choice for actinomycosis is:**
    a. Itraconazole
    b. Tetracycline
    c. Penicillin
    d. Posaconazole

45. **The words 'Sunray fungus' refer to:**
    a. Actinomycosis
    b. Actinic elastosis
    c. Actinic keratosis
    d. Actinomadura

46. **Which of the following drugs is not effective for nocardial infections?**
    a. Rifampicin
    b. Gentamycin
    c. Penicillin
    d. Cotrimoxazole

47. **The best oral treatment of pityriasis versicolor is with:**
    a. Ketoconazole
    b. Griseofulvin
    c. Terbinafine
    d. Fluconazole

48. **The first line oral treatment of dermatophyte infections is:**
    a. Ketoconazole
    b. Itraconazole
    c. Terbinafine
    d. Fluconazole

49. **Which of the following conditions is associated with hyphae of *Malassezia furfur*?**
    a. Seborrheic dermatitis
    b. Pityriasis versicolor
    c. Pityriasis alba
    d. Pityriasis rosea

50. **Which of the following conditions is not associated with *Malassezia furfur*?**
    a. Seborrhoeic dermatitis
    b. Pityriasis versicolor
    c. Pityriasis alba
    d. Pityrosporum folliculitis

51. ***Rhinosporidium seeberi* causes:**
    a. Rhinoscleroma
    b. Lobomycosis
    c. Nasal polyp
    d. Rhinosporidiosis

52. ***Rhinosporidium seeberi* is a:**
    a. Fungus
    b. Yeast
    c. Parasite
    d. Bacterium

53. **Scutulum is the diagnostic finding of:**
    a. Grey patch
    b. Favus
    c. Kerion
    d. Black dot

54. **The diagnostic finding of favus is:**
    a. Exclamation mark hair
    b. Scybala
    c. Scutulum
    d. Easy pluckability of hair

55. **All the following are used in treatment of pityriasis versicolor, *except*:**
    a. Ketoconazole
    b. Griseofulvin
    c. Selenium sulphide
    d. Clotrimazole

56. **Wood's lamp is used in the diagnosis of:**
    a. Tinea capitis
    b. Candida albicans
    c. Histoplasma
    d. Cryptococcus

57. **'Dhobi's itch' is known as:**
    a. Tinea corporis
    b. Tinea cruris
    c. Tinea barbae
    d. Tinea capitis

58. **A boggy swelling over scalp with easily pluckable hair in a child, the investigation done is:**
    a. Giemsa staining
    b. Bacterial culture
    c. KOH preparation
    d. Gram staining

59. **All is true about Madura foot *except*:**
    a. Swollen infiltrated foot
    b. Sinus formation
    c. Invasion of bone and destruction
    d. Fever, malaise

60. **The causative organism of trichomycosis axillaris is a:**
    - a. Bacterium
    - b. Fungus
    - c. Virus
    - d. Parasite

61. **Which of the following infections is also known as ringworm?**
    - a. Nummular eczema
    - b. Herpes simplex
    - c. Annular impetigo
    - d. Tinea corporis

62. **Clotrimazole and nystatin are both:**
    - a. Topical antifungals
    - b. Anti itch creams
    - c. Topical antibiotics
    - d. Used to treat eczema

63. **Which of the following organisms does not cause tinea capitis?**
    - a. Epidermophyton
    - b. Microsporum
    - c. Trichophyton rubrum
    - d. Trichophyton violaceum

64. **Which of the following drugs is effective in the treatment of pityriasis versicolor:**
    - a. Ketoconazole
    - b. Metronidazole
    - c. Griseofulvin
    - d. Oral steroids

65. **All of the following antimicrobials are used topically *except*:**
    - a. Clotrimazole
    - b. Griseofulvin
    - c. Nystatin
    - d. Miconazole

Chapter 7

Cutaneous Fungal Infections

ANSWERS

1-d,	2-c,	3-d,	4-d,	5-b,	6-d,	7-a,	8-a,	9-d,	10-b,
11-d,	12-b,	13-b,	14-d,	15-d,	16-d,	17-d,	18-c,	19-d,	20-d,
21-b,	22-c,	23-d,	24-d,	25-d,	26-a,	27-d,	28-b,	29-c,	30-c,
31-c,	32-d,	33-c,	34-c,	35-c,	36-c,	37-d,	38-d,	39-d,	40-d,
41-a,	42-b,	43-d,	44-c,	45-a,	46-c,	47-d,	48-c,	49-c,	50-c,
51-d,	52-c,	53-b,	54-c,	55-b,	56-a,	57-b,	58-c,	59-d,	60-a,
61-d,	62-a,	63-a,	64-a,	65-b					

Viral Infections

MOLLUSCUM CONTAGIOSUM

This is a common cutaneous viral infection seen principally in children and occasionally as a sexually transmitted disease in adults; it is caused by the molluscum virus (a DNA virus of the pox group).

Patient Profile

Usually young children acquire this infection by skin-to-skin contact while playing. Adults may acquire it through sexual or non-sexual contact. Occurrence of widespread extragenital lesions of molluscum contagiosum in an adult is a marker of immunodeficiency, e.g. human immunodeficiency virus (HIV) disease, leukemia.

Morphology

Smooth, shiny, pearly white or yellowish dome shaped papule with a central umbilication represents a classic lesion (Figs 8.1 and 8.2). Early lesions lack central umbilication. Yellow cheesy material can be expressed from the centre of a fully developed lesion.

Distribution

In children, face, extremities (exposed sites) and trunk are involved in that order of frequency, Sexually acquired infections involve the male/female genital and perigenital regions (Fig. 8.3). When widespread, HIV infection, as an underlying factor, has to be ruled out. Due to spread by autoinoculation, lesions tend to be aggregated in one region.

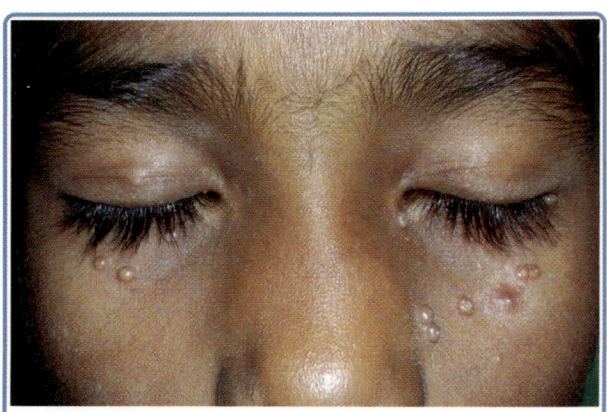

Fig. 8.1: Molluscum contagiosum—umbilicated papules in a child on face

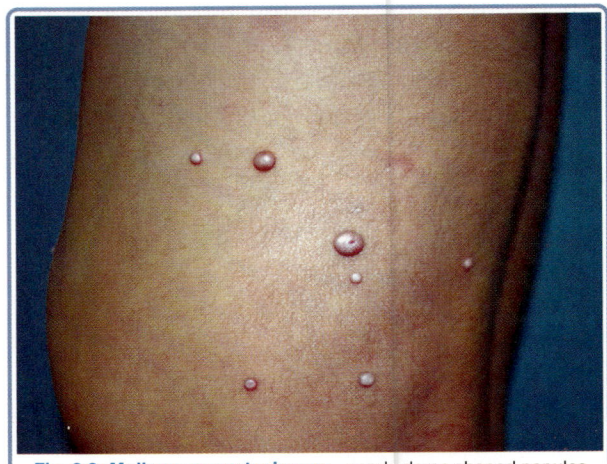

Fig. 8.2: Molluscum contagiosum—pearly dome shaped papules and nodules of Molluscum contagiosum

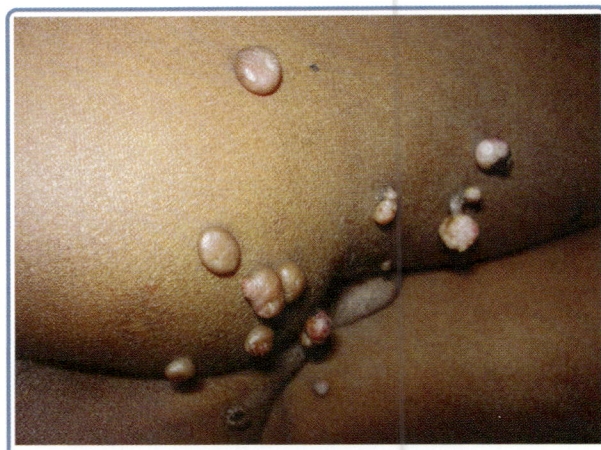

Fig. 8.3: Perianal molluscum contagiosum—lesions exclusively limited to genitals or perianal area should raise possibility of sexual abuse

Diagnosis

Morphology is characteristic. Diagnosis can be established by preparing a smear of the cheesy material expressed from a lesion. When stained with Giemsa stain. Intracytoplasmic molluscum bodies (Henderson Paterson bodies) are seen within epithelial cells.

Treatment

As there is no antiviral medicine against the molluscum virus, the principle of therapy is to destroy all virus infected cells. This may be done, under topical anaesthesia with EMLA by extracting lesions with a sharp instrument (small curette or tiny forceps or hypodermic needle). Cryotherapy or ablation laser is another alternative. For numerous lesions, inducing inflammation with application of phenol or trichloroacetic acid under medical supervision once a week is more practicable. This is thought to stimulate immunity leading to resolution of lesions. Milder irritants like 5% potassium hydroxide may be used on alternate days with similar effects, but have the benefit of application at home. Topical 5% imiquimod cream applied on alternate days is a fairly effective immunostimulant but the effect occurs slowly over 6–12 weeks. Recurrence is common with all forms of therapy. Oral levamisole once or twice a week or microneedling or diphenylcyclopropanone (DPCP) therapy has also been used to stimulate immunity.

Treatment Modalities in Molluscum Contagiosum

- Extraction under topical anaesthesia with sharp instruments (small curette, tiny forceps and hypodermic needle)
- Cryotherapy
- Diathermy or Laser ablation
- Application of phenol or trichloroacetic acid
- Topical imiquimod cream 5%
- Topical KOH 5% or 10%
- Oral levamisole
- Topical immunomodulators like DPCP

Summary: Molluscum contagiosum, caused by a poxvirus, is transmitted among children through close contact and in adults through sexual contact. Its smooth, dome shaped, pearly white and shiny papules with central umbilication are characteristic. Numerous extragenital mollusca in adults are a marker for HIV infection. Extraction, curettage and cryo or chemical cautery are options for therapy. Topical imiquimod is moderately effective.

VERRUCAE (WARTS)

Human papillomavirus (HPV) infections are collectively called verrucae or viral warts. According to the site affected these may be dry (verruca vulgaris, verruca plana and palmoplantar warts) or moist warts (condyloma acuminata) (Fig. 8.4).

VERRUCA VULGARIS (COMMON WART)

Commonest of the HPV induced cutaneous hyperplasias, it is transmitted either by direct contact or through fomites.

Patient Profile

Older children and young adults are affected most commonly. Immunodeficiency, as in HIV infection or lymphoma may present as widespread verrucae (generalised verrucosis) although most cases of widespread warts do not have general immuno-deficiency. Lesions are asymptomatic except when situated in the periungual region.

Morphology

Grayish white, skin coloured or occasionally hyperpigmented, rounded, extremely rough surfaced (keratotic) papules (or when large, nodules or plaques) situated on normal skin typify this infection (Figs 8.5 and 8.6). It is common for the infection to begin as a single lesion and then spread by autoinoculation leading to multiple lesions. Some warts tend to have a narrow base or stalk and a projecting, pedunculated profile. When only one such soft, pedunculated and thread like lesion is observed it is termed as filiform wart. When a bunch of these arise from a common base the structure resembles fingers of a hand and is called as a digitate wart. Linear plaques due to autoinoculation (pseudo-Koebner phenomenon) occur infrequently (Figs 8.7 and 8.8).

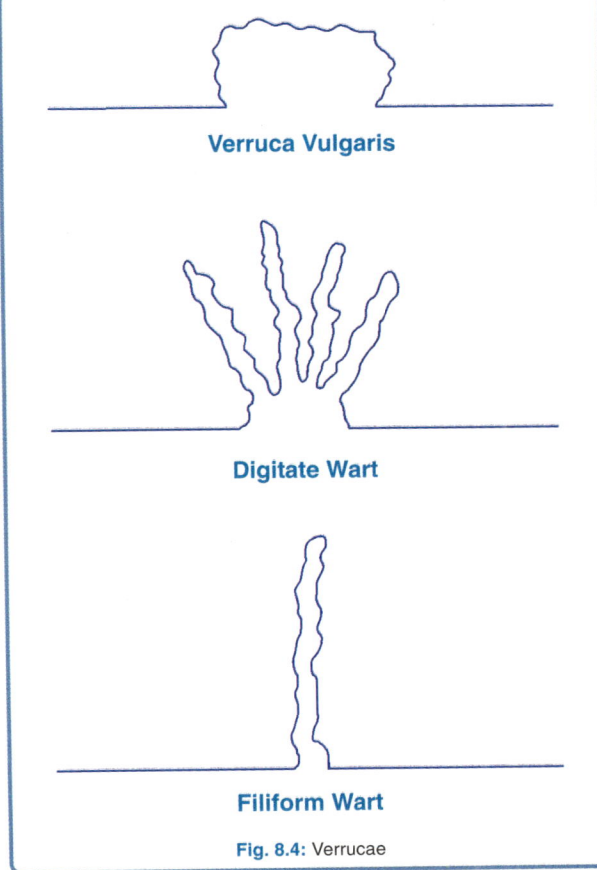

Verruca Vulgaris

Digitate Wart

Filiform Wart

Fig. 8.4: Verrucae

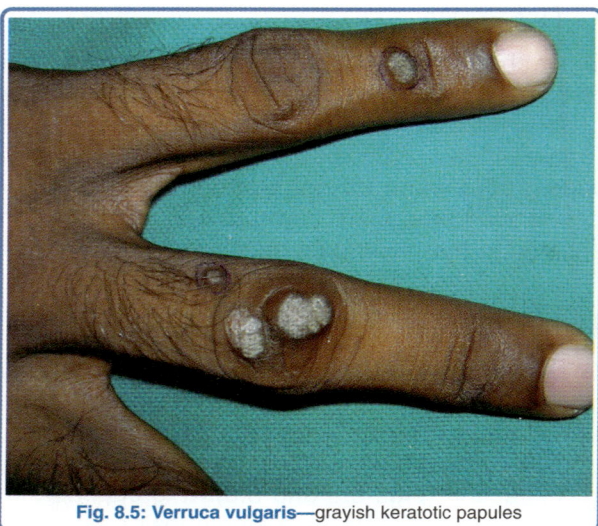

Fig. 8.5: **Verruca vulgaris**—grayish keratotic papules

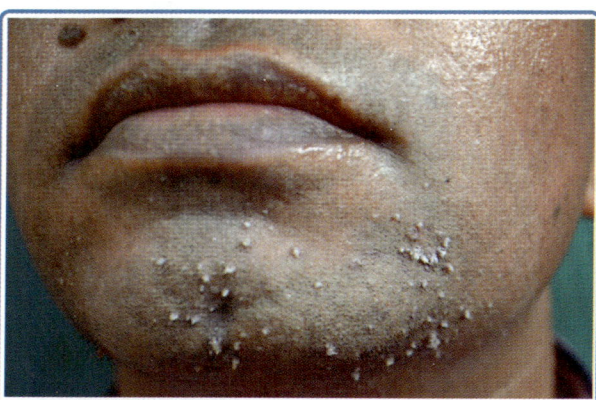

Fig. 8.6: **Verruca vulgaris**—filiform warts in beard region commonly spread while shaving

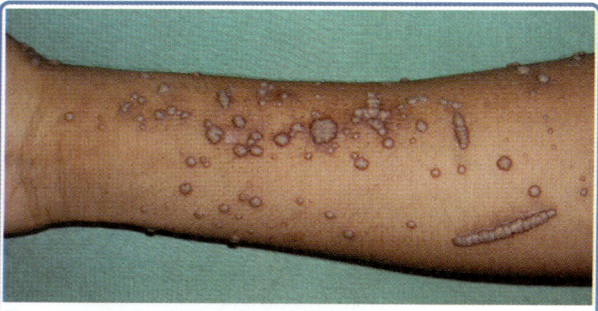

Fig. 8.7: **Verruca vulgaris**—unusually numerous with pseudo-Koebner phenomenon

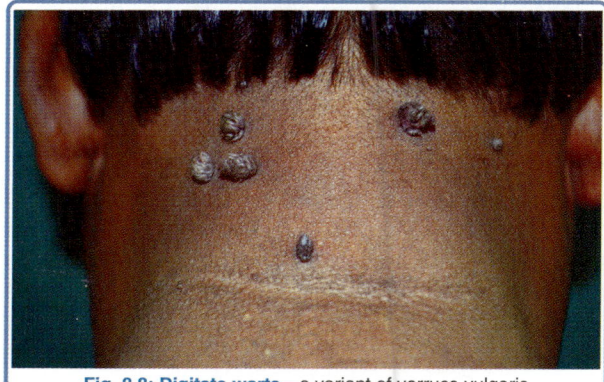

Fig. 8.8: **Digitate warts**—a variant of verruca vulgaris

become filiform or digitate. Filiform and digitate warts also occur over scalp, axillae, groins, perineum genitals and perianal region.

Diagnosis

It is based on clinical grounds. Biopsy is rarely necessary. Demonstration of viral particles and DNA typing is a sophisticated investigation possible only in a research setup.

Therapy

As effective antiviral agents are unavailable, all virus-infected cells need to be destroyed to ensure complete eradication of infection. This may be done by electrodessication or cryotherapy or an ablative laser (carbon dioxide laser). Alternatively, application of a strong keratolytic solution consisting of salicylic acid 16.7%, lactic acid 16.7% in a base of flexible collodion twice a day for 2–4 weeks may be used. Care has to be taken to avoid irritant dermatitis of surrounding skin by protecting it with petroleum jelly. Other therapies that have been used in cases with recurrences include topical cantharidine, topical 5-fluorouracil, diphenylcyclopropanone (DPCP). Non-specific stimulants like levamisole or BCG therapy or autoinoculation interferons and autologous HPV vaccines have all been used. Spontaneous resolution is not uncommon (Table 8.1).

Distribution

Commonest sites of verruca vulgaris include dorsa of fingers and hands, as well as toes and feet. Elbows, knees and extensors of extremities are also affected frequently. Periungual (round the nails) and subungual (under the nail plate) warts are painful and may hamper work. Involvement of face and neck is common in male adults probably because they contract the infection by sharing shaving blades. In these locations, warts tend to

Clinical Presentations of Human Papilloma Virus Infections
Verruca vulgaris/Common wart
Filiform wart
Digitate wart
Plain wart/Verruca plana
Palmoplantar wart
Mosaic wart
Condyloma acuminata

Summary: Common warts (verrucae vulgaris) are caused by HPV that gets transmitted by contact or fomites among the young. Asymptomatic, grayish, rough, dry and sessile papules based on normal looking skin characterise the disease. Hands, feet, face and neck are common sites. Electrocautery, cryotherapy and topical salicylic acid are usually effective.

OTHER VARIETIES OF WARTS

Verruca Plana (Plain Wart, Juvenile Wart)

This uncommon variety of warts is encountered in children and young adults. Grouped, skin coloured or brownish, flat topped, smooth surfaced (less keratotic as compared to verruca vulgaris) papules over face (Fig. 8.9), dorsa of hands and feet, forearms (Fig. 8.10) and shins characterise this condition. Pseudo-Koebner phenomenon is common (Fig. 8.9). Lesions are asymptomatic and tend to persist for years or spread slowly. Therapy with chemical cautery or light electrodessication is usually successful. Spontaneous resolution may occur after several years.

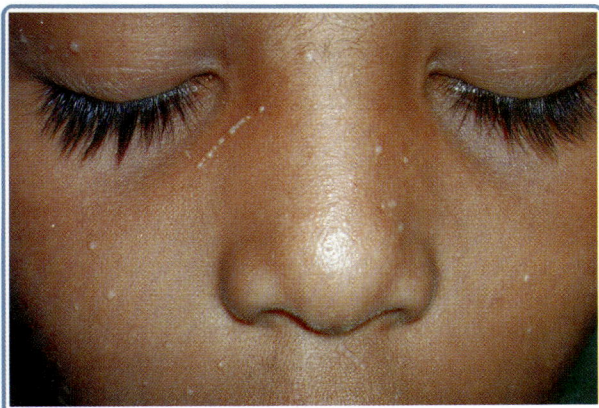

Fig. 8.9: Verruca plana—asymptomatic barely elevated grayish papules with pseudo-Koebner phenomenon

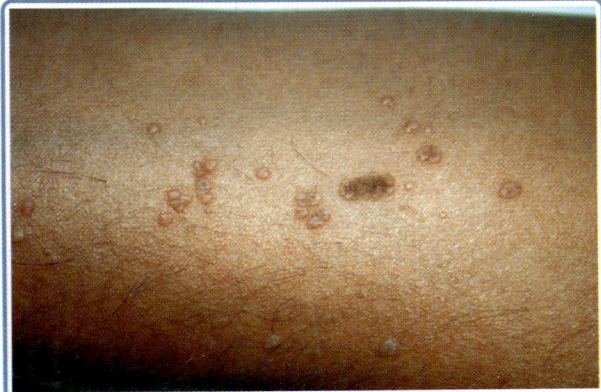

Fig. 8.10: Plain warts—flat topped papules, some of them coalescing to form plaques

Palmoplantar Warts

Clinical features

These warts, being present on pressure bearing palmoplantar thick skin that is also sensitive, grow within the skin rather than project out like common warts. Hence, the lesions are seen as painful, gray coloured, rounded, single or multiple indurated papules and plaques. The lesions are rough to the feel and are often surrounded by a collar of thicker skin. Paring the top part of a lesion with a sterile blade reveals black dots on its surface.

Diagnosis

As against callosities, which are an effect of persistent friction on palmoplantar skin, the normal dermatoglyphic lines are lost within the more lesion. Warts can be differentiated from corns by paring the surface which reveals black dots that represent thrombosed vessels. In corns, paring the top reveals a white soft keratin core, which is cone shaped. Corns are tender on vertical pressure whereas warts are tender when picked up between fingers and pressed side to side.

Therapy

Treatment of palmoplantar warts requires persistent efforts. Repeated paring following application of 20–40% salicylic acid under occlusion is a frequently used remedy. Topical application of 16.7% each of salicylic acid and lactic acid in a collodion base is effective for small lesions. Cryotherapy and ablative lasers are useful options in resistant cases.

> Electrocautery is relatively contraindicated in palmoplantar warts due to the fear of producing painful scars on pressure areas. Topical glutaraldehyde, DPCP, intralesional bleomycin and podophyllin under occlusion are some other less commonly used therapies.

CONDYLOMA ACUMINATA (GENITAL WARTS, VENEREAL WARTS)

These are transmitted sexually with an incubation period of a few weeks to 6 months.

Patient Profile

Being sexually transmitted, young adult males practising unsafe sex and, less commonly females, are the usual patients.

Chapter 8

Viral Infections

Morphology

Soft, pink or grayish blue, moist, exophytic, conical papules are the earliest lesions (Figs 8.11–8.14). Multiple lesions are a rule and their coalescence and enlargement may lead to pedunculated, soft, pink and cauliflower like masses. Large lesions on the undersurface of prepuce are prone to develop secondary bacterial infection. Trauma may lead to haemorrhage. Lesions that exceed 3 cm in diameter should preferably be biopsied, before treatment, to rule out squamous cell carcinoma.

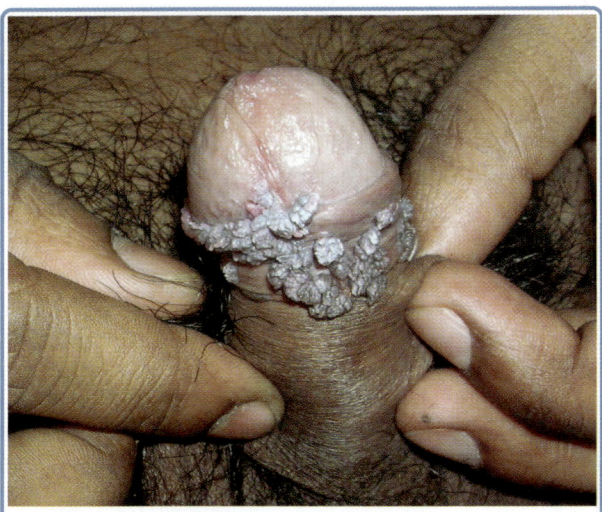

Fig. 8.11: Condyloma acuminata—multiple gray and pink conical papules over penis

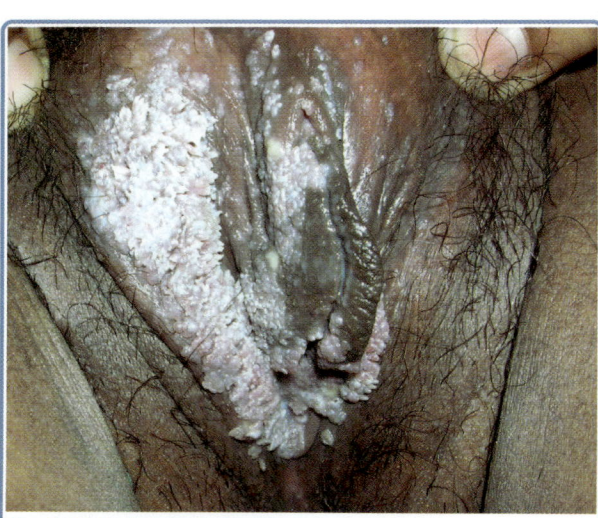

Fig. 8.12: Genital warts (condyloma acuminata)—numerous pinkish gray pointed papules and plaques over vulva

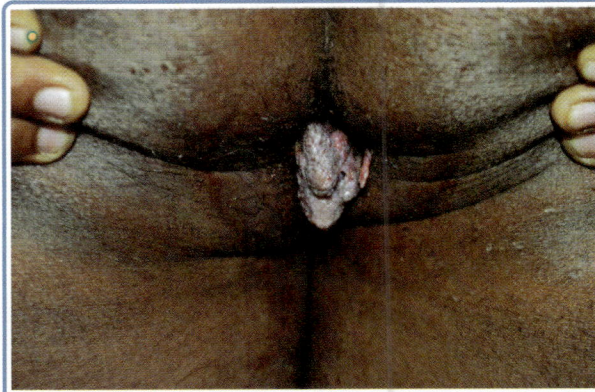

Fig. 8.13: Condyloma acuminata—exuberant pink fleshy growth around anus. Biopsy may be necessary in such cases to rule out malignancy

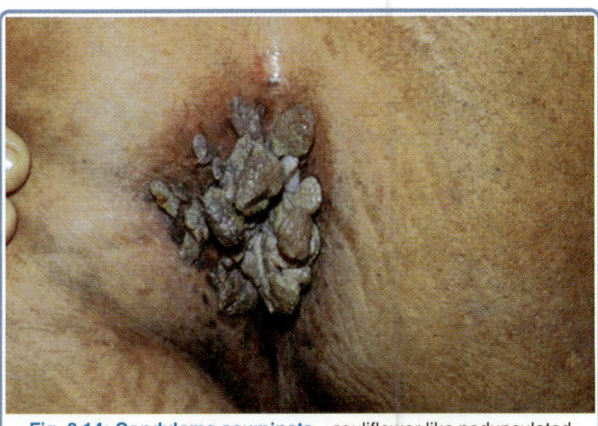

Fig. 8.14: Condyloma acuminata—cauliflower like pedunculated outgrowths

Distribution

They occur over moist regions of the body viz. mucosae and body folds. Commonest sites of affection are prepuce, shaft and glans of penis. Contiguous skin of scrotum, inner thighs, pubis, perineum, perianal region, anus and urethral meatus may also be involved.

Therapy

Podophyllin 20%, in tincture of benzoin, is the therapy of choice. The active component, podophyllotoxin can also be used in 5% concentration with reduced chances of side effects.

Podyphyllotoxin can be used by patients at home whereas podophyllin must be applied by a doctor every time because of the likelihood for irritant dermatitis if it spreads to surrounding normal skin. After protecting the surrounding parts with petroleum jelly, podophyllin is applied carefully to the skin lesions. The solution is than allowed to dry and the patient instructed to wash it off after 4–6 hours. Application may be repeated after one week. Podophyllin is contraindicated during pregnancy.

Chapter 8

Viral Infections

Alternative treatment modalities include electrocautery or cryotherapy for larger lesions and application of trichloroacetic acid for smaller lesions. Topical 5% imiquimod cream is a slow acting but effective mode of treatment for multiple or recurrent condyloma acuminata. The cream needs to be used 3 times weekly for 8–12 weeks.

Summary: Condyloma acuminata are caused by a human papilloma virus that is transmitted by sexual contact. Early lesions are pink conical papules. Pink, fleshy, pedunculated and cauliflower like growths are seen in advanced cases. Topical podophyllin (20%) or podophyllotoxin (5%) are usually effective. Topical imiquimod cream or cryotherapy are used for resistant cases.

TABLE 8.1: Treatment modalities in verruca

Type of therapy	Options
Ablation	• Diathermy or radio-frequency ablation • Cryotherapy • CO_2 laser ablation
Topical agents	• Application of strong keratolytics like salicylic acid, trichloroacetic acid • Topical retinoic acid over plain warts • Topical 5-fluorouracil • Topical imiquimod • Topical cantharidine • Topical podophyllin in genital warts • Topical contact sensitisers (DPCP)
Intralesional	• Intralesional bleomycin • Intralesional MMR vaccine, PPD
Systemic	• Oral levamisole • Oral zinc supplementation

MMR, measles, mumps and rubella; PPD, purified protein derivative

VARICELLA (CHICKENPOX, PRIMARY INFECTION WITH VARICELLA-ZOSTER VIRUS)

A common viral affection that is transmitted as airborne droplet infection, presents with an exanthem (rash) as well as an enanthem (mucosal lesions). After an incubation period of about 10–14 days constitutional symptoms begin. Severity of constitutional disturbance varies greatly and it may be absent in young children. Chickenpox is infective from the prodromal period until the formation of crusts in all lesions.

Morphology

Skin lesions are pruritic and appear in crops. They begin as erythematous macules that rapidly turn into papules and then vesicles within a few days (Fig. 8.16). Initial vesicles have clear fluid and a wide erythematous halo that is easily apparent in fair skinned persons and is responsible for the so-called 'dew drop on a rose petal' appearance (Fig. 8.15). Over the next 4–5 days the fluid may turn turbid thus forming vesiculo-pustules. Vesicles develop umbilications in the centre that later turn into thin crusts. Secondary bacterial infection with pyogenic organisms is a common complication. At a given time, one is able to observe a variety of lesions, i.e. macules, papules, vesicles, pustules. Hence, the rash of varicella is described as being polymorphous.

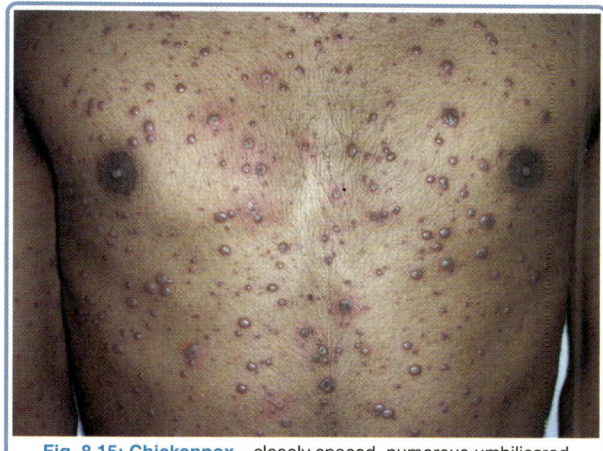

Fig. 8.15: Chickenpox—closely spaced, numerous umbilicated vesicles on erythematous base

Distribution

Trunk is predominantly affected. Proximal extremities, face and oral mucosa commonly have scattered lesions. Other cutaneous and mucosal sites may be affected in patients with severe infections.

Diagnosis

Scraping the floor or roof of the vesicles to make a smear (Wright's or Giemsa stain) is a useful procedure that reveals multinucleated epithelial giant cells and acantholytic cells. These findings are common for other infections caused by herpes virus, i.e. herpes zoster [secondary attack of varicella-zoaster virus (VZV) infection] and herpes simplex (both primary and secondary). High or rising serum titres of antibodies to VZV can be diagnostic.

Chapter
8

Viral Infections

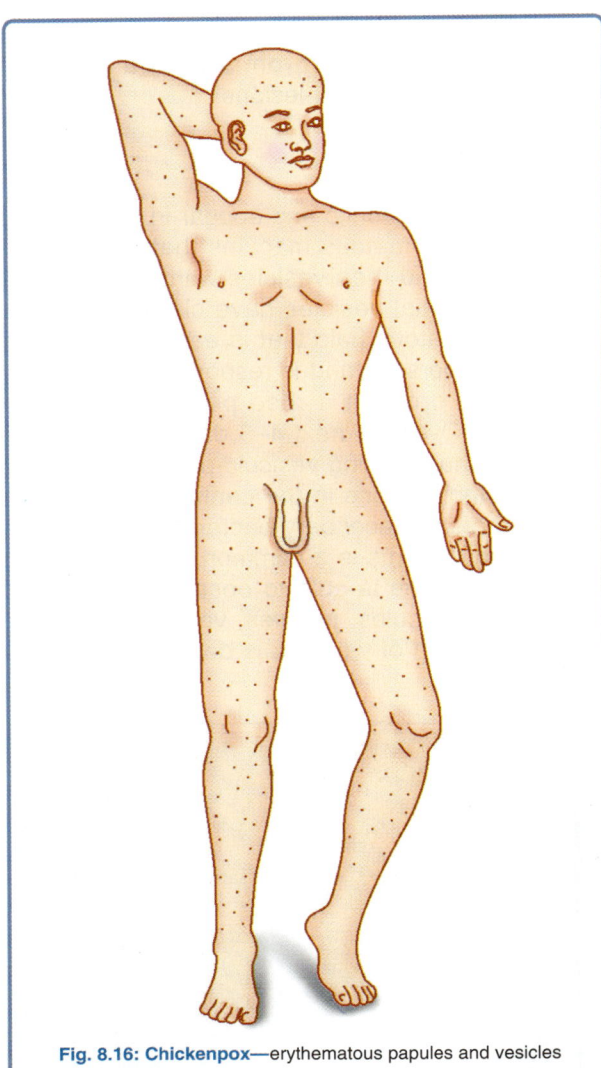

Fig. 8.16: Chickenpox—erythematous papules and vesicles

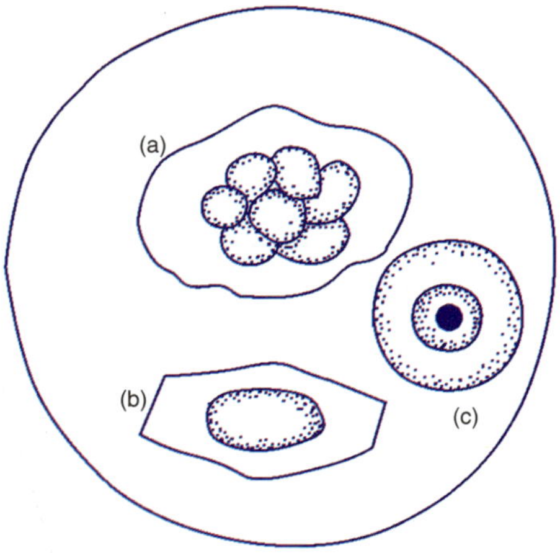

(a) Herpes infected multinucleated epithelial giant cell
(b) Herpes infected keratinocyte
(c) Acantholytic keratinocyte

Fig. 8.17: Tzanck smear

Viral culture from vesicle fluid requires a specialised set-up. Virus may also be demonstrated by immuno-fluorescence of smears (Fig. 8.17).

Treatment

In most instances chickenpox is a self-limiting infection. Antiviral therapy is used (acyclovir 800 mg orally 5 times a day) for 5 days for uncomplicated varicella and for 10 days in some specific situations like:

- Immuno-compromised host.
- Complications like cerebellar ataxia, Reye's syndrome, encephalitis and pneumonitis.
- Haemorrhagic, gangrenous and ulcerative lesions.

Children may be treated with only symptomatic therapy in the form of antihistamines to control itching, antibiotics to control secondary bacterial infection, if any, and paracetamol for fever. Adults are more likely to have complicated disease and hence need antiviral therapy. However, when begun within 24 hours of appearance of rash, oral acyclovir may modify the course of the disease and make its features milder. Many a times antiviral therapy is started late in the course of the disease to promote healing of skin lesions and prevent complications like scarring. Valacyclovir and famciclovir have pharmacokinetic advantages over acyclovir.

Summary: Chickenpox is a manifestation of initial infection with VZV. It is common in children, who usually have a mild, self-limiting disease. Clear coloured fluid containing vesicles with surrounding erythema are characteristic. Papules umbilicated vesicles and pustules also occur. Complications include bacterial infection, pneumonitis and encephalitis. Oral acyclovir is used for 5–7 days to control severity and promote healing. Longer courses are used in immunocompromised persons or for complications.

HERPES ZOSTER

Herpes Zoster (Reactivation or Secondary Attack of Varicella-Zoster Virus Infection)

After an attack of varicella, the virus of varicella remains dormant in the neurons of posterior root ganglia and becomes reactivated at times when body immunity is low. During this reactivation the virus travels along nerve twigs and causes skin lesions that are usually restricted to a region innervated by that nerve segment.

Factors that precipitate an attack of herpes zoster include unusual stress, or an immuno-compromised state like HIV disease or lymphoma, systemic administration of immunosuppressives or steroids or irritation of nerve roots due to trauma, surgery or tumours. Patient remains infective till skin lesions get crusted. Since the virus of varicella and zoster are the same, a patient with herpes zoster can transmit the infection to a previously unexposed child causing varicella. However, since herpes zoster represents reactivation rather than reinfection, contact with a case of varicella does not result in herpes zoster but in varicella (Fig. 8.18, Table 8.2).

Patient Profile

Males and females are affected equally. Elderly individuals are common victims. However, it is not uncommon in middle aged or even young adults. Young adults are affected more frequently in the HIV era. Zoster in a young adult male is considered a marker for HIV infection and it is necessary to consider screening such patients for HIV infection.

History

It is common for pain and hyperaesthesia to precede the skin lesions in the affected segments. Hence, patients with zoster commonly present to specialists other than dermatologists with complaints of pain in extremities, chest, abdomen, back, ear or tooth or headache. Pain may be mild or even absent in younger individuals but is usually severer in the elderly. Pain precedes skin lesions by a few days. Prodromal symptoms of fever and malaise are noted in occasional cases. Skin lesions appear in one to three crops over 3–5 days.

Morphology

Grouped tense vesicles containing clear fluid that have a base or a halo of erythema and oedema

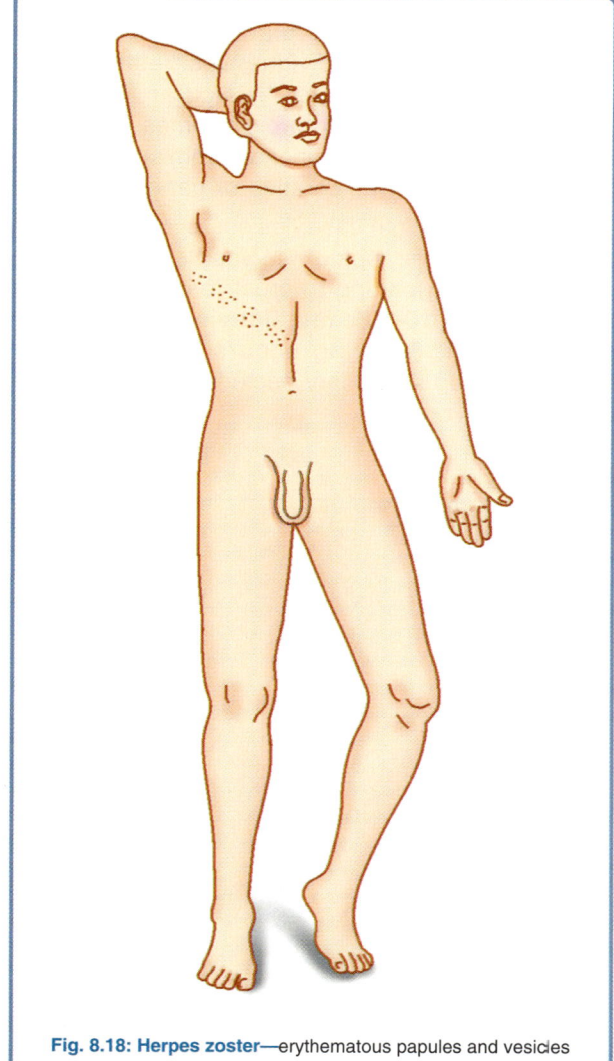

Fig. 8.18: Herpes zoster—erythematous papules and vesicles

are seen in the developed stage of the disease (Fig. 8.19). Erythematous macules, papules and papulovesicles in grouped configuration constitute

TABLE 8.2 : Syndromes associated with herpes zoster	
Syndrome	**Features**
Herpes zoster ophthalmicus	VZV reactivation affects the ophthalmic division of the trigeminal nerve and subsequently the eye causing severe eye pain and can lead to vision loss
Ramsay Hunt syndrome	VZV in any of the zoster zones with facial palsy and auditory symptoms (e.g. tinnitus, deafness, vertigo, nystagmus and ataxia)
Crocodile tears syndrome	Gustatory lacrimation during the recovery from Ramsay Hunt syndrome
Ogilvies syndrome	Acute colonic pseudoobstruction due to VZV
Complex regional pain syndrome (CRPS)	Syndrome characterised by pain, tenderness, dystrophic skin changes, swelling, stiffness in joints and vascular instability following herpes infection

the earlier lesions. In severe cases, such groups of vesicles are so closely placed as to become confluent (Fig. 8.20). Individual vesicles may also coalesce forming bullae. Vesicular fluid may become haemorrhagic or turbid at times (Figs 8.21 and 8.22). Rarely, in immunocompromised patients, the lesions may turn ulcerative or gangrenous.

In a stereotypical case, lesions evolve over one week and then the tops of the vesicles become dry and depressed leading to crust formation. Crusts fall off within 10–15 days leaving behind dyspigmentation. Scarring occurs only when the lesions develop secondary bacterial infection or are unusually severe.

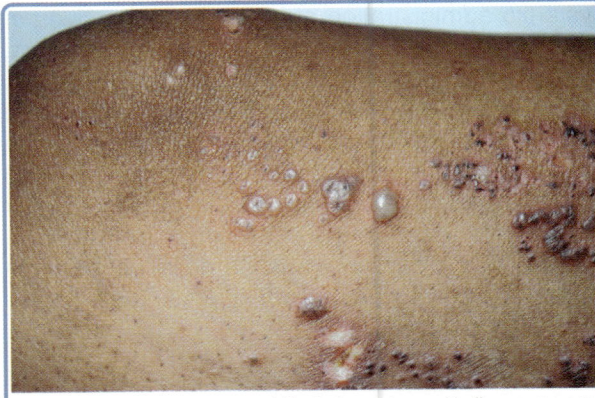
Fig. 8.21: Herpes zoster—umbilicated vesicles and bullae, some are haemorrhagic

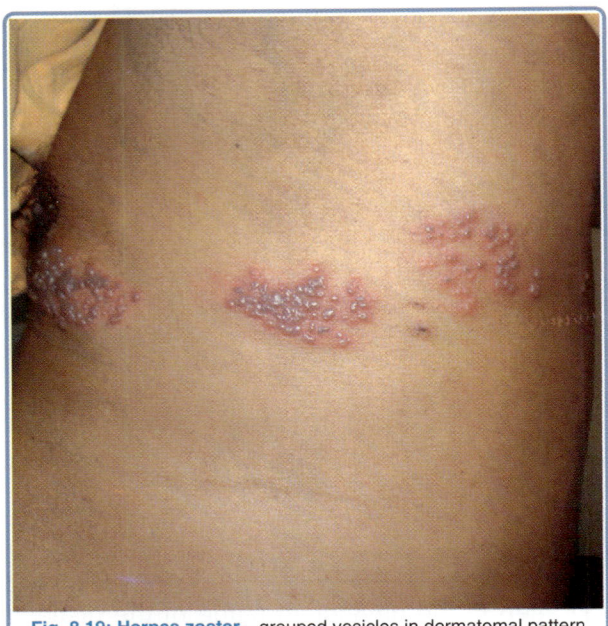
Fig. 8.19: Herpes zoster—grouped vesicles in dermatomal pattern

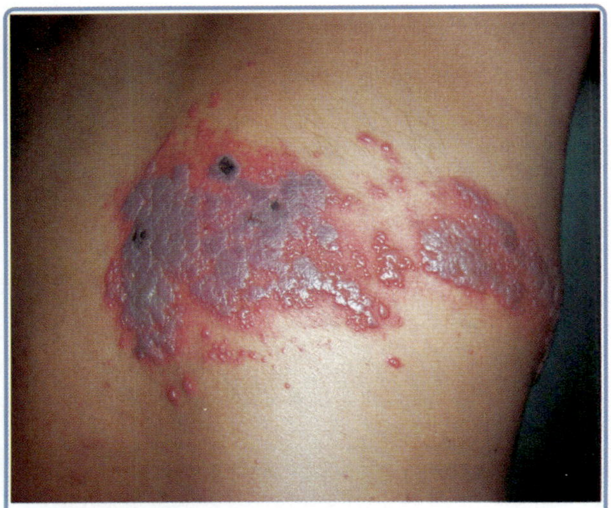

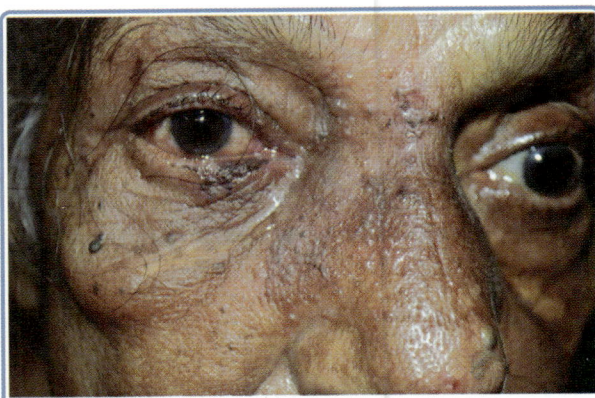
Fig. 8.22: Herpes zoster—herpes zoster affecting the ophthalmic branch of the trigeminal nerve. Lesions on tip of nose are indicative of eye involvement

Distribution

Zoster involves one or two contiguous nerve segments. Hence, the lesions are arranged in a unilateral segmental distribution either across the trunk or along an extremity. A few lesions outside the involved segment do not signify dissemination. Commonly involved segments include divisions of trigeminal nerve and segments supplying the trunk (T3–L1).

Complications of Herpes Zoster

Common complications of zoster include secondary bacterial infection, scarring and postherpetic neuralgia. Postherpetic neuralgia is common in the elderly and may be prevented by early administration of antivirals. When severe, it may disturb sleep and needs to be treated with analgesics or antiepileptics.

Other complications may be related to:

- **Morphology:** Bullous, confluent, haemorrhagic, ulcerative and gangrenous lesions in immunocompromised patients.

Fig. 8.20: Herpes zoster—coalescing vesicles on erythematous background. Note sharp delineation of lesions at midline

Chapter
8

Viral Infections

- **Distribution:** Multisegmental zoster, disseminated zoster involving the skin and viscera in that immunocompromised.

- **Segment affected**

  Ophthalmic: Keratoconjunctivitis, glaucoma, extraocular muscle palsy, delayed cerebral angiitis leading to hemiplegia.

  Facial: Facial palsy, deafness, vertigo (Ramsay Hunt syndrome).

  Upper cervical: Unilateral paralysis of diaphragm.

- **Systemic:** Myelitis, meningoencephalitis, and radiculitis.

Therapy

Being a self-limiting viral infection, a mild case of zoster with no pain and only one or two clusters of vesicles does not automatically warrant antiviral therapy. However, systemic antiviral agents are a must for patients with underlying immune deficiency or cases with unusually dense, deep or disseminated or painful lesion. For typical cases, oral acyclovir 800 mg 5 times a day shortens the course of zoster and leads to faster healing of lesions. It needs to be administered early in the course of the disease (within 2–3 days of the eruption) to be of significant benefit to the patient. Oral famciclovir or valaciclovir have the advantage of a more convenient dosing. If begun within 24 hours of starting of lesions, antivirals reduce the severity of attack and lessen the chance of post-herpetic neuralgia.

> **Summary:** Herpes zoster is due to reactivation of the dormant Varicella-Zoster virus under conditions of stress. Grouped vesicles on an erythematous, oedematous base in a unilateral segmental pattern are typical. Branches of the trigeminal nerve are commonly affected. Ophthalmic branch involvement can lead to keratoconjunctivitis. Other complications are post herpetic neuralgia and, in immunocompromised persons, visceral dissemination. Oral or intravenous acyclovir is particularly useful for such patients.

HERPES SIMPLEX

This viral infection caused by a DNA virus, herpes simplex virus (HSV), is known for its tendency to recur. HSV infections are transmitted by close personal skin and mucosal contact. HSV type I affects the oral, ocular and nasal mucosae whereas HSV type II, being transmitted sexually, affects the genitalia.

Primary and Secondary Attacks

Initial infection, which occurs in childhood with HSV I and in adulthood with HSV II, is called a primary attack whereas subsequent recurrences due to reactivation of dormant virus are termed as secondary attacks.

Primary attacks are severer in terms of extent of morphology of lesions as well as the duration of disease. Severity of infection reduces gradually with every recurrence. Severer attacks (e.g. primary) are accompanied by regional lymphadenopathy.

Chance of recurrence in a particular case is unpredictable and in many instances the infection does not recur or is subclinical. Factors known to precipitate a recurrence include trauma, fever, sunburn, surgery and stress.

Morphology

Whatever the site of affection, morphology of HSV infections remains similar. Lesions begin as erythematous macules that progress within hours to papules and clear coloured vesicles, 2–5 mm in diameter, with a halo of erythema and oedema. Lesions are invariably arranged in grouped configuration (Figs 8.23 and 8.24). As against herpes zoster, the lesions are not restricted to a dermatome and commonly cross the midline. In frictional and moist regions, like the mucosae and body folds, intact vesicles are rarely observed. Tiny tender, grouped erosions that tend to coalesce are seen in these regions. Skin lesions take 1–2 weeks to heal in primary infections (Fig. 8.25) and 3–5 days in secondary infections. Healing occurs without scarring.

Herpes Simplex Virus I

Common presentations of primary HSV I infection are herpetic gingivostomatitis and herpetic

Chapter 8

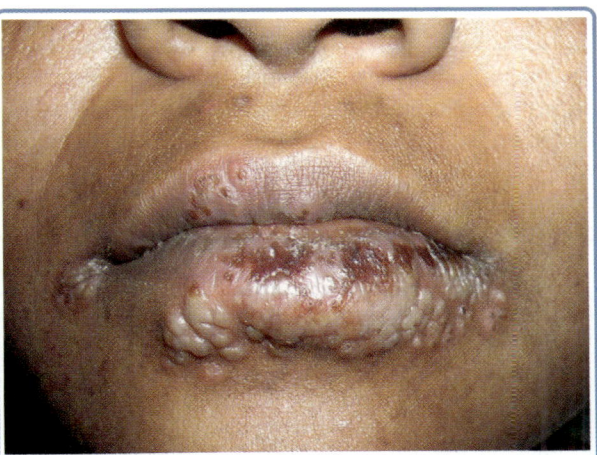

Fig. 8.23: Primary herpes labialis—grouped vesicles on a base of erythema and oedema

Viral Infections

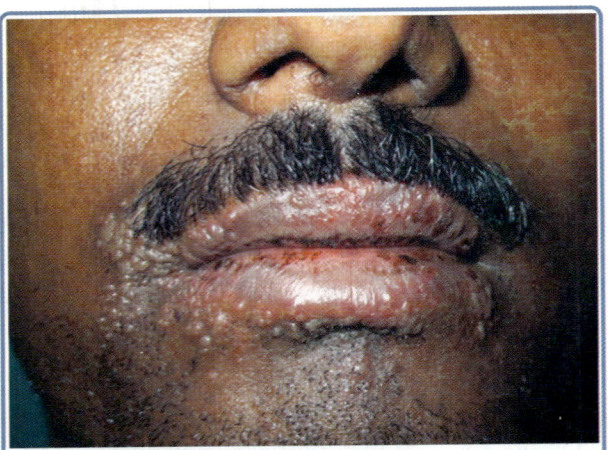

Fig. 8.24: Primary herpes simplex—severe involvement of lips and extension to nose

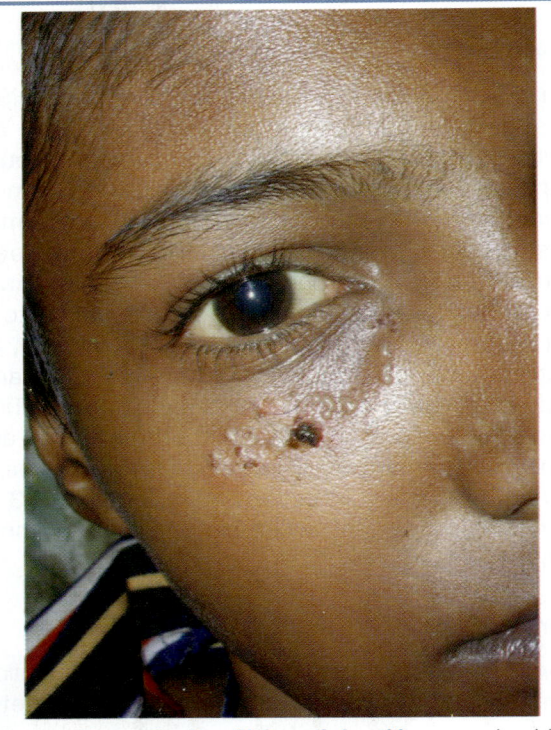

Fig. 8.25: Herpes simplex with herpetic keratitis—grouped vesicles in periocular location with haziness of cornea

keratoconjunctivitis. Secondary HSV I infections characteristically affect the lips (herpes labialis). Accidental HSV I infections include herpetic whitlow, that is characterised by painful vesicles over fingers of dentists or paramedical personnel due to contact with active lesions.

> Herpetic gingivostomatitis presents as extensive painful erosions of the oral cavity that hinder feeding in older infants and preschool children. Vesicular lesions in the perioral area may coexist. Herpetic keratoconjunctivitis, manifests as conjunctivitis with painful dendritic corneal erosions. Periocular skin lesions may be associated. Corneal opacities are uncommon.

Herpes Simplex Virus II

Primary and secondary syndromes of HSV II are known as herpes genitalis. This sexually transmitted disease is notorious for its recurrences and the pain and discomfort that ensues from it. Accidental infection of foetus during passage through birth canal may lead to disseminated and visceral HSV II infection that frequently results in death or disability.

> Herpes simplex virus infections in immunocompromised patients (e.g. in HIV disease) are severe in terms of morphology, extent and duration. Hence, the lesions may turn bullous, haemorrhagic, gangrenous or ulcerative. They may be numerous, extensive, generalised or involve the viscera (encephalitis, hepatitis and pneumonitis) or they may last for several weeks or even months.

Investigations

Smear of vesicular fluid stained with Wright's stain [Tzanck smear (Fig. 8.17)] reveals multinucleated epithelial giant cells peculiar to all infections caused by herpes viruses. Establishing the diagnosis by viral culture or a rising litre of serum antibodies is of academic importance. Presence of anti HSV immunoglobulin M (IgM) antibodies is suggestive of primary infection.

Therapy

Please *see* under herpes labialis and genitalis.

> Development of primary genital herpes during the last 6 weeks of pregnancy is an indication for caesarean section as foetus lacks protection of maternal antibodies in this circumstance. Section should be performed before or within 4 hours of rupture of membrane.

Summary: Herpes simplex virus I causes stomatitis and keratoconjunctivitis and HSV II causes genital infections that are transmitted sexually. The virus has a tendency to remain dormant and cause recurrences at frequent intervals. Grouped vesicles on erythematous bases characterise the disease. Regional lymphadenopathy is common. Lesions last for about 1–2 weeks. Smear of vesicular fluid shows multinucleated epithelial giant cells. Oral acyclovir does not prevent recurrences but hastens healing of lesions.

HERPES LABIALIS

This infection is caused by HSV type I and only uncommonly by HSV II (less than 10%). Primary attack of HSV I involving the oral cavity (herpetic gingivostomatitis) usually occur in early childhood.

Recurrence (secondary attacks) of dormant HSV infection in future presents as herpes labialis. Subclinical (without signs or symptoms) or mild primary infections are well documented. Hence, a patient may present with recurrent herpes labialis without a prior history suggestive of a primary attack.

Common factors precipitating recurrences include fever, common cold and unusual stress. Most patients 'feel it coming' as skin lesions are typically preceded by paraesthesia.

Morphology

Small (2–5 mm), grouped and clear coloured vesicles based on erythema represent fully developed lesions (Figs 8.23 and 8.25). Early lesions are grouped red macules and papules. Later, vesicles may dry and forms crusts or may burst and ooze fluid or lead to erosions (Figs 8.26 and 8.27). Occasionally their fluid may turn pustular or haemorrhagic. Over mucosae, vesicles either burst or are deroofed, leaving behind grouped red erosions that have a tendency to coalesce.

Distribution

Although, skin and vermillion of lower and upper lips are classically affected, inner labial mucosa commonly displays tiny grouped erosions. In severe cases buccal, gingival and lingual mucosae and perioral skin are also affected. Regional lymphadenopathy is commonly in severe cases.

Investigations

Please *see* under herpes simplex.

Therapy

Recurrent herpes labialis is essentially a mild, self-limiting disease and the patient is usually bothered about the cosmetic appearance more than pain or discomfort. Oral administration of acyclovir 200 mg 5 times a day during the period of premonitory symptoms may shorten the severity and course of an attack. Later, prevention of secondary bacterial infection by a topical antibacterial is the only consideration. Primary attacks are severe and need treatment with oral acyclovir 200 mg 5 times a day for 5 days. Immunocompromised cases may need a longer course of acyclovir. Oral famciclovir and valaciclovir have the advantage of twice daily dosing. Topical acyclovir is popular but is not shown to have significant benefit.

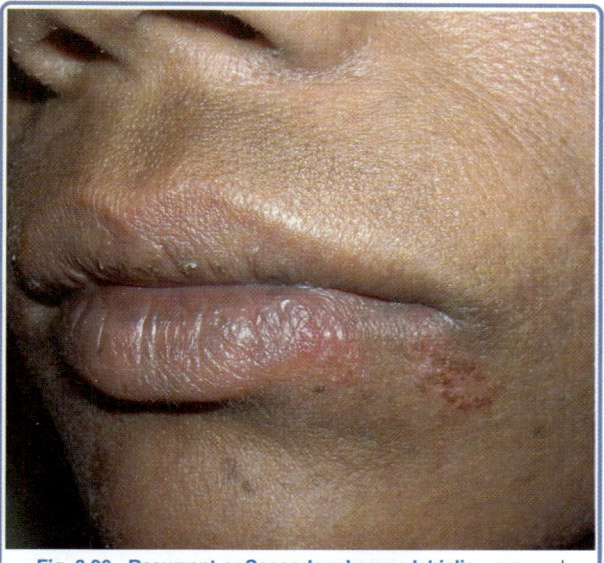

Fig. 8.26 : Recurrent or Secondary herpes labialis—grouped vesicles and erosions with thin crusts. Note lack of oedema

> **Summary:** Caused by HSV I, herpes labialis usually represents secondary attack following initial herpetic gingivostomatitis. Attacks are precipitated by fever, trauma or stress. Grouped vesicles on a base of erythema on or around the lips, including their mucosal aspects, are characteristic. Regional lymphadenopathy is common in severe episodes. Therapy is symptomatic for this self-limiting disorder. Oral acyclovir, used early, shortens duration of disease.

HERPES GENITALIS

This is one of the commonest sexually transmitted diseases in India. 90% infections are caused by HSV II and the rest by HSV I. Common incubation period is about 5–7 days. Primary infections are more severe than secondary attacks that may occur at intervals of every few months or even weeks.

Patient Profile

Young adults are the commonly affected. Males are affected more often than females probably due to

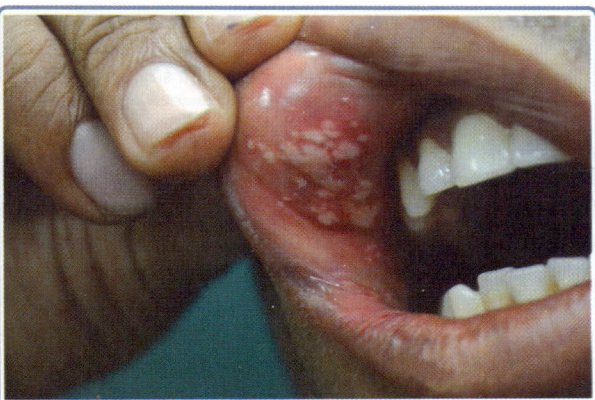

Fig. 8.27: Herpes simplex—herpes simplex involving oral mucosa

Chapter 8

Viral Infections

higher likelihood of reporting and the lesions being hidden in females. Primary infections tend to be more symptomatic in females and may cause urinary retention due to the severe pain.

> **Clinical implication:** Unusually severe, ulcerative or non-healing lesions of herpes genitalis are a marker for underlying HIV infection. Counselling for safe sex practices and if the patient consents, screening for HIV infection is advised for all patients with a history of unsafe sex practices.

Morphology

This is similar to herpes labialis. However, intact vesicles (Fig. 8.28) are difficult to find over genitalis and most of the lesions are erosions.

Distribution

Prepuce, glans and shaft of penis are the commonest sites in males (Fig. 8.29). Pubis, perineum and inner thighs may be involved in both sexes in primary attacks or in the immunocompromised. Labia minora and majora are common sites in women (Fig. 8.30). Vaginal introitus and mucosa, cervix and vestibule may also be affected.

Investigations

Please *see* under herpes simplex.

Therapy

Oral acyclovir 200 mg 5 times a day for 5 days hastens healing. If taken very early in an attack (e.g. during prodrome or on first day) it substantially reduces duration and severity. For primary attacks and severe secondary attacks (particularly in

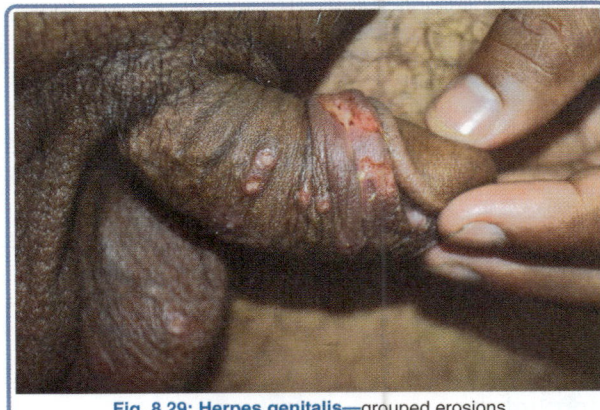

Fig. 8.29: Herpes genitalis—grouped erosions

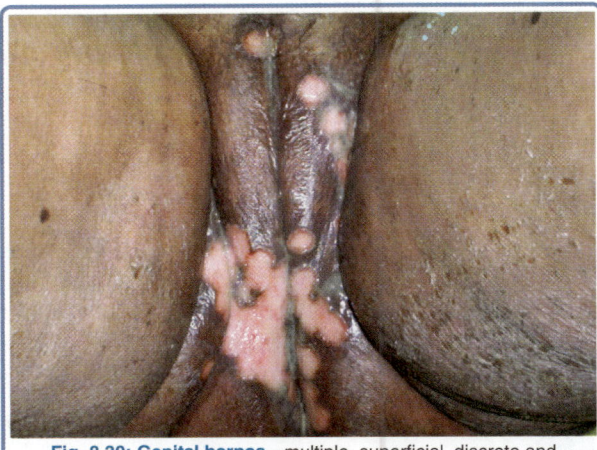

Fig. 8.30: Genital herpes—multiple, superficial, discrete and coalescing ulcers with polycyclic outline

immunocompromised cases) the duration of therapy may be extended to 10 days. Oral famciclovir and valaciclovir have the advantage of twice daily dosing.

> Immunocompromised cases with dissemination to other organs may need intravenous acyclovir 250 mg 6 hourly to control the infection. Interferons are claimed to have given results in prevention of recurrences. For patients who get frequent recurrences (2 or more attacks in a month) long-term suppressive therapy with oral acyclovir 400 mg twice a day for 6–12 months prevents recurrences during therapy and is claimed to have reduced frequency of recurrences subsequently. However, such long-term therapy is not recommended routinely for all cases because of the risk of development of acyclovir resistant strains.

Avoidance of sex in the presence of lesions, at least till a week after erosions have reepithelialised, is necessary, if transmission to partner is to be prevented. Due to substantial prevalence of asymptomatic shedding, use of barrier contraceptive will ensure prevention of transmission to partner. Antiviral therapy is ineffective if lesions are more than a few days old. As dormant virus resides in sacral ganglia therapies based on removal or destruction of involved skin are ineffective.

Chapter 8

Viral Infections

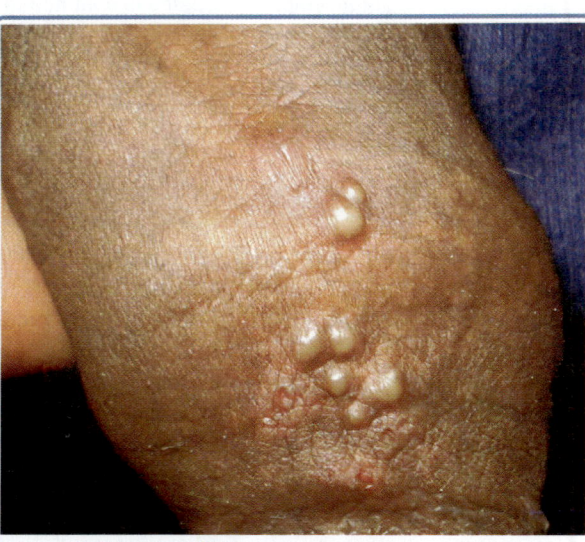

Fig. 8.28: Herpes genitalis—clustered vesicles are initial lesions of herpes. However, they usually break down and form erosions

Summary: Caused by HSV II, a primary attack of herpes genitalis tends to be severe with regional lymphadenopathy. Secondary attacks are common and are precipitated by trauma of intercourse or stress. Grouped erosions or vesicles on a base of erythema on glans, prepuce or the shaft of penis are characteristic. Oral or topical acyclovir, used early, may shorten the duration of disease but does not prevent recurrences. Oral acyclovir is especially useful in the immunoincompetent and may be used as a long term suppressive measure if recurrences are frequent and troublesome.

VIRAL EXANTHEMS

A plethora of viruses including rubella (others being coxackie, echovirus and adenovirus groups and even HIV) cause a syndrome of fever, rash, mucositis, constitutional symptoms and signs with or without lymphadenopathy. The rash usually appears after two to three days of fever and may consist of erythematous macules (Fig. 8.31) or/and papules which may become partly or wholly confluent. Sometimes the rash, being largely asymptomatic, may go unnoticed as it may be mistaken for flush due to fever. The rash affects the body in cephalocaudal direction and lasts for 2–4 days, usually healing without any postinflammatory pigmentation.

The main differential diagnosis of such a viral exanthems is a maculopapular eruption induced by drugs taken for initial fever. However, the drug rash is more pruritic, more oedematous and scaly and tends to last for 1–2 weeks. Blood counts may show eosinophilia and biopsy shows denser infiltrate of lymphocytes and eosinophils (Table 8.3).

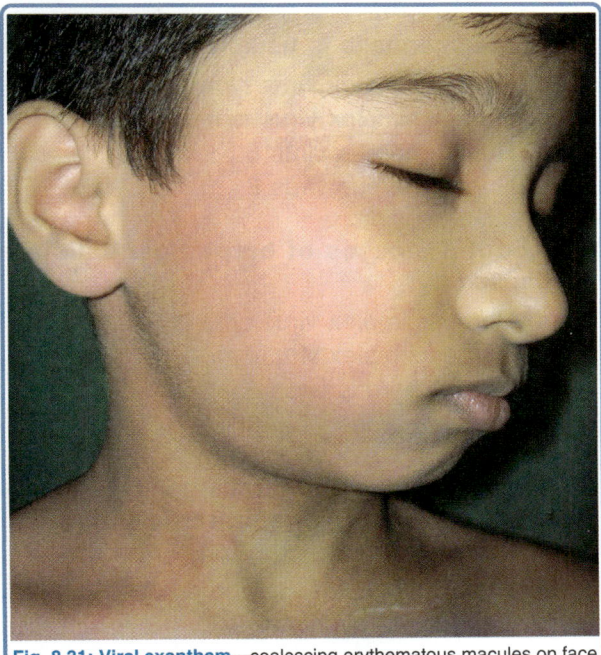

Fig. 8.31: Viral exanthem—coalescing erythematous macules on face and neck

EXANTHEMS

Any sudden widespread erythematous eruption on skin is termed as an exanthem. Traditionally, the term is used for describing viral rashes. However, other conditions resembling viral rashes (e.g. maculopapular drug eruption) also cause an exanthem. Similar erythematous eruption on mucosae is termed as an enanthem. Although, maculopapular eruption is the most common presentation, an exanthem may also be vesicular, e.g. chickenpox. Although, most exanthems are monomorphous or have just one or two types of skin lesions. Some conditions like chickenpox are characterised by three or more types of skin lesions (polymorphous, e.g. macules, papule and vesicles in chickenpox).

The commonest of the viral exanthems is measles. However, many other viruses can cause rash resembling measles (morbilliform rash). These rashes are not easy to distinguish from maculopapular drug eruption. However, clinical features and investigations are helpful for making such a distinction (Table 8.3).

The rash of measles is preceded by an enanthem (Koplik spots). These are punctuate whitish spots that appear a couple of days before the exanthem when the child is febrile and therefore looking for them is helpful in early diagnosis of measles. The rash consists of ill defined erythematous macules and slightly elevated papules that tend to coalesce. The rash tends to heal with scaling and pigmentation.

TABLE 8.3 : Distinguishing viral exanthem and maculopapular drug rash		
Parameter	Viral exanthema	Drug rash
Age	Common in young	Common in elderly
Associated fever	Common	Uncommon
Pruritus	Mild or Absent	Moderate or Severe
Drug history	May be absent	Present
Evolution of rash	Cephalocaudal	Begins on trunk
Constitutional symptoms	Common	Less common
Enanthem	Common	Less common
Lymphadenopathy	Common	Uncommon
Blood counts	Lymphocytosis	Eosinophilia
Skin biopsy	Sparse lymphocytic infiltrate, vascular change	Moderate infiltrate of lymphocytes, eosinophils, necrotics, spongiosis, parakeratosis
Devolution	Subsides in 3–5 day	Subsides in 1–2 weeks after withdrawal of drug

Chapter 8

Viral Infections

MCQs

1. **The causative organism of chickenpox is:**
   a. Herpes simplex virus type 1
   b. Herpes simplex virus type 2
   c. Varicella-zoster virus
   d. Human herpes virus 8

2. **The appearance of fully evolved lesions of chickenpox is described as:**
   a. Grouped vesicles
   b. Umbilicated papules
   c. Few drops on rose petal
   d. Dew drops on rose petal

3. **The distribution of chickenpox rash is described as:**
   a. Central
   b. Centripetal
   c. Centrifugal
   d. Peripheral

4. **The morphology of chickenpox rash is:**
   a. Papular
   b. Vesicular
   c. Monomorphic
   d. Polymorphic

5. **The incubation period of chickenpox is:**
   a. 3 days
   b. 7 days
   c. 11 days
   d. 21 days

6. **Chickenpox is infective till the time:**
   a. No more crops appear
   b. All crusts fall off
   c. All the lesions get crusted
   d. No more vesicles form

7. **Most lesions of the rash of chickenpox heal:**
   a. Without scarring
   b. With varioliform scars
   c. With pitted scars
   d. With atrophy

8. **Children exposed to a patient with herpes zoster may develop:**
   a. Chickenpox
   b. Primary herpes simplex
   c. Herpes zoster
   d. Herpetic whitlow

9. **Ramsay Hunt syndrome is a variant of herpes zoster that affects the:**
   a. Sacral nerve plexus
   b. Posterior root ganglion
   c. Geniculate ganglion
   d. Trigeminal ganglion

10. **Hutchinson's sign in herpes zoster ophthalmicus refers to skin lesions over:**
    a. Upper eyelid
    b. Lower eyelid
    c. Tip of nose
    d. Root of nose

11. **Initial infection with the Varicella zoster virus (VZV) results in:**
    a. Herpes zoster
    b. Herpes labialis
    c. Herpes genitalis
    d. Chickenpox

12. **Vesicles of herpes zoster are distributed:**
    a. Uniformly all over the body
    b. Centripetally, mainly affecting trunk
    c. Centrifugally, mainly affecting face and limbs
    d. Unilaterally, in area supplied by one or two nerve segments

13. **The first attack of herpes simplex infection is termed as:**
    a. Mother patch
    b. Mother attack
    c. Primary attack
    d. Primary chancre

14. **A viral infection that is notorious for recurrence is:**
    a. Herpes zoster
    b. Herpes simplex
    c. Herpes iris
    d. Chickenpox

15. **Herpes genitalis is usually caused by:**
    a. Herpes simplex virus type II
    b. Herpes simplex virus type I
    c. Human herpes virus 6
    d. Human herpes virus 8

16. **About 5% cases of herpes genitalis are caused by:**
    a. Herpes simplex virus type II
    b. Herpes simplex virus type I
    c. Human herpes virus 6
    d. Human herpes virus 8

17. **The morphology of herpes genitalis that is most commonly encountered in clinical practice is:**
    a. Grouped papules
    b. Umbilicated papules
    c. Grouped vesicles
    d. Grouped erosions

18. The most discomforting symptom in herpes genitalis is:
    a. Severe itching
    b. Burning pain
    c. Embarrassing spots
    d. Continuous discharge

19. Over a period of years, recurrences of herpes genitalis go on:
    a. Reducing in severity
    b. Reducing in duration
    c. Reducing in frequency
    d. All of the above

20. About 5% cases of herpes labialis are caused by:
    a. Herpes simplex virus type II
    b. Herpes simplex virus type I
    c. Human herpes virus 6
    d. Human herpes virus 8

21. All of the following precipitate a recurrence of herpes labialis except:
    a. High fever   b. Sunlight
    c. Trauma   d. Lipstick usage

22. The initial infection with herpes simplex virus type 1 infection usually occurs during:
    a. Infancy   b. Childhood
    c. Adolescence   d. Sexual activity

23. Herpes infections are characterised by:
    a. Upper epidermal vesicle
    b. Midepidermal vesicle
    c. Lower epidermal vesicle
    d. Subepidermal vesicle

24. The prodromal stage of herpes zoster may present as:
    a. Toothache   b. Backache
    c. Earache   d. Any of these

25. Premonitory symptoms of herpes genitalis include all except:
    a. Pain   b. Burning
    c. Itching   d. Blisters

26. All of the following are complications of herpes zoster except:
    a. Constipation
    b. Photophobia
    c. Radicular pain
    d. Diaphragmatic paralysis

27. Serious complications of herpes zoster ophthalmicus occur due to involvement of the:
    a. Nasociliary nerve
    b. Supraorbital nerve
    c. Supratrochlear nerve
    d. Zygomatic nerve

28. A herpetic vesicle shows on histopathology:
    a. Paget cells
    b. Acantholytic cells
    c. Multinucleated Langhan's giant cells
    d. Virchow cell

29. A herpetic vesicle shows on histopathology:
    a. Multinucleated foreign body giant cells
    b. Multinucleated epithelial giant cells
    c. Multinucleated Langhan's giant cells
    d. All of the above

30. The organism causing verruca vulgaris is:
    a. Human papillomavirus
    b. Molluscum contagiosum virus
    c. Human herpes virus 6
    d. Human herpes virus 8

31. Which of the following is not a type of viral wart?
    a. Flat wart   b. Common wart
    c. Seborrhoeic wart   d. Juvenile wart

32. Which of the following is not a type of viral wart?
    a. Condyloma acuminata
    b. Condyloma lata
    c. Venereal wart
    d. Genital wart

33. Which of the following is a common site of verruca vulgaris?
    a. Hands   b. Back
    c. Chest   d. Scalp

34. Which type of wart is not seen over face?
    a. Mosaic warts
    b. Verruca vulgaris
    c. Verruca plana
    d. Filiform wart

35. Which of the following therapies is recommended for common warts?
    a. 20% salicylic acid under occlusion
    b. Glutaraldehyde soaks
    c. Oral imiquimod
    d. Salicylic acid lotion

Chapter
8

Viral Infections

36. **Which one of the following is not a recommended therapy for verruca plana?**
    a. Electrofulguration
    b. Paring
    c. Topical imiquimod
    d. Salicylic acid lotion

37. **What is a complication of overzealous electrosurgery for verrucae?**
    a. Depigmentation
    b. Deeper inoculation
    c. Secondary infection
    d. Systemic dissemination

38. **Which is a common side effect of cryotherapy for warts?**
    a. Depigmentation   b. Hypothermia
    c. Secondary infection   d. Gangrene

39. **Which one of the following is not used for treating viral warts?**
    a. Lactic acid
    b. Dinitrochlorobenzene
    c. Liquid nitrogen
    d. Glycolic acid

40. **The organism causing condyloma acuminata is:**
    a. Human papillomavirus
    b. Herpes simplex virus
    c. Epstein–Barr virus
    d. Human herpes virus 8

41. **Which of the following is a first line of therapy for condyloma acuminata?**
    a. Podophyllin   b. Salicylic acid
    c. Electrofulguration   d. Paring

42. **A rare complication of condyloma acuminata is:**
    a. Systemic dissemination
    b. Secondary infection
    c. Bleeding
    d. Squamous cell carcinoma

43. **Podophyllin is contraindicated in:**
    a. Childhood   b. Hypertension
    c. Diabetes mellitus   d. Pregnancy

44. **The organism causing oral hairy leukoplakia is:**
    a. Human papillomavirus
    b. Herpes simplex virus
    c. Epstein-Barr virus
    d. Human herpes virus 8

45. **The organism causing molluscum contagiosum is a:**
    a. Human papilloma virus
    b. Epstein–Barr virus
    c. Picorna virus
    d. Pox virus

46. **Molluscum contagiosum usually affects the:**
    a. Face   b. Scalp
    c. Palms   d. Back

47. **Facial lesions of molluscum contagiosum occur usually in:**
    a. Infants   b. Children
    c. Adolescents   d. Adults

48. **Typical morphology of molluscum contagiosum lesion is:**
    a. Acuminate papules
    b. Umbilicated papules
    c. Umbilicated vesicles
    d. Acuminate vesicles

49. **The colour of lesions of molluscum contagiosum is typically described as:**
    a. White   b. Golden yellow
    c. Pearly white   d. Gray

50. **A common site for molluscum contagiosum in adults is:**
    a. Face   b. Scalp
    c. Hands   d. Genitals

51. **The molluscum bodies are seen within the:**
    a. Dermis   b. Giant cells
    c. Nucleus   d. Cytoplasm

52. **Which of the following is not true for molluscum contagiosum:**
    a. It is caused by a DNA virus
    b. It usually resolves by itself
    c. Lesions heal without scarring
    d. Lesions never enlarge beyond 1 cm

53. **Following one is not a preferred mode of therapy for molluscum contagiosum:**
    a. Curetting
    b. Potassium hydroxide
    c. Imiquimod
    d. Electrocautery

54. **Which of the following viral infections is sexually transmitted?**
    a. Verruca vulgaris
    b. Chickenpox
    c. Molluscum contagiosum
    d. Rubella

55. Hand, foot and mouth disease is caused by a:
a. Herpes virus
b. Influenza virus
c. Epstein–Barr virus
d. Coxsackie A virus

56. Koplik's spots are seen first over:
a. Sole
b. Palate
c. Lips
d. Buccal mucosa

57. The rash of rubella usually lasts for:
a. 3 days
b. 5 days
c. 7 days
d. 10 days

58. Which of the following viral infections are not vertically transmitted to the foetus or newborn?
a. Condyloma acuminata
b. Chickenpox
c. Rubella
d. Verruca vulgaris

59. A 25-year-old lady with 9 months amenorrhoea and in labour but without rupture of membranes was detected to have active lesions of herpes genitalis. What would be your choice of management?
a. Lower segment caesarean section (LSCS)
b. Vaginal delivery
c. Vaginal delivery with antiviral cover
d. Delay labour till herpes lesions heal

60. Herpes infections in HIV infection are all except:
a. Persistent
b. Ulcerative
c. Papular
d. Widespread

61. Pseudo-Koebner phenomenon is seen in:
a. Molluscum contagiosum
b. Verruca vulgaris
c. Both (a) and (b)
d. None of the above

62. Herpes zoster is most commonly seen in:
a. Thoracic region
b. Cervical region
c. Lumbar region
d. Ophthalmic region

63. Shingles is the other name for:
a. Herpes simplex
b. Varicella
c. Herpes zoster
d. Herpes labialis

64. Eczema herpeticum is caused by:
a. Herpes simplex virus
b. Varicella
c. Cytomegalovirus
d. Human papilloma virus

65. Drug of choice for herpes zoster is:
a. Vidarabine
b. Acyclovir
c. Idoxuridine
d. Cidofovir

66. Morbilliform eruption is seen in:
a. Scarlet fever
b. Mumps
c. Toxic shock syndrome
d. Measles

67. Exanthems are caused by all except:
a. Malaria
b. Typhoid
c. Measles
d. Rubella

ANSWERS

1-c,	2-d,	3-b,	4-d,	5-c,	6-c,	7-a,	8-a,	9-c,	10-c,
11-d,	12-d,	13-c,	14-b,	15-a,	16-b,	17-d,	18-b,	19-d,	20-a,
21-d,	22-b,	23-b,	24-d,	25-d,	26-a,	27-a,	28-b,	29-b,	30-a,
31-c,	32-b,	33-a,	34-a,	35-d,	36-b,	37-c,	38-a,	39-d,	40-a,
41-a,	42-d,	43-d,	44-c,	45-d,	46-a,	47-b,	48-b,	49-c,	50-d,
51-d,	52-d,	53-d,	54-c,	55-d,	56-d,	57-a,	58-d,	59-a	60-c,
61-c,	62-a,	63-c,	64-a,	65-b,	66-d,	67-a			

Eczemas

Definition

Eczemas are a group of aetiologically unrelated conditions that have similar clinical morphology. They have been defined as a pattern of skin inflammation that has characteristic morphologies in acute, subacute and chronic phases (Table 9.1) viz.:

Acute Phase

Erythema, oedema, vesiculation, oozing and crusting (Fig. 9.1).

Subacute Phase

Erythematous, hyperpigmented plaques with scaling and crusting (Figs 9.2–9.5).

Chronic Phase

Lichenification (a combination of thickening, hyperpigmentation and prominent skin markings) (Fig. 9.6).

The term dermatitis is usually used synonymously with eczema. The word eczema should preferably

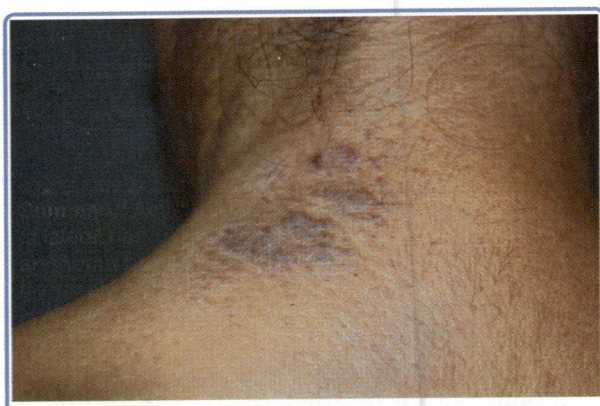

Fig. 9.3: Subacute eczema—erythematous scaly papules and plaques due to nickel allergy

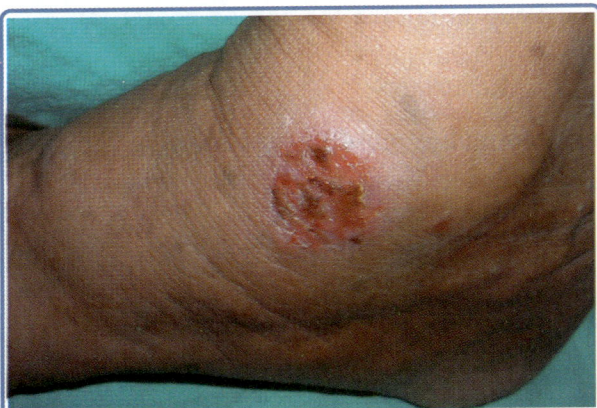

Fig. 9.1: Nummular eczema—coin shaped, plaque with oozing and crusting

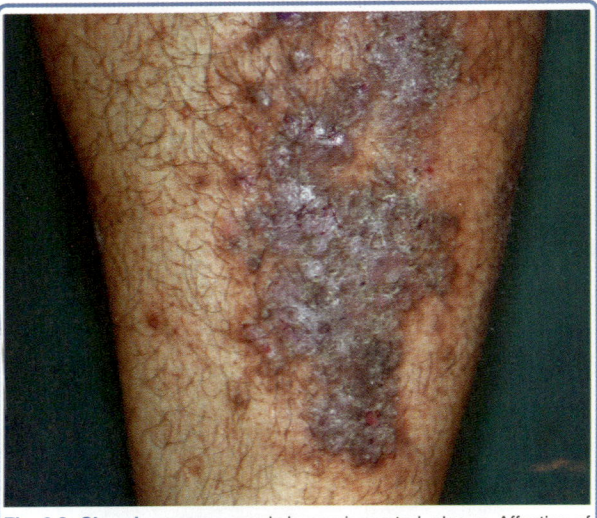

Fig. 9.2: Chronic eczema—scaly hyperpigmented plaque. Affection of lower leg and foot is common in adult atopic dermatitis

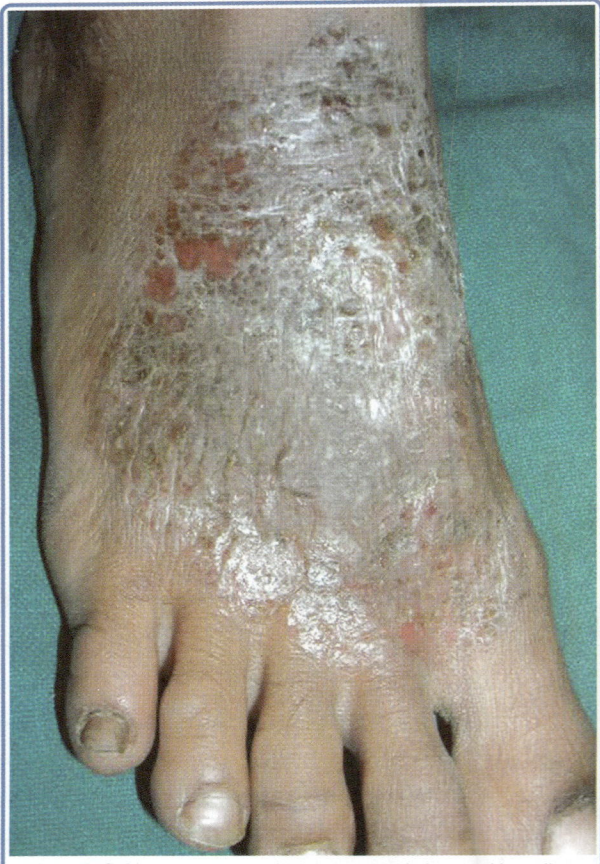

Fig. 9.4: Subacute eczema—hyperpigmented plaque with scaling, crusting and erosions

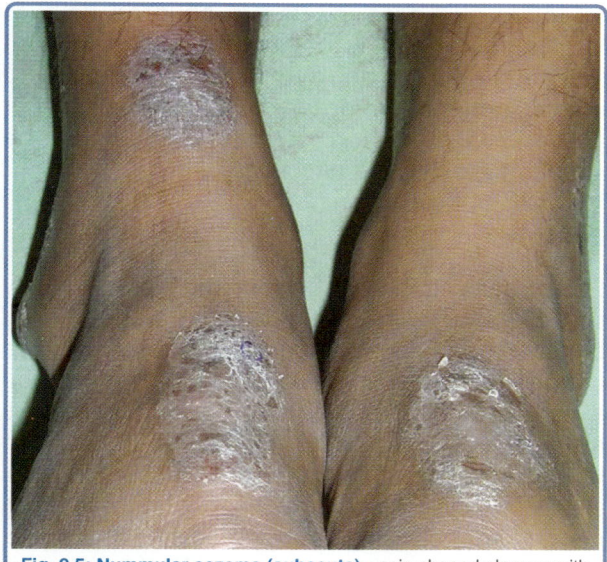

Fig. 9.5: Nummular eczema (subacute)—coin shaped plaques with minimal oozing and scaling

not be used without a preceding qualifying term as in contact allergic eczema or xerotic eczema. Histopathologically, this group of conditions is typified by epidermal intercellular oedema (spongiosis).

TABLE 9.1: Classification of eczema	
Exogenous	**Endogenous**
• Irritant contact dermatitis	• Atopic dermatitis
• Photodermatitis	• Seborrhoeic dermatitis
• Allergic contact dermatitis	• Nummular eczema
• Infective dermatitis	• Asteatotic eczema
• Eczematous drug eruptions	• Stasis dermatitis
	• Pompholyx
	• Juvenile plantar dermatosis

AETIOLOGIC GROUPING OF ECZEMAS

Exogenous Eczemas

An external cause for the eczema is identifiable and when this is removed, eczema does not recur. Contact dermatitis is the prototype of exogenous eczemas.

Endogenous Eczemas

An internal cause or an inherent property of the skin is responsible for the occurrence of eczema. Prime example is seborrhoeic dermatitis.

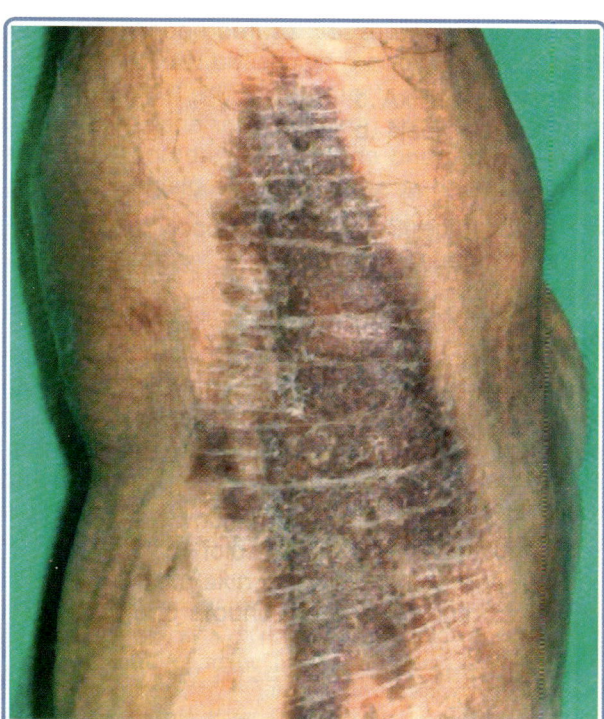

Fig. 9.6: Lichen simplex chronicus—hyperpigmented itchy plaque with prominent skin markings. Note hypopigmentation of surrounding skin as a side effect of application of potent steroid cream over surrounding normal skin

Combined Eczemas

Some eczemas may have an exogenous as well as an endogenous component, e.g. xerotic eczema precipitated by cold and dry winter climate and excessive use of soap in a person who has dry type of skin—dry skin is endogenous component whereas climate and soap usage are exogenous components. Hence, eczemas may frequently have a multifactorial aetiology.

Most subacute and chronic eczemas are perpetuated by itch-scratch-itch cycle. Itching in eczemas induces a scratching response which in turn leads to more itching.

TREATMENT OF ECZEMAS

It is a myth that eczemas are incurable. Most patients with eczemas can be cured with a systematic approach. Common aspects of managing eczemas are covered here (Table 9.2).

General Principles of Therapy

In order to bring about rapid resolution and more importantly to prevent future relapses it is extremely important to explain to the patient the causes that underlie initiation and perpetuation of the disease and advise her or him to take corrective measures. Measures specific for each variety of eczema are discussed with their clinical features. Apart from this, the principles of managing eczema remain similar and they depend on the extent and chronicity of the condition. The more acute an eczema the more bland and drying should be the topical agent used.

Topical Therapy

Acute

Topical open wet compresses with diluted (1:10000) KMnO$_4$ (Condy's solution) administered by placing a soaked layered cotton cloth over the lesions is cooling, relieves pruritus, removes crusts and reduces erythema and oozing. Similarly, soaking in Condy's solution is effective for hands and feet.

> Involvement of more than 20% body area is better treated with, drying and cooling and calamine lotion. Soaps should be avoided while bathing. Systemic steroids are often necessary when extensive involvement is present. Once the acute phase is brought under control with bland lotions, topical steroid lotions may be used.

Subacute

Topical steroid creams are highly effective. Topical mometasone or fluticasone are moderately potent, effective and safe for use in children or over intertriginous areas for several weeks. Potent steroids should be avoided over face and intertriginous areas for fear of causing atrophy or striae. Systemic steroids may occasionally be needed for extensive affections.

Chronic

Potent (fluocinolone or beclomethasone) or highly potent (clobetasol propionate or halobetasol or betamethasone dipropionate) topical steroids are usually effective. However, their use should be avoided in children, over face or on intertriginous areas. For resistant cases, efficacy of steroids can be raised by combining them with a keratolytic agent (salicylic acid) or the use of an occlusive plastic film (occlusive therapy) for a period of 4–8 hours following steroid application. Residual lesions can be injected with intralesional depot preparation of a steroid like triamcinolone acetonide 5 mg/mL. Intralesional injection may be repeated after 4–6 weeks, if needed.

Use of Non-steroidal Agent

Introduction of non-steroidal agents, i.e. calcineurin inhibitors like tacrolimus and pimecrolimus has provided new options for topical treatment of eczemas especially in moderate and recurrent

TABLE 9.2 : Topical steroids			
Drug	**Potency**	**Advantage**	**Disadvantage**
Halobetasol propionate Clobetasol propionate	Most potent	Useful for thick, lichenified dermatoses	If overused (> 15 days) commonly induces skin atrophy. Applied over large regions, for prolonged periods, can lead to systemic absorption effects.
Betamethasone dipropionate	Highly potent	Same as above	Same as above
Mometasone furoate Fluticasone propionate oint	Potent Potent	Safe for long term use and in children, once daily use, low chance of atrophy	Relatively expensive Prolonged use on face or flexures may cause sensitive and thin skin
Beclomethasone dipropionate Fluocinolone acetonide Betamethasone valerate	Moderately potent	Useful for most steroid responsive conditions	If used for many months can induce skin atrophy esp. on flexures/face or in children.
Clobetasone butyrate Hydrocortisone butyrate Fluticasone propionate cream	Mild potency	Low chance of HPA suppression and lower atrophogenic potential allows use in children and on face in adults	Lower effectivity
Hydrocortisone	Least potent	Can be used safely for indications where patient misuse (overuse) is expected	Low effectivity

cases or when topical steroids are contraindicated, e.g. on face, genitals, flexures or in children.

Clinical implication: Long term topical use of potent or very potent corticosteroids with or without occlusive therapy or intralesional injection may lead to skin atrophy, striae, ulceration, hypopigmentation and telangiectasiae especially on face, neck, breasts and intertriginous (body folds) areas and in children. Frequent injections of intralesional steroids can lead to systemic absorption and consequent systemic side effects of steroids. However, systemic absorption and its effects may also be seen with long term use of topical potent steroids.

Systemic Treatment of Eczemas

This is necessary in moderate to severe cases. Apart from oral antihistamines, short courses oral steroids are frequently used. For patients needing frequent courses of oral steroids, oral immuno-suppressive agents like azathioprine or cyclo-sporine may be considered with appropriate blood monitoring.

Summary: Eczema or Dermatitis is a pattern of inflammation of skin induced by many unrelated causes. The causes may be in the body (endogenous eczemas), e.g. seborrhoeic dermatitis or atopic dermatitis or in the environment (exogenous eczemas), e.g. contact dermatitis, drug induced dermatitis. Most eczemas are curable if removal of the cause can be ensured. Localised eczemas can be controlled with topical therapy. Acute eczemas are best treated initially with bland cooling creams or solutions. Subacute and chronic eczemas respond well to topical steroids. Oral antihistamines and steroids may be used when necessary, the latter only occasionally and with caution.

CONTACT DERMATITIS

This dermatitis induced by contact with an external agent may be an irritant contact dermatitis (due to a direct irritant effect of the agent) or may be an allergic contact dermatitis (due to delayed, type IV hypersensitivity reaction).

Contact irritant dermatitis is caused by many chemicals in their undiluted forms. Common examples include lysol, hydrochloric acid and over the counter preparations containing salicylic acid. Burning, rather than itching, of affected skin is followed in minutes to hours by erythema, oedema, vesicles, pustules or bullae. Reddish brown discolouration of the skin may occur. Washing with plenty of cold water and open cold compresses relieves pain and reduces oedema during the acute phase of inflammation. Later topical steroid applications hasten healing.

Cumulative contact irritant dermatitis due to repetitive contact with detergents or soaps (alkalis) or spices or vegetable or fruit juices is one of the commonest forms of eczema seen in housewives. Over a period of months, the skin of palms and fingers becomes dry, rough, thick, erythematous and scaly. Fissures (cracks) may occur later. In addition to topical emollients and steroids, long term avoidance of soaps and detergents is essential to get back the skin to normal.

Contact allergic dermatitis (CAD) is a type IV (cell mediated) hypersensitivity reaction to a plethora of antigens in the environment. Morphology of lesions in CAD varies according to whether it is acute, subacute or chronic. However, it is usually the distribution that offers a clue to the contactant (Figs 9.7–9.9).

Contant allergic dermatitis is an important occupational disease. Occupations like masons (due to cement), beauticians (due to hair dye) and workers in paint, plastic and chemical industries are at risk. Occupational CAD affects hands as a rule. Dorsa of fingers and hands are affected more severely than palmar aspects. Some cases of industrial dermatitis are, however, caused by contact irritant dermatitis to acids, alkalies or solvents.

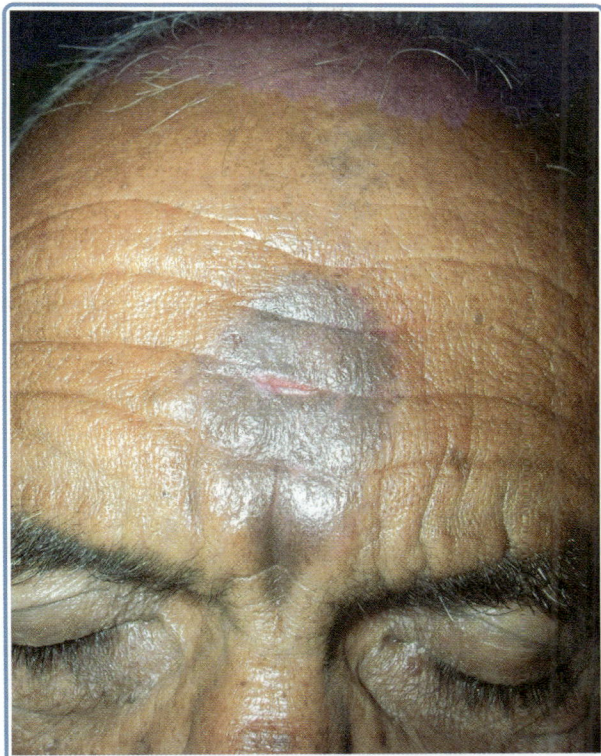

Fig. 9.7: Allergic contact dermatitis to sandalwood paste— erythematous oedematous hyperpigmented plaque

Chapter
9

Eczemas

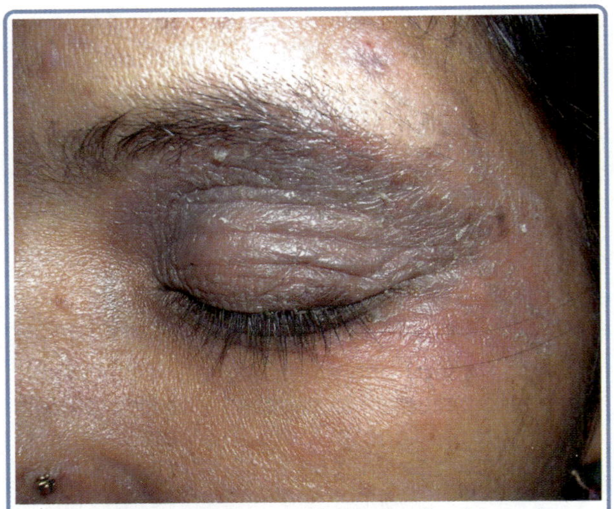

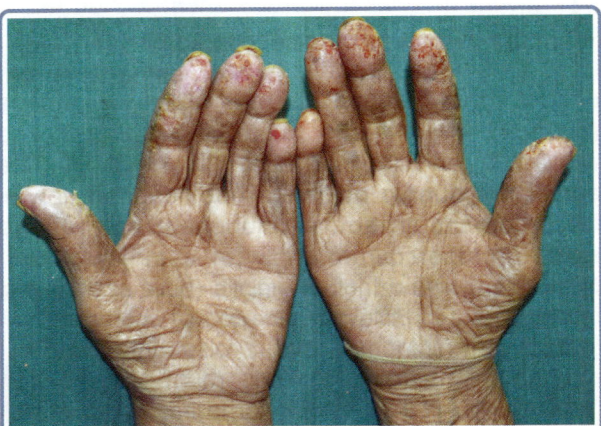

Fig. 9.8: Allergic contact dermatitis due to nail polish—erythema, scaling and pigmentation of eyelid

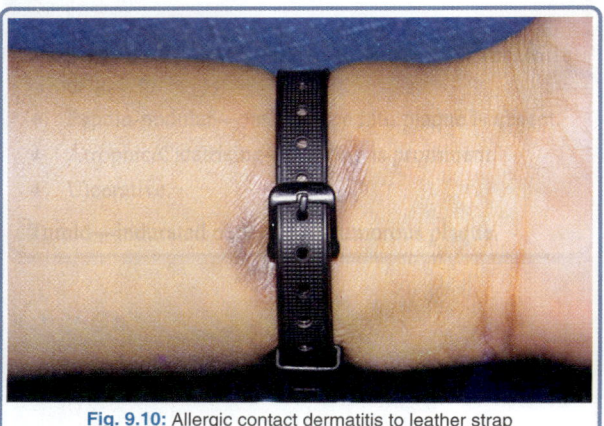

Fig. 9.9: Allergic contact dermatitis in a florist—preferentially affecting tips of fingers

Contact allergic dermatitis can also occur due to a variety of substances in ordinary environment. Contact with artificial jewellery or any white metallic substance (nickel), leather goods (chrome) (Fig. 9.10), plastic (formaldehyde), hair dye (para-phenylene diamine) can cause dermatitis in sensitised individuals. Iatrogenically, CAD may occur due to topical formulations of antibacterials like nitro-furazone or neomycin. CAD can virtually occur at any body site depending on the mode of contact. Sometimes contact allergic dermatitis may be caused by daily use articles like soaps, fragrances, cosmetics, nail polish, preservatives or bases in creams. A detailed inquiry into possible contactants is necessary to rule out contact allergic dermatitis.

Occasionally, CAD can be caused by airborne allergens, e.g. pollens or industrial dust. Such a dermatitis can be widespread but tend to preferentially involve exposed parts (face, distal extremities) and flexures (axillae). Some allergens (e.g. musk fragrance) induce a sensitivity to sunlight, i.e. photoallergic contact dermatitis.

Parthenium dermatitis (Figs 9.11 and 9.12): An airborne allergen that is the commonest cause of photoallergic contact dermatitis in India is parthenium. This antigen from the plant parthenium hysterophorus (congress grass) can induce disabling widespread dermatitis. The grass grows wild over unused land and is virtually omnipresent in many parts of India, making the life of the victim miserable. Severe cases need treatment with oral steroids or immunosuppressants.

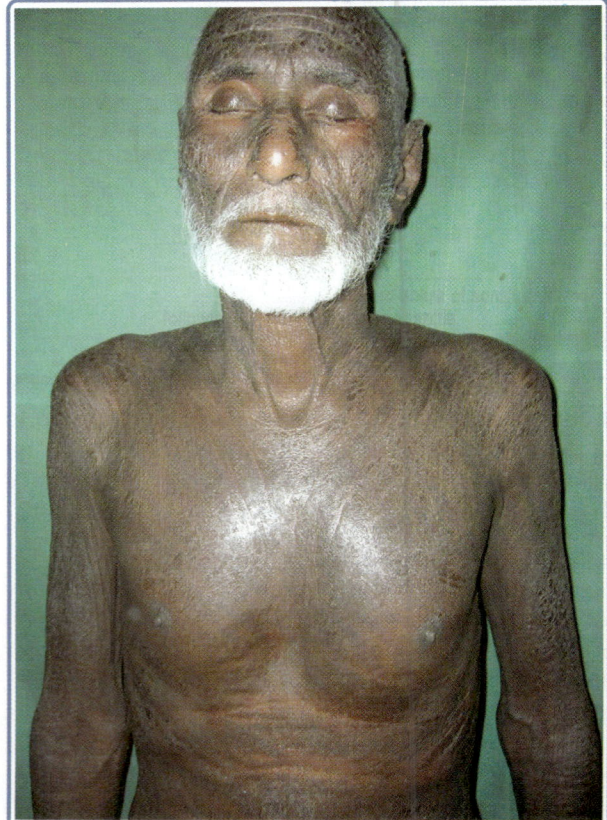

Fig. 9.11: Airborne contact dermatitis to parthenium leading to erythroderma—diffuse generalised erythema and scaling

Fig. 9.10: Allergic contact dermatitis to leather strap

Diagnosis

Taking detailed history and keeping a high index of suspicion are essential for diagnosis.

The diagnosis of CAD can be confirmed with patch testing. A measured amount and concentration of the suspected allergen is applied, under occlusion, to the patient's back and the reaction read after 48 hours. Positive test is indicated by oedematous papules or vesicles at the site of application of the patch. Avoidance of contactant is a must for cure of CAD. Occupational contact dermatitis can be prevented by a change of job or the method of work or a change in the job material. Alternatively, contact with the allergen may be avoided by use of protective wear (e.g. gloves or clothing) or use of a barrier cream containing dimethicone.

Special Patterns of Contact Allergic Dermatitis

Apart from eczematous pattern other morphologies like depigmented patches (contact leucoderma due to contact with chemicals in plastics or rubber), hyperpigmented patches (pigmented contact dermatitis due to cosmetics or lichenoid rash due to photo developers, etc.

> **Summary:** Contact dermatitis due to irritants like acids or alkalis manifests as burning, erythema, vesicles or bullae. Cumulative contact irritant dermatitis affects hands due to repeated contact with detergents. Contact allergic dermatitis is a type IV hypersensitivity reaction to environmental antigens. It may affect any body site and may be acute or chronic. Detailed history and sites of affection usually offer a clue about the contactant. Common alltergens are industrial chemicals, plants (parthenium), metals (nickel), leather (chrome) and plastics (formaldehyde). Diagnosis can be confirmed by patch testing. Avoidance of allergen is necessary for cure of contact allergic dermatitis.

SEBORRHOEIC DERMATITIS

It is an endogenous form of dermatitis that is seen in individuals who commonly have hyperactive sebaceous glands (oily skin). It has been suggested that it is an abnormal response to heavy colonisation of the skin by the lipophilic yeast Malassezia.

> **Clinical Implication:** Unresponsive seborrhoeic dermatitis can be brought under control with systemic antifungals.

Patient Profile

The condition begins in early adulthood. Being extremely common in its mildest form as dandruff

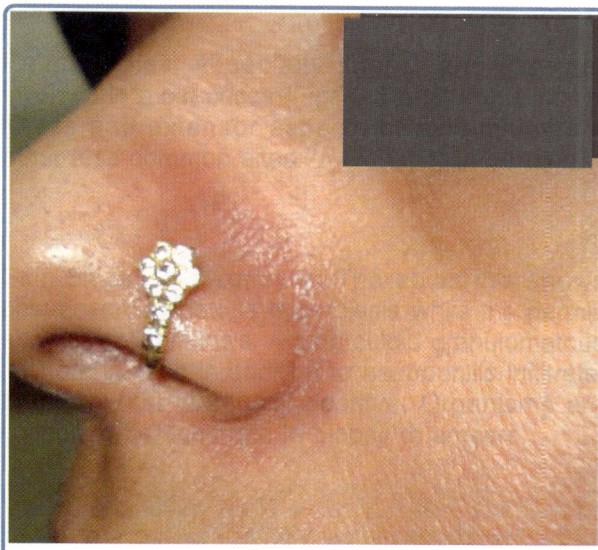

Fig. 9.12: Seborrhoeic dermatitis—erythema and minimal scaling in paranasal fold

(pityriasis sicca), it is observed during the second to fourth or the fifth decade. Males are more commonly and more severely affected, a reflection probably of androgenic control of sebaceous glands. Milder variety is common during infancy (cradle cap).

Morphology

Lesions are hardly seen in early disease unless pointed out by the patient. Tiny erythematous macules and papules topped with a yellowish oily scale are the stereotypical lesions. In severe cases, fusion of adjacent lesions results in red patches and plaques covered with thick, yellowish white and greasy scales. Psoriasis can be distinguished from seborrhoeic dermatitis by its dry, silvery white scale and the presence of Auspitz sign. Moreover, unlike seborrhoeic dermatitis psoriasis tends to spread beyond scalp margins.

Distribution

This is more distinctive than morphology. Scalp and face are involved as a rule. Eyebrows, eyelashes, glabella, paranasal (Fig. 9.12), nasolabial (Fig. 9.13), infralabial and postauricular folds, mustache and beard regions in males and external auditory meatus are preferentially affected. However, any part of face may be involved. Mid-chest, mid-back, axillae, groins, submammary fold (in women), periumbilical, genital, perineal and perianal regions may also be affected. Uniregional affections have been termed individually as pityriasis sicca (scalp), otitis externa (ext. aud. meat.), squamous blepharitis (eyelid margins), etc.

Chapter
9

Eczemas

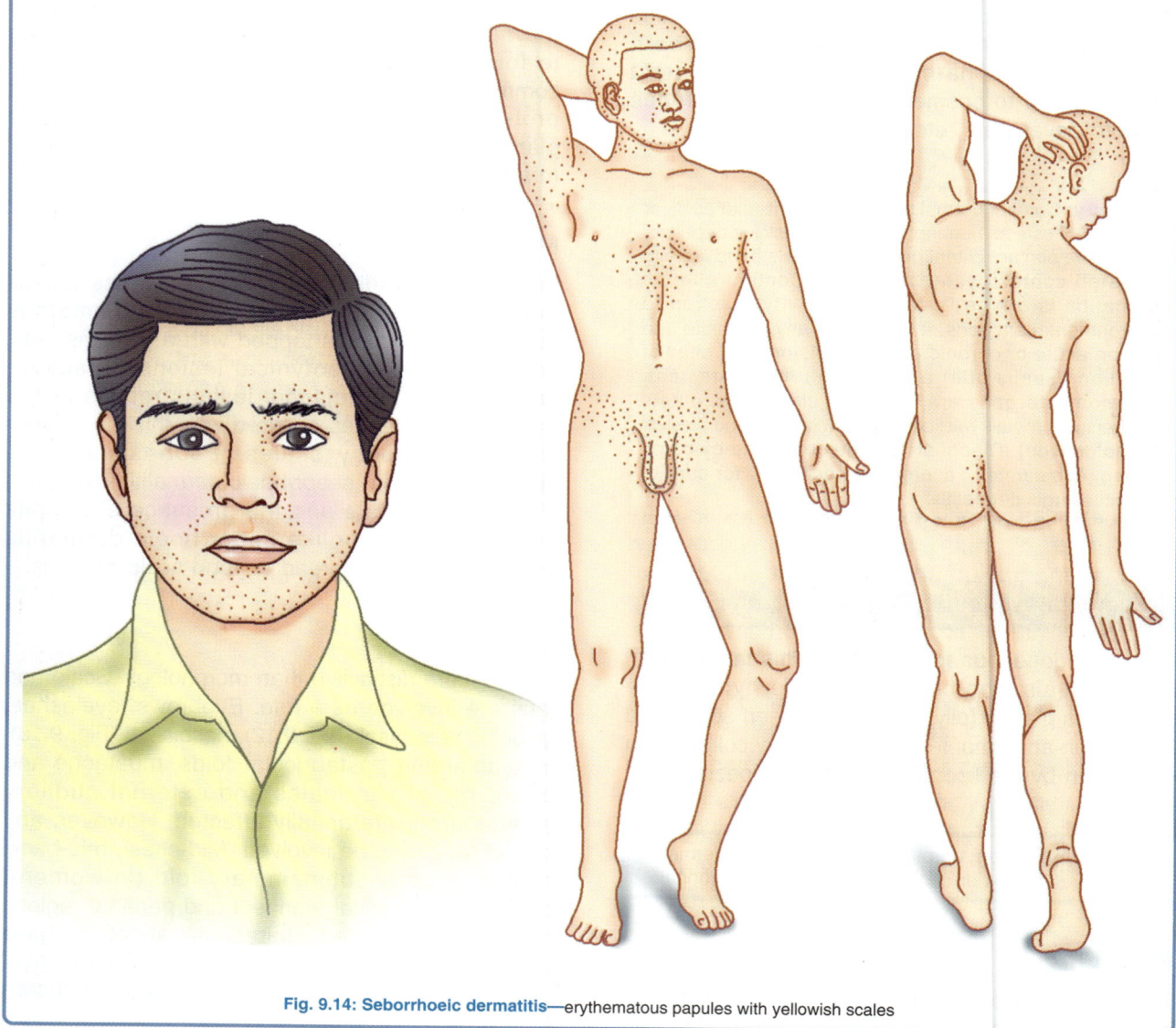

Fig. 9.13: Seborrhoeic dermatitis—ill defined erythema and scaling accentuated in nasolabial folds and eyebrows

Diagnosis

This is based on clinical features. Biopsy is rarely necessary. Symptoms are frequently more prominent than signs. Typical distribution serves as a clue.

> Severe seborrhoeic dermatitis of scalp can be distinguished from scalp psoriasis by being pruritic, with diffuse involvement of sclap, failure to extend beyond scalp margins, and the scales being yellowish and oily rather than silvery white and dry. Moderate to severe seborrhoeic dermatitis may be a manifestation of underlying HIV infection (Fig. 9.15).

Therapy

Mild to moderate scalp affection responds well to regular use of a **shampoo** containing antifungals

Fig. 9.14: Seborrhoeic dermatitis—erythematous papules with yellowish scales

Chapter
9

Eczemas

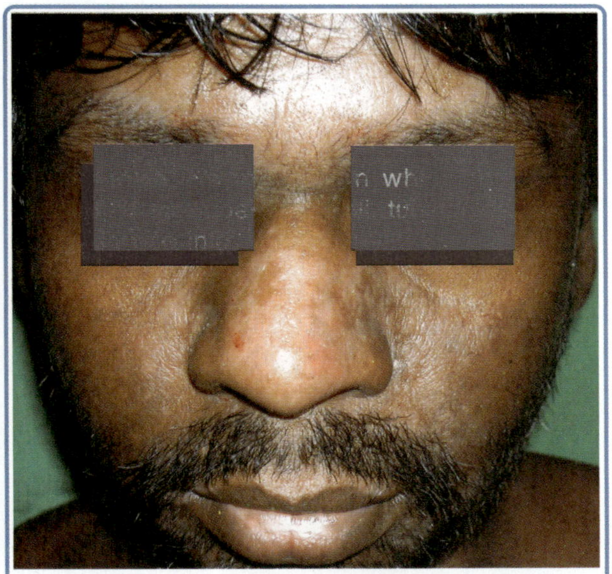

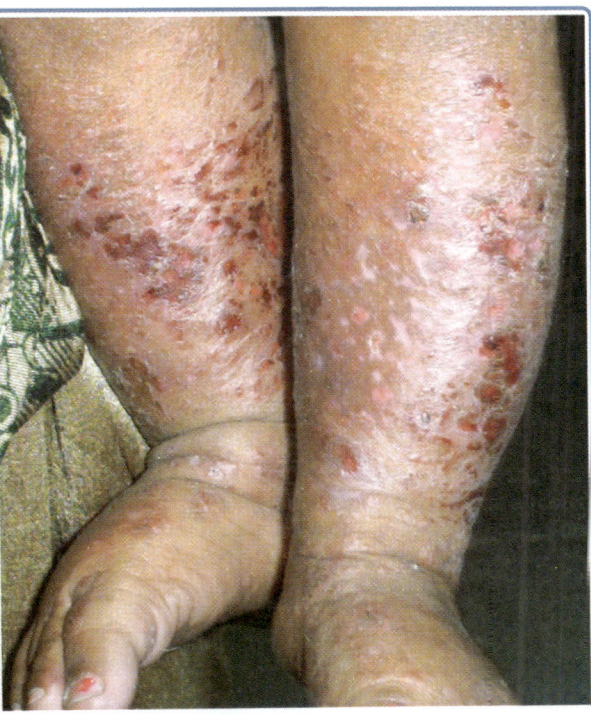

Fig. 9.15: Severe Seborrhoeic dermatitis in HIV seropositive

like zinc pyrithionate, cyclopirox or ketoconazole with or without topical **antifungal lotions** or gels containing ketoconazole or clotrimazole or miconazole. Shampoos containing coal tar are useful for severe disease. Oral antibiotics (doxycycline) and vitamin B2—riboflavin are of some help. Oral antihistamines may reduce pruritus.

Application of strong topical steroid (e.g. betamethasone, fluocinolone) over face is avoided for fear of causing skin atrophy, photosensitivity and telangiectasia, and inducing perioral dermatitis. Unresponsive seborrhoeic dermatitis can be controlled with oral itraconazole 100 mg od for 10–14 days or fluconazole 150 mg once a week for 4–6 weeks. When uncontrolled disease results in erythroderma, systemic steroids may be required to bring it under control.

Summary: Seborrhoeic dermatitis is an endogenous eczema that is probably due to abnormal body response to the commensal yeast malassezia. Young adult males are typically affected. Red papules topped by yellowish greasy scales are characteristic. Lesions may coalesce to involve large areas or form thick scales. Face, scalp, central trunk and flexures are classically involved. Topically, antifungals and shampooing are useful. Systemic itraconazole or fluconazole are occasionally needed to control the disease and steroids necessary for erythrodermic disease.

ATOPIC DERMATITIS

Along with allergic rhinitis, bronchial asthma (endogenous) and hay fever, atopic dermatitis constitutes atopy, a condition of altered reactivity to common and mild environmental stimuli. Common stimuli like changes in environmental temperature or contact with woolen clothing induces pruritus in these patients thereby initiating the itch-scratch-itch cycle which perpetuates the disease.

Patient Profile

Personal and family history of an atopic state (asthma, allergic rhinitis, hay fever, allergic conjunctivitis and persistent or relapsing dermatitis) is usually observed. Presentation is common in childhood. Over the years, the condition tends to improve, so that it is seen less commonly in adults. Both sexes are equally affected.

Clinical Features

Infantile phase

Morphologic features of acute or subacute eczema are observed over the face and extremities of an infant (Fig. 9.16). Other body parts are affected in severe cases (Fig. 9.17a).

Childhood phase

Excoriated papules, papulovesicles and features of subacute eczema are seen over extensors and flexures of extremities up to the age of 10 years. Face and trunk are involved uncommonly (Fig. 9.18). Lesions resemble prurigo due to insect bite allergy.

Fig. 9.16: Atopic dermatitis (infantile phase)—erythema, scaling and crusted erosions

Chapter
9

Eczemas

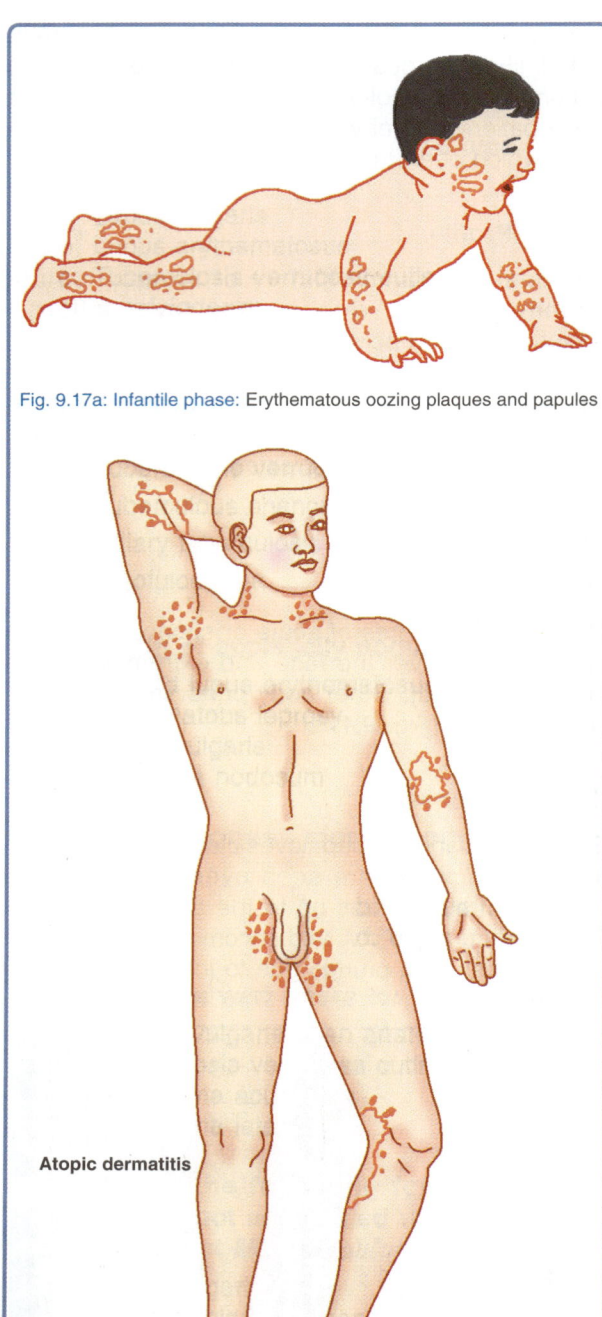

Fig. 9.17a: Infantile phase: Erythematous oozing plaques and papules

Atopic dermatitis

Fig. 9.17b: Adolescent phase: Lichenified plaques and erythematous papules

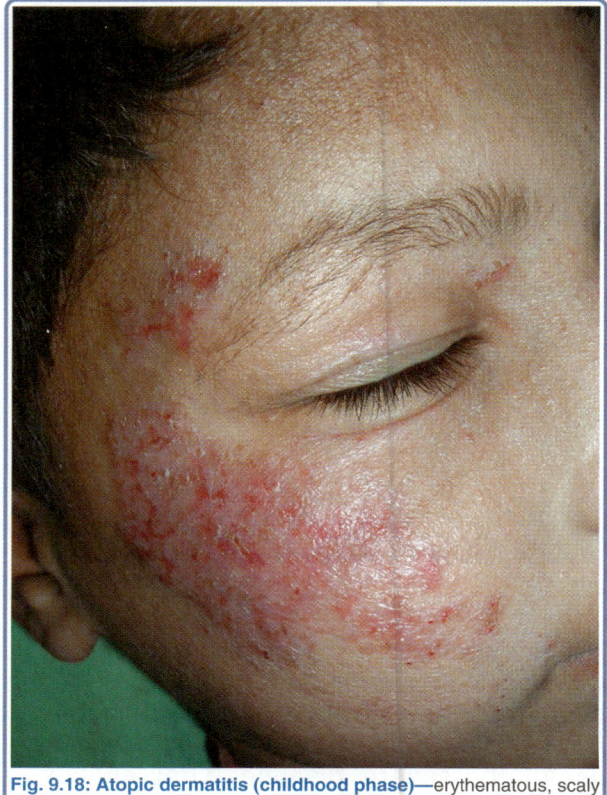

Fig. 9.18: Atopic dermatitis (childhood phase)—erythematous, scaly lesions

Adolescent and adulthood phase

Features of chronic eczema (lichenification) are present on the flexures of extremities (antecubital, popliteal fossae, axillae, wrists, and ankles). Lesions begin as itchy erythematous oozing patches and gradually turn into lichenified plaques (Fig. 9.17b).

Diagnosis

It is based on three cardinal features of atopic dermatitis:

- present or past, personal or family history of atopy,
- presence of severe pruritus and
- persistent or relapsing eczema.

Minor markers of atopic state include hyperlinear palmar creases, pityriasis alba, extra infraorbital fold, spring catarrh, keratoconus and anterior subcapsular cataracts. Serum immunoglobulin E (IgE) is frequently raised; peripheral eosinophilia is common.

Therapy

Since common environmental stimuli induce pruritus in these patients, the aim is to minimise such stimuli and promote the use of bland, soothing and moisturising creams containing paraffin or squalene. Hence, exposure to soap and other chemicals (including topical medicaments), synthetic and woolen clothes, too hot or too cold environs should be minimum.

Topically, a mild corticosteroid like hydrocortisone is preferred for long term usage although a potent steroid may be needed for 1–2 weeks initially to break the itch-scratch-itch cycle and resolve lichenified plaques. Oral antihistamines including sedative antihistaminics like hydroxyzine or cetirizine are helpful adjuncts. Occasionally, a case with widespread persistent lesions may need a short course of systemic steroids or immuno-suppressants to induce remission.

Summary: Atopic dermatitis is a component of atopy, i.e. an abnormal reactivity to common environmental stimuli like contact with wool or synthetic fibres, dust, animal or plant products. These persons react with severe pruritus, acute weeping eczema of face in infancy and chronic lichenified flexural eczema in adults. Extensors of limbs are involved during infancy and childhood. Therapy involves avoidance of irritants and precipitating factors and the use of moisturisers and mild topical steroids.

INFANTILE ECZEMA (ECZEMA IN INFANTS)

Common causes of eczema in infants include the following:

● **Atopic dermatitis**

Seen usually in bottle fed infants with a personal history of lactose intolerance and a family history of atopy, this disorder presents as acute eczematous lesions involving the face and, when severe, extremities (Figs 9.19 and 9.20) and even trunk. The condition tends to worsen during winter and in the latter half of the first year of life. When severe, it may result in exfoliative dermatitis.

● **Seborrhoeic dermatitis**

This is noted during the first half of infancy, most commonly in a mild form as a 'cradle cap' (Fig. 9.21). This is an extremely common condition that is seen as yellowish, thick, oily and adherent scales over the vertex. Uncommonly, it may present as widespread

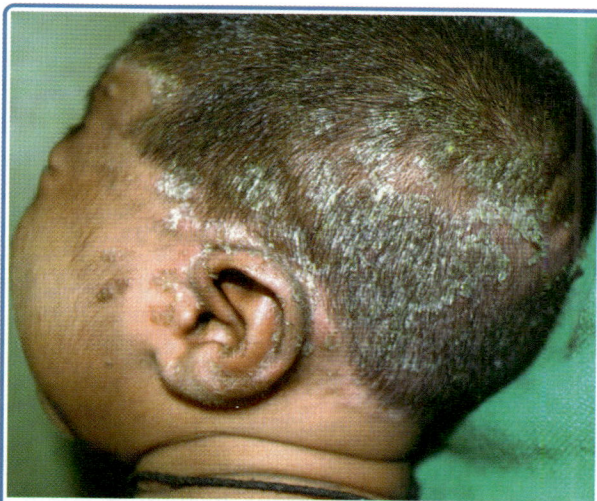

Fig. 9.20: Atopic dermatitis—diffuse erythema and scaling of scalp in a young child. Differentiation from seborrhoeic dermatitis may be difficult

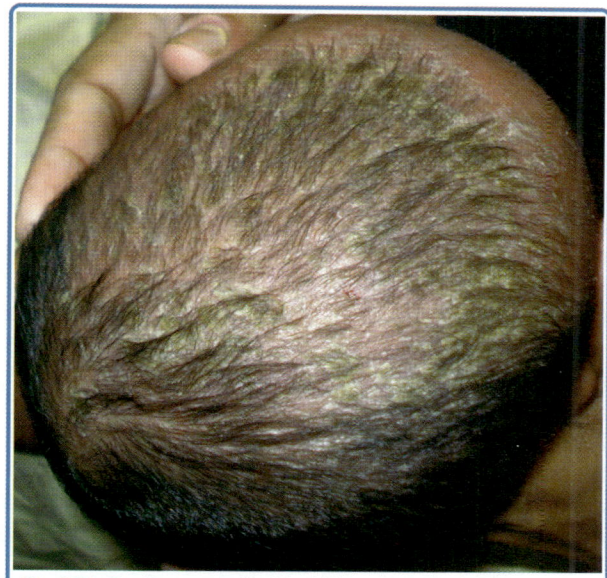

Fig. 9.21: Cradle cap—yellowish, thick scales with slight erythema in an infant

diffuse erythema covered with yellowish flaky scales and, at times, groups of vesicles and pustules with consequent oozing and crusting over other seborrhoeic areas and flexures. Rarely generalised exfoliative dermatitis occurs.

● **Xerotic eczema**

Ill-defined patches of dry erythema and fine scaling over cheeks and extensors of extremities are the initial features. As the lesions progress, oozing, crusting and fissuring develop. Lesions worsen in winter and with the use of a soap. Extensors of body are preferentially affected.

● **Napkin dermatitis**

Please *see* section on 'napkin dermatitis'.

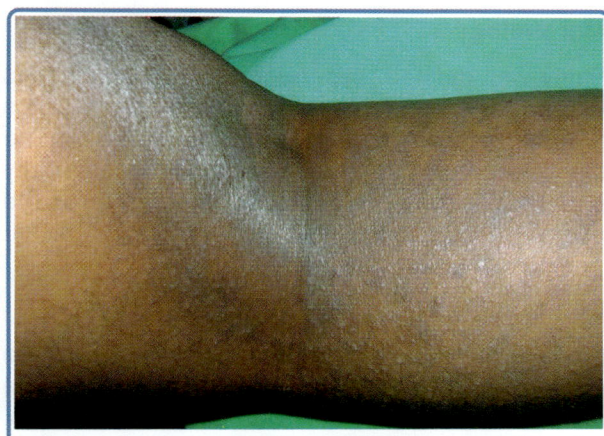

Fig. 9.19: Atopic dermatitis in an adult—hyperpigmentation and thickening of skin due to constant rubbing

Chapter
9

Eczemas

- ### Contact allergic dermatitis

  This is uncommon in infants, due to either reduced exposure or to poorly developed immunity. It should still be suspected if a dermatitis fails to respond to apparently adequate measures. More commonly, contact irritant dermatitis occurs in infants due to topical agents that may not produce an irritant dermatitis in adults, e.g. various over the counter preparations containing rubefacients, counterirritants, antiseptics and oils.

- ### Secondary eczematisation

  Development of eczematous change as a complication of scabies in infants is seen occasionally in untreated disease or following irritation due to topical antiscabietics. Face and extremities are usually affected. Palms and soles show burrows.

Therapy of Infantile Eczema

Mild to moderately severe eczema with limited distribution responds well to correction of cause and use of emollients with topical steroids. Milder steroids like clobetasone (not clobetasol) or hydrocortisone are preferred in infants due to their thin skin. Compresses are helpful in wet eczema whereas moisturisers are helpful in xerotic eczema as well as the dry skin that frequently accompanies atopic dermatitis. Unresponsive and widespread lesions may be treated with an initial short course of a stronger topical steroid like mometasone or fluticasone or when severe with even an additional short course of systemic steroids tapered over 5–10 days.

Summary: Eczema in infancy may be due to atopic dermatitis or seborrhoeic dermatitis or less frequently, xerotic eczema and napkin dermatitis. Contact allergic dermatitis is rare in infancy but contact irritant dermatitis may be seen. Acute eczema of face and extremities with positive family history of atopy is seen with atopic dermatitis. Greasy scales over erythema with accentuation in seborrhoeic distribution are features of seborrhoeic dermatitis. Xerotic eczema is a dry eczema of face and extensors that occurs in winter. Mild topical steroids should preferably be used. Stronger topical steroids and systemic steroids may be used in short courses in extensive or severe disease.

NAPKIN DERMATITIS

This form of dermatitis is encountered in infants who are not attended to with the necessary frequency of change of napkins. Persistent contact with urine and faeces, with consequent moisture may not only damage the skin and compromise its defenses, but also alter the normal bacterial flora. Urealytic bacteria from faeces act on urine to release ammonia, which is thought to be irritating to the skin.

Clinical differential diagnosis is candidiasis that tends to affect the inguinal flexures and intergluteal cleft whereas napkin dermatitis leads to erythema, oedema and erosions of the contours of buttocks and inner thighs, sparing flexures. Therapy consists of ensuring that the baby remains dry and the use of soothing and protective creams (zinc cream) or a mild topical steroid (hydrocortisone or desonide).

Summary: Napkin dermatitis affects the rounded contours of buttocks in infants due to prolonged contact with urine. The erythema, oedema and erosions spare the flexures. Keeping the baby dry and using zinc cream or hydrocortisone is helpful.

LICHEN SIMPLEX CHRONICUS (CHRONIC LICHENIFIED DERMATITIS, CIRCUMSCRIBED NEURODERMATITIS)

This is the result of persistent rubbing and scratching of an area of the skin. The initiating cause for the pruritus could be a transient chemical or mechanical irritation or even an allergic contact dermatitis or underlying atopy. At times, it may be the result of a habit tic and is then termed as circumscribed neurodermatitis. Whatever the initiating cause the itch-scratch-itch cycle perpetuates the condition.

Patient Profile

Most patients are adults, although atopic children are occasionally affected. Both sexes are equallly affected.

Morphology

Fairly well defined, hyperpigmented thick plaques with prominence of normal crisscross skin markings are characteristic of this conditions (Fig. 9.6). The skin becomes thickened and may occasionally show tiny crusts or erosions, indicative of the effects of scratching.

Distribution

Most of the sites of affection are those that are easy to rub or scratch and exposed to the environment. Hence, dorsa of feet, ankles, wrists, extensor forearms and posterior neck are the some of the common sites.

Chapter

9

Eczemas

Diagnosis

Ruling out contact dermatitis is an important consideration, as otherwise, relapse is likely.

Therapy

Since the itch-scratch-itch cycle is primarily responsible for perpetuating the condition, realisation by the patient about this phenomenon is essential. Potent topical corticosteroids break the cycle by relieving pruritus. Fluocinolone acetonide or beclomethasone dipropionate or betamethasone valerate creams are effective for milder cases. Oral antihistamines may be used initially to relieve pruritus.

Resistant cases may be treated with clobetasol or halobetasol propionate or betamethasone dipropionate. Efficacy of topical steroids can be enhanced combining them with 3–6% salicylic acid ointment or by occluding the area for 6–8 hours, with a plastic film, after the steroid application. Residual lesions may be injected with triamcinolone acetonide suspension. When using potent topical steroids or intralesional steroids, the patient must be observed regularly by the doctor to detect any signs of skin atrophy due to steroids. Mometasone and fluticasone are fairly potent steroids with lesser chance of inducing skin atrophy.

Summary: Lichen simplex chronicus is a plaque of chronic lichenified dermatitis that results from persistent rubbing of an area, as an end result of any localised eczema or a habit tic. Prominence of skin markings, hyperpigmentation and thickening are features of lichenification. Potent topical steroids like clobetasol or betamethasone with or without salicylic acid and if needed under plastic film occlusion, are effective. Resistant lesions respond to intralesional steroid injection. Mometasone and fluticasone are potent and safe topical steroids.

XEROTIC ECZEMA (WINTER ECZEMA)

A result of excessive drying of the skin, this is common in the cool and dry climates of central and northern India. Overzealous use of a strong alkaline soap is an added causative factor (Fig. 9.22).

Patient Profile

Individuals with the 'dry' skin type are predisposed. Elderly persons and children are frequently affected. Rarely, it may be a manifestation of an underlying systemic disorder like hypothyroidism or lymphoma. Genetic traits like atopy or ichthyosis may be associated.

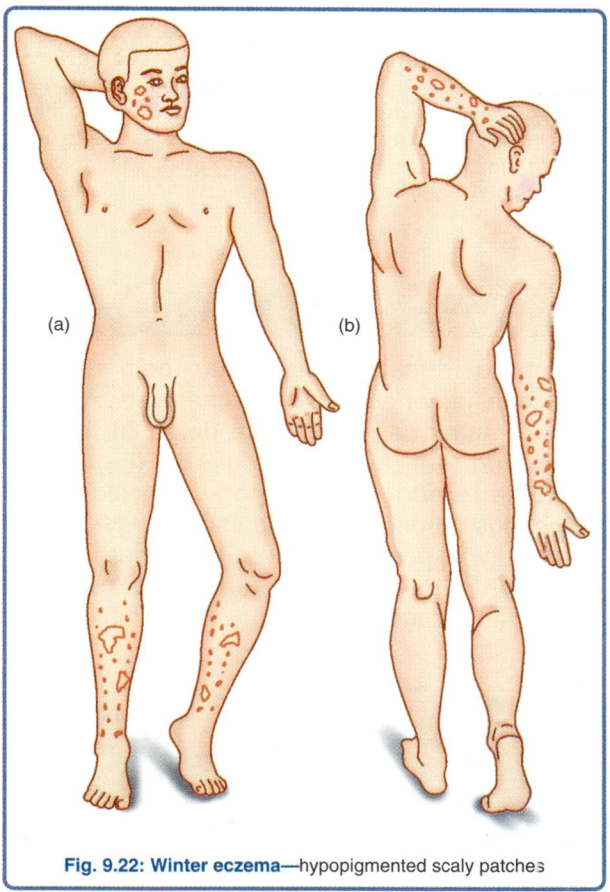

Fig. 9.22: Winter eczema—hypopigmented scaly patches

Morphology

Ill-defined, rounded, dry, scaly and hypopigmented patches are the initial lesions. Later, crusting, oozing and fissuring overlie these patches which turn erythematous and oedematous.

Distribution

Extensors of the extremities and face are the preferred sites. Extensors of forearms and arms, shins, lateral thighs and back are thus affected. Cheeks and sides of face are commonly involved in children.

Therapy

Avoidance of soap or sparing use of a mild soap (glycerin containing or neutral or moisturising soap) and frequent application of a cold cream (oil based) or vanishing cream (water based) impoves most patients. Occlusive and moisturising agents like white soft paraffin, liquid paraffin, lactic acid or urea are the active components of most of these creams. Topical steroids are useful in bringing about rapid resolution in a severe case. However, correction of predisposing factors is essential for maintaining remission.

Chapter **9**

Eczemas

Summary: Individuals with 'dry type' of skin, especially eldelry and children, tend to develop xerotic eczema during winter. Dry, hypopigmented, ill-defined patches with fine scales over extensors and face are typical. Oozing, crusting and fissuring occurs later. Avoidance of soap and use of moisturisers improves most cases. Mild topical steroids may be used to bring it under control with rapidity.

NUMMULAR ECZEMA

It is characterised by nummular (coin shaped) areas of acute or subacute eczema over extensors of extremities especially, the dorsa of fingers, hands and feet (Figs 9.1 and 9.5), (Fig. 9.23]. Combined endogenous (atopy, dry skin) and exogenous (strong soaps, contact allergy) factors are usually responsible. Correction of these factors along with the use of a topical steroid and moisturiser induce remission.

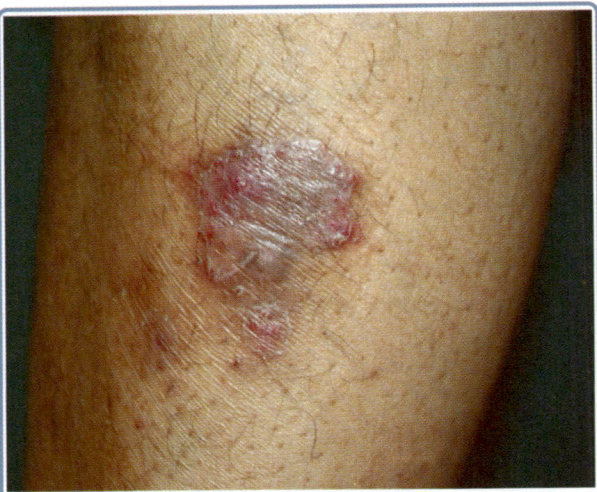

Fig. 9.23: Dry nummular eczema is common in winter. Needs differentiation from psoriasis

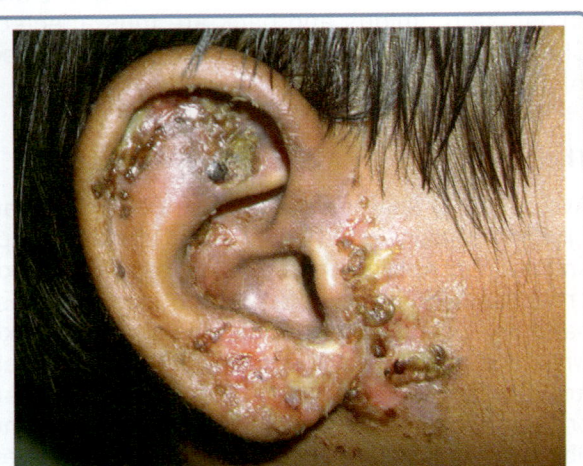

Fig. 9.25: Bacterial eczema—vesiculopustules, erosions with purulent discharge and seropurulent crusts

STASIS ECZEMA

This eczema occurs around the ankles in a setting of venous stasis of legs (Fig. 9.24). Stasis pigmentation, varicose veins or ulcer accompany the eczema lesions. Leg elevation, elastic stockings to support venous drainage, avoidance of antiseptics and antibiotics that may irritate and sensitise the skin and a topical steroid cream are necessary.

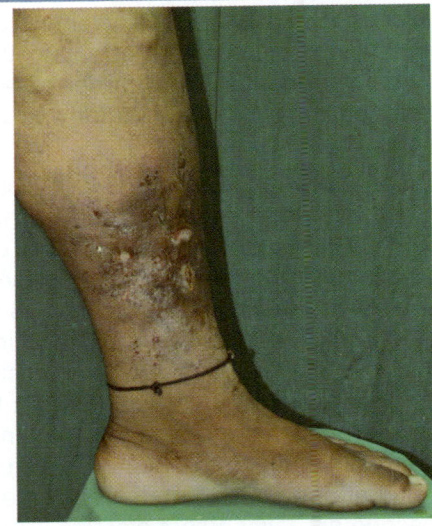

Fig. 9.24: Varicose eczema and ulceration—crusted papules and superficial ulcers on background of erythematous hyperpigmented plaque in a patient with varicose veins

BACTERIAL ECZEMA (INFECTIVE ECZEMA)

This follows persistent drainage of pus on to the surrounding normal skin, from a discharging lesion, like an abscess or osteomyelitis. The affected skin shows features of acute eczema with prominent purulent crusts (Figs 9.25 and 9.26). Oral and topical antibacterials to treat the initiating pyogenic infection are essential. Rest of the treatment is that of acute eczema.

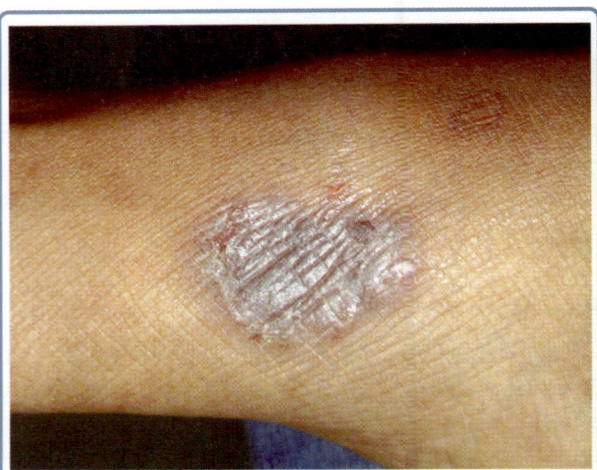

Fig. 9.26: Nummular eczema with superimposed secondary bacterial infection—purulent crusts are indicative

MCQs

1. **Which of the following is a form of endo-genous eczema?**
   a. Contact allergic dermatitis
   b. Contact irritant dermatitis
   c. Cumulative contact irritant dermatitis
   d. Atopic dermatitis

2. **Which of the following is not an exogenous eczema?**
   a. Irritant dermatitis
   b. Phototoxic dermatitis
   c. Photoallergic dermatitis
   d. Pompholyx

3. **Which of the following eczema changes its appearance with increasing age?**
   a. Contact allergic dermatitis
   b. Contact irritant dermatitis
   c. Seborrhoeic dermatitis
   d. Atopic dermatitis

4. **All of the following are phases of atopic dermatitis *except*:**
   a. Infantile   b. Childhood
   c. Adolescent   d. Geriatric

5. **Atopic dermatitis in adults preferably affects:**
   a. Face
   b. Scalp
   c. Antecubital and popliteal fossae
   d. Elbows and knees

6. **Infantile atopic dermatitis preferentially affects:**
   a. Face
   b. Scalp
   c. Flexures of extremities
   d. Hands and feet

7. **Atopic dermatitis in young children pre-ferentially affects:**
   a Face
   b. Scalp
   c. Flexures of extremities
   d. Extensors of extremities

8. **The circulating immunoglobulin raised in atopic dermatitis is:**
   a. IgA   b. IgE
   c. IgG   d. IgM

9. **Under the umbrella term 'atopy' are included all of the following *except*:**
   a. Childhood asthma   b. Allergic rhinitis
   c. Atopic dermatitis   d. Contact dermatitis

10. **All of the following should be avoided in atopic dermatitis *except*:**
    a. Woolen clothes
    b. Strong soaps
    c. Alcohol consumption
    d. Oil application

11. **Atopic dermatitis in adults presents usually as:**
    a. Lichenified plaques
    b. Oozing plaques
    c. Plaques studded with pustules
    d. Papules topped by vesicles

12. **Atopic dermatitis in infants presents commonly as:**
    a. Lichenified plaques
    b. Oozing plaques
    c. Plaques studded with pustules
    d. Nodules studded with pustules

13. **A non-steroidal topical agent that helps in improving atopic dermatitis is:**
    a. Calcipotriol   b. Tacrolimus
    c. Anthralin   d. Tazarotene

14. **One of the associations of atopic dermatitis is:**
    a. Seborrhoeic dermatitis
    b. Psoriasis
    c. Lichen planus
    d. Urticaria

15. **Which of the following is not usually advised in atopic dermatitis?**
    a. Avoidance of strong soap
    b. Emollients
    c. Drying lotions
    d. Soothing baths

16. **All of the following are common sites for lichen simplex chronicus *except*:**
    a. Dorsa of feet
    b. Nape of neck
    c. Trunk
    d. Antecubital fossae

Chapter 9

Eczemas

17. **All of the following are features of atopic dermatitis in an adult** *except*:
    a. Oozing plaques
    b. Lichenified plaques
    c. Affection of flexures
    d. Family history of atopy

18. **Lichenification is a combination of following morphological features** *except*:
    a. Hyperpigmentation
    b. Thickening of skin
    c. Prominence of dermatoglyphic lines
    d. Prominence of skin markings

19. **Seborrhoeic dermatitis of scalp needs to be differentiated from:**
    a. Psoriasis
    b. Pityriasis rosea
    c. Pityraisis versicolor
    d. Photodermatitis

20. **Another name for seborrhoeic dermatitis of scalp is:**
    a. Pityriasis versicolor
    b. Pityriasis rosea
    c. Pityriasis sicca
    d. Pityriasis lichenoides

21. **Seborrhoeic dermatitis is believed to be due to overgrowth of:**
    a. *Staphylococcus aureus*
    b. *Streptococcus hemophilus*
    c. *Trichophyton capitis*
    d. Malassezia

22. **Seborrhoeic dermatitis is associated with increased activity of:**
    a. Apocrine sweat glands
    b. Eccrine sweat glands
    c. Sebaceous glands
    d. Mucinous glands

23. **Which of the following sites is not affected in seborrhoeic dermatitis?**
    a. Palms and soles
    b. Eyebrows
    c. Nasolabial folds
    d. Back

24. **Scales in seborrhoeic dermatitis are:**
    a. Silvery
    b. Thick
    c. Yellowish
    d. Collarette

25. **Nummular dermatitis commonly affects the:**
    a. Forearms and hands
    b. Palms and soles
    c. Back
    d. Flexures

26. **Contact allergic dermatitis commonly affects the:**
    a. Forearms and legs
    b. Hands and Palms
    c. Back
    d. Extensor of limbs

27. **A typical site of affection in contact dermatitis due to nail polish allergy is:**
    a. Eyelids
    b. Neck
    c. Hands
    d. Back

28. **Contact allergy to this metal is common in ladies:**
    a. Nickel
    b. Silver
    c. Gold
    d. Platinum

29. **Contact allergic dermatitis is due to Coombs and Gell hypersensitivity of:**
    a. Type I
    b. Type II
    c. Type III
    d. Type IV

30. **Hair dye allergy is due to the chemical:**
    a. Para-propylene diamine
    b. Para-phenylene diamine
    c. Para-tertiary butyl phenol
    d. Para-methylene diamine

31. **Which is not a common site for nickel allergy?**
    a. Ears
    b. Scalp
    c. Forearms
    d. Neck

32. **Contact leucoderma refers to occurrence of:**
    a. Spread of leucoderma through skin-to-skin contact
    b. Contact allergic dermatitis leading to leucoderma
    c. Chemical induced irritant dermatitis leading to leucoderma
    d. Leucoderma at the site of contact of chemicals

33. **Dermatitis from detergents is usually due to:**
    a. Irritant contact dermatitis
    b. Cumulative irritant contact dermatitis
    c. Contact allergic dermatitis
    d. Photocontact allergic dermatitis

34. **A test that can prove contact allergic dermatitis is:**
    a. Skin prick test
    b. Skin patch test
    c. Skin biopsy
    d. Skin confocal microscopy

35. Patch test is read after:
a. 24 hours
b. 48 hours
c. 2 weeks
d. 4 weeks

36. This cream is useful for prevention of contact dermatitis:
a. Steroid cream
b. Barrier cream
c. Calcipotriol cream
d. Emollient cream

37. While managing contact dermatitis, this must be avoided:
a. Oral antihistamines
b. Oral steroids
c. Allergen
d. Topical steroids

38. Morphology of this contact dermatitis resembles burns:
a. Irritant contact dermatitis
b. Cumulative irritant contact dermatitis
c. Contact allergic dermatitis
d. Photoallergic contact dermatitis

39. Seborrhoeic dermatitis is associated with:
a. Lipid storage disorders
b. Diabetes mellitus
c. Hypertension
d. Parkinson's disease

40. The itch that rashes, is:
a. Atopic dermatitis
b. Insect bite
c. Seborrhoeic dermatitis
d. Tinea cruris

41. All of the following about atopic dermatitis are true, *except*:
a. Pruritus
b. Chronic relapsing course
c. Mica like scales
d. Xerosis

42. Most common cause of airborne contact dermatitis in india is:
a. Parthenium
b. Celery
c. Crysophilus
d. Chrysanthemum

43. Coin shaped eczema is:
a. Nummular eczema
b. Atopic eczema
c. Infantile eczema
d. Seborrhoeic dermatitis

Chapter 9

Eczemas

ANSWERS

1-d,	2-d,	3-d,	4-d,	5-c,	6-a,	7-d,	8-b,	9-d,	10-d,
11-a,	12-b,	13-b,	14-a,	15-c,	16-c,	17-a,	18-c,	19-a,	20-c,
21-d,	22-c,	23-a,	24-c,	25-a,	26-a,	27-a,	28-a,	29-d,	30-b,
31-b,	32-d,	33-b,	34-b,	35-b,	36-b,	37-c,	38-a,	39-d,	40-a,
41-c,	42-a,	43-a							

Acne Vulgaris and Rosacea

ACNE VULGARIS

This condition is so common in adolescence that it may be considered physiological to have a few lesions of acne vulgaris at some time during adolescence and young adulthood. However, incidence of acne is low in some countries (e.g. Japan) indicating that perhaps genetic make-up of a person plays some role in pathogenesis.

Etiology

Underlying factors include:

- **Androgens:** Spurt in androgen production during puberty and adolescence is responsible for increased activity of sebaceous glands. Early onset of puberty may lead to earlier onset of acne.

- **Follicular keratinisation:** Abnormality of keratinisation of the hair follicles plays an important role in the pathogenesis of acne. Mechanism of this abnormality is ill understood.

- *Propionibacterium acnes:* These commensal bacteria are markedly increased in number, in subjects with acne. Other microbes like staphylococci and pityrosporum are inconsistently isolated from acne lesions.

- **Heredity:** Excessive sebaceous gland activity is probably due to variation in end organ response to androgens and this may be genetically controlled. Hence, patients with severe acne frequently have parents with acne scars. Acne prevalence is much less in mongoloid races.

Pathogenesis

The non-inflammatory papules of acne are primarily due to abnormal follicular keratinisation. It is hypothesized that the resultant formation of keratotic plugs at follicular ostia leads to obstruction to the flow of sebum and dilation of the follicle (Fig. 10.1).

Inflammatory papules and pustules of acne develop from non-inflammatory lesions. Follicular obstruction in combination with excess sebum production may lead to internal rupture of the follicular wall. This brings the dermis into contact with several proteases and lipases, leading to acute inflammation.

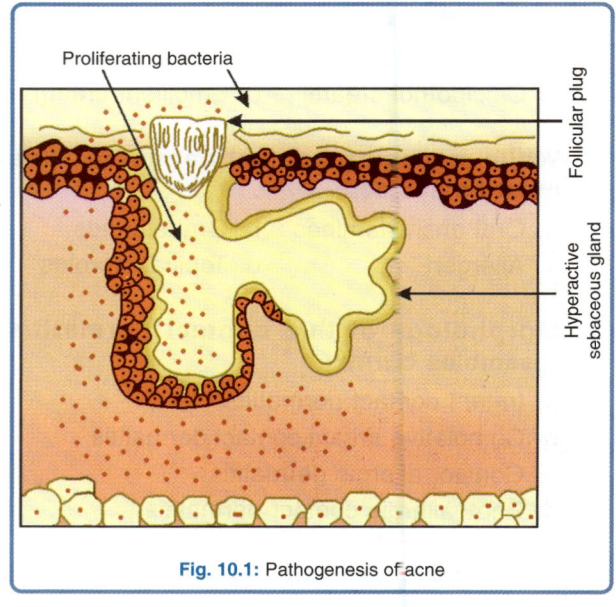

Fig. 10.1: Pathogenesis of acne

Raised bacterial count in skin of patients with acne, adds to the inflammation as bacteria break down fatty acids in the sebum to short chain fatty acids that initiate inflammation.

When inflammation is acute and severe, it leads to formation of tiny abscesses (clinically seen as pustules) within and around follicles. Healing of such follicular and perifollicular microabscesses results in the long standing and distressing sequalae of acne, i.e. acne scars. When deep, these larger abscesses may form pseudocysts that tend to run a longer course than the pustules. In the severest variety of acne, numerous such pseudocysts, draining sinuses and hypertrophic scars are seen.

Patient Profile

Adolescents and young adults are typically affected. However, the stress of city life and increased use of cosmetics may lead acne to persist in middle age of may even rarely begin during middle age. Men are more severely affected than women. If acne begins during middle age in a woman or when unusually severe acne is seen in a woman, an endocrinologic cause should be sought. Contact with oil and oily preparations (e.g. oil based make-up moisturisers or even oily sunscreens) tend to aggravate acne. Hot and humid environment and resultant sweating may exacerbate acne. Premenstrual flare of acne in women is well known.

Morphology

According to clinical severity, a simplified grading of acne is of the following types:

- **Grade I (non-inflammatory acne, comedonal acne):** Skin coloured papules (whiteheads, closed comedones), 1–2 mm in diameter (Fig. 10.2), with a central whitish dot representing a follicular opening, are the earliest lesions of acne. Little larger, conical papules with a central dilated follicular pore that houses a black plug are called blackheads or open comedones (Figs 10.3–10.5). A few erythematous papules may also be present at this stage.

- **Grade II (papulopustular acne):** Multiple erythematous, conical, follicular papules, 2–4 mm in diameter, some of these topped by tiny pustules (Figs 10.6–10.10), are observed. Sometimes, follicular pustules may predominate.

- **Grade III (papulonodular acne):** A few larger (more than 5 mm) indurated erythematous nodules are present. Larger and deeper pustules may also occur.

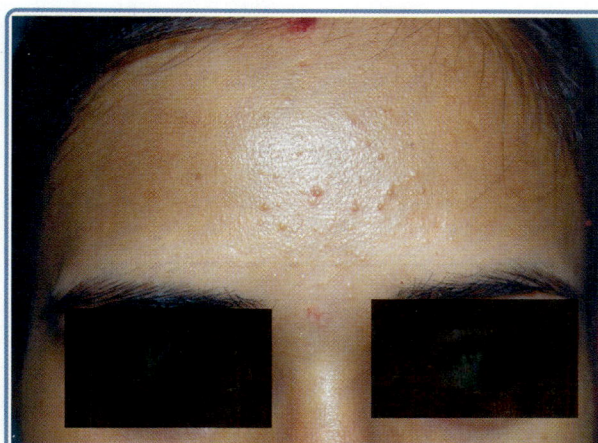

Fig. 10.2: Mild acne—skin coloured papules, i.e. whiteheads (closed comedones)

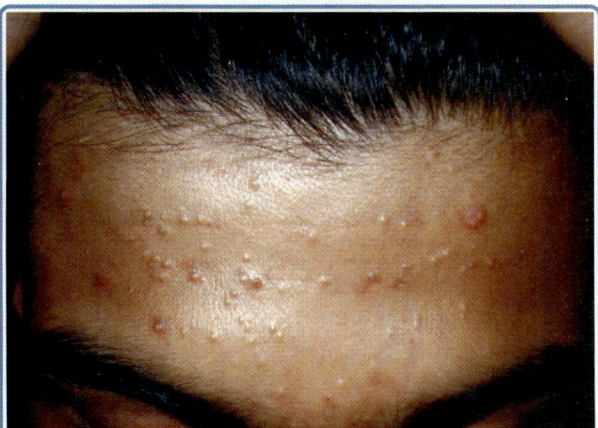

Fig. 10.3: Moderate acne—closed comedones and erythematous papules. Skin coloured papules (whiteheads) and a few papules with central black plugs (blackheads)

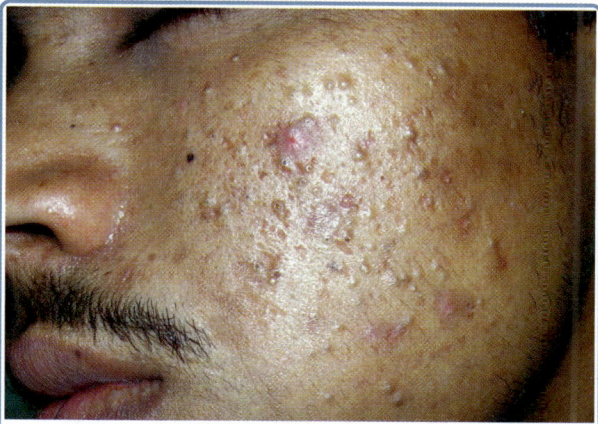

Fig. 10.4: Acne vulgaris—closed comedones (whiteheads) and pitted scars

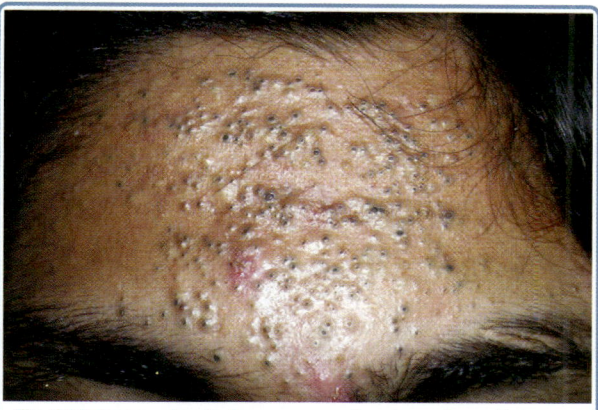

Fig. 10.5: Acne vulgaris (severe comedonal acne)—multiple open comedones with black plugs

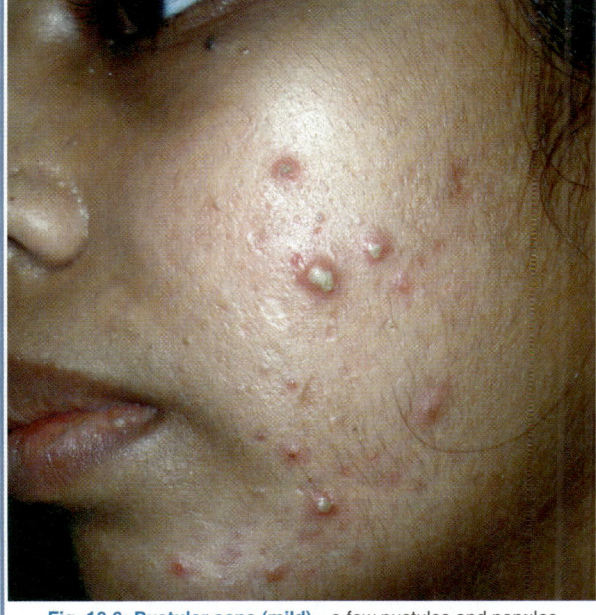

Fig. 10.6: Pustular acne (mild)—a few pustules and papules

- **Grade IV (nodulocystic acne):** Large skin coloured and erythematous indurated nodules and their sequelae characterise this stage. Such painful nodules progress slowly to form

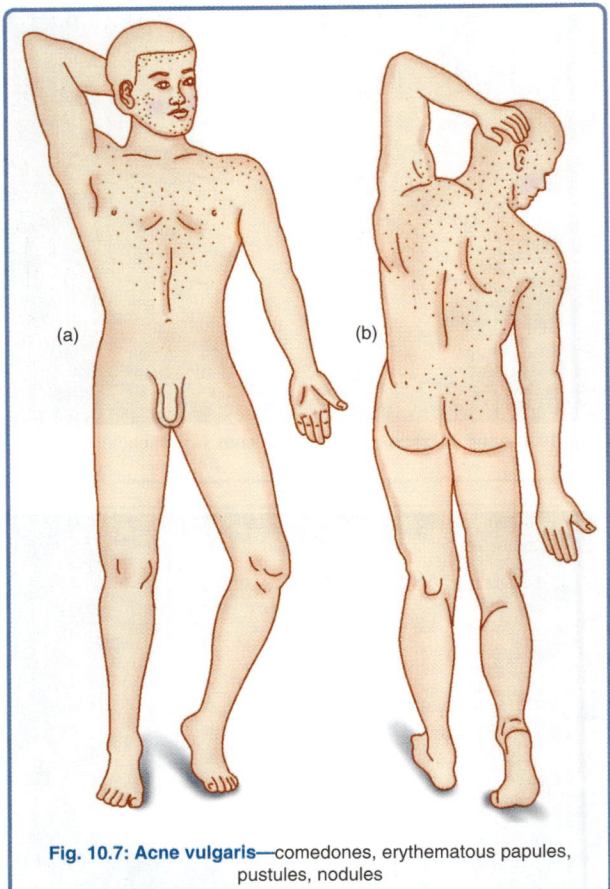

Fig. 10.7: Acne vulgaris—comedones, erythematous papules, pustules, nodules

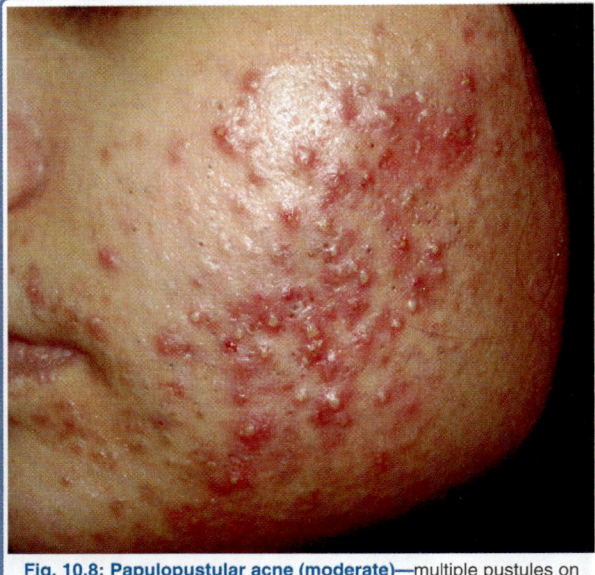

Fig. 10.8: Papulopustular acne (moderate)—multiple pustules on erythematous background and closed comedones

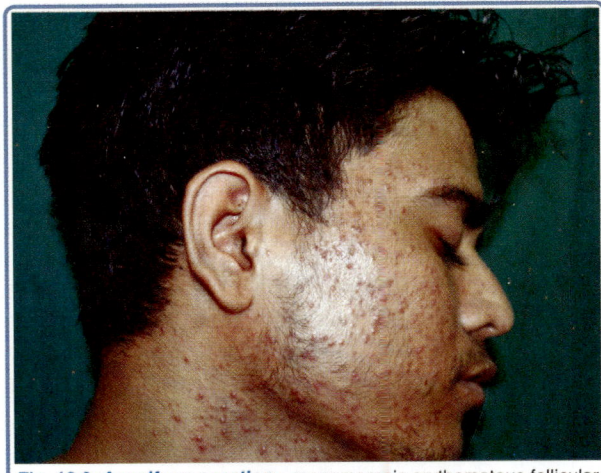

Fig. 10.9: Acneiform eruption—monomorphic erythematous follicular papules

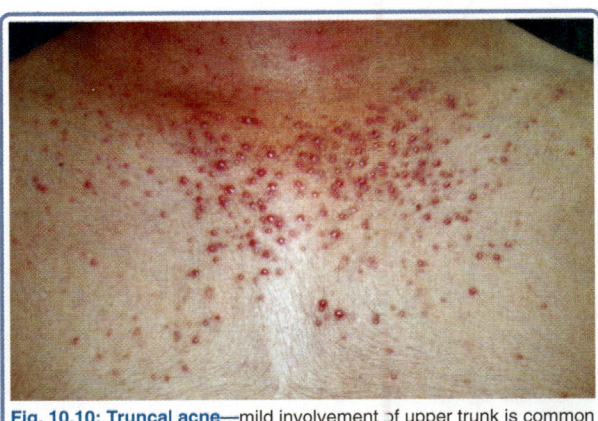

Fig. 10.10: Truncal acne—mild involvement of upper trunk is common in acne vulgaris

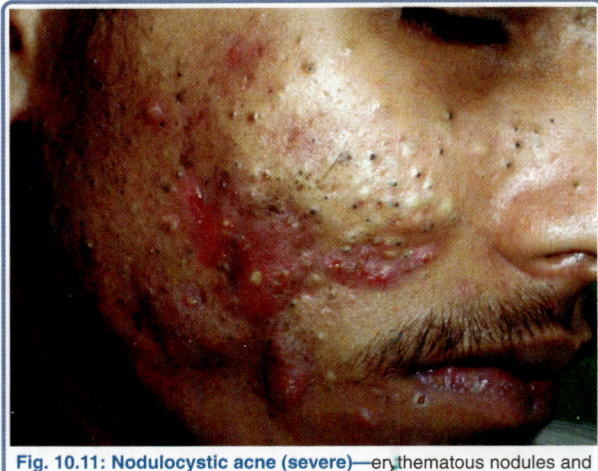

Fig. 10.11: Nodulocystic acne (severe)—erythematous nodules and multiple open comedones

painless cystic swellings (Figs 10.11 and 10.12) that ultimately rupture and heal with scars. Sometimes such scarring may be hypertrophic and be then associated with discharging sinuses with interconnecting sinus tracts (Figs 10.13 and 10.14). Large open comedones are common. Such severe nodulocystic acne has been termed as acne conglobata.

In severe grades of acne, lesions representing milder grades are usually present.

Distribution

Forehead, cheeks, nose and chin are the affected areas on face. Although, face is involved in most

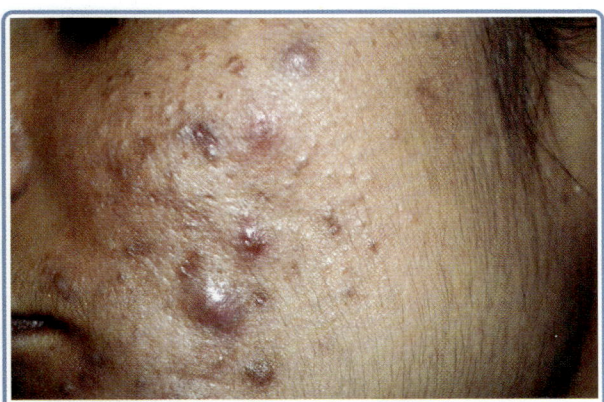

Fig. 10.12: Acne vulgaris (moderate)—occasional nodule in papular acne

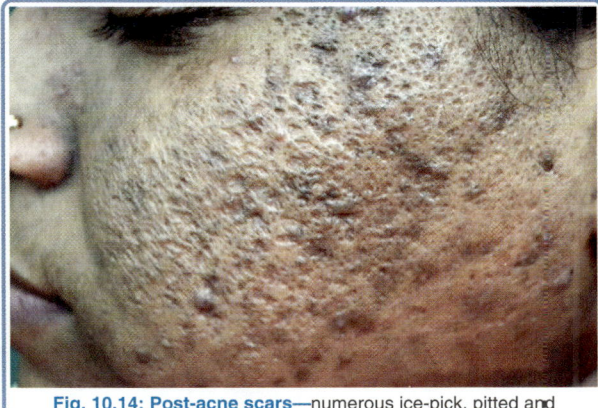

Fig. 10.14: Post-acne scars—numerous ice-pick, pitted and variolliform scars following acne

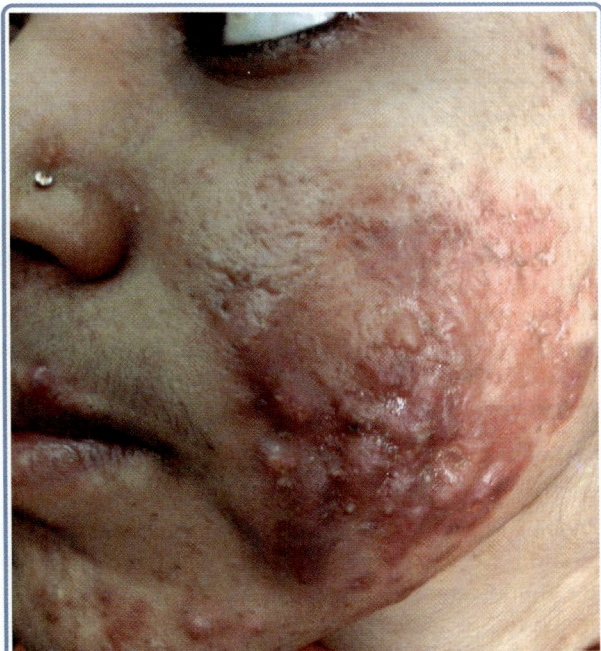

Fig. 10.13: Nodulocystic acne (severe)—erythematous nodules and pus discharging sinuses, healing with scarring. Severe acne is uncommon in women

cases, other regions like upper back, chest, shoulders and upper arms frequently bear some lesions. Lower back and buttocks are also affected in the nodulocystic and conglobate variety.

Complications of Acne

- Psychological impact of acne on the personality development of an adolescent or on job performance of a young adult is tremendous.
- Large painful nodules are uncomfortable enough, but their progression to abscesses, cysts and discharging sinuses can be disabling.
- Facial scarring due to acne vulgaris is an important complication because of its cosmetic importance and psychological sequelae. Several types of scars seen in patients with

acne include pitted scars, ice pick scars, varioliform scars, atrophic scars, hypertrophic scars, keloidal scars, bridge like scars, etc.

- Systemic symptoms rarely accompany severe acne (acne fulminans). Fever, myalgia, arthralgia have been described.

Treatment

General advice for a case of acne has always included frequent (2–4/day) washing of face with antibacterial soap and water. This is believed to reduce facial oiliness, check bacterial count, soften comedones and cause mild peeling that helps in opening follicular ostia. Special soaps for acne sometimes contain abrasive cleaners. Controlling possible contributing factors like hot and humid environment, of contact with oil or hyper-androgenism in women is essential.

Topical Therapy

Topical agents are aimed at either correcting the defect in keratinisation (adapalene, retinoic acid 0.025–0.05%) or checking bacterial count (clindamycin 1%, erythromycin 2%) or both (**benzoyl peroxide** 2.5–5%, sulphur 2%, resorcinol 1%). Topical adapalene and retinoic acid are preferred in patients with comedonal and papular acne whereas other agents are preferred in papulopustular acne. These agents may be combined to increase efficacy. Most of the agents do not cause any side effect other than skin irritation. Retinoic acid can cause photosensitivity (hence, applied at night) as well as initial worsening of skin lesions (Table 10.1).

Clinical implication: Initiation of therapy with retinoic acid and benzoyl peroxide must be done with a lower concentration and cream or gel may be washed off after a short time to avoid irritation. As the tolerance of skin increases higher concentrations can be used and left over the skin for longer periods.

Chapter
10

Acne Vulgaris and Rosacea

TABLE 10.1 : Topical therapy of acne

Agent	%	Action	Side Effect	Indication
Benzoyl peroxide	5%	Antibacterial Comedolytic	Irritation	Grade I–III
Adapalene	0.1%	Comedolytic	Less irritating as compared to retinoic acid	Grade I–III
Retinoic acid (tretinoin)	0.05%	Comedolytic	Irritation, photosensitivity	Grade I–III
Erythromycin	2–4%	Antibacterial	Contact allergy	Grade II–III
Clindamycin	1%	Antibacterial	Contact allergy	Grade II–III
Calamine lotion or cream with added :				
Sulphur	2%	Peeling agents	Irritation	Grade I–III
Salicylic acid	1%			
Resorcinol	1%			

Systemic Therapy

Patients with grade I acne and those with few inflammatory papules and pustules do not need any systemic therapy except vitamin A 25000–50000 IU daily orally. Dose should not exceed 1 lac units per day, else hypervitaminosis A could occur (Table 10.2).

Antibacterials

Tetracycline 250 mg QDS or doxycycline 100 mg OD or cotrimoxazole 1 tablet BD or erythromycin 250 mg QDS have comparable efficacy in conrolling acne that exceeds Grade II in severity. These agents have to be administered over extended periods varying from 2–6 months according to disease severity and patient response. Minocycline 50 mg BD has also given excellent results. Oral azithromycin 250 mg BD for 3 consecutive days every fortnight or month is also effective. Dapsone 100 mg OD is useful for Grade IV acne. Combining antibacterials with retinoids may prevent bacterial resistance.

Oral Retinoids

Isotretinoin 0.2–0.5 mg/kg body weight/day is better reserved for the treatment of moderate to severe acne (Grade II–IV). It reduces sebum secretion and affects resolution of existing lesions probably through its effect on follicular keratinisation and anti-inflammatory action. Because of its terato-genicity, it is absolutely contraindicated in women of childbearing age without proper counselling, and adequate contraceptive precaution. Women on isotretinoin should avoid pregnancy during treatment and up to 2 months after stoppage of isotretinoin.

Antiandrogens

Cyproterone acetate, 2 mg. In combination with ethinyl oestradiol 35 microgram, given cyclically (like oral contraceptives), is very effective in women not desiring conception. Side effects of oestrogens may be minimised by reducing the amount of ethinyl oestradiol to 20 mcg. Other oestrogen contraceptives were used in the past for the control of acne. However, they are now rarely used for this indication alone.

Other Modalities of Therapy

These are used occasionally and include aspiration of acne cysts and their injection with triamcinolone acetonide suspension, application of dry ice (CO_2) or exposure to ultraviolet light to induce peeling. Scars that follow acne can be dealt with, once control of the disease is achieved. Dermabrasion, excision, collagen injection, chemical peels and lasers are some of the methods used to improve acne scars.

Summary: Acne vulgaris is a common disorder of adolescence and young adults. Heredity, androgens, follicular occlusion, excess sebum production and proliferation of propionibacterium acnes, all play their role in its pathogenesis. Skin coloured follicular papules with central plugs (comedones), erythematous papules, nodules, pustules and cysts characterise the disease. Cheeks, forehead, chin, nose, neck, back and chest are the sites involved.

Topical antibacterials like benzoyl peroxide, erythromycin, clindamycin and topical adapalene or retinoic acid are effective in the control of mild to moderate acne. Oral antibacterials like tetracycline,

TABLE 10.2 : Systemic therapy of acne			
	Dose	**Main side effects**	**Indication**
Antibacterials			Grade II–IV
Tetracycline	250 mg QDS	Gastritis, candidiasis, diarrhoea and drug eruptions	
Doxycycline	100 mg OD	Gastritis	
Erythromycin	250 mg QDS	Gastritis hepatitis	
Azithromycin	250 mg BD x 3 days		
Minocycline	50–100 mg BD	Hyperpigmentation	
Cotrimoxazole	1 tab BD	Drug eruptions	
Anti-inflammatory antibacterial			
Dapsone	100–200 mg OD	Anaemia, drug eruptions	Grade V
Sebostatic (antiandrogens)			
Cyproterone	2 mg with cyclical oestrogen	Breakthrough bleeding, vaginal candidiasis	Grade II–IV in women
Sebostatic, keratostatic and anti-inflammatory (retinoids)			
Isotretinoin	10–20 mg OD for 8–12 weeks	Teratogenicity, hyperlipidaemia, dry skin and mucosae, hepatotoxicity	Grade II–IV in men

doxycycline, cotrimoxazole or erythromycin, given over many weeks, help in resolution of unresponsive or severer grades of the disease. Oral contraceptive pills, antiandrogens are options in females whereas oral isotretinoin is reserved for males with severe acne.

ROSACEA (ACNE ROSACEA)

A facial eruption in middle aged men and women, rosacea is quite unrelated to acne vulgaris. Facial flushing is a forerunner of rosacea in many instances. Aetiology of rosacea is not fully known. However, in addition to the role played by the mite Demodex folliculorum, factors that induce facial flushing also play a part in the pathogenesis of rosacea. Demodex folliculorum, a normal inhabitant of the follicular canal in humans, is increased in number in patients with rosacea. An associated change in the bacterial flora is also noted.

Patient Profile

Although, women are more commonly affected, rosacea occurs in males as well. Premenopausal or menopausal episodes of flushing may predispose to the occurrence of rosacea. Other exacerbating factors include sunlight and excess consumption of hot and coffeine containing beverages, spicy foods and alcoholic beverages.

Distinctly common in the midle aged, rosacea can sometimes affect younger adults.

Morphology

Bright red, easily blanchable, ill defined 2-5 mm macules, papules, some of them topped by tiny pustules, characterise this disease. (Fig. 10.16). A fixed flush of the rest of the face may accompany the lesions. In males, persistent affection of nose is associated with overgrowth of fibrofatty tissue that distorts the normal shape of nose (rhinophyma) (Figs 10.17 and 10.18).

Distribution

Both malar regions are usually involved symmetrically. Forehead, chin, nose and lips are also commonly affected. Uncommonly, lesions may extend to preauricular region, ears, neck and upper trunk. Conjunctivitis may also occur.

Therapy

Therapy is based on elimination of exacerbating factors mentioned above, and administration of antibacterial agents. Tetracycline 250 mg QDS, azithromycin 500 mg OD or roxithromycin 150 mg BD or doxycycline 100 mg OD are equally effective in short courses.

Chapter 10

Acne Vulgaris and Rosacea

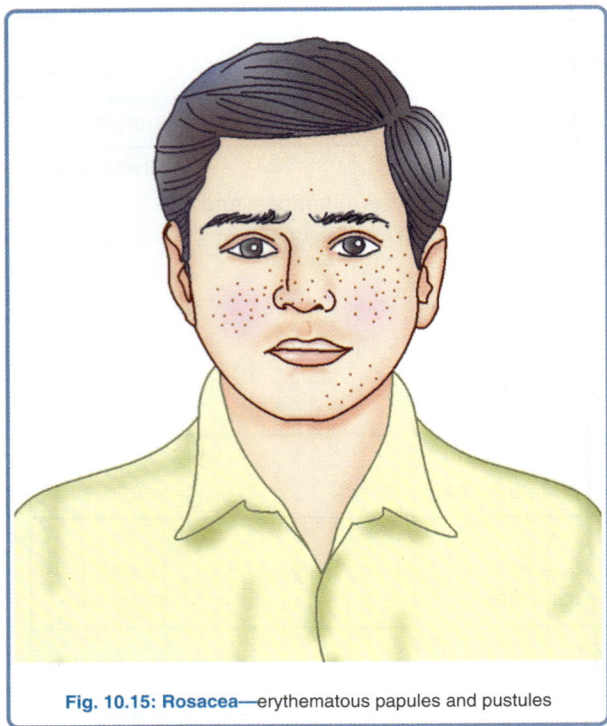

Fig. 10.15: Rosacea—erythematous papules and pustules

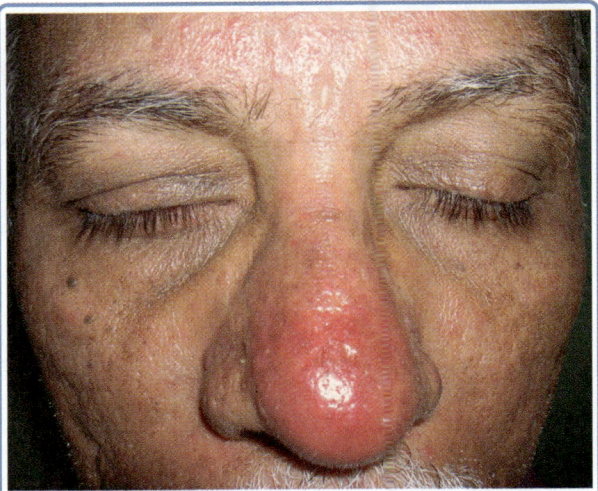

Fig. 10.17: Rhinophyma (early)—erythema, swelling and distortion of shape of nose

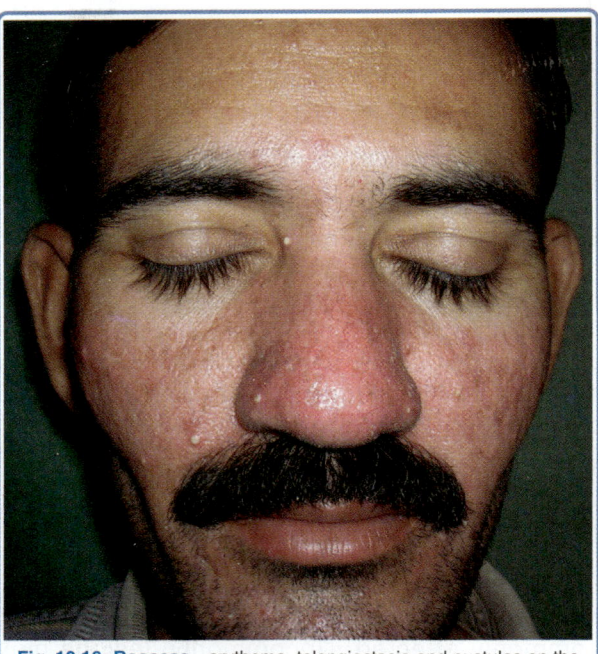

Fig. 10.16: Rosacea—erythema, telangiectasia and pustules on the nose and malar areas

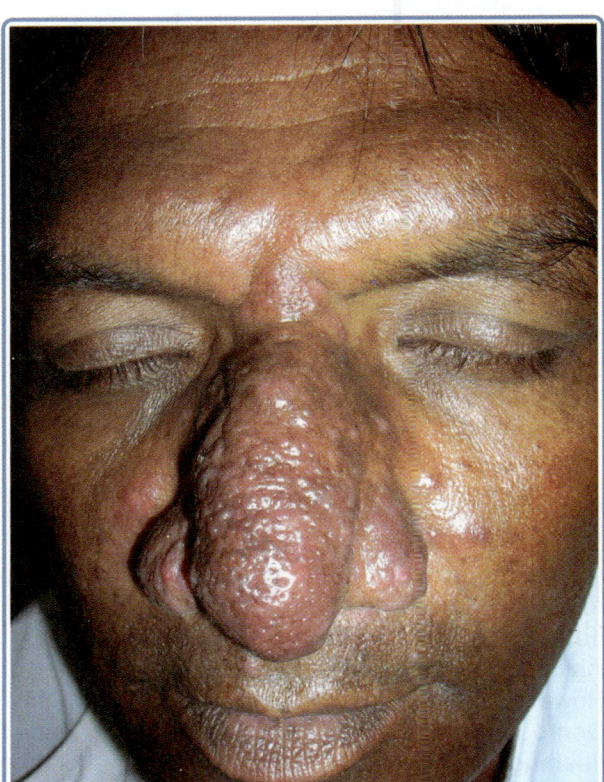

Fig. 10.18: Rhinophyma (advanced)—deformed and thickened nose along with erythematous papules and papulopustules

Topically, metronidazole 1% gel are effective. Topical steroids are contraindicated in general in rosacea. However, a milder steroid like hydrocortison 1% can be used to hasten improvement. Use of stronger topical steroids will temporarily clear the disease which rebounds after steroids are stopped. Besides, use of stronger topical steroids on face may result in skinatrophy.

Summary: Rosacea is unrelated to acne. Typically, it affects middle aged ladies. A facial eruption of bright red papules with a flare of erythema and topped by tiny pustules characterises the disease. Avoidance of sunlight, hot spicy foods, caffienated and alcoholic beverages is helpful. Topical benzoyl peroxide or metronidazole can control milder disease whereas systemic antibacterials like tetracycline or azithromycin are needed for severer cases. Topical 1% hydrocortisone may be used but stronger steroids are contraindicated due to the fear of rebound exacerbation and skin atrophy.

Perioral Dermatitis

An eruption of erythematous macules, papules, some of them topped with pustules, affecting the perioral region characterises this condition. A stereotypical patient is one who has been applying a fluorinated potent or moderately potent topical steroid over face. Discontinuation of steroid usage and a course of oral antibacterial like tetracycline or azithromycin is effective.

Topical Steroid Abuse on Face

Stronger and fluorinated topical steroids either alone or in combination with anti-acne agents on fairness creams have been used indiscriminately as a quick fix solution for all facial rashes including acne, rosacea or facial pigmentation problems like melasma. Use of these agents for more than a few weeks may result in what is described as 'steroid dermatitis'. Patients typically complain of a steroid dependent rash with extremely sensitive skin and photosensitivity. This type of skin is difficult to manage as withdrawal of the steroid cream results in worsening of earlier symptoms, sunscreens and soothing creams may help.

Chapter
10

Acne Vulgaris and Rosacea

MCQs

1. **Bacterial agent contributing to acne pathogenesis is:**
   a. Bacteroides
   b. Propionibacterium acnes
   c. Pityrosporum ovale
   d. Corynebacterium tenuis

2. **Topical antibiotic agents helpful in acne are all except:**
   a. Clindamycin
   b. Dapsone
   c. Erythromycin
   d. None of the above

3. **A teenager girl with moderate acne also complains irregular menses, the drug of choice in this patient will be:**
   a. Oral isotretinoin
   b. Oral acitretin
   c. Oral minocycline
   d. Cyproterone acetate and oestrogen pill

4. **For a 24-year-unmarried female with nodulocystic acne on face and back, the treatment of choice would be:**
   a. Acitretin
   b. Isotretinoin
   c. Doxycyclin
   d. Azithromycin

5. **Drugs capable of causing acne are:**
   a. Steroids
   b. Isoniazid
   c. Antiepileptics
   d. All of the above

6. **Acne vulgaris is due to involvement of:**
   a. Sebaceous gland
   b. Pilosebaceous unit
   c. Eccrine gland
   d. Apocrine gland

7. **Comedones are seen in:**
   a. Acne vulgaris
   b. Lichen planus
   c. Adenoma sebaceum
   d. Acne rosacea

8. **Rhinophyma is seen in:**
   a. Acne vulgaris
   b. Acne rosacea
   c. Seborrhoeic dermatitis
   d. Rhinosporidiosis

9. **Rhinophyma is associated with:**
   a. Septal deviation of nose
   b. Sweat gland hypertrophy
   c. Mucous gland hypertrophy
   d. Sebaceous gland hypertrophy

10. **Rosacea is characterised by all except:**
    a. Telangiectasia
    b. Pustules
    c. Papules
    d. Comedones

11. **Parasitic infestation commonly associated with rosacea:**
    a. Demodicosis
    b. Sarcoptes scabies
    c. Ascariasis
    d. Pediculosis capitis

12. **General advice to a patient with acne is all except:**
    a. Frequent washing of face
    b. Self removal of comedones
    c. Gentle padding of the wet face
    d. Avoid frequent touching of the lesions

13. **Retinoic acid should be applied at which time of the day?**
    a. Early morning before work
    b. Morning and evening
    c. Night
    d. Afternoon

14. **Retinoid dermatitis can be avoided by:**
    a. Using higher concentrations to allow development of tolerance
    b. Keeping it overnight
    c. Gradually increasing the concentration and duration of contact
    d. Mixing it with benzoyl peroxide

15. **First line agent for grade 4 acne is:**
    a. Oral contraceptives
    b. Oral isotretinoin
    c. Oral antibiotics
    d. Combination treatment

16. **Which of the following lesions of acne usually do not scar?**
    a. Comedones
    b. Pustules
    c. Nodules
    d. None of these

17. **A 40-year-old male presents with papulo-pustular lesions on the face and photosensitivity. The likely diagnosis is:**

    a. Rosacea
    b. Acne fulminans
    c. Lupus erythematosus
    d. Acne vulgaris

18. **Treatment of acne in pregnant women is:**

    a. Oral doxycycline
    b. Oral isotretinoin
    c. Oral contraceptives
    d. Topical clindamycin

19. **While starting a female patient on oral isotretinoin, it is important to discuss the following aspects:**

    a. Contraception
    b. Family or Personal history of hyperlipidaemia
    c. Compliance to therapy
    d. All of the above

ANSWERS

1-b,	2-d,	3-d,	4-b,	5-d,	6-b,	7-a,	8-b,	9-d,	10-d,
11-a,	12-b,	13-c,	14-c,	15-b,	16-a,	17-a,	18-d,	19-d	

Urticaria and Angioedema

URICARIA

Aetiology

Aetiologic classification is shown in Table 11.1.

Immunologic urticaria

Urticaria is commonly a type I hypersensitivity reaction (immunoglobulin E) mediated immediate hypersensitivity] of the skin to a variety of exogenous and endogenous antigens. Vascular dilation, the resultant dermal oedema and pruritus are caused by the release of histamine and other mediators from mast cells consequent upon binding of IgE antibodies to the antigens over cell surfaces. The causative antigens may be:

- **Exogenous**
  - ❑ **Ingestants**

    This includes drugs like sulphonamides, chloroquine and nonsteroidal anti-inflammatory drugs (NSAIDs) and foods like seafood, colouring agents (tartrazine), eggs, meat, spices and some vegetables, etc.

  - ❑ **Inhalants**

    Pollens, plant hair and animal dander.

  - ❑ **Injectants**

    Drugs like penicillins, insulin.

  - ❑ **Contactants**

    Bee stings, bug bites, animal dander, excreta and plants.

- **Endogenous**
  - ❑ **Infections—Bacterial**

    Upper respiratory tract infection, urinary tract infection and cholecystitis.

  - ❑ **Infestations**

    Helminthiasis, amoebiasis and giardiasis.

  - ❑ **Systemic diseases**

    Systemic lupus erythematosus.

Non-immunologic urticaria

Several of the above mentioned exogenous agents like animal and plant products or certain drugs like morphine, codeine, atropine, thiamine, pilocarpine, quinine or aspirin induce urticaria through non-immunologic mechanisms, e.g. morphine, atropine are histamine liberators.

TABLE 11.1: Aetiologic classification of urticaria
Spontaneous Urticarias
Acute urticaria
Chronic urticaria
Contact urticaria
Autoimmune Urticaria
Physical Urticarias
Dermographism
Delayed pressure urticaria
Vibratory angioedema
Cholinergic urticaria
Solar urticaria
Heat urticaria
Cold urticaria
Aquagenic urticaria
Angioedema without Wheals

Physical urticaria

Some cases of urticaria are mediated through a different mechanism, e.g. dermographism (Fig. 11.1) which is induced by trauma. Uncommonly, urticaria may be induced by cold (cold urticaria), sweating (cholinergic urticaria), sunlight (solar urticaria), pressure (pressure urticaria), or contact with water (aquagenic urticaria). These cases of urticaria are collectively termed as physical urticarias.

Autoimmune urticaria

Urticaria lasting more than 6 weeks is termed as chronic urticaria. About 30% cases of chronic

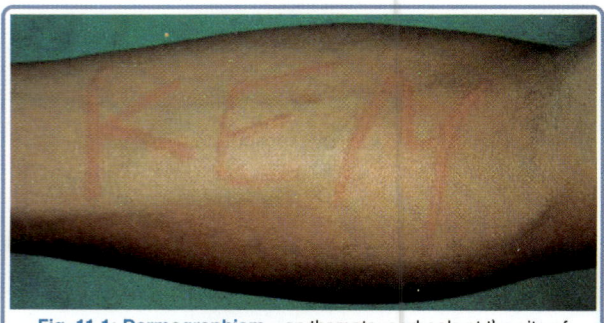

Fig. 11.1: Dermographism—erythematous wheals at the site of stroking of the skin

urticaria are due to a circulating antibody and these are termed as autoimmune urticaria.

Morphology

Lesions begin as pruritic ill defined erythematous macules or patches. They rapidly develop (within minutes) to form the typical lesions (called 'wheals') that are pale red oedematous papules or plaques with a brighter red periphery (Figs 11.2 and 11.3). Wheals are rounded or oval and closely placed lesions that may coalesce to form various shapes and sizes from a few mm to 20 cm (Fig. 11.4). A characteristic feature of wheals is that they are transient, lasting individually for less than 4–8 hours, although the condition may persist with appearance of new wheals.

Distribution

Any part of the body may be affected. Trunk is involved more commonly than extremities or face but, in a patient, it is common to obtain a history of involvement of various body regions. Mucosae may

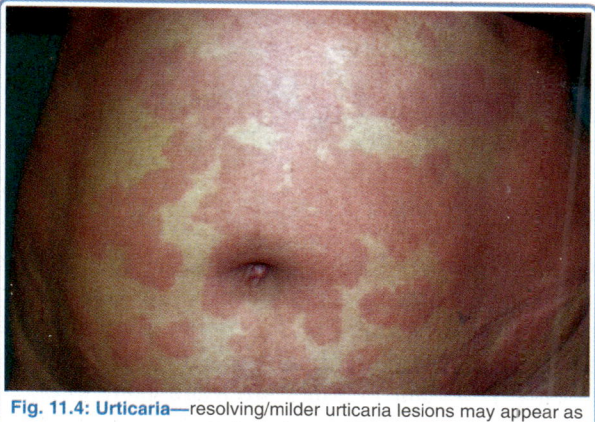

Fig. 11.4: Urticaria—resolving/milder urticaria lesions may appear as erythematous patches

also become swollen, lips being the commonest region affected.

Systemic Symptoms

Rhinitis, difficulty in breathing, sensation of heaviness in chest, wheezing and abdominal pain may accompany the skin lesions and are indications for urgent treatment to avoid the complication of laryngeal oedema.

Investigations

A detailed history is probably more important than a battery of investigations in the detection of a causative agent. However, in many instances of chronic urticaria (lasting more than 6 weeks) it is extremely difficult to pinpoint the allergen. A urine and stool analysis and a complete blood count should be done as screening investigations for any infections or infestations.

Allergy tests

Allergy testing may be done by intradermal scratch test or as estimation of levels of serum IgE directed specifically at each allergen (specific IgE). Both methods are equally unreliable with respect to the clinical relevance of results and are relatively expensive. Hence, although popular with patients, allergy testing is of help only to a minority of urticaria patients.

Tests for physical urticaria

These involve producing physical conditions of cold, heat, pressure, exercise or contact with water to induce lesions and urticaria.

Autologous serum skin test

Patients with autoimmune urticaria are allergic to a component of their blood. This can be

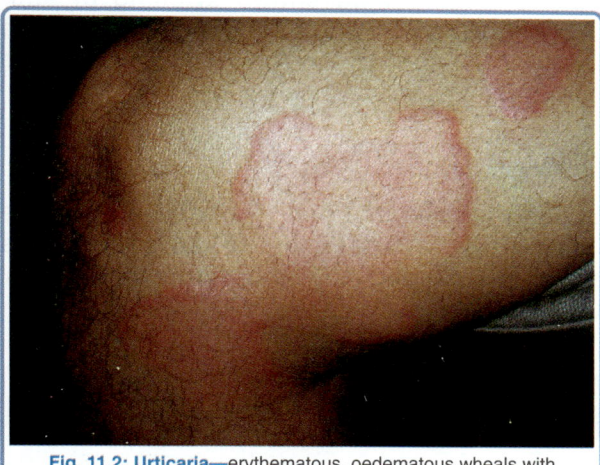

Fig. 11.2: Urticaria—erythematous, oedematous wheals with erythematous flare

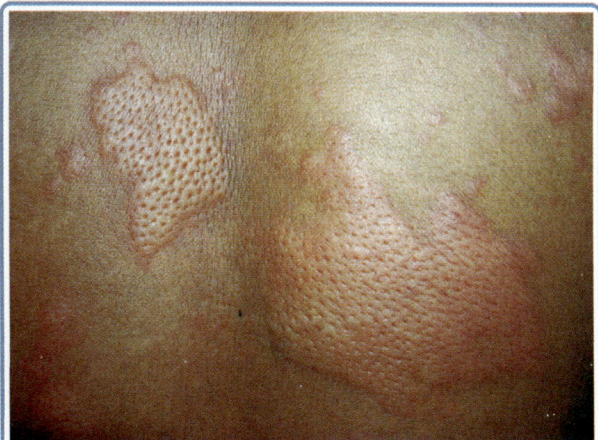

Fig. 11.3: Urticaria—erythematous plaques with peau-de-orange appearance

demonstrated by autologous serum skin test (ASST) in which urticarial wheal develops when a patient is injected with his/her own serum. Antithyroid antibodies have been used as a surrogate marker for autoimmune urticaria with limited utility.

Therapy

Acute urticaria should be attended to immediately, since this is usually a manifestation of a systemic type I hypersensitivity response and may be accompanied by laryngeal oedema and bronchospasm. The latter features are more likely to occur when angioneurotic oedema accompanies urticaria. For acute widespread urticaria, unaccompanied by bronchospasm. intramuscular antihistamines (e.g. pheniramine maleate) should be given initially and if there is no relief, be followed, after 1–2 hours, with intramuscular or intravenous hydrocortisone. If there is no response, intramuscular or subcutaneous adrenaline (0.5 mL of 1:1000 solution) brings about prompt relief. Cases with bronchospasm should be treated immediately with hydrocortisone and adrenaline in the above mentioned doses. Milder cases can be controlled with oral antihistamines.

TABLE 11.2: Antihistamines commonly used in dermatology

Group	Drug	Dose
Sedative	Pheniramine	25 mg TDS
	Hydroxyzine	10 mg TDS
	Cetirizine	10 mg OD or BD
	Loratidine	10 mg OD or BD
Non-sedative	Levocetirizine	5–10 mg/day
	Desloratidine	10–20 mg/day
	Fexofenadine	180 mg OD or BD
	Mizolastine	10 mg BD

An earnest attempt must be made to detect responsible endogenous or exogenous allergens and avoid them. Failing this, mild acute urticaria as well as chronic urticaria can usually be kept in check with oral antihistamines. Pheniramine maleate, 25 mg tds, is a frequently used drug. However, others like hydroxyzine, diphenhydramine and cyproheptadine are equally effective. If sedation is to be avoided, desloratidine or fexofenadine can be used. Such preventive treatment may extend to many weeks or even months for chronic urticaria if a treatable cause can't be found.

Summary: Urticaria is a Type I hypersensitivity reaction to a variety of internal (e.g. bacterial infections and parasitic infestations) and external (foods, drugs, insects, plant and animal products) allergens. A sudden but transient (lasting for a few hours) pruritic eruption of rounded or oval pale coloured papules and plaques with a halo of erythema is diagnostic. Any part of the body may be affected. Therapy includes avoidance of known allergens and oral antihistaminics like pheniramine maleate, hydroxyzine, loratidine or fexofenadine. Severe, acute urticaria responds to parenteral antihistamines, steroids and, if needed, subcutaneous adrenaline.

ANGIOEDEMA

Pathogenesis of this condition is similar to urticaria. However, it affects extremities, face, periorificial regions and mucosae. Please *see* the section on urticaria for aetiology and pathogenesis (page 130). Compared to urticaria, angioedema is, more commonly mediated through IgE antibodies against inciting allergen or is drug induced and sudden in onset. While urticaria lesions show oedema in the dermis angioedema shows swelling of subcutaneous fat of limbs and mucocutaneous junctions. Hereditary angioedema is rare and is due to C1 esterase deficiency.

Morphology

Sudden, diffuse and non-tender swelling of the involved parts is alarming to the patient. The swelling is soft and may be pale or erythematous. Urticarial wheals may co-exist.

Distribution

Bilateral affection is not uncommon. Eyelids and lips (Figs 11.5 and 11.6) are the commonest sites.

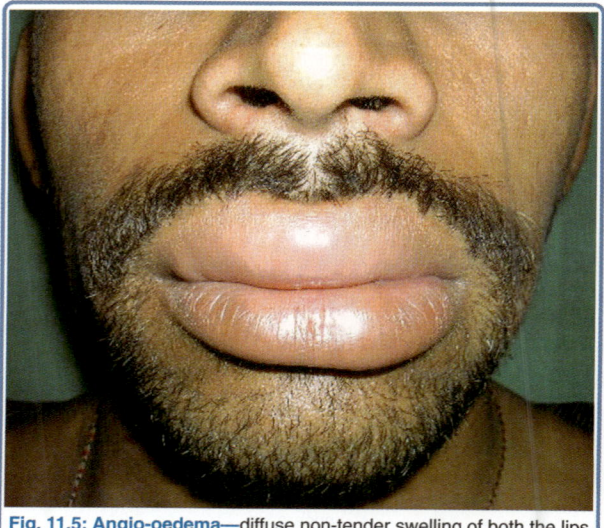

Fig. 11.5: Angio-oedema—diffuse non-tender swelling of both the lips

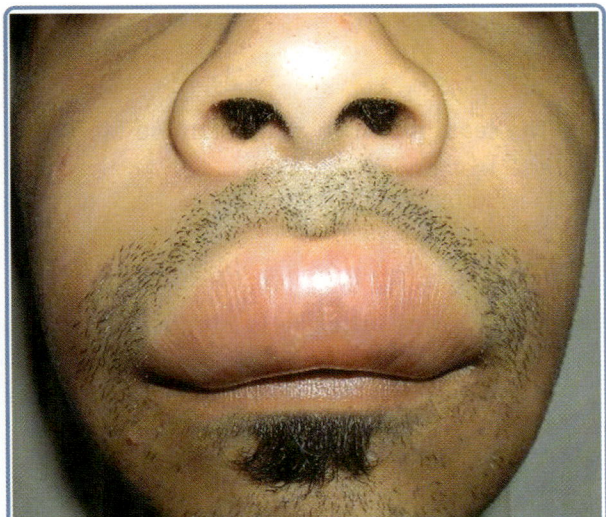

Fig. 11.6: Angio-oedema—marked painless swelling of the upper lip and face

Marked eyelid swelling can lead to chemosis with inability to open the eye. Lip and face involvement leads to distortion of face. Hands, forearms, feet, scrotum, vulva and penis may be affected, The most dangerous manifestation of angioneurotic oedema is the involvement of laryngeal mucosa.

Complications

Laryngeal oedema may occur suddenly and lead to obstruction of airway. This may end fatally, if not treated promptly with subcutaneous adrenaline and, if needed, tracheostomy. Involvement of bronchial mucosa also results in airway obstruction that manifests as wheezing and breathing difficulty.

Therapy

This is same as that for acute urticaria.

Summary: Urticaria and angioedema are aetiologically one condition. Involvement of subcutaneous tissue of limbs, mucosae, and mucocutaneous junctions leads to diffuse swelling and is termed as angioedema. By contrast urticaria involves only the dermis. Breathlesness, when associated with angioedema, indicates laryngeal or tracheobronchial mucosal affection and has to be treated urgently. It responds to parenteral antihistamines, steroids and, if needed, subcutaneous adrenaline.

For recurrent severe angioedema with breathing difficulty, it is safer to have quick access to adrenaline subcutaneous injections.

Chapter 11

Urticaria and Angioedema

MCQs

1. **The characteristic lesion of urticaria is:**
   a. Erythema
   b. Vesicle
   c. Prurigo-like papule
   d. Wheal

2. **For urticaria to be termed as chronic urticaria, it should have lasted at least:**
   a. 15 days
   c. 6 months
   b. 6 weeks
   d. 1 year

3. **Exogenous urticaria may be caused by all of the following except:**
   a. Ingestants
   b. Inhalants
   c. Contactants
   d. Infections

4. **Physical urticarias include all of the following except:**
   a. Cold urticaria
   b. Pressure urticaria
   c. Dermographism
   d. Contact urticaria

5. **Systemic symptom associated with urticaria may be:**
   a. Fever
   b. Pruritus
   c. Breathing difficulty
   d. Diarrhoea

6. **Endogenous urticaria may be due to all of these except:**
   a. Bacterial infections
   b. Parasitic infestations
   c. Viral infections
   d. Systemic lupus erythematosus

7. **All of these drugs are frequent causes of urticaria except:**
   a. Penicillins
   b. Insulin
   c. Aspirin
   d. Erythromycin

8. **This NSAID is less likely to cause urticaria than others:**
   a. Ibuprofen
   b. Diclofenac
   c. Indomethacin
   d. Paracetamol

9. **The least sedative antihistamine is:**
   a. Fexofenadine
   b. Hydroxyzine
   c. Levocetirizine
   d. Cetirizine

10. **This type of urticaria is mediated through IgE:**
    a. Type I hypersensitivity associated urticaria
    b. Autoimmune urticaria
    c. Physical urticarias
    d. Dermographism

11. **Severe acute urticaria not responding to injectable antihistamine therapy needs to be treated with:**
    a. Intramuscular atropine
    b. Intravenous adrenaline
    c. Intravenous hydrocortisone
    d. Intravenous ranitidine

12. **Angio-oedema with breathing difficulty should be immediately treated with:**
    a. Intravenous antihistamine
    b. Intravenous adrenaline
    c. Intramuscular adrenaline
    d. Subcutaneous adrenaline

13. **A common site for angioedema is:**
    a. Lips
    b. Genitals
    c. Arm
    d. Scalp

14. **A site not affected in angioedema is:**
    a. Eyelids
    b. Face
    c. Back
    d. Feet

15. **The worst complication of angioedema is:**
    a. Bronchospasm
    b. Laryngeal oedema
    c. Angina
    d. Pulmonary oedema

16. **A 26-year-old man developed itchy weals all over the body since 5 days. On enquiry he had been treated with metronidazole and diphenoxylate for colcky abdominal pain and bulky stools 6 weeks back with partial relief. What is the most probable cause for his urticaria?**
    a. Amoebiasis
    b. Diphenoxylate
    c. Metronidazole
    d. Urticaria pigmentosa

17. **A characteristic clinical feature of urticaria that helps it distinguish from other conditions is:**
    a. Extremely itchy
    b. Transient lesions
    c. Heal without leaving behind any mark
    d. All of the above

18. **A 2-year-old girl is brought with generalised urticaria since 2 days. On enquiry there was history of pica while playing in the garden and use of a deworming agent 2 months back. The most likely cause for her urticaria is:**
    a. Helminthiasis
    b. Atopy
    c. Deworming agent
    d. Allergy to grass pollen

19. **A pathognomonic feature of urticaria is:**
    a. Nonpruritic
    b. Bullous
    c. Evanescent
    d. Macular

20. **A man takes peanut and develops tongue swelling, stridor, hoarseness of voice, what is the probable diagnosis:**
    a. Angio-oedema
    b. Foreign body in bronchus
    c. Parapharyngeal abscess
    d. Acute urticaria

21. **Physical urticaria includes:**
    a. Dermographism
    b. Urticaria pigmentosa
    c. Chronic idiopathic urticaria
    d. Autoimmune urticaria

22. **A patient has recurrent urticaria while doing exercise and on exposure to sunlight, the most likely cause:**
    a. Chronic idiopathic urticaria
    b. Heat urticaria
    c. Solar urticaria
    d. Cholinergic urticaria

Chapter
11

Urticaria and Angioedema

ANSWERS

1-d,	2-b,	3-d,	4-d,	5-c,	6-d,	7-d,	8-d,	9-a,	10-a,
11-c,	12-d,	13-a,	14-c,	15-b,	16-a,	17-d,	18-a,	19-c,	20-a,
21-a,	22-d								

Papulosquamous Diseases

Papulosquamous diseases are an aetiologically unrelated group of disorders that have one common clinical feature viz. the predominant morphology of lesions is papulosquamous, i.e. papules or plaques covered with scales. The list includes psoriasis, lichen planus, pityriasis rosea, seborrhoeic dermatitis (*see* Chapter 9, page 109), drug eruptions, pityriasis rubra pilaris and secondary syphilis (*see* Chapter 14, page 167).

PSORIASIS

A skin and joint disease with multifactorial aetiology, psoriasis affects 1–2% of the general population. Pustular and erythrodermic psoriasis may pose a threat to life whereas widespread skin and joint affection is disabling. However, these complications are uncommon (Fig. 12.1).

Aetiology

Exact cause is unknown, though the current thinking is that psoriasis is one of the commonest autoinflammatory diseases occurring in humans. Familial occurrence suggests genetic predisposition. Mechanical, chemical or radiation trauma can initiate or worsen psoriasis (Koebner phenomenon). Drugs like chloroquine, lithium, beta-blockers, and non-steroidal anti-inflammatory drugs (NSAIDs) can worsen or induce psoriasis. Withdrawal of systemic corticosteroids in a patient of psoriasis can precipitate an attack of erythrodermic or generalised pustular psoriasis. Usually, summer improves psoriasis and winter worsens it.

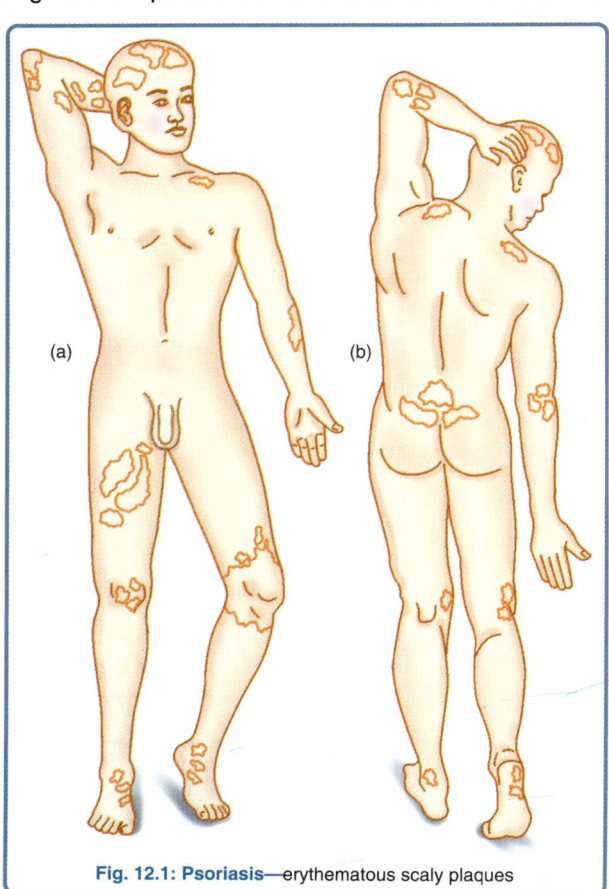

Fig. 12.1: Psoriasis—erythematous scaly plaques

Various Types of Papulosquamous Disorders
• Psoriasis
• Eczemas
• Pityriasis rosea
• Lichen planus
• Reiter's disease
• Pityriasis rubra pilaris
• Parapsoriasis
• Secondary syphilis

Clinical implication: Nonsteroidal anti-inflammatory drugs should be used under close supervision in treating psoriatic arthritis. Systemic corticosteroids are generally contra-indicated in psoriasis. They may probably be used only when severe erythrodermic or pustular psoriasis does not come under control with other therapeutic approaches. Chloroquine should be used in psoriatics only when necessary.

Pathology

The epidermal rete ridges show regular test tube shaped hyperplasia and neutrophilic infiltration of the epidermis as well as papillary vascular dilatation. Accelerated epidermal turnover and deficient keratinocyte maturation (seen as parakeratosis) result in visible exfoliation of the skin (scaling). Vascular changes lead to erythema whereas dense neutrophilic infiltrate may lead to sterile (non-infective) intraepidermal pustules in pustular psoriasis. In classical psoriasis, a micropustule in upper epidemis is associated with spongiosis (spongiform pustule of Kogoj) and in stratum corneum it is associated with parakeratosis (Munro's microabscesses). Recent research reveals psoriasis to be an autoinflammatory disease mediated by T-lymphocytes which stimulate epidermal proliferation and attract neutrophils to epidermis thus explaining the major findings in pathology of psoriasis.

Patient Profile

Most patients are young or middle aged adults although, no age is exempt. Males are affected a little more frequently than females.

Morphology

Initial lesion of psoriasis is a barely elevated, erythematous papule topped by a whitish scale. Sometimes, scales may not be evident unless the surface is stroked or scratched.

Papules may enlarge or coalesce to form plaques. Thus, fully established psoriasis consists of well-defined rounded erythematous plaques covered with thick silvery scales (Fig. 12.2).

When the scales are removed, pinpoint bleeding is visible on the involved skin (Auspitz sign). When psoriasis is unstable, lesions can be induced by mechanical or other types of truama (Koebner phenomenon). Most commonly this is seen as linear arrangement of psoriasis papules within scratch marks. The papules may coalesce and form linear plaques.

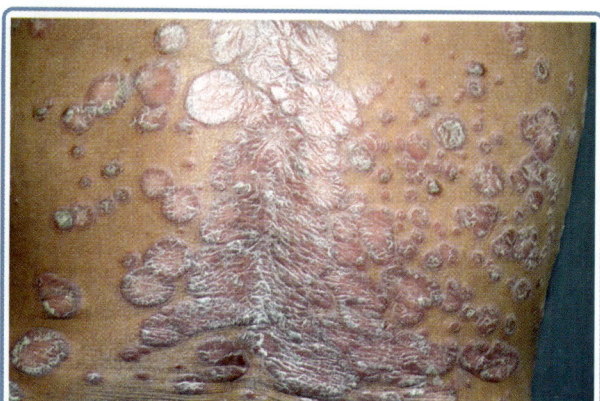

Fig. 12.2: Psoriasis—eruption of scaly papules and plaques over back

Variations in Morphology and Configuration	
Follicular psoriasis	: Lesions begin as follicular papules.
Linear psoriasis	: Linear plaques.
Annular/Figurate psoriasis	: Ring shaped or other figurate : pattern plaques.
Pustular psoriasis	: Superficial pustules on a background of erythema

Distribution

Classic plaque type of psoriasis (psoriasis vulgaris) affects elbows, knees, extensors of extremities,

scalp and sacral region in a symmetric pattern (Figs 12.3 and 12.4). Palms and soles are involved commonly.

Variations in Distribution

Scalp psoriasis: Asymptomatic plaques with thick silvery scales have a tendency to extend beyond scalp margins (Fig. 12.5).

Palmoplantar psoriasis: Symmetric erythematous patches covered with thick and large scales affecting palms and soles is the typical presentation. If untreated painful fissures supervene and affect day to day activities (Figs 12.6 and 12.7).

Nail psoriasis: Nails are involved secondary to affection of nail matrix or nail bed. Numerous pits in the nail plate and subungual hyperkeratosis (accumulation of soft keratin under the nail plate) are the commonest manifestations of nail psoriasis (Fig. 12.8).

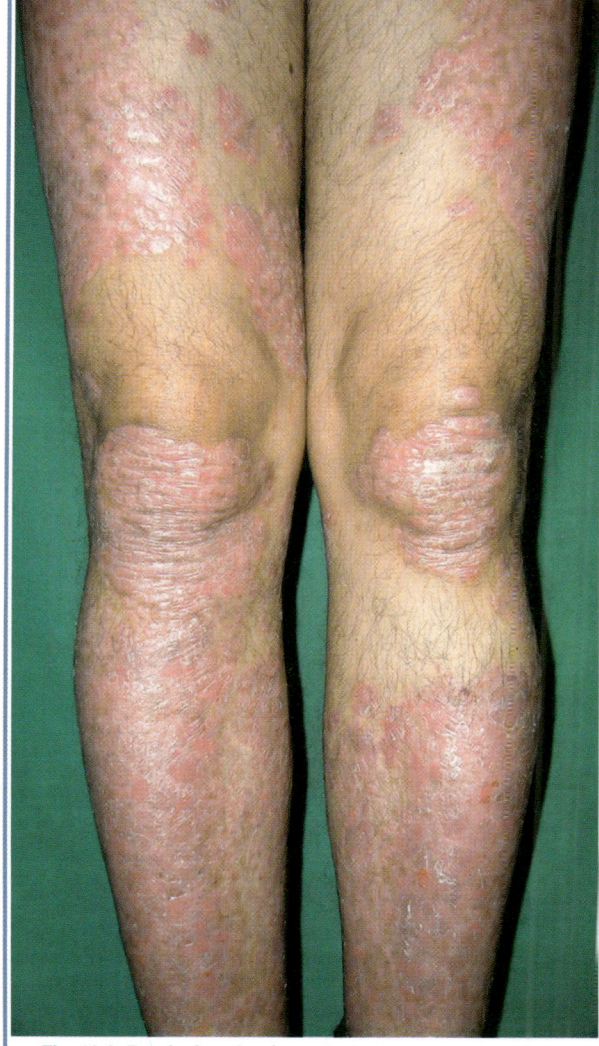

Fig. 12.3: Psoriasis vulgaris—well defined scaly erythematous plaques over extensors

Chapter
12

Papulosquamous Diseases

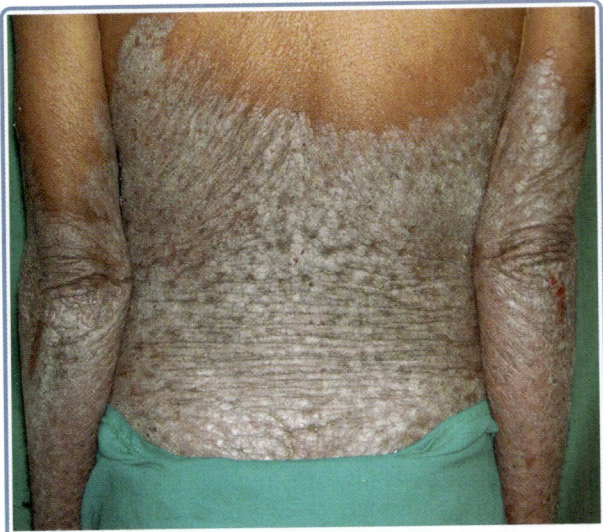

Fig. 12.4: Psoriasis vulgaris—large plaques with thick silvery white scales

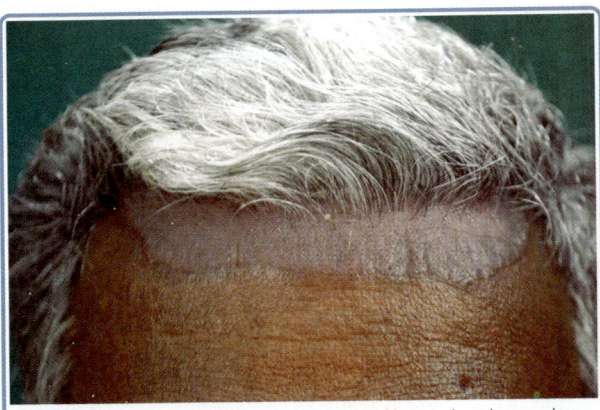

Fig. 12.5: Scalp psoriasis tends to extend beyond scalp margins

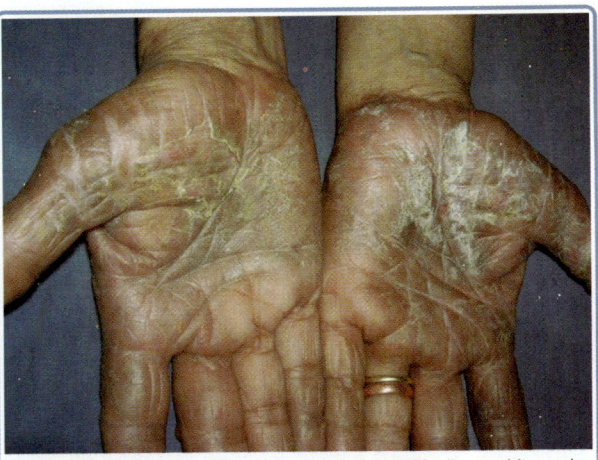

Fig. 12.6: Palmar psoriasis—erythema plaques with silvery white scales

> Other features of nail psoriasis include separation of nail plate from the nail bed (onycholysis), oil spots and a nail plate that becomes thick, yellow-brown, fragile and deformed (dystrophic).

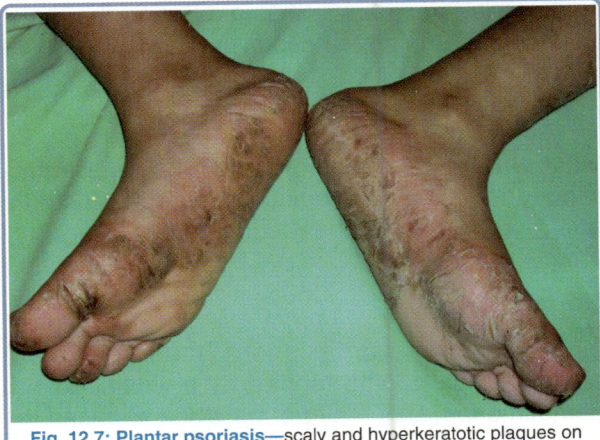

Fig. 12.7: Plantar psoriasis—scaly and hyperkeratotic plaques on both soles

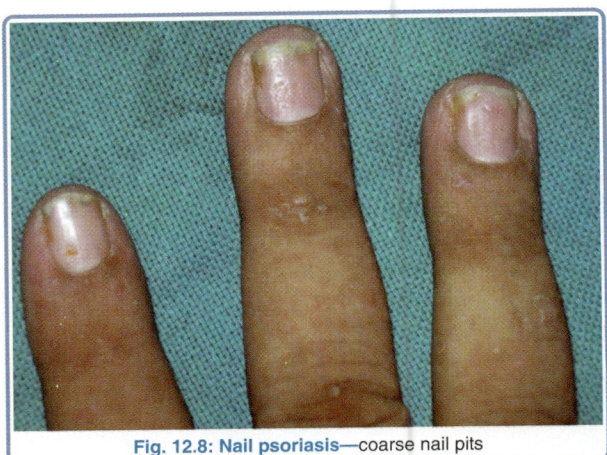

Fig. 12.8: Nail psoriasis—coarse nail pits

Variations in Morphology and Distribution

Guttate psoriasis: This variant is common in children and has the best prognosis. Guttate (drop like) papules topped with white scale appear all over the body, especially the trunk. Lesions resolve within 1–2 months.

Sebopsoriasis: Lesions occur in the distribution pattern of seborrhoeic dermatitis and tend to have yellowish rather than silvery scales.

Erythrodermic psoriasis: Affection of most or all of the body seen as widespread or whole body erythema and scaling (Fig. 12.9).

Flexural psoriasis (inverse psoriasis): Erythematous well defined plaques over axillae and groins without prominent scaling.

Pustular psoriasis: Crops of pustules based on erythema. Distributional subtypes of pustular psoriasis include (Fig. 12.10):

- **Localised palmoplantar pustular psoriasis**
- **Generalised pustular psoriasis:** This is the life-threatening variant, the patient being febrile and toxic as waves of pustules based on tender

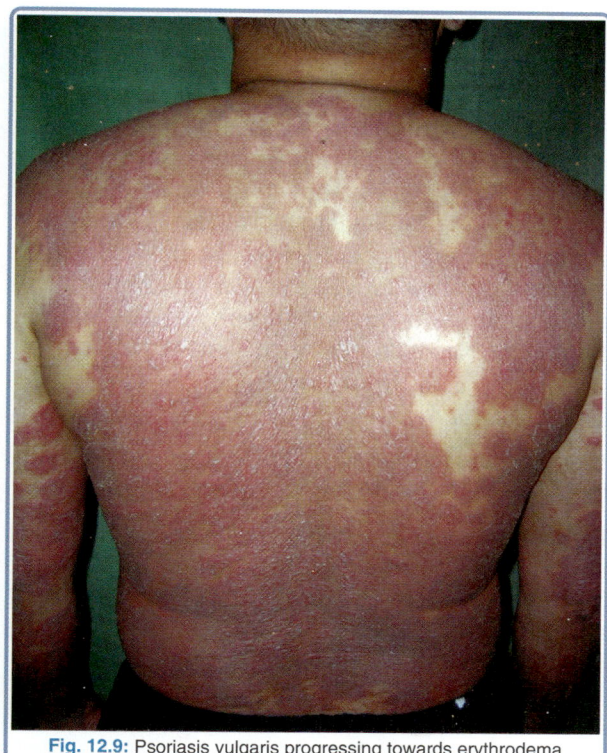

Fig. 12.9: Psoriasis vulgaris progressing towards erythrodema

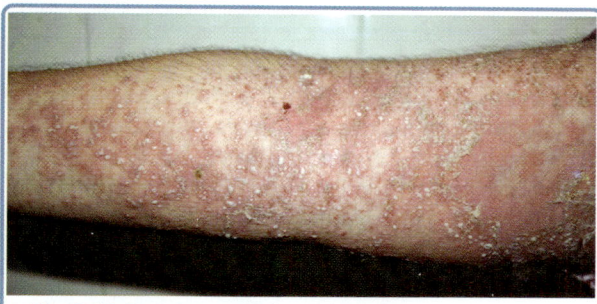

Fig. 12.10: Pustular psoriasis—ill-defined erythematous patches topped with pustules

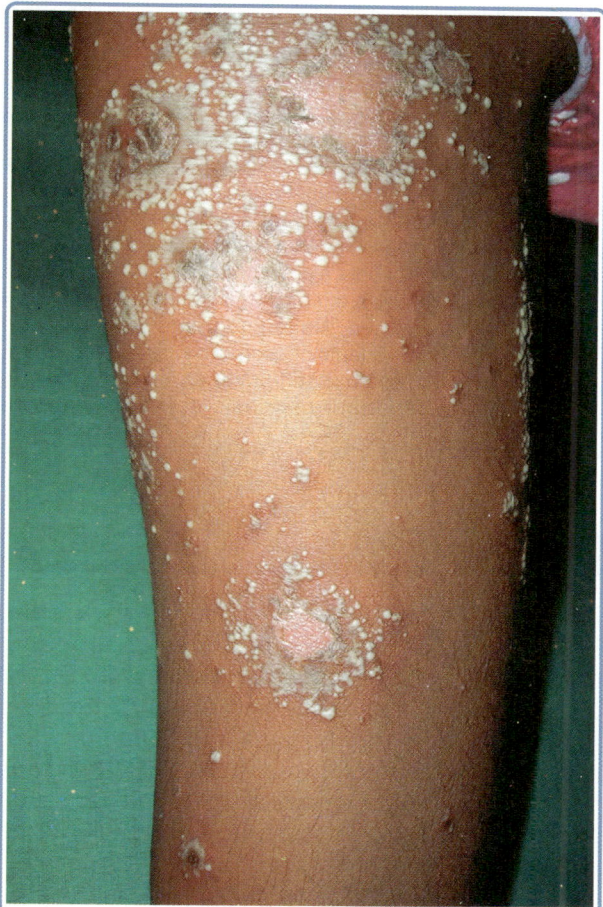

Fig. 12.11: Pustular psoriasis—sterile pustules on erythematous background

erythema appear all over the body (Figs 12.11 and 12.12). Hypocalcaemia and hypoproteinaemia are common.

Psoriatic Arthritis

About 15% of psoriatics develop arthritis sometime during their life. Although, classic psoriatic arthritis affects distal interphalangeal joints, this variety is uncommon. More commonly, psoriatic arthritis involves a few large joints (oligoarticular) or may mimic rheumatoid arthritis.

Complications

Complications of psoriasis are eminently those of erythroderma. Complications of pustular psoriasis are mentioned above. Arthritis leads to disability.

Patients are depressed and withdraw from social activities. Alcohol abuse, obesity, diabetes

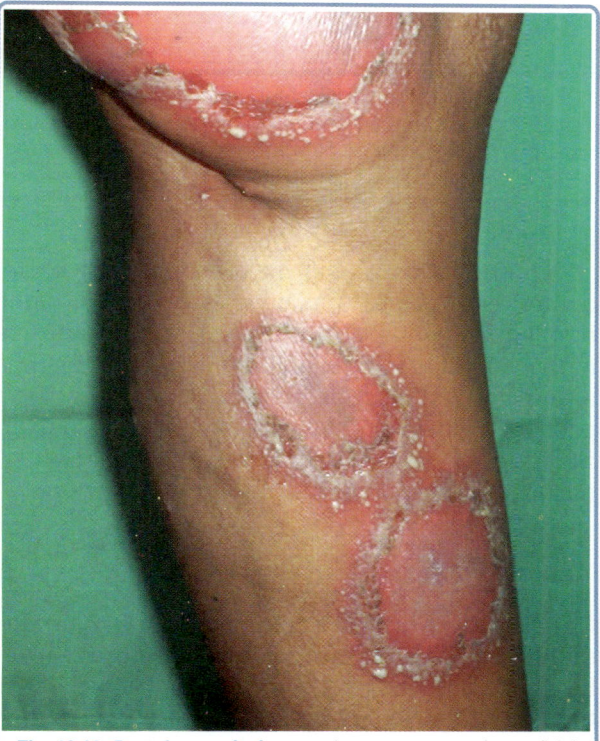

Fig. 12.12: Pustular psoriasis—annular arrangement of superficial pustules on a background of erythema

and ischaemic heart disease are common than the general population.

Summary: Psoriasis is an autoimmune papulosqamous disorder that represents an inflammation pattern of the skin to external (trauma) or internal (drugs) stimuli in a predisposed (genetic) individual. Erythematous papules and plaques covered with thick silvery white scales are the classical lesions. Koebner's phenomenon and Auspitz sign are present. Extensors of limbs and trunk and scalp are preferentially affected. Nails and joints may also be affected. Important variants of psoriasis include guttate (in children, widespread but self-limiting), erythrodermic, sebopsoriasis, pustular psoriasis and arthropathic psoriasis.

TREATMENT OF PSORIASIS

Psoriasis is widely believed to be incurable. However, it can be brought under control and, usually heals with prolonged remissions. Correction of overweight, avoidance of trauma or irritating agents including strong soaps and detergents and avoidance of smoking and alcoholic beverages helps in halting progression. Sunlight and sea bathing improve psoriasis except in the photosensitive patients.

Psoriasis is said to be unstable based on the presence of Koebner phenomenon, bright erythema, pustules or eruption of many new lesions especially guttate lesions over short period.

Clinical implication: Topical tar, anthralin, potent topical steroids and psoralen and ultraviolet A (PUVA) therapy are relatively contraindicated for unstable psoriasis for fear of worsening it or precipitating pustular psoriasis.

Unstable psoriasis may be brought under control with liberal applications of topical bland emollients (white soft paraffin) and supportive therapy. Oral methotrexate, retinoids, cyclosporine and even systemic steroids can control unstable psoriasis. However, systemic steroids are usually avoided for the fear of precipitating pustular psoriasis upon withdrawal.

Topical Therapy

Emollients: White soft paraffin and liquid paraffin soothe the skin, trap moisture, restore barrier function to some extent and help in removal of thick scales by softening them. They also potentiate the action of sunlight and ultraviolet light by improving their penetration.

Keratolytics and humectants: Salicylic acid 3–10% and urea 10–20% help in resolution of stable plaques by their keratolytic and humectant properties.

Steroids: Potent topical steroids like halobetasol, betamethasone dipropionate or clobetasol propionate form the first line of therapy for localised stable and thick plaques of psoriasis especially in the flexural variety. However, after 2–4 weeks they should be replaced by safer topical steroids like mometasone or fluticasone to prevent atrophy of surrounding skin as well as side effects of systemic absorption.

Coal tar: Stable but resistant plaques are best managed with 5–10% coal tar with or without UV-B exposure (or sunlight). Coal tar is available as lotion or paste or in shampoos.

Dithranol: Alernatively, 0.1–1% dithranol, applied carefully over the plaques and left only for 15–30 minutes, can be used with good results. It is available as a paste or ointment and can be combined with topical steroids.

Clinical implication: Dithranol is highly irritant if applied over normal skin or on lesions of unstable psoriasis and hence, it should be used under close medical supervision.

Calcipotriol: This vitamin D analogue is effective in inducing remissions of loclaised plaques. Used alone it may be irritating and is usually combined or alternated with topical steroids in stable plaques.

Systemic Therapy

Widespread psoriasis needs systemic agents in addition to topical therapy.

Methotrexate: Three doses of 2.5–5 mg oral methotrexate at 12 hourly intervals administered every week are extremely effective. Hepatic and renal diseases are relative contraindications. Close monitoring of blood counts and hepatic function is essential. Methotrexate is best suited for long-term therapy of widespread psoriasis.

Psoralen and ultraviolet A therapy: Oral 8-methoxy-psoralen 30 mg on alternate days followed up with ultraviolet-A (UVA) (320–400 nm) exposure constitutes psoralen and ultraviolet A (PUVA) therapy. PUVA therapy is best suited for stable psoriasis that is widespread and is not responding adequately to emollients and other topical agents.

Ultraviolet-B phototherapy: Narrow band ultraviolet-B (UVB) phototherapy comprises exposure to UVB light of 311 nm, which clears stable widespread psoriasis. No additional medications (like psoralens) are needed, making it safe even for pregnant women, children and the elderly. High cost of the light limits its widespread use in India. Broad band UVB phototherapy is comparatively less effective but is also less expensive.

Steroids: Systemic steroids should only be used in life-threatening situations in erythrodermic and pustular psoriasis to bring them under control with rapidity.

Retinoids: Acitretin, 25–50 mg per day orally, is another option for the treatment of recalcitrant widespread psoriasis. It is absolutely contra-indicated in pregnancy and must be avoided in women of child bearing age.

Cyclosporine: This immune modulator is useful in controlling erythrodermic and resistant psoriasis. However, it is expensive and nephrotoxic. It is best reserved for acute exacerbations.

Biologic therapy for psoriasis: In recent years many biologic injectable drugs targeting tumor necrosis factor alpha (TNFα) (infliximab, adalinumab and etanercept) or interleukin 17 (secukinumab) have been introduced and provide an effective and safe option for treatment of psoriasis. Pre-existing latent infections like human immunodeficiency virus (HIV), hepatitis and tuberculosis are contraindications for these drugs. However, it must be explained to the patients that biologics are not curative but only control psoriasis.

> **Summary:** Emollients, weight reduction, and avoidance of trauma and alcohol are helpful in control of psoriasis. Unstable psoriasis is managed with topical emollients and supportive therapy. If erythroderma or pustular lesions supervene, systemic methotrexate, steroids, acitretin and cyclosporin are the available options. Stable plaque type psoriasis responds to topical potent steroids or coal tar or anthralin or, if extensive, to systemic PUVA therapy or UVB phototherapy, methotrexate, cyclosporine or biologics like etanercapt or secukinumab provide adequate.

PITYRIASIS ROSEA

This exanthem is proposed to be caused by a virus though the condition is not contagious and a virus has not been isolated. However, its seasonal occurrence in young adults and children, presence of a primary lesion, occasional prodromal symptoms, spontaneous resolution within 6 weeks and rarity of second attacks are all pointers to a viral aetiology.

Patient Profile

Young adults, adolescents and children are preferentially affected. Uncommonly, it may occur in the elderly or the middle aged. Both sexes are affected equally.

Morphology

A sudden eruption of oval or circular, erythematous, barely elevated plaques with central clearing and fine scaling typifies pityriasis rosea. It is common for a single large lesion (mother plaque) to precede the generalised eruption by 2–7 days. Lesions begin as macules and progress to form papules that keep on expanding at the periphery and clear in the center, thereby resulting in annual (ring shaped) plaques (Fig. 12.13). Fine scales can be seen attached to the inner border of the ring shaped lesion forming a 'collarette' (Fig. 12.14). Oval lesions arranged symmetrically along the ribs give rise to a 'fir tree or Christmas tree' pattern (Fig. 12.15)

Distribution

Trunk and proximal extremities (covered parts) are principally affected. Face and distal extremities

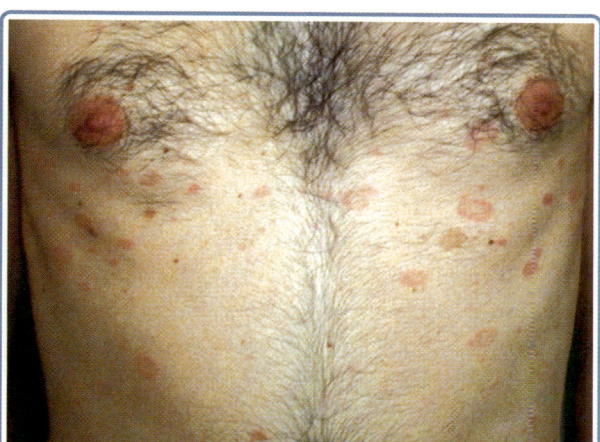

Fig. 12.13: Pityriasis rosea—sudden eruption of erythematous scaly annular plaques over trunk

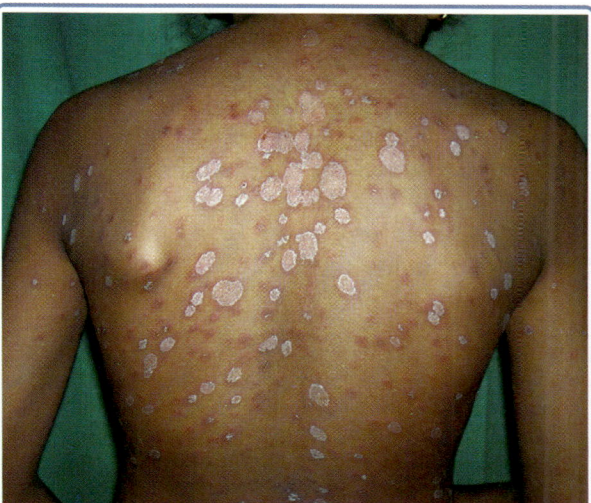

Fig. 12.14: Pityriasis rosea—annular erythematous plaques with fine collarette scale

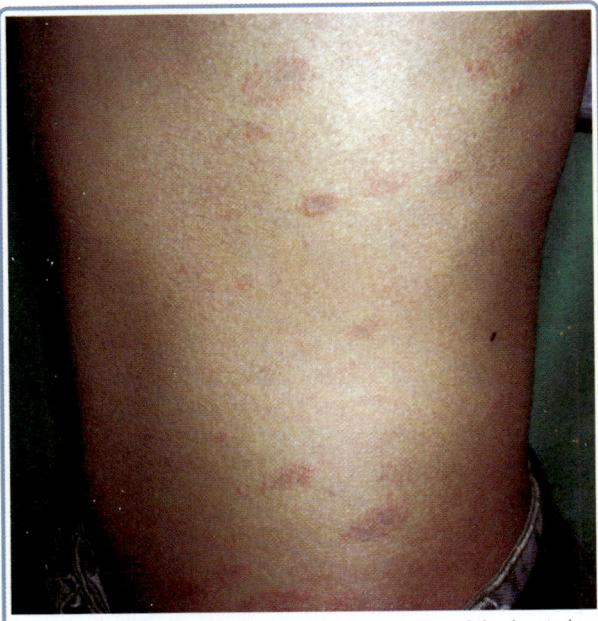

Fig. 12.15: **Pityriasis rosea**—oval erythematous, subtly elevated, plaques with fine scales arranged along the ribs

are involved in severe cases or in the inverse variety.

Variations in morphology or distribution of pityriasis rosea include

- **Papular** – no or scant scales.
- **Psoriasiform** – thick scales resembling psoriasis.
- **Vesicular** – vesicles are also present.
- **Localised** – only one region (e.g. axilla) is involved.
- **Inverse** – extremities and face involved, trunk spared.

Diagnosis

It is based on clinical features, skin biopsy being necessary only uncommonly.

Therapy

Being a self-limiting viral infection, therapy is supportive. Avoidance of irritating agents and soaps, use of soothing creams and, if pruritus is present, topical steroids are helpful. The eruption resolves without any therapy within 4–6 weeks. Second attacks are rare.

Summary: Pityriasis rosea is a viral exanthem with minimal prodromal symptoms. It affects the young and is seasonal. Initial lesion (mother plaque) is an annular erythematous plaque with fine collarette scales. Within a few days, it is followed by numerous smaller but similar lesions, round or oval, arranged along the ribs. Lesions are non-pruritic and occur over the trunk or proximal extremities. Self-healing withi 4–6 weeks is a rule.

LICHEN PLANUS

A common inflammatory disorder of the skin, lichen planus is an autoimmune disease characterised by a dense, band like (lichenoid) infiltrate in the upper dermis.

Patient Profile

Young adults are commonly affected. However, no age is exempt. Both sexes are affected equally. In older adults lichen planus must be distinguished from lichenoid drug eruption. Such eruption may be caused by antipsychotics, antituberculous, antidiabetics, antimalarials or antiepileptics. Careful history, differences in morphology and distribution and biopsy are need for differentiation.

Morphology

Flat topped, polygonal, violaceous, erythematous, 2–10 mm papules covered with scanty scales are characteristic (Figs 12.16 and 12.17). Application of oil to the surface of the papules demonstrates fine crisscross white lines termed as Wickham's striae. Initial lesions are tiny 1–2 mm skin coloured micro-papules whereas later, coalescence of lesions may lead to formation of large (2–5 cm) plaques

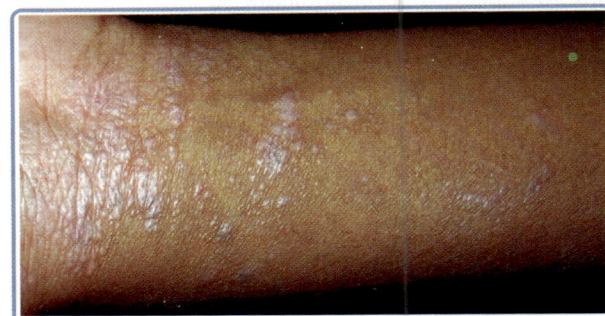

Fig. 12.16: **Lichen planus**—violaceous, itchy, flat topped papules

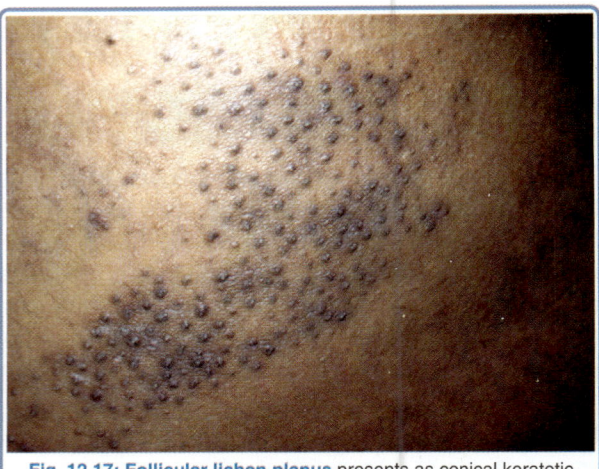

Fig. 12.17: **Follicular lichen planus** presents as conical keratotic hyperpigmented papules

(Figs 12.18–12.20). Occurrence of lesions within scratch marks (Koebner phenomenon) is an indication of activity of disease.

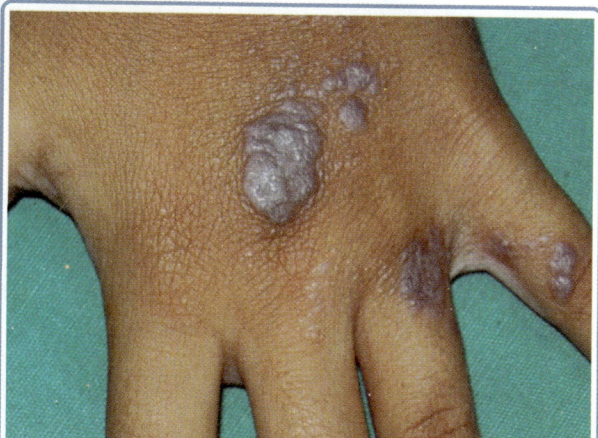

Fig. 12.18: Lichen planus—violet coloured, polygonal, flat topped papules and plaques

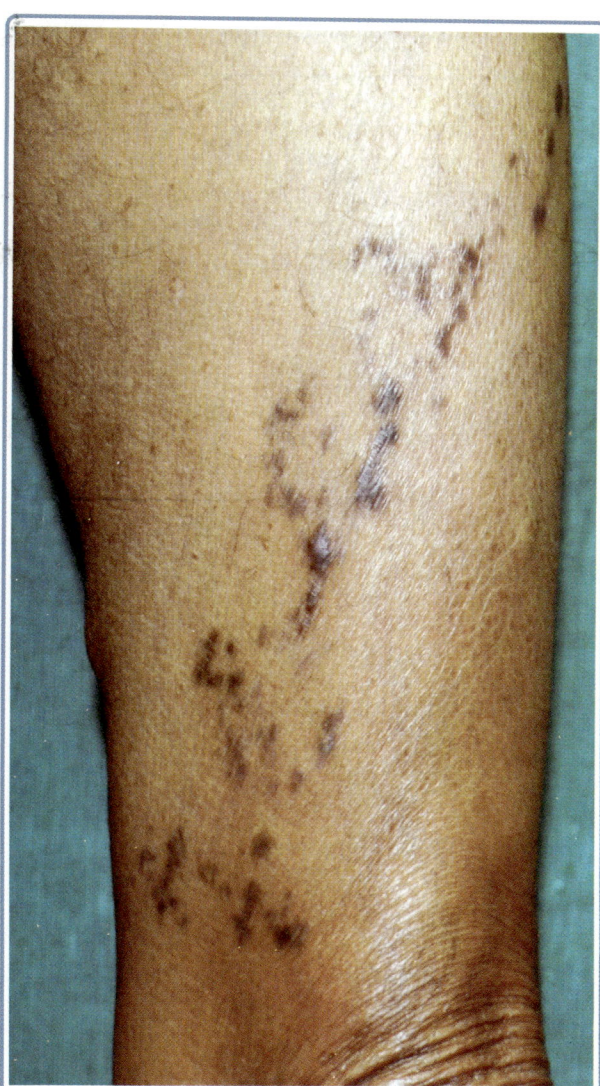

Fig. 12.19: Linear lichen planus—lichen planus lesions in unilateral segmental distribution

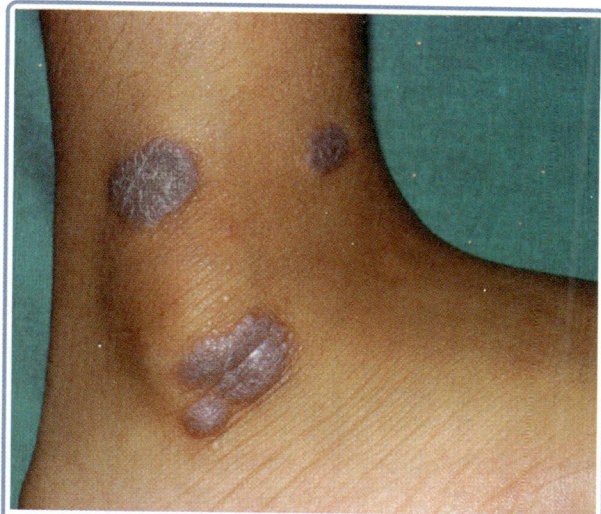

Fig. 12.20: Lichen planus—close up of lesions over ankle

Variations in the morphology and configuration of lichen planus include:

- Annular—ring like.
- Vesicular and bullous.
- Linear.
- Hypertrophic—large thick plaque on shin, ankle or foot (Fig. 12.21).
- Atrophic—macular (flat) lesions.
- Follicular—conical papules with central keratin plug. A common consequence of this type is scarring alopecia of scalp (Graham-little syndrome)

Distribution

Flexor aspects of wrists and forearms, shins, ankles, dorsa of feet, anterior thighs and flanks are sites of predilection. Oral, especially buccal mucosa, lips and genitalia are also commonlly affected (Fig. 12.22).

Variations in lichen planus based on distribution include:

- **Acute widespread,** involving most of the areas mentioned.
- **Chronic localised,** common around ankles and wrists (Figs 12.16, 12.20 and 12.21).
- **Segmental,** involves a unilateral linear segment of the trunk or limbs.
- **Oral** papules arranged in an annular or lacelike pattern (Figs 12.22 and 12.23).
- **Nail:** Thin striated nails with pterygium (extension of proximal nail fold on to the nail bed with dystrophy of nail plate in that focus) (Fig. 12.24).

Therapy

Oral antihistaminics like levocetirizine or desloratidine may help to relieve pruritus. Other

Chapter 12

Papulosquamous Diseases

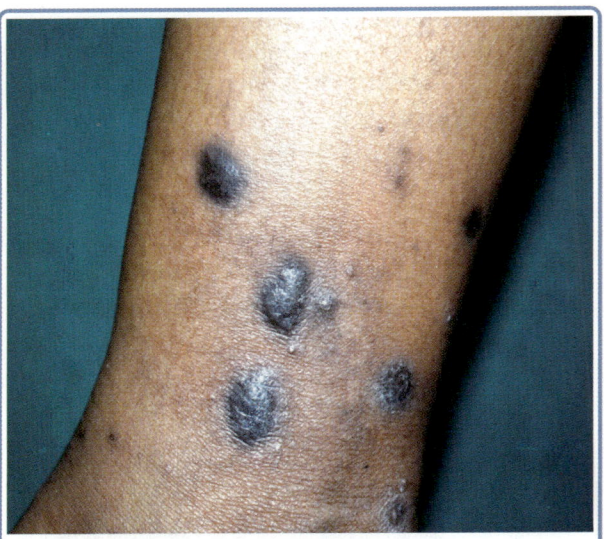

Fig. 12.21: Lichen planus—hypertrophic lichen planus is common on lower legs and ankle

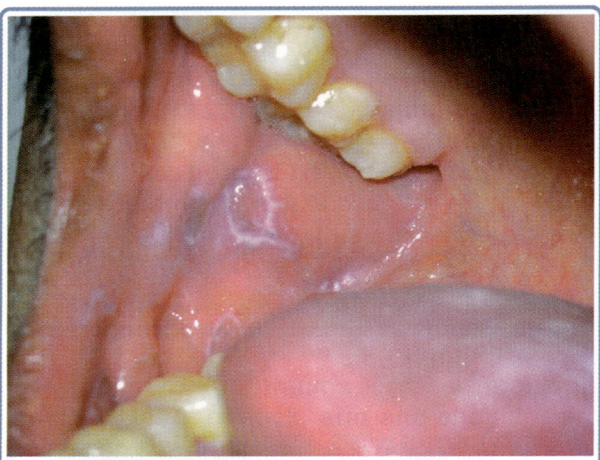

Fig. 12.22: Oral lichen planus—whitish annular plaques and papules on buccal mucosa

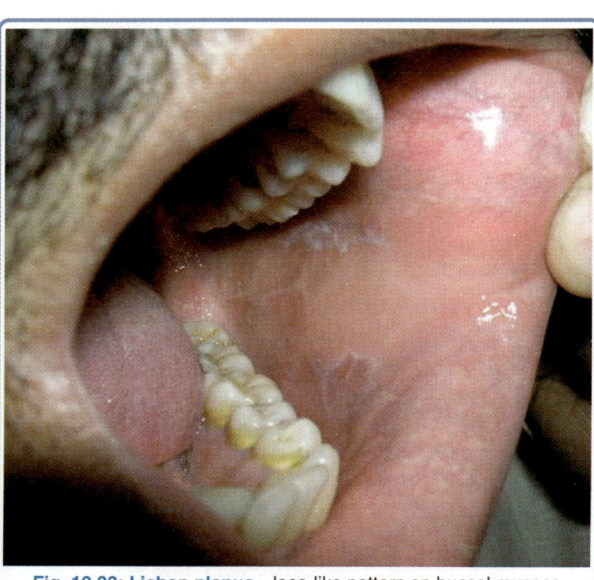

Fig. 12.23: Lichen planus—lace-like pattern on buccal mucosa

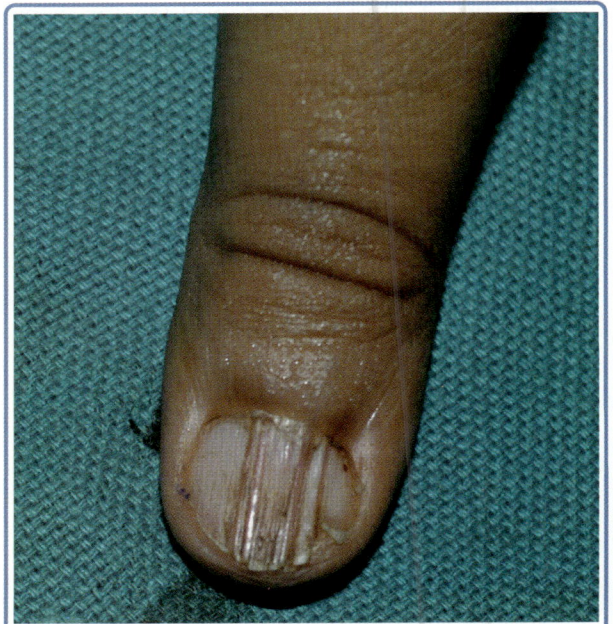

Fig. 12.24: Nail lichen planus—longitudinal ridging with extension of nail fold onto the nail plate (pterygium)

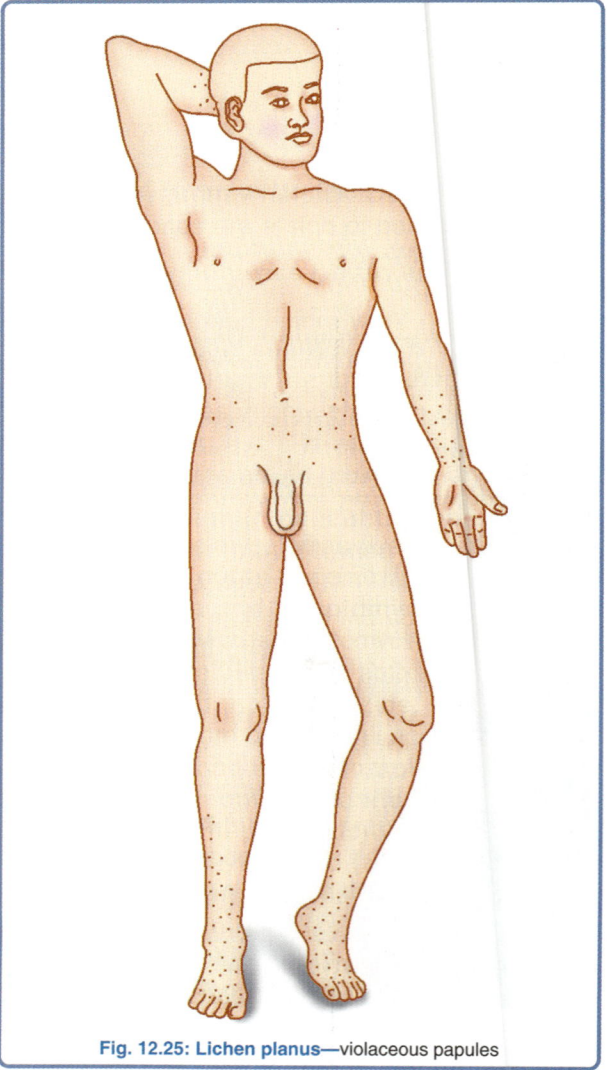

Fig. 12.25: Lichen planus—violaceous papules

Chapter 12

Papulosqamous Diseases

than this, topical steroids suffice for localised lesions. Potent corticosteroids like fluocinolone acetonide, betamethasone valerate are effective for ordinary lesions. Hypertrophic lesions need stronger steroids like clobetasol or halobetasol propionate or intralesional injections of triamcinolone acetonide. Patient needs to be monitored for side effects of potent topical steroids like atrophy or depigmentation.

Widespread lichen planus is an indication for systemic steroids or immunosuppressants. All contraindications to systemic steroids or immuno-suppressants should be ruled out. Prednisolone, 20–30 mg per day, tapered over 4–6 weeks, brings about resolution of existing lesions. Lesions resolve with pigmentation that may last for many months or even a year. Dapsone has also been found to be useful. Other non-steroidal options include acitretin, cyclosporine and methotrexate. However, side effects of these drugs must be looked for during the therapy.

Summary: Lichen planus is an autoimmune disease that affects the young and middle aged adults. An eruption of pruritic, erythematous, polygonal, flat topped papules with a violaceous hue and scanty scale characterise the disease. A typical case has Wickham's striae (crisscross whites lines) and Koebner phenomenon (induction of lesions by trauma). Flexors of wrists and forearms, thighs, shins, ankles, oral and genital mucosae are affected frequently. Variants include hypertrophic, annular and linear lesions. Biopsy is diagnostic. Topical and intra-lesional steroids are effective for localised lesions. Widespread disease frequently requires systemic steroid or immunosuppressive therapy.

REITER'S DISEASE

It is characterised by a triad of conjunctivitis, arthritis and urethritis. Symptoms start following an episode of diarrhoea or urinary tract infections caused by *Shigella flexneri*, *Salmonella typhimurium*, *Yersinia enterocolitica*, *Campylobacter jejuni*, or *Chlamydia trachomatis*. Persons with human leukocyte antigen B27 (HLA B27) phenotype and HIV infection are more prone to develop Reiter's disease. Skin lesions include crusted, scaly lesions which can resemble psoriatic plaques, but are usually more hyperkeratotic than psoriatic lesions (Figs 12.26 and 12.27). These lesions when they occur on the penis are known as circinate balanitis (Fig. 12.28) and hyperkeratotic lesions occurring on palms and soles as keratoderma blenorrhagicum. Weight bearing joints of lower extremities are commonly affected, also plantar fasciitis can occur. Joint involvement if

untreated, may lead to severe mutilating deformities (Figs 12.26 and 12.27).

Treatment includes antibiotic therapy with doxycycline or tetracycline for diarrhoea and urethritis. Joint involvement can be managed

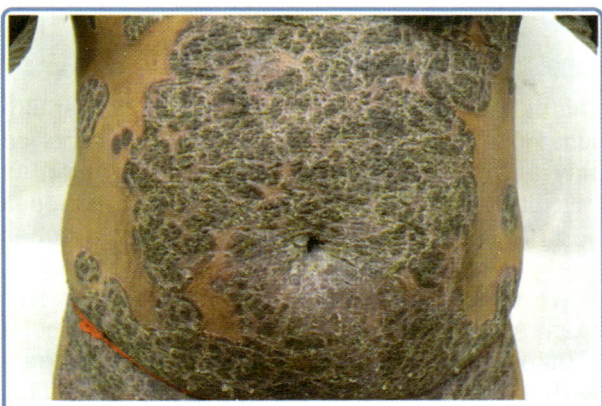

Fig. 12.26: Reiter's disease—psoriasiform plaques with thick keratotic scales

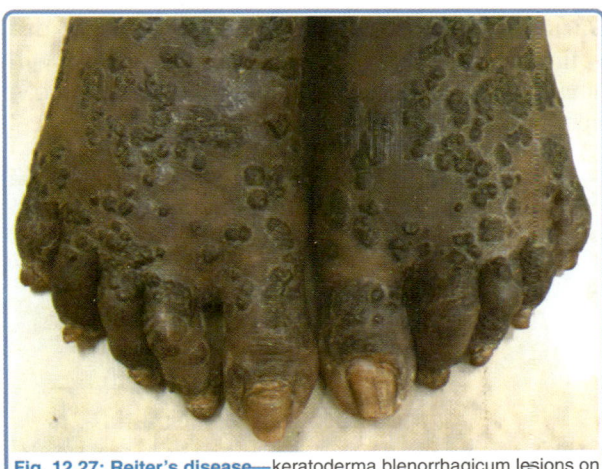

Fig. 12.27: Reiter's disease—keratoderma blenorrhagicum lesions on feet with nail changes

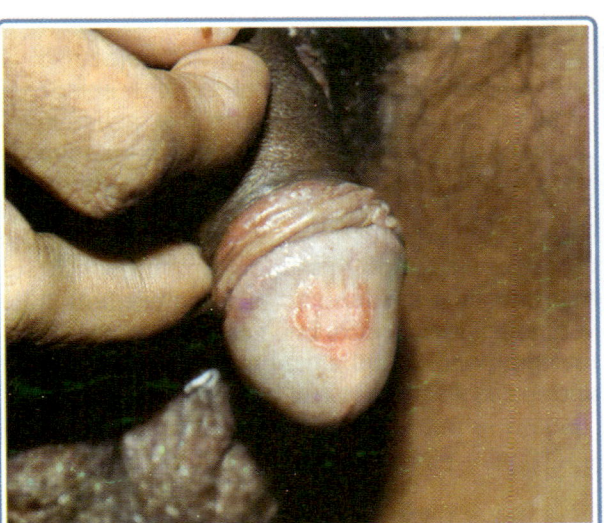

Fig. 12.28: Circinate balanitis in Reiter's disease—erythematous annular plaque on the glans

Chapter
12

Papulosquamous Diseases

symptomatically with NSAIDs. More severe type of joint or skin involvement requires drugs like methotrexate, sulphadiazine and retinoids like isotretinoin or acitretin. Plantar fasciitis can be managed with steroid injections in plantar fascia.

PITYRIASIS RUBRA PILARIS

This is seen as generalised non-pruritic papulo-squamous rash resembling psoriasis. This condition may affect adults or children. Lesions begin as follicular papules that coalesce and form plaques (Fig. 12.29). Coalescence of adjacent patches finally results in generalised erythroderma. However, a few islands of sparing are commonly seen. Auspitz sign is negative. Keratotic follicular papules over dorsa of proximal interphalangeal (PIP) joints have characteristic 'nutmeg crater' feel. Palms and soles show yellowish thickening. Biopsy is helpful to differentiate it from psoriasis. In spite of the erythroderma, the patient is fairly comfortable. Various therapies (high dose vitamin A, oral retinoids, methotrexate) have been used with limited success. Pityriasis rubra pilaris may resolve spontaneously after several years.

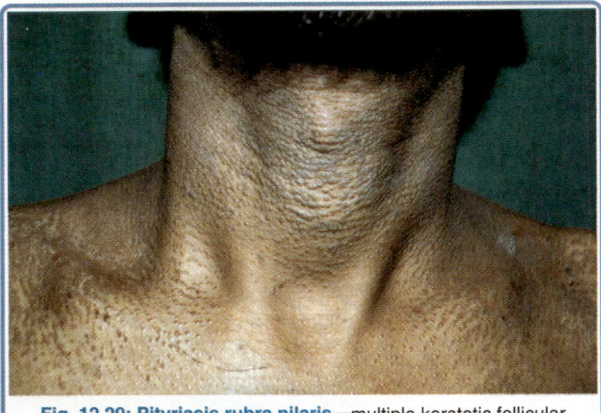

Fig. 12.29: Pityriasis rubra pilaris—multiple keratotic follicular papules in a young male

PARAPSORIASIS

This term describes a group of papulosquamous disorders that clinically resemble psoriasis. Pityriasis lichenoides and pityriasis lichenoids et varioliformis acuta (PLEVA) display guttate (drop-like) lesions while parapsoriasis and plaque presents as scaly patches and plaques.

Pityriasis Lichenoids

This may occur as chronic and acute variants viz. pityriasis lichenoids chronica and PLEVA (Fig. 12.30A and B).

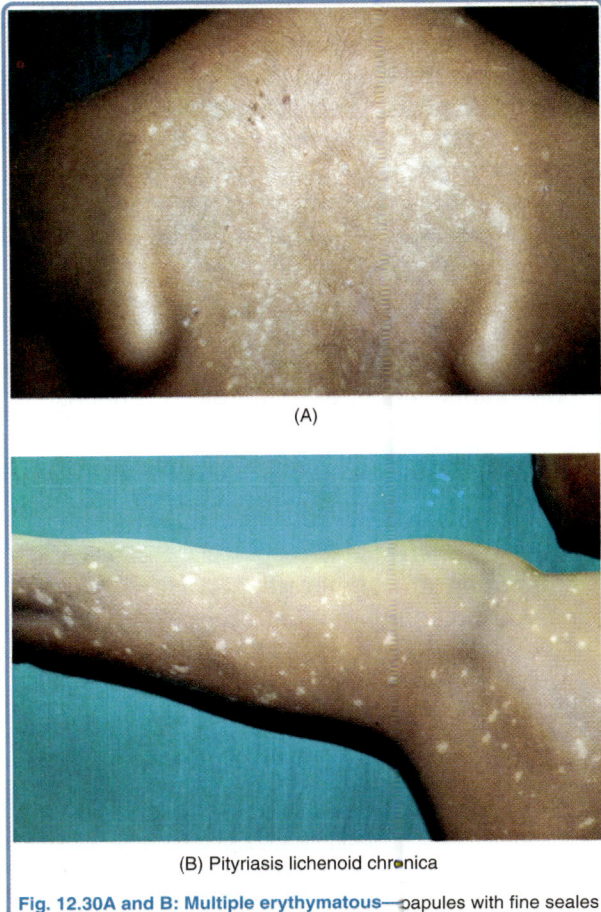

(A)

(B) Pityriasis lichenoid chronica

Fig. 12.30A and B: Multiple erythymatous—papules with fine seales leaving behind hypopigmentation in a symmetric distribution

Pityriasis lichenoids chronica occurs as a generalised, non-pruritic papulosquamous eruption of long duration. While individual lesions heal with post-inflammatory hypopigmentation, new lesions continue to appear. Biopsy is helpful in reaching the diagnosis. Response to tetracycline or dapsone is variable.

Pityriasis lichenoids et varioliformis acuta presents as a sudden onset generalised papulo-vesicular rash especially involving the trunk and proximal limbs in adolescents or young adults. Constitutional disturbance may be associated. The vesicles may be haemorrhagic, commonly turn into pustules and later heal leaving behind varioliform scars. Response to treatment is unsatisfactory.

Mycosis Fungoides

Mycosis fungoides is the commonest type of cutaneous T-cell lymphoma. It evolves very slowly over a period of several years to several decades. The lesions usually progress orderly through the patch stage and plaque stage to tumour stage and eventually involve the whole of the body (erythrodermic stage) (Figs 12.31 and 12.32). Initially, the lesions are seen as patches of

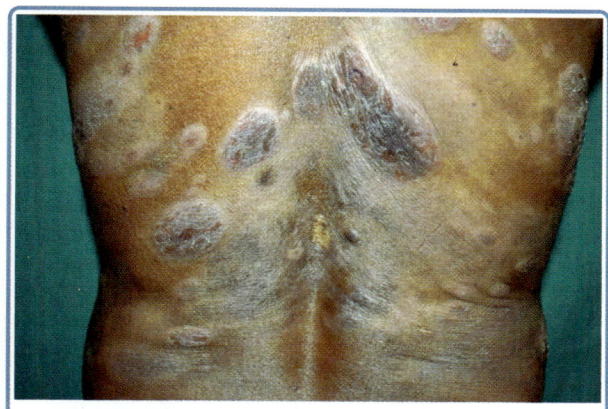

Fig. 12.31: Mycosis fungoides—scaly patches and plaques (cutaneous T-cell lymphoma)

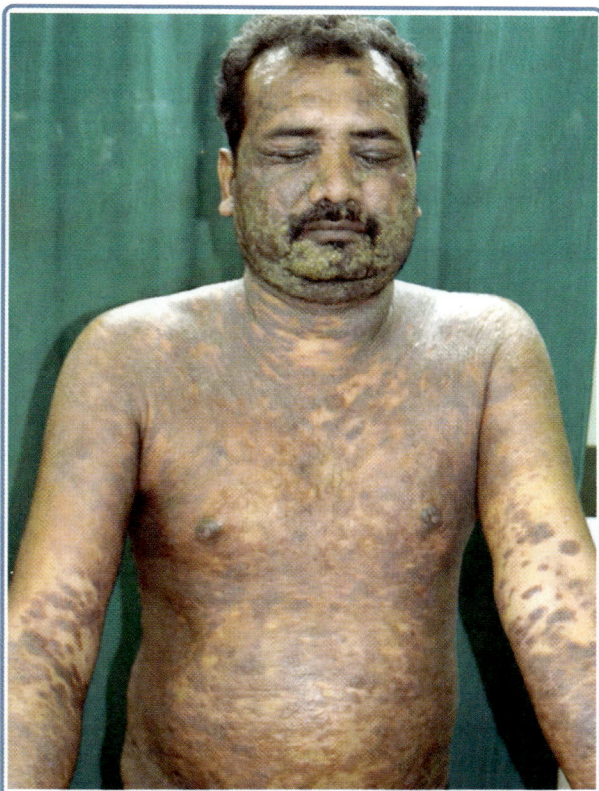

Fig. 12.32: Erythorodermic mycosis fungoids—coalescent hyperpigmented erythematous and atrophic plaques and patches in mycosis fungiodes leading to erythroderma

over the plaques and thereafter the disease progresses relatively faster with involvement of the liver, spleen, lymph nodes and peripheral blood.

In early cases the skin biopsy shows moderately dense patchy upper dermal infiltrate of lymphocytes that focally infiltrate the epidermis without much spongiosis. All systemic tests on blood lymph nodes or bone marrow, at this stage, are negative. At a slightly later plaque stage collections of lymphocytes in epidermis (pautrier's microabscess) appear and are diagnostic.

In advanced cases, the skin biopsy as well as the peripheral blood show the classical 'mycosis cell' a large lymphocyte with large convoluted or irregular nucleus. Ultrasonography of abdomen, lymph node biopsy and bone marrow may be necessary in the advanced cases to stage the lymphoma. Treatment of the patch and plaque stage involves administering PUVA therapy or electron beam therapy. The later stages require chemotherapy (Fig. 12.33A and B).

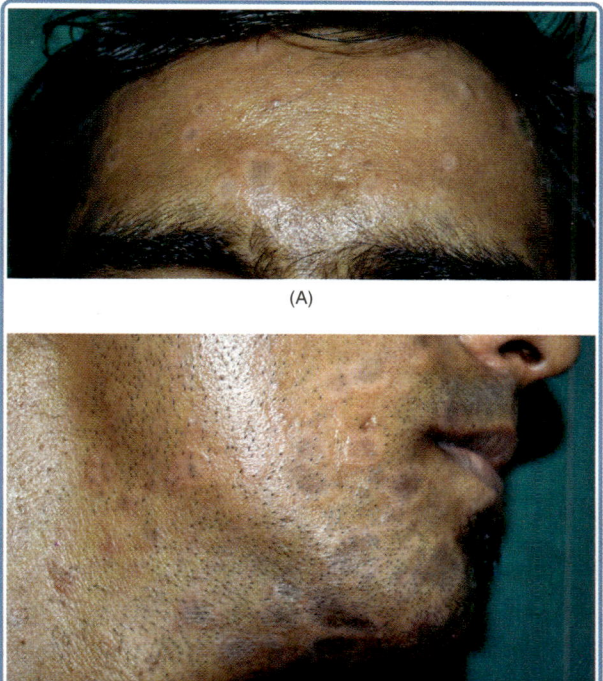

(A)

(B)

Fig. 12.33A and B: Annular papulosquamous lesions over face in secondary syphilis

poikiloderma (combination of alternating hypo-pigmentation and hyperpigmentation with atrophy and telangiectasia) that over several years progress to subtly elevated pruritic plaques with scant scales and later into infiltrated erythematous plaques. Slowly nodules and tumours supervene

Chapter
12

Papulosquamous Diseases

MCQs

1. **Whitish coloured lines on surface of lesions of lichen planus are called:**
   a. Wickham's striae
   b. Whiting striae
   c. Winchester lines
   d. Auspitz lines

2. **The colour of typical lichen planus lesions is:**
   a. Red
   b. Violet
   c. Pink
   d. Brown

3. **The outline of lichen planus lesions is:**
   a. Circular
   b. Square
   c. Polygonal
   d. Triangular

4. **The shape of lichen planus lesions is:**
   a. Rounded
   b. Conical
   c. Hemispherical
   d. Flat topped

5. **The typical pattern of lichen planus lesions in the mouth is:**
   a. Linear
   b. Lace like
   c. Serpiginous
   d. Geographic

6. **Commonest sites of affection of lichen planus is:**
   a. Bony prominences
   b. Extensors of limbs
   c. Flexors of limbs
   d. Exposed surfaces

7. **Which of the following conditions is extremely itchy?**
   a. Psoriasis
   b. Lichen planus
   c. Pityriasis rosea
   d. Discoid lupus erythematosus

8. **Lichen planus usually does not affect:**
   a. Mouth
   b. Ankles
   c. Wrists
   d. Back

9. **Lesions of lichen planus heal with:**
   a. Hypopigmentation
   b. Hyperpigmentation
   c. Depigmentation
   d. Scarring

10. **Drug that does not cause lichen planus like eruption is:**
    a. Chloroquine
    b. Chlorpropamide
    c. Chlorpromazine
    d. Chloramphenicol

11. **The aetiology of lichen planus is:**
    a. Fungal infection
    b. Viral infection
    c. Autoimmune
    d. Developmental

12. **Which of the following is not a variant of lichen planus?**
    a. Hypertrophic
    b. Pustular
    c. Annular
    d. Linear

13. **Psoriasis vulgaris affects all of the following *except*:**
    a. Sacrum
    b. Axillae
    c. Knees
    d. Scalp

14. **The scales in psoriasis are:**
    a. Collarette
    b. Silvery
    c. Thin
    d. Powdery

15. **Scales in psoriasis are:**
    a. Easy to remove
    b. Thick
    c. Silvery
    d. All of these

16. **Sterile pustules are seen in:**
    a. Impetigo
    b. Pustular folliculitis
    c. Pustular psoriasis
    d. Pustular lesions of tinea capitis

17. **Generalised pustular psoriasis is sometimes associated with:**
    a. Hypouricaemia
    b. Hypocalcaemia
    c. Hypercalcaemia
    d. Hyperglycaemia

18. **Which of the following variant of psoriasis is life threatening?**
    a. Psoriasis vulgaris
    b. Generalised plaque type
    c. Generalised pustular psoriasis
    d. Inverse psoriasis

19. **Inverse psoriasis refers to occurrence of psoriasis lesions over:**
    a. Soles and palms
    b. Flexures
    c. Sun-exposed areas
    d. Lower half of the body

20. **Which of the following signs over nail plate is highly suggestive of nail psoriasis?**
    a. Longitudinal ridges
    b. White bands
    c. Red bands
    d. Irregular pits

21. **Psoriatic arthropathy typically involves:**
    a. Metacarpophalangeal joints
    b. Proximal interphalangeal joints
    c. Distal interphalangeal joints
    d. Large joints

22. **Commonly, psoriasis lesions get worse in:**
    a. Summer
    b. Monsoon
    c. Winter
    d. No particular season

23. **Which of the following is helpful for control of psoriasis?**
    a. Avoiding alcohol
    b. Avoiding smoking
    c. Avoiding trauma
    d. All of these

24. **The Auspitz sign refers to occurrence of:**
    a. New lesions at sites of trauma
    b. Bleeding at sites of trauma
    c. Pinpoint bleeding at sites of trauma
    d. Pinpoint bleeding on removal of scale

25. **Occurrence of new lesions at sites of non-specific trauma in psoriasis is called:**
    a. Auspitz sign
    b. Wickham's striae
    c. Isotopic phenomenon
    d. Koebner phenomenon

26. **A variant of psoriasis associated with preceding streptococcal infection is:**
    a. Psoriasis vulgaris
    b. Pustular psoriasis
    c. Guttate psoriasis
    d. Annular psoriasis

27. **Guttate psoriasis refers to:**
    a. Exanthem of drop-size lesions of psoriasis
    b. Generalised psoriasis
    c. Childhood psoriasis
    d. Psoriasis associated with streptococcal gut infection

28. **The type of psoriasis that typically occurs in children is:**
    a. Inverse psoriasis
    b. Guttate psoriasis
    c. Pustular psoriasis
    d. Erythrodermic psoriasis

29. **Isomorphic phenomenon refers to:**
    a. Occurrence of linear lesions in psoriasis
    b. Exacerbation of disease following stress
    c. Exacerbation of psoriasis following trauma
    d. New lesions of pre-existing skin disease at sites of non-specific trauma

30. **Napkin psoriasis occurs in:**
    a. Neonates
    b. Infants and young children
    c. Older children
    d. Young ladies who overuse napkins

31. **The type of psoriasis which responds best to topical steroids is:**
    a. Flexural psoriasis
    b. Scalp
    c. Palms and soles
    d. Pustular psoriasis

32. **Psoriasis area severity index (PASI index) takes into account morphologic severity and extent of lesions on the body. PASI for a worst case of psoriasis is about:**
    a. 15–30
    b. 30–60
    c. 60–75
    d. 80–100

33. **Psoriasis patients rarely develop:**
    a. Plaques
    b. Papules
    c. Pustules
    d. Vesicles

34. **Oral steroids are contraindicated in:**
    a. Lichen planus
    b. Psoriasis vulgaris
    c. Pityriasis rosea
    d. Pemphigus vulgaris

35. **Which of the following drugs are not used for psoriasis?**
    a. Methotrexate
    b. Calcipotriol
    c. Cyclosporine
    d. Cyclophosphamide

36. **Which of the following nutrients are significantly lost from skin in erythroderma?**
    a. Fats
    b. Proteins
    c. Carbohydrates
    d. Calcium

37. **Which of the following is not a complication of erythroderma?**
    a. Hypothermia
    b. Concealed pyrexia
    c. Hypertension
    d. Renal failure

38. **Standard dose of methotrexate for psoriasis is:**
    a. 2.5 mg daily
    b. 15 mg daily
    c. 2.5 mg weekly
    d. 15 mg weekly

39. **All of the following are contraindications for methotrexate therapy in psoriasis *except*:**
    a. Past history of hepatitis
    b. Alcohol abuse
    c. Pustular psoriasis
    d. Obesity

40. **Most common side effect of methotrexate in psoriasis therapy is:**
    a. Hepatotoxicity
    b. Nephrotoxicity
    c. Nausea
    d. Diarrhoea

Chapter **12**

Papulosquamous Diseases

41. The most prominent inflammatory cell in the epidermis in psoriasis is:
a. Neutrophil
b. Eosinophil
c. Plasma cell
d. Histiocyte

42. A striking characteristic of the histopathology of psoriasis is:
a. Marked hyperkeratosis
b. Spongiosis
c. Basal vacuolar change
d. Regular epidermal hyperplasia

43. A striking characteristic of histopathology of lichen planus is:
a. Perivascular infiltrate
b. Nodular infiltrate
c. Band like infiltrate
d. Diffuse infiltrate

44. The type of acanthosis seen in lichen planus is described as:
a. Test tube shaped
b. Pseudoepitheliomatous
c. Confluent
d. Saw tooth

45. The type of epidermal hyperplasia seen in psoriasis is:
a. Irregular
b. Pseudoepitheliomatous
c. Saw tooth
d. Test tube shaped

46. The classical histopathologic change in a psoriatic lesion is:
a. Neutrophilic spongiosis
b. Orthokeratosis
c. Saw tooth hyperplasia
d. Dyskeratosis

47. Which of the following is least likely to exacerbate psoriasis?
a. Smoking
b. Sunlight
c. Metoprolol
d. Alcohol consumption

48. Which of the following drugs does not exacerbate pre-existing psoriasis?
a. Lithium
b. Chloroquine
c. Metoprolol
d. Enalapril

49. Disadvantage of PUVA therapy over NB-UVB therapy for psoriasis is:
a. Shorter remission periods
b. Shorter exposure times

c. No logistics problems affecting compliance
d. More eye protection is needed

50. Psoriatic arthritis of the distal interphalangeal joints occurs more often with:
a. Flexural psoriasis
b. Nail psoriasis
c. Scalp psoriasis
d. Psoriasis vulgaris

51. Pityriasis rosea is probably due to a:
a. Viral infection
b. Bacterial infection
c. Fungal infection
d. Allergic response

52. The organism suspected to be responsible for pityriasis rosea is:
a. Hepatitis B virus
b. Herpes simplex virus type 1
c. Human herpes virus 7
d. Epstein-Barr virus

53. The configuration of lesions in pityriasis rosea is:
a. Annular
b. Linear
c. Grouped
d. Figurate

54. The type of scale in pityriasis rosea is described as:
a. Collarette
b. Micaceous
c. Furfuraceous
d. Fish like

55. The duration of rash of pityriasis rosea is about:
a. 3–5 days
b. 1 week
c. 2 weeks
d. 6 weeks

56. The pattern of distribution of rash in pityriasis rosea is:
a. Centrifugal
b. Centripetal
c. Christmas tree like
d. Banyan tree like

57. The course of pityriasis rosea is:
a. Chronic and persistent
b. Relapses and remissions
c. Severe and life threatening
d. Short and self-resolving

58. The initial lesion in pityriasis rosea is termed as:
a. First plaque
b. Mother plaque
c. Primary stage
d. Indeterminate patch

59. Second attacks of pityriasis rosea are:
a. Common
b. Frequent
c. Uncommon
d. Rare

Chapter 12

Papulosqamous Diseases

60. **Important feature of psoriasis is:**
    a. Crusting
    b. Scaling
    c. Oozing
    d. Blistering

61. **Auspitz sign is classically seen in:**
    a. Plaque psoriasis
    b. Pustular psoriasis
    c. Lichen planus
    d. Inverse psoriasis

62. **Itchy purple papule followed by hyper-pigmentation on resolution is seen in:**
    a. Addison's disease
    b. Seborrhoeic keratosis

    c. Hyperthyroidism
    d. Lichen planus

63. **40-year-old female has violaceous papules and pterygium of nails. The likely diagnosis is:**
    a. Psoriasis
    b. Pemphigus
    c. Lichen amyloidosis
    d. Lichen planus

64. **Annular herald patch is seen in:**
    a. Psoriasis
    b. Pityriasis alba
    c. Pityriasis rosea
    d. Nocardiasis

Chapter
12

Papulosquamous Diseases

ANSWERS

1-a,	2-b,	3-c,	4-d,	5-b,	6-c,	7-b,	8-d,	9-b,	10-d,
11-c,	12-b,	13-b,	14-b,	15-d,	16-c,	17-b,	18-c,	19-b,	20-d,
21-c,	22-c,	23-d,	24-d,	25-d,	26-c,	27-a,	28-b,	29-d,	30-b,
31-a,	32-c,	33-d,	34-b,	35-d,	36-b,	37-c,	38-d,	39-c,	40-c,
41-a,	42-d,	43-c,	44-d,	45-d,	46-a,	47-b,	48-d,	49-d,	50-b,
51-a,	52-c,	53-a,	54-a,	55-d,	56-c,	57-d,	58-b,	59-d,	60-b,
61-a,	62-d,	63-d,	64-b						

Pigmentary Disorders

PIGMENTARY SYSTEM

Melanocytes, the cells that produce melanin pigment, are located in the basal layer of epidermis and distribute melanin in packets called melanosomes to surrounding keratinocytes through long branching cytoplasmic process called dendrites. Pigmentary disorders may be caused by alterations in melanocyte structure or functions. Thus, absence of melanocytes through auto-immune damage is seen in vitiligo whereas affected function leads to albinism. Melasma occurs due to melanocyte stimulation from hormones and sunlight.

ALBINISM

Oculocutaneous albinism is an autosomal recessively transmitted disorder of melanin synthesis. Melanin is the pigment responsible for normal skin colour and hence, even though the number of melanocytes is normal in albinism, defective melanin synthesis leads to white or light coloured skin and eyes. As per the type of defect, the pigment maybe totally or partially absent.

Clinical Features

The disorder usually presents at birth although, when mild, it may go unnoticed in infancy. Affected individual has pale skin, white hair, nystagmus, photo-phobia and red coloured irides at birth (Fig. 13.1).

A refractive error is commonly associated. Ophthalmic examination reveals a red reflex, pale retina and prominent retinal vessels. As age advances, eye colour, photophobia, nystagmus as well as skin and hair colour may improve marginally. Adult patients commonly show some pigmented melanocytic nevi over the pale skin. Persistent sun exposure results in solar keratoses and solar elastosis by early adulthood. Squamous and basal cell carcinomas (Fig. 13.2) as well as melanomas are commoner in albinos than in the general population.

> **Differential diagnosis:** Universal vitiligo is distinguished from albinism by the absence of eye involvement and by its acquired nature. Most patients with albinism are otherwise normal, exceptions being the rare Chediak Higashi Syndrome and Wiscott Aldrich Syndrome. Some aminoacidurias (e.g. phenylketonuria) present as pale coloured hair and skin and must be ruled out as they are managed differently.

Treatment

In absence of effective therapy, protection from sunlight to prevent skin and eye cancers is the most important consideration. This may be achieved with protective clothing, use of sunscreening lotions, umbrella or a suncap. Common sunscreens include zinc, para amino benzoic acid and titanium dioxide. A sunscreen with high sun protection factor (SPF) more than 40 is recommended. Avoiding sunburns with all of these

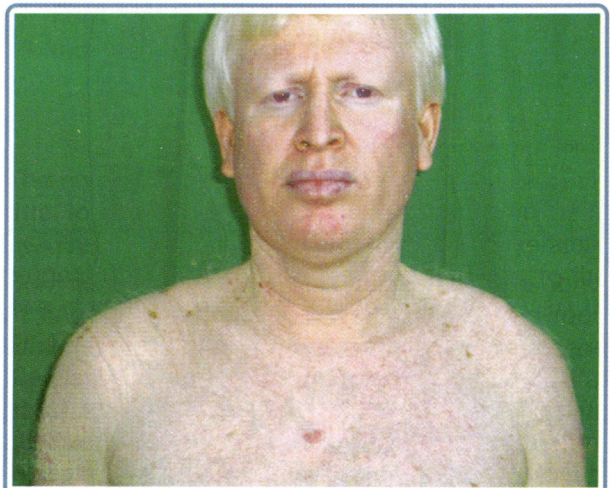

Fig. 13.1 : Oculocutaneous albinism—absence of melanin pigment in the skin, hairs and iris

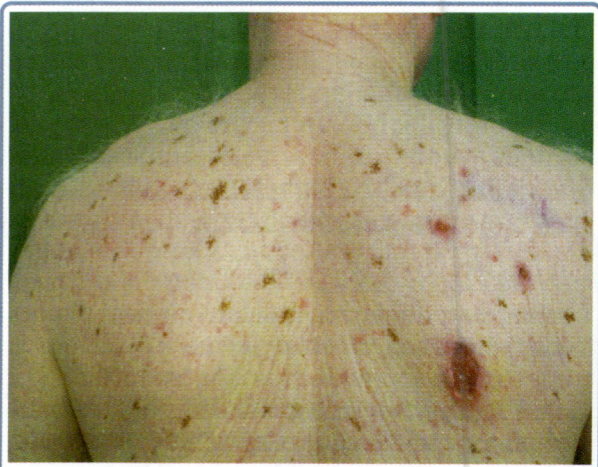

Fig. 13.2: Squamous cell carcinoma (arrow) and actinic keratoses in a case of oculocutaneous albinism—non-healing ulcer with indurated base

measures and avoiding peak time (noon) sun exposure are vital in preventing cancers over the long term. Modern sunscreens are a mixture of physical sunscreens like micronised titanium dioxide or zinc oxide along with broad spectrum chemical sunscreens like octinoxate avobenzone, salicylates and para-amino benzoic acid (PABA) esters. Sunscreen quantity must be adequate and they need to be reapplied frequently. Sunscreens are not completely waterproof. Correction of refractive errors and use of photoprotective sun glasses with side shields improves eye symptoms. Genetic counselling should be offered to patients with this autosomal recessive disorder.

Summary: Oculocutaneous albinism is an autosomal recessively transmitted defect in melanin synthesis. Skin and hair are white and irides, red. Nystagmus, refractive errors and photophobia are usual. Over the years, the skin develops solar keratoses and elastosis due to sun damage. Management comprises photo-protection of skin and eyes, correction of refractive errors and genetic counselling.

VITILIGO

This pigmentary disorder of unknown cause is characterised by depigmented or hypopigmented patches that result from absence or reduction in melanocytes (Fig. 13.3). **Leucoderma**, a term used for vitiligo in non-medical literature, is different from vitiligo. The term leucoderma is applied to depigmented patches of known causes, e.g. following burns, contact with chemicals like phenols or catechols or following an inflammatory skin disease. As opposed to vitiligo, it does not progress after the cause is removed.

The most accepted theory for pathogenesis of vitiligo is the autoimmune hypothesis. This states that vitiligo is due to a T-cell directed attack on epidermal melanocytes. Finding of lymphocytic infiltrate on skin biopsy, association of vitiligo with other autoimmune disorders like thyroid disorders, lichen planus, alopecia areata, etc., affection of extracutaneous melanocytes in patients with vitiligo and response of vitiligo to steroids and immunosuppressants all support the autoimmune theory.

Clinical Profile

About 1–2% of the general population has vitiligo. Vitiligo begins commonly in the second to fourth decade. It is less common in children and the elderly. Both sexes are affected equally. Family

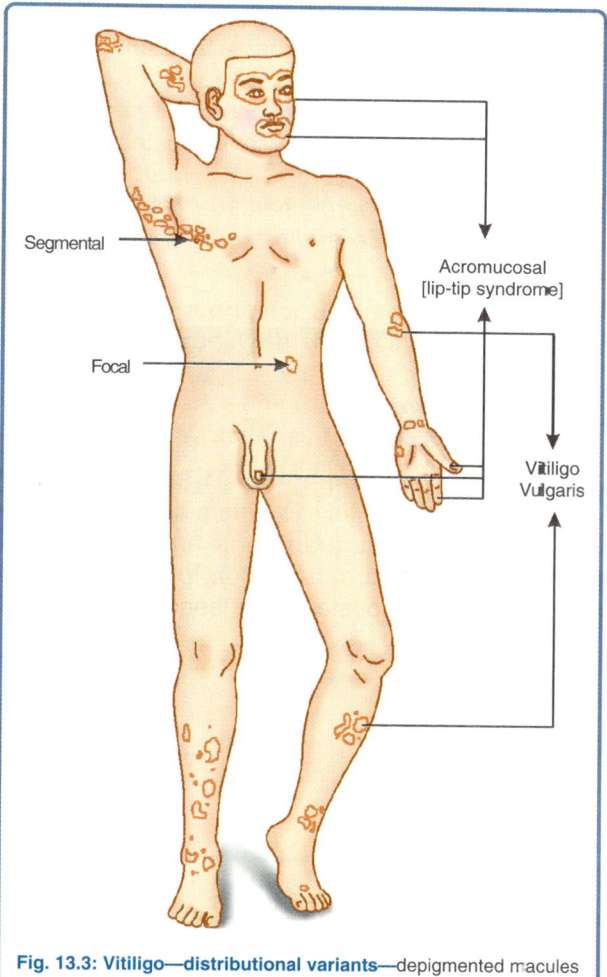

Fig. 13.3: Vitiligo—distributional variants—depigmented macules and patches

history of vitiligo is present in only about 25% of cases. Most patients with vitiligo are otherwise normal and do not need any investigations. However, there is an increased incidence of other autoimmune diseases like autoimmune thyroid dysfunction, Addison's disease, alopecia areata and lichen planus in patients with vitiligo (Table 13.1).

TABLE 13.1: Types of vitiligo	
Localised	Focal
	Segmental
	Acrofacial
	Mucosal
Generalised	Vitiligo vulgaris
	Universalis

Morphology

Depigmented, milky white or hypopigmented (light coloured) macules and patches that are sometimes

Chapter **13**

Pigmentary Disorders

sharply demarcated from the surrounding normal coloured skin typify the disease. The affected skin is otherwise normal except for a little erythema of patches on sun exposed regions due to heightened sensitivity to sunlight. Hair within a patch may turn white (leucotrichia) (Fig. 13.4). Margins of the patches may be hyperpigmented (stable lesion) or hypopigmented (spreading lesion) or normal in colour.

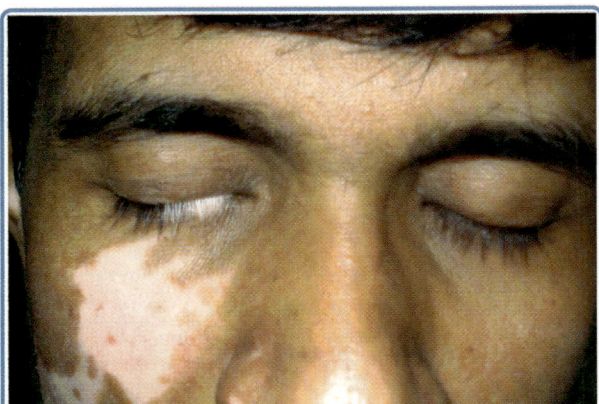

Fig. 13.4: Leucotrichia in segmental vitiligo—depigmented hair over a depigmented patch of vitiligo on the cheek and lower eyelid

Clinical Implication: Margins of vitiligo patches are a good indicator of the activity of the disease. Hyperpigmented margins are a sign of stability or recovery whereas hypopigmented margins are a sign of activity. A margin of normal colour is an indication that the disease is stabilising. Hyperpigmentation may also be seen around follicles within a patch and this is a sign of recovery.

Distribution

According to the extent of involvement, vitiligo can be classified into:

- **Localised focal or regional:** A few patches over one body region, has best prognosis.
- **Dermatomal** patches limited to the region of one or two nerve segments (Fig. 13.5).
- **Vulgaris:** Widespread and symmetrical patches involving extremities and trunk. Common sites of affection include shins, forearms, palms, soles, elbows, knees, lips, eyelids (Figs 13.6 and 13.7), upper trunk, genitals, axillae and groins.
- **Acro-orificial:** Involves acral (Fig. 13.8) (fingers, toes, palms and soles) and periorificial (lips, perioral, periocular and glans penis) areas; carries poor prognosis.
- **Universal:** Total or near total affection of the whole body, has poor prognosis.

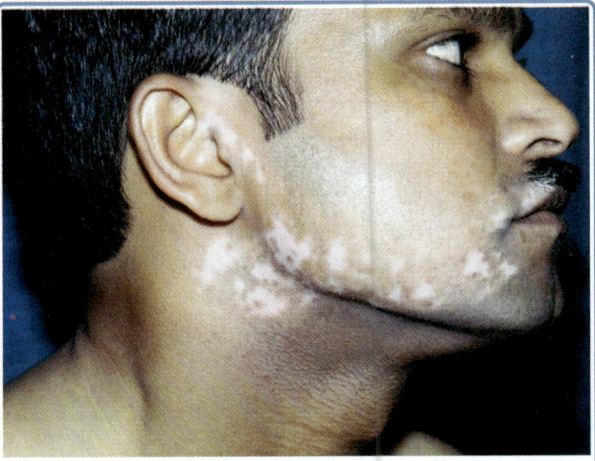

Fig. 13.5: Segmental vitiligo—depigmented macules in segmental distribution

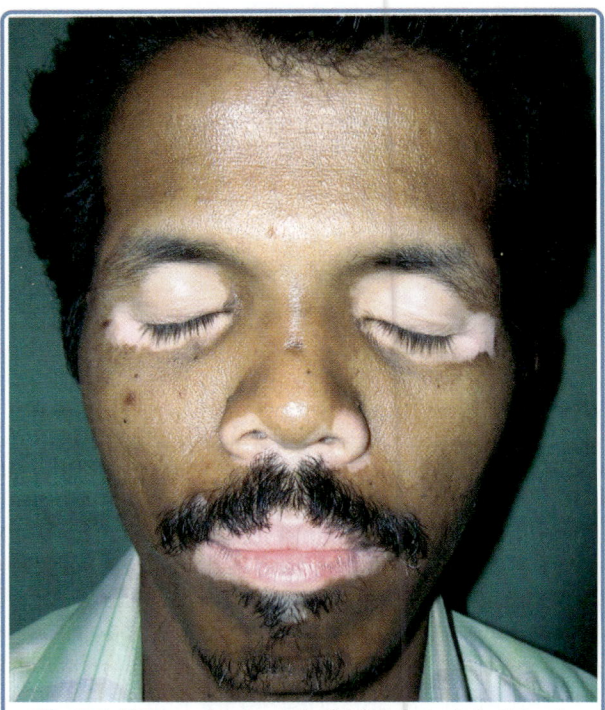

Fig. 13.6: Vitiligo vulgaris—periorificial depigmented patches in symmetric pattern

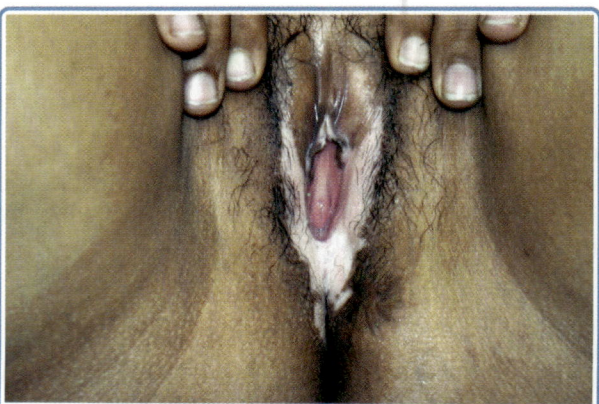

Fig. 13.7: Mucocutaneous vitiligo of female genitalia. Needs to be differentiated from secondary leucoderma due to lichen sclerosus et atrophicus and lichen simplex chronicus

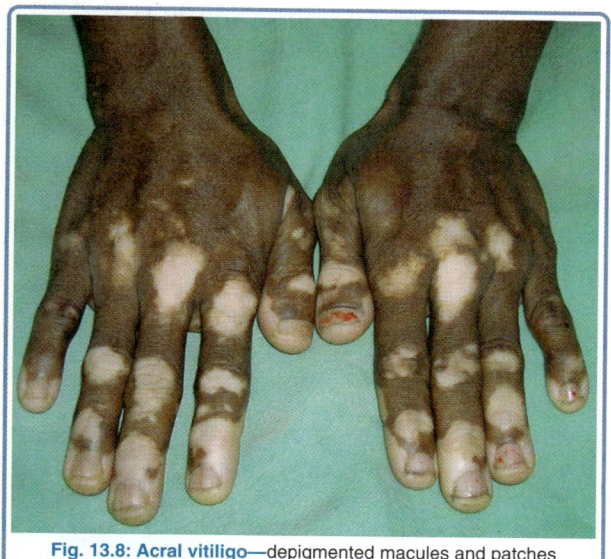

Fig. 13.8: Acral vitiligo—depigmented macules and patches

Differential Diagnosis

Leprosy patches rarely become depigmented (milky white) and usually have impaired sensations. Hypopigmented (but not depigmented) patches of pityriasis versicolor are covered with powdery scales that get accentuated on stroking the affected skin. Leucoderma due to contactants can be suspected based on its characteristic sites, e.g. dorsa of feet due to chappals (Fig. 13.9), central forehead due to bindi.

Therapy

Explanation of the non-infectious and cosmetic nature of the disease is necessary. Treatment of

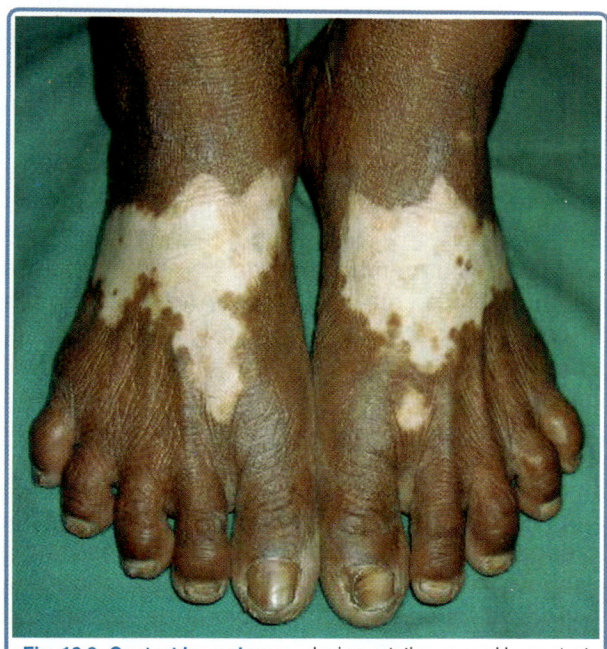

Fig. 13.9: Contact leucoderma—depigmentation caused by contact with chemicals in plastic footwear

this asymptomatic benign disease is important due to the great social stigma associated with the disease. Modality of therapy is decided by the distribution and progress of the disease as well as patient's convenience and preference. No therapy is uniformly effective and the chances of complete repigmentation are smaller in acromucosal type and in patients with more than 50% body area involvement. Localised and unstable vitiligo of short duration may respond to a moderately potent **topical steroid** like mometasone or fluticasone. **Topical psoralen and ultraviolet A (PUVA)** therapy is effective once such patches become stable. Progress of rapidly spreading, unstable and widespread vitiligo may be arrested by administration of small doses of **systemic steroids**. However, caution must be exercised to avoid their adverse effects. Oral immunosuppressants like azathioprine, methotrexate or cyclosporin may be used as steroid substitutes with careful monitoring. Once the disease stops spreading, multiple patches, with > 20% body area involvement, are best managed with ultraviolet light therapy. Topical beta fibroblast growth factor and pseudocatalase have shown some benefit.

Once the disease is static and only small areas of depigmentation remain, dermatosurgical techniques **like mini punch grafting, shave grafting and suction blister grafting or tattooing** can be used to treat these residual patches. Melanocyte culture and autografts probably offer a ray of hope to cases with widespread vitiligo that are resistant to other therapies.

Punch Grafting

Punch grafting is a procedure used for surgical treatment of small patches of stable vitiligo. Just like other types of skin grafting it works on the principle of donor dominance. Small pieces of normal skin are taken from donor area with the help of a cylindrical skin biopsy punch and grafted onto holes made in the affected skin by a similar instrument. At a time multiple skin grafts of size 2–2.5 mm are taken from normal skin and placed at regular distance on the affected skin so as to cover a large lesion. Once the graft has taken up, pigmentation from the grafts spreads to the surrounding affected skin leading to repigmentation in about 3–6 months. The main problems with the procedure are graft failure, irregular surface (cobblestoning) and irregular pigmentation. However, its main advantage that it is a simple procedure and can be used to treat large areas of the skin. Follicular grafts have also been used to good effect (Table 13.2).

Chapter 13

Pigmentary Disorders

TABLE 13.2: Treatment modalities for vitiligo	
Topical agents	Steroids—clobetasol 0.05%, mometasone 0.1%, fluticasone 0.05%
	Topical PUVA
	Topical beta fibroblast growth factor and pseudocatalase
	Placental extract
Systemic agents	Oral or Injectable cortico-steroids
	Oral PUVA
	Immunosuppressants like azathioprine, methotrexate and cyclosporine
Surgical	Punch grafting
	Shave grafting
	Suction blister grafting
	Non-cultured melanocyte grafting
	Follicular unit transplant

Suction Blister Grafting

This procedure is best suited for small residual areas of depigmentation over cosmetically important regions. A suction machine is used to raise blisters over normal coloured skin. The roof of these blisters is grafted onto dermabraded depigmented patches. Repigmentation takes 1–2 months after the procedure.

Summary: Vitiligo is an autoimmune disease directed against melanocytes. Common age of onset is between 15–35 years. Lesions are well defined, milky white (depigmented) macules or patches. Vitiligo may be localised, regional (or segmental), generalised, universal (affecting all the skin surface) or acromucosal. Because of the social stigma it carries, treatment of this benign condition is important. Unstable (spreading) vitiligo is controlled with systemic steroids. Once static, localised patches can be treated with topical steroids or topical PUVA and then residual areas surgically grafted whereas generalised lesions need systemic PUVA therapy for repigmentation.

PUVA THERAPY

PUVA Therapy for Vitiligo

Psoralen and ultraviolet A (PUVA) therapy comprises topical or systemic administration of psoralen followed by irradiation with ultraviolet A

(320–400 nm) light. Psoralens are a group of plant derived chemicals (furocoumarins) that sensitise the skin to ultraviolet rays thereby stimulating melanocyte function and their regeneration. PUVA therapy is contraindicated in pregnant women and young children as well as in individuals with hepatic or renal damage.

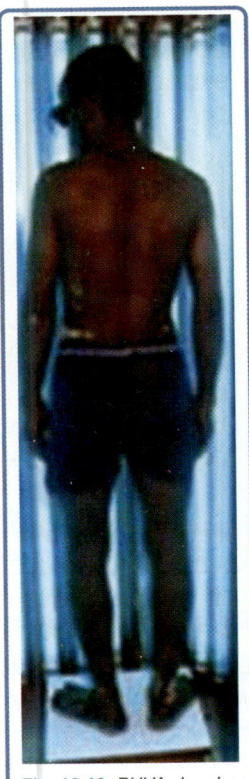
Fig. 13.10: PUVA chamber

Sunlight can also be used (PUVASOL therapy) instead of an artificial source of UVA. However, due to variables like time of day, clouds and inadvertent exposure it is difficult to monitor the exact exposure dose with sunlight. This increases the chances of phototoxicity (sunburn). In spite of this, sunlight remains the cheapest and easily available source of UVA (Table 13.3).

Topical PUVA therapy involves careful application of 0.01–0.1% solution of trimethylpsoralen or B-methoxypsoralen over the affected skin, protecting the surrounding skin with a sunscreen. Ultraviolet exposure is given after 20–30 minutes of application. Avoidance of further exposure is necessary to avoid sunburn. Therapy is repeated every alternate or third day with gradual increase of exposure. A few small patches of vitiligo respond well to topical PUVA therapy over 2–4 months.

Systemic PUVA therapy consists of oral ingestion of trimethylpsoralen or methoxalen 20–30 mg to be followed, after 2 hours, by ultraviolet exposure. It is important to avoid further sun exposure as also to protect eyes with sunglasses (ultraviolet protective glasses). Therapy is repeated on alternate days with a graded increase in ultraviolet (UV) exposure. Widespread sable vitiligo takes 6–12 months to respond to this treatment.

Side Effects of PUVA Therapy

Oral psoralens may cause nausea and vomiting. Over-exposure (phototoxicity) to UVA leads to erythema, oedema, vesiculation, pain and tenderness of the involved skin. Hyperpigmentation of the surrounding normal skin is the commonest side effect. In white skinned people, after many months or years of use, skin damage due to UV

TABLE 13.3 : Comparison of psoralen and ultraviolet A vs narrow-band ultraviolet B

Psoralen and ultraviolet A (PUVA)	Narrow-band ultraviolet B (NBUVB)
Cannot be used in pregnancy, lactation, childhood and liver failure	Can be used in pregnancy, lactation, childhood and liver failure
Increased photosensitivity hence cannot be used for people working outdoors	Safer as no photosensitive agent used
Dosing is in terms of minutes	Dosing in terms of seconds It has to be frequently adjusted and exact
Accidental overexposure may lead to mild sunburn	Accidental overexposure may lead to severe sunburn
Strict photoprotection of skin and the eyes needed even outside the chamber	No photoprotection of skin and eyes needed outside the chamber
Relatively inexpensive	Expensive

radiation may lead to skin ageing, solar elastosis, solar keratoses and squamous cell carcinoma. Long term use is also fraught with the danger of developing cataracts, unless eyes are protected during therapy.

PUVA Therapy in Other Disorders

Systemic PUVA therapy constitutes an important therapeutic option in psoriasis. It is indicated in patients with chronic, stable, plaque type psoriasis involving > 25% body surface area that is unresponsive to topical therapy. Oral psoralen tablets are followed up with UVA exposure as in vitiligo, on alternate days.

Topical as well as systemic PUVA therapy has been used successfully in unresponsive alopecia areata, especially when whole scalp or whole body is affected. Other disorders in which PUVA therapy is occasionally used are pityriasis rosea, atopic dermatitis, mycosis fungoides and guttate parapsoriasis.

Narrow-band Ultraviolet B Phototherapy

Irradiation with ultraviolet B spectrum (290–320 nm) is useful for treatment of several skin diseases including vitiligo and psoriasis. Since no drug needs to be taken along with it, the therapy has become more popular than PUVA for widespread stable vitiligo and psoriasis. Of the UVB spectrum, the narrow band between 311–313 is maximally effective in the treatment of psoriasis. Such narrow band UVB phototherapy (311–313 nm) gives comparable results in other dermatoses responsive to PUVA therapy. However, it is safer than PUVA therapy as no photosensitising drug (psoralen) needs to be taken before exposure to the radiation.

Hence, no photoprotection for the eye and skin is needed outside the chamber. UVB phototherapy is safe during pregnancy, lactation and in childhood and old age.

Disadvantages of UVB phototherapy are that it is comparatively expensive and requires 2–3 clinic visits per week. Psoriasis that clears with UVB phototherapy frequently relapses unless maintenance exposures are given.

Targeted Ultraviolet B Phototherapy and Excimer Laser

These equipment help by giving targeted irradiation to the affected patches in a controlled fashion. Since surrounding normal skin is not exposed, tanning does not occur and doses can be increased in a quicker updosing regime giving faster response. Due to these advantages such therapy is likely to be the gold standard in treatment of localised stable vitiligo.

Summary: PUVA stands for psoralen with ultraviolet A (320–400 nm) irradiation. Sunlight can be substituted as a source of UVA light (PUVASOL therapy). For localised lesions of vitiligo, psoralens may be applied locally and then followed up with local UVA irradiation (local PUVA). Systemic PUVA therapy consists of oral psoralens (20–30 mg/dose), followed 2 hours later with UVA irradiation. PUVA therapy is quite effective in inducing pigmentation in vitiligo and causing resolution of psoriasis plaques in cases unresponsive to topical agents. Alopecia areata, parapsoriasis, mycosis fungoides and pityriasis rosea also respond to PUVA therapy. Side effects of PUVA include phototoxicity, hyperpigmentation, solar elastosis, cataracts and, in white skinned individuals, squamous cell carcinoma. UVB phototherapy is a safer alternative to PUVA therapy but is relatively expensive

Chapter

13

Pigmentary Disorders

DIFFERENTIAL DIAGNOSIS OF HYPOPIGMENTED PATCH

Most patients presenting with this complaint are worried about the diagnoses of leprosy and vitiligo. Hence, sympathetic attention and careful assessment of this complaint are essential. Other common causes of hypopigmented patches include pityriasis versicolor, pityriasis alba, postinflammatory hypopigmentation and nevus depigmentosus.

Differential Diagnosis of Hypopigmented Patch

- Leprosy
- Vitiligo
- Nevus depigmentosus
- Pityriasis versicolor
- Post-inflammatory hypopigmentation
- Pityriasis alba
- Lichen sclerosus et atrophicus

Leprosy

Although, hypopigmented patches can occur in any variety of leprosy they are more common in the indeterminate, tuberculoid and borderline tuberculoid varieties. Patches in these types are only a few in number, sharply demarcated, may be dry, slightly scaly, atrophic and anaesthetic. Reddish, hypopigmented patch of indeterminate leprosy may or may not be hypoaesthetic or dry. Towards the lepromatous pole patches become numerous, symmetrical, shiny, less dry and with normal sensations.

Sweat function is reduced in leprosy lesions as compared with unaffected skin on opposite side of the body. It may be measured by bromophenol blue paper or by injection of pilocarpine after painting with iodine and powdering with starch. Histamine test checks the spinal reflex arc which is damaged in leprosy. Injection of histamine does not elicit a flare in leprosy. Skin biopsy demonstrates a granulomatous infiltrate in leprosy. Skin smears are positive in borderline lepromatous and lepromatous leprosy.

In contrast to vitiligo, leprosy patches almost never turn depigmented (milky white). Other features of leprosy, e.g. plaques, nodules or regional nerve thickening may also be present. In cases of doubt, leprosy patches can be distinguished from others by sweat test, histamine test or a skin smear/biopsy.

Vitiligo

Although, depigmentation is more characteristic of vitiligo, evolving patches of vitiligo are hypopigmented. As opposed to leprosy, vitiligo patches may show variation in colour within or between patches. Other than lightening of skin colour vitiligo patches do not exhibit any other abnormality. Sensations are preserved and sweating, unaffected. Biopsy shows reduced or absent melanocytes. Wood's lamp examination accentuates vitiligo and nevus depigmentosus macules while those due to other causes are not accentuated. Dermoscopy and biopsy are supplementary for diagnosis of vitiligo.

Nevus Depigmentosus

This, usually solitary, birthmark is seen as an irregularly shaped, sharply demarcated, hypopigmented or depigmented patch. Skin is otherwise normal and the condition remains stable although the patch may grow proportionately with the growth of the child.

Pityriasis Versicolor

The numerous, discrete as well as coalescing, hypopigmented patches covered with powdery scales are typical of pityriasis versicolor. Early lesions as well as satellite lesions tend to be perifollicular. Upper trunk, neck and axillae are common sites. In lesions with scant scales, where demonstration of fungi under the microscope is difficult, preserved sensations and sweat function help in differentiation from leprosy. Scaly lesions show yellowish fluorescence on Wood's lamp.

Post-inflammatory Hypopigmentation

Several inflammatory disorders like tinea corporis, candidiasis, Xerotic eczema, polymorphous light eruption may heal with hypopigmentation. Past history of reddish skin lesions and preserved sensations and sweat function distinguish post-inflammatory hypopigmentation from patches of leprosy.

Pityriasis Alba

This benign hypopigmentation disorder of childhood causes concern because of its predominant involvement of face. Current opinion is to classify it as a form of mild subacute eczema affecting predominantly the sensitive skin of face in children (Fig. 13.11).

Clinically, poorly defined rounded hypopigmented macules and patches that bear scanty fine scales

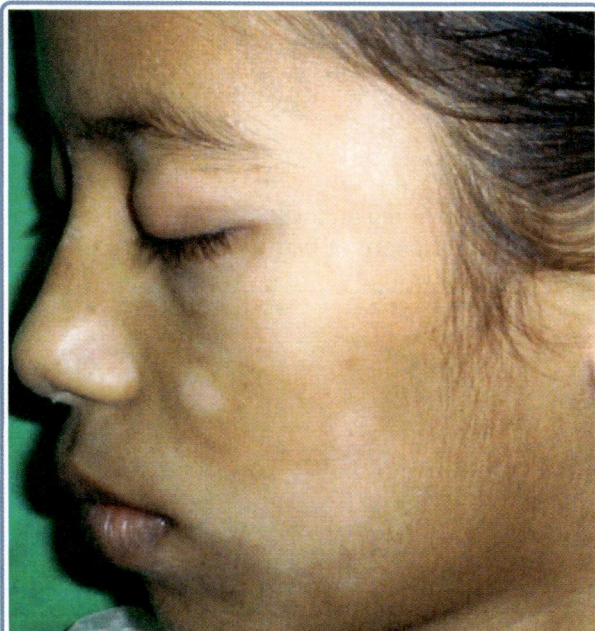

Fig. 13.11: Pityriasis alba—hypopigmented patches with barely appreciable scaling

characterise the condition. The condition responds to avoidance of all irritating agents (e.g. soaps) and application of a soothing and moisturising cream or a mild corticosteroid like hydrocortisone.

Summary: Differential diagnosis of a hypopigmented patch includes leprosy, vitiligo, pityriasis alba, pityriasis versicolor and postinflammatory hypopigmentation. Leprosy patches can be distinguished by their atrophy and reduced or absent sensations and sweating as well as enlarged nerves. Biopsy is confirmatory. Vitiligo patches are frequently depigmented (as against leprosy) but the skin is otherwise normal. Pityriasis versicolor presents as scaly hypopigmented macules and patches on the trunk of young adults. Scaling becomes prominent on scratching the lesions and fungi can be demonstrated under the microscope. Postinflammatory hypopigmentation follows an inflammatory process and lacks scaling. Pityriasis alba affects the face of children as ill defined hypopigmented macules and patches with fine scaling. Woods lamp examination and dermoscopy are helpful tools.

Differentiation of pityriasis alba from indeterminate leprosy is done on the basis of preserved sensations, sweat function, biopsy or observation with a therapeutic trial of a soothing cream.

DIFFERENTIAL DIAGNOSIS OF HYPERPIGMENTATION

Hyperpigmentation may be due to increased melanin in the epidermis or in the dermis.

Epidermal melanin appears brown or brownish black whereas dermal melanin appears blue or bluish black.

Clinical approach to a case of hyperpigmentation depends on whether it is localised, widespread or generalised as well as if it is dermal or epidermal or combined.

Localised

Common examples include:

Epidermal

Melasma—face, during or after pregnancy

Café au lait spots—any part of the body (Figs 13.12 and 13.13)

Freckles—face, in very fair skinned persons (Fig. 13.14)

Junctional melanocytic nevi-palms, soles, genitalia, in children and young adults.

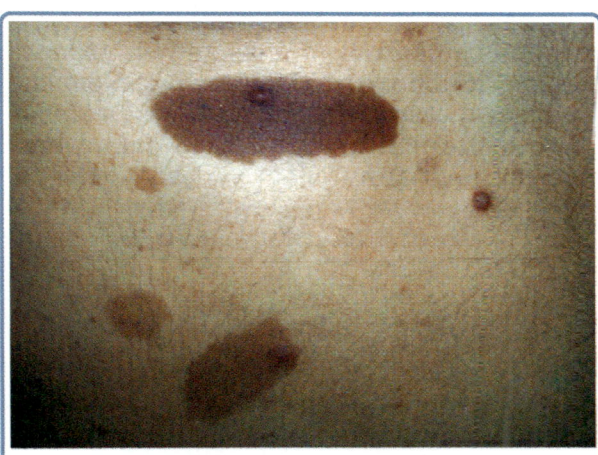

Fig. 13.12: Neurofibromatosis—multiple cafe au lait spots and papulonodules are characteristic

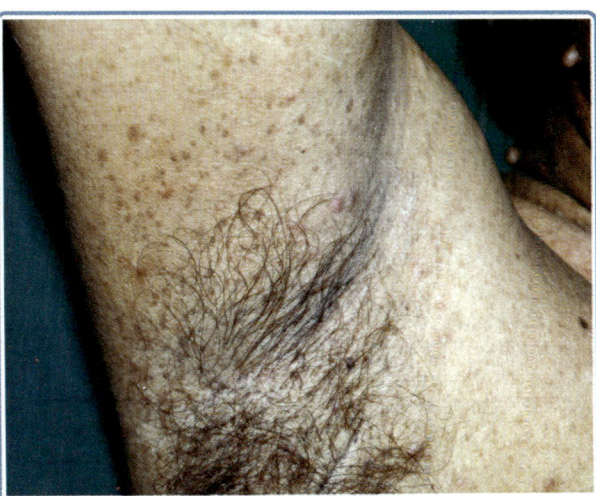

Fig. 13.13: Axillary freckling (Crowe's sign) is a feature of neurofibromatosis

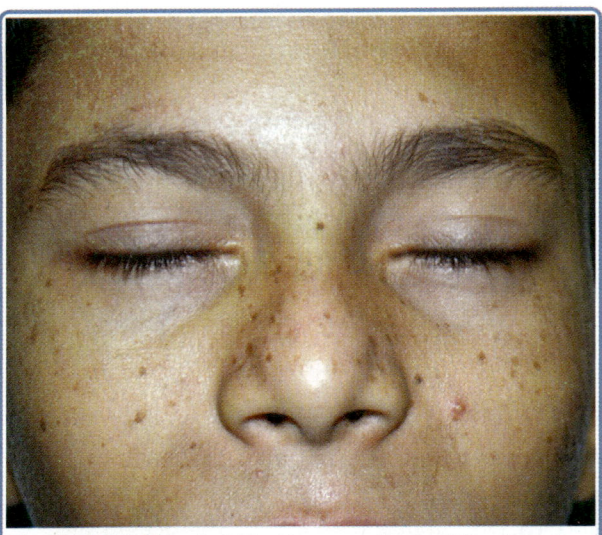

Fig. 13.14: Freckles—facial freckles presenting in childhood may be a manifestation of neurofibromatosis

Postinflammatory hyperpigmentation following eczema, dermatophytosis.

Dermal

Mongolian spots—sacrum, back of infants and young children.

Postinflammatory hyperpigmentation following lichen planus, fixed drug eruption (Figs 13.20 and 13.21).

Combined

Congenital melanocytic nevi—any site, present at birth.

Melanoma—hands and feet, variegated colour, slow growing macule or patch, young adults progresses to nodule which may ulcerate.

Widespread (Involving More than One Region)

> Although, this is the commonest presentation of cutaneous melanoma in Indians (acral lentiginous melanoma), melanoma is much more common in white skinned in whom it affects sun exposed skin.

Epidermal

Café au lait spots of neurofibromatosis: Presence of more than 5 cafe au lait spots of more than 1.5 cm diameter in an infant and more than 5 cm diameter in an adult suggests a diagnosis of neurofibromatosis (Fig. 13.12).

Postinflammatory hyperpigmentation following a widespread dermatosis, e.g. psoriasis.

Dermal

Post-inflammatory hyperpigmentation following widespread lichen planus, fixed drug eruption.

Combined

Giant congenital melanocytic nevus—involves large part of body, present at birth (Fig. 13.14A and B).

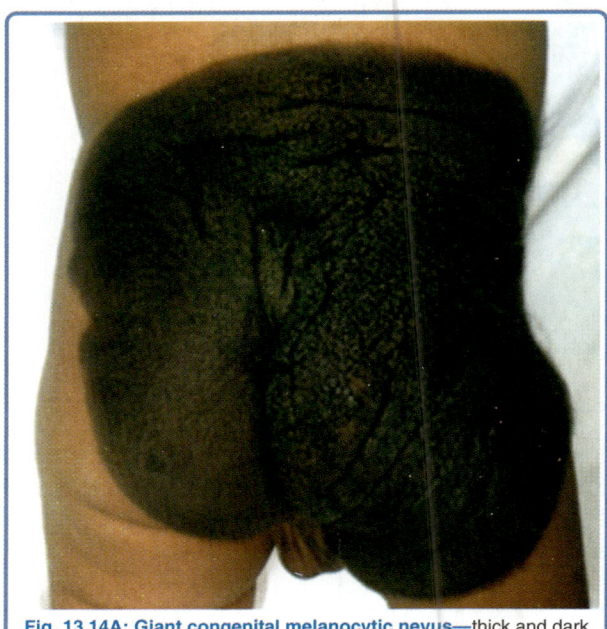

Fig. 13.14A: Giant congenital melanocytic nevus—thick and dark nevi may be hairy or have cerebriform pattern as seen here

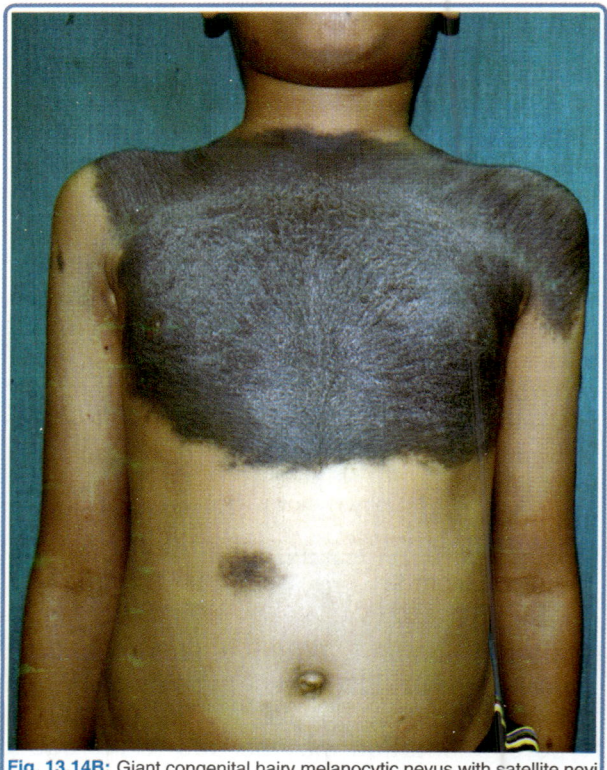

Fig. 13.14B: Giant congenital hairy melanocytic nevus with satellite nevi

Generalised

Epidermal

Suntan—exposed parts, uniform brown colour, 2–5 days after exposure.

Addison's disease—exposed parts, bony prominences, mucosae and brown-black colour.

Summary: Hyperpigmentation of skin may be generalised or localised. It may also be classified as epidermal, dermal or combined. Common causes of hyperpigmentation include melanocytic nevi, cafe au lait spots, mongolian spots, freckles, melasma (Fig. 13.15), post-inflammatory hyperpigmentation and the diffuse pigmentation involving sunexposed regions due to suntan or in Addison's disease.

MELASMA (PREGNANCY MASK)

This is the commonest cause of hyperpigmentation of face in women (Fig. 13.16).

Types of Melasma
• Centrofacial (63%)
• Malar (21%)
• Mandibular (16%)

Patient Profile

Although, most patients are women, men are occasionally affected. Hormonal changes are thought to underlie this disorder which frequently appears in the latter half of pregnancy or postpartum. Oral contraceptives have also been implicated in its causation in some cases.

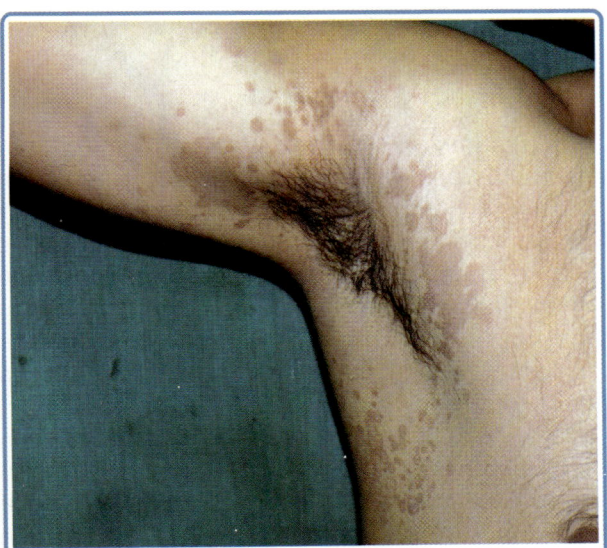

Fig. 13.15: Hyperpigmented pityriasis versicolor—hyperpigmented macules with fine scales made prominent on stroking (scratch sign)

Morphology

Grouped, well defined, 2–5 mm, light to dark brown macules tend to coalesce in the centre resulting in bigger brown patches (Figs 13.16–13.19). Macules remain more or less discrete at the periphery which becomes irregular in outline.

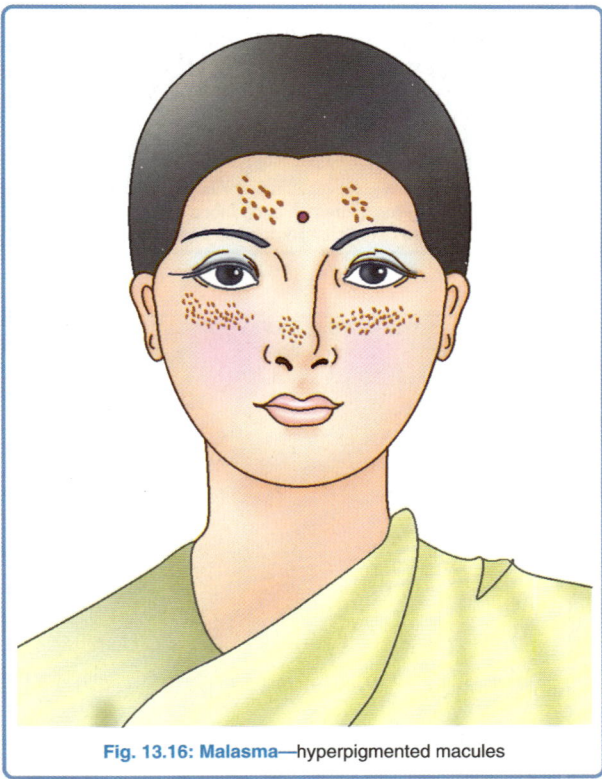

Fig. 13.16: Malasma—hyperpigmented macules

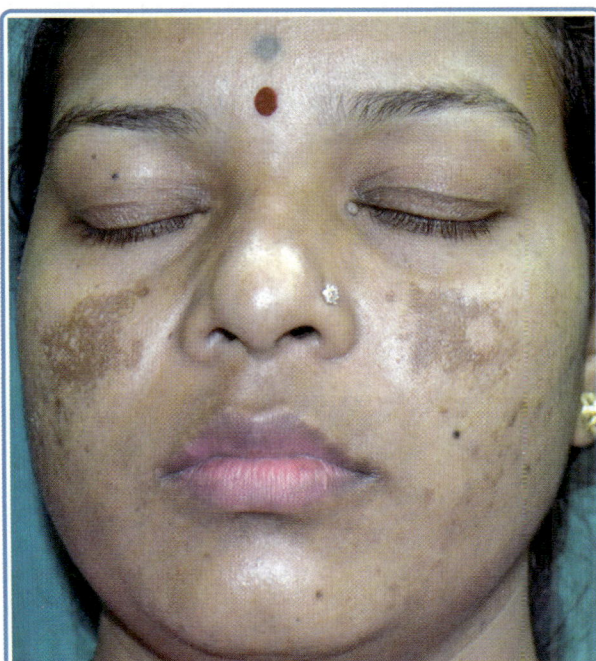

Fig. 13.17: Melasma—brown blotchy reticulate hyperpigmentation in symmetric pattern over cheeks

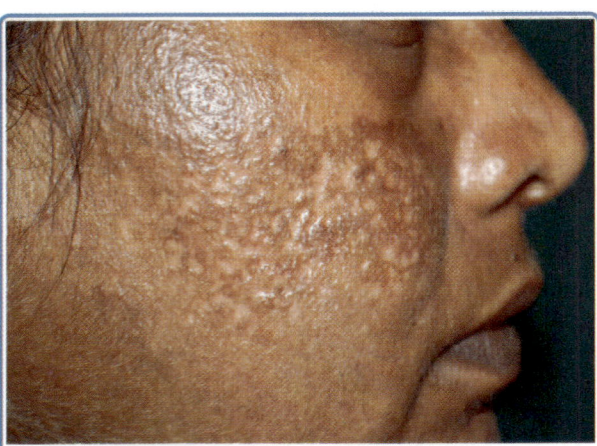

Fig. 13.18: Melasma—melasma with exogenous ochronosis seen with overuse of topical hydroquinone creams

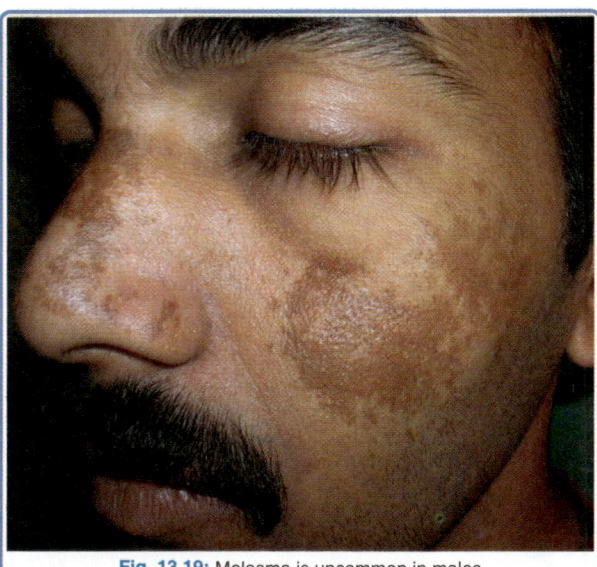

Fig. 13.19: Melasma is uncommon in males

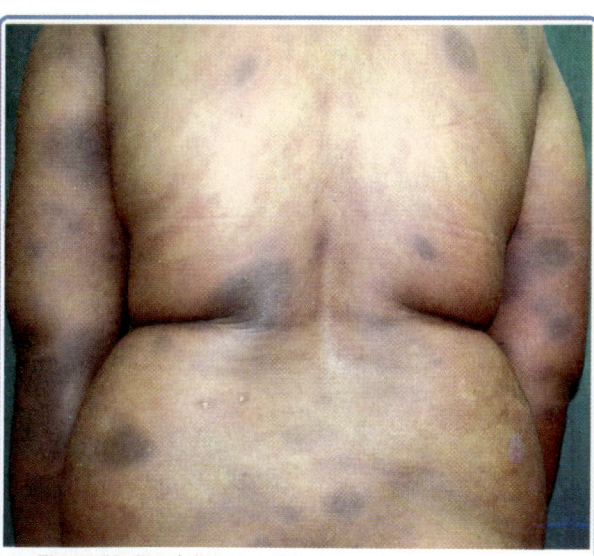

Fig. 13.20: Fixed drug eruption—discrete slate gray coloured hyperigmented patches with or without erythematous halo

Distribution

Symmetrical affection of malar regions and nose is typical. Sides of face, forehead and chin are involved in severe cases.

Therapy

Avoidance of sunlight and application of a sunscreen (PABA or titanium dioxide or calamine) is helpful. Topical application of 2–5% hydroquinone or 20% azelaic acid cream over many months leads to lightening of the dark patches. However, complete clearing is exceptional. Chemical peels are, claimed to be useful, if used at regular intervals. However, they should be used with caution since they may, by themselves induce hyperpigmentation in some cases.

> **Summary:** Melasma commonly begins in young ladies during pregnancy. Multiple, brown, coalescing macules over cheeks and nose in symmetric fashion are characteristic. Avoidance of sunlight, use of a sunscreen, 2–5% hydroquinone, and chemical peels help in improving the pigmentation.

Post-inflammatory Hyperpigmentation

Such pigmentation is light to dark brown when it is epidermal and grey-brown to bluish-grey, if it is dermal. It commonly follows inflammatory diseases like tinea corporis, acne, eczema or psoriasis and is reversible over time. Pigmentation for lichen planus or fixed drug eruption is dermal, grey-blue in colour and takes much longer to resolve. Skin lightening agents like hydroquinone or kojic acid improve the epidermal hyperpigmentation disorders.

Lichen Planus Pigmentosus

This uncommon brown-grey hyperpigmentation resembles post-inflammatory hyperpigmentation following lichen planus but is not preceded by any popular lichen planus lesions (Fig. 13.21). Biopsy is needed to demonstrate activity of disease. Unlike lichen planus it affects the face, neck, upper limbs and upper trunk more dominantly and spares mucosae. It is autoimmune in nature and causes much distress due to its cosmetic concerns. Treatment is unsatisfactory partial response is seen with immunomodulators like dapsone, hydroxy-chloroquine, cyclosporin and methotrexate, but due care must be exercised to avoid side effects. Sunprotective measures and skin lightening creams are partially effective.

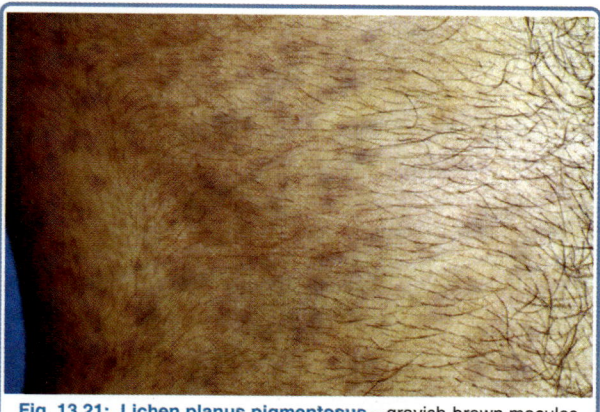

Fig. 13.21: **Lichen planus pigmentosus**—grayish-brown macules appear de novo in lichen planus pigmentosus

Abuse of Fairness Creams

Patients seeking 'fair skin' must be discouraged from joining the race for fairness as our skin pigment melanin is the protective umbrella that saves us from the harmful effects of ultraviolet radiation in sunlight. This is evident from the increased incidence of skin cancer among fair skinned caucasians who have migrated to tropical climates. Many fairness creams also contain steroids which damage the skin or hydroquinone in higher concentrations which causes ochronosis. Use of such creams for longer duration is not recommended.

MCQs

1. **Factors for induction of melasma include all of the following *except*:**
   a. Sunlight
   b. Ageing
   c. Pregnancy
   d. Drugs

2. **The commonest site of affection of melasma is:**
   a. Nose
   b. Cheeks
   c. Forehead
   d. Chin

3. **Topical drug used for treatment of melasma includes:**
   a. Tretinoin
   b. Benzoyl peroxide
   c. Trimethylpsoralen
   d. Clindamycin

4. **Addisonian pigmentation does not affect:**
   a. Palmar creases
   b. Knuckles
   c. Scalp
   d. Oral cavity

5. **Drug used for oral treatment of melasma is:**
   a. Hydroxychloroquine
   b. Prednisolone
   c. Trimethylpsoralen
   d. None of the above

6. **Most common skin malignancy occurring in albinism is:**
   a. Squamous cell carcinoma
   b. Melanoma
   c. Basal cell carcinoma
   d. Adenocarcinoma

7. **Commonest variety of albinism is transmitted as:**
   a. Autosomal recessive
   b. Autosomal dominant
   c. X-linked recessive
   d. X-linked dominant

8. **The enzyme that is deficient in albinism is:**
   a. Tryptase
   b. Phenylalanine hydroxylase
   c. Tyrosinase
   d. Tyrosine reductase

9. **Café au lait macules are a typical feature of:**
   a. Osler Weber Rendu disease
   b. Von Reckling Hausen disease
   c. Hansen's disease
   d. Park Weber syndrome

10. **All of the following are features of neuro-fibromatosis *except*:**
    a. Adenoma sebaceum
    b. Café au lait macules
    c. Acoustic neuroma
    d. Phaeochromocytoma

11. **The side effect of psoralen therapy that occurs with long term use is:**
    a. Skin blistering
    b. Fixed drug eruption
    c. Skin tanning
    d. Skin ageing

12. **Vitiligo is differentiated from leucoderma by:**
    a. Loss of sensations
    b. Loss of pigmentation
    c. Absence of prior inflammation
    d. Absence of scarring

13. **This type of vitiligo is least likely to spread:**
    a. Vitiligo vulgaris
    b. Segmental vitiligo
    c. Focal vitiligo
    d. Leucoderma

14. **The most accepted theory for pathogenesis of vitiligo is:**
    a. Neural theory
    b. Toxic theory
    c. Autotoxic theory
    d. Autoimmune theory

15. **Acromucosal vitiligo does not affect:**
    a. Lips
    b. Penis
    c. Axillae
    d. Toes

16. **Prevalence of vitiligo in general population is:**
    a. 1–2%
    b. 2–4%
    c. 4–5%
    d. 5–8%

17. **Therapy of choice for stable widespread vitiligo is:**
    a. PUVA therapy
    b. Punch grafting
    c. Oral steroids
    d. UVB phototherapy

18. **Which of the following is used as a source of ultraviolet light for treatment of vitiligo?**
    a. Wood's lamp
    b. Diathermy lamp
    c. Sunlight
    d. Tungsten lamp

19. **Contact leucoderma commonly occurs due to contact with:**
    a. Flowers
    b. Plastic
    c. Plants
    d. Colours

20. **Preferred surgical corrective therapy for stable small residual patches of vitiligo is:**
    a. Punch grafting
    b. Suction blister grafting
    c. Split thickness grafting
    d. Flap surgery

21. **Commonest side effect of topical PUVA therapy is:**
    a. Nausea
    b. Cataract
    c. Phototoxicity
    d. Allergic dermatitis

22. **In PUVA therapy, correct interval for ultraviolet exposure after psoralen ingestion is:**
    a. 30 minutes
    b. 60 minutes
    c. 120 minutes
    d. 180 minutes

23. **Commonest side effect of systemic PUVA therapy is:**
    a. Nausea
    b. Hepatotoxicity
    c. Phototoxicity
    d. Cataract

24. **All of the following commonly present as a hypopigmented patch *except*:**
    a. Pityriasis versicolor
    b. Pityriasis alba
    c. Pityriasis rosea
    d. Leprosy

25. **Most common presentation of pityriasis versicolor is:**
    a. Hypopigmented patches
    b. Hyperpigmented patches
    c. Erythematous patches
    d. Mixture of all colours

26. **Vitiligo is differentiated from leprosy patches based on:**
    a. Presence of sensations
    b. Chalky white colour
    c. Lack of nerve enlargement
    d. All of the above

27. **A 4-year-old child is brought with asthma and ill defined scaly white patches on cheeks. The most likely diagnosis is:**
    a. Vitiligo
    b. Pityriasis alba
    c. Pityriasis versicolor
    d. Indeterminate leprosy

28. **A 28-year-old woman complains of recent onset of asymptomatic well defined brown pigmented macules and patches over cheeks and nose. The most likely diagnosis is:**
    a. Fixed drug eruption
    b. Sunburn
    c. Melasma
    d. Lichen planus

29. **A 12-year-old child developed asymptomatic chalky white patches around nails and eyes. The most likely diagnosis is:**
    a. Pityriasis alba
    b. Vitiligo
    c. Contact leucoderma
    d. Pityriasis versicolor

30. **A 2-year-old boy is brought with multiple asymptomatic rounded light brown patches all over the body. He has a high chance of developing:**
    a. Giant congenital melanocytic nevi
    b. Epidermal nevi
    c. Neurofibromatosis
    d. Tuberous sclerosis

31. **A common site for fixed drug eruption is:**
    a. Abdomen
    b. Hand
    c. Scalp
    d. Back

32. **The colour of post-inflammatory hyperpigmentation following fixed drug eruption is:**
    a. Black
    b. Blue
    c. Slate-gray
    d. Brown

33. **Café au lait spots are a sign of:**
    a. Tuberous sclerosis
    b. Neurofibromatosis
    c. Birth asphyxia
    d. Neurolipomatosis

34. **Crowe's sign in neurofibromatosis relates to occurrence of:**
    a. Adenoma sebaceum
    b. Neurofibromas
    c. Café au lait spots
    d. Axillary freckling

35. **As per Crowe's rule the minimum number of café au lait spots needed for diagnosis of neurofibromatosis is:**
    a. 4
    b. 5
    c. 6
    d. 10

36. **Hyperpigmented lesions are seen in all *except*:**
    a. Melasma
    b. Pitiriasis alba
    c. Lichen planus pigmentosus
    d. Urticaria pigmentosa

Chapter 13

Pigmentary Disorders

37. **The commonest type of vitiligo is:**
    a. Vulgaris
    c. Acrofacial
    b. Segmental
    d. Facial

38. **Most common internal disease associated with vitiligo is:**
    a. Addison's disease
    b. Thyroid disease
    c. Vitamin D deficiency
    d. Diabetes mellitus

39. **Diffuse form of hyperpigmentation is seen in:**
    a. Vitamin B_{12} deficiency
    b. Ectopic ACTH secretion
    c. Addison's disease
    d. All the above

40. **17-year-old girl with acne has been taking a drug for last 2 years. She now presents with blue-black pigmentation of nails. The likely medication causing above pigmentation is:**
    a. Tetracycline   b. Minocycline
    c. Doxycycline   d. Azithromycin

				ANSWERS					
1-b,	2-b,	3-a,	4-c,	5-d,	6-a,	7-a,	8-c,	9-b,	10-a,
11-d,	12-c,	13-b,	14-d,	15-c,	16-a,	17-d,	18-c,	19-b,	20-b,
21-c,	22-c,	23-a,	24-c,	25-a,	26-d,	27-b,	28-c,	29-b,	30-c,
31-b,	32-c,	33-b,	34-d,	35-c,	36-b,	37-a,	38-b,	39-d,	40-b

Drug Eruptions including Erythema Multiforme and its Variants

DRUG ERUPTIONS

Patient Profile

Drug eruptions are less likely to occur in children and pregnant women. Most patients are adults, male or female. Elderly individuals are more likely to develop an eruption due to drugs.

General Characteristics

A drug eruption appears usually within the first 2–3 weeks of starting a drug. Most commonly, it appears within the first few days and at times within hours of drug ingestion. Most eruptions are pruritic and have a tendency to heal spontaneously on withdrawal of the offending drug.

Therapy of Drug Eruptions

Withdrawal of the causative or suspected drug/ drugs and oral antihistamines and topical soothing lotions suffice for most of the eruptions. Patients with widespread eruptions (drug induced exfoliative dermatitis) or severe eruptions (blistering fixed drug

TABLE 14.1: Common eruptions due to drugs

Fixed drug eruption	:	NSAIDs, sulphonamides and tetracyclines, phenolphthalein and ciprofloxacin
Maculopapular rash (Figs 14.1 and 14.2A and B)	:	Ampicillin and other penicillins, NSAIDs, antiepileptics, sulphonylureas, anti-hypertensives, nevirapine and efavirenz
Urticaria	:	NSAIDs, penicillins and cephalosporins, vaccines, contrast media, insulin and other hormones
Acneiform	:	INH, glucocorticoids, androgens, iodides and bromides
Erythema multiforme and Stevens Johnson syndrome	:	Sulphonamides and penicillins, NSAIDs, rifampicin, antiepileptics, sulphones and nevirapine
Photodermatitis	:	NSAIDs, tetracyclines and sulphonamides, phenothiazines, thiazides and sulphonylureas
Erythroderma	:	Sulphonamides, penicillins, NSAIDs, antiepileptics and gold
Lichen planus like eruption	:	Chloroquine, gold, anti-tuberculous drugs, anti-epileptics and phenothiazines
Toxic epidermal necrolysis	:	NSAIDs, antituberculous drugs, penicillins, antiepileptics, sulphonamides allopurinol

TABLE 14.2: Common drugs that cause eruptions

Sulphonamides and Co-trimoxazole	:	Fixed drug eruption, erythema multiforme and Stevens Johnson syndrome
Aspirin and NSAIDs	:	Urticaria, maculopapular rash, fixed drug eruption, erythema multiforme and Stevens Johnson syndrome
Penicillins	:	Urticaria, maculopapular rash
Tetracyclines	:	Fixed drug eruption, photodermatitis
INH and steroids	:	Acneiform eruption
Chloroquine, phenothiazines and sulphonylurea	:	Lichenoid eruption, photodermatitis
Barbiturates, phenytoin	:	Maculopapular eruption, lichenoid eruption and acneiform eruption
Quniolones	:	Fixed drug eruption, photodermatitis and Stevens Johnson syndrome
Antiretrovirals	:	Maculopapular rash, erythema multiforme and Stevens Johnson syndrome

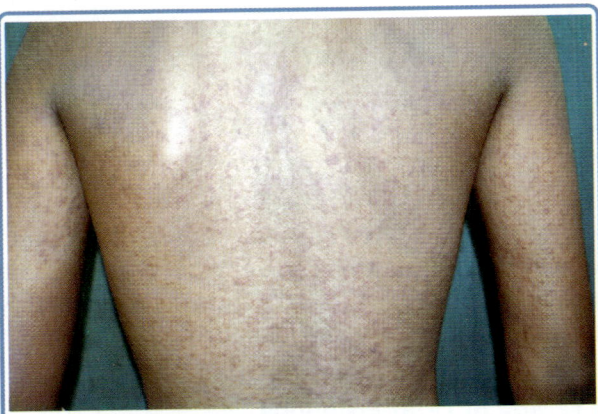

Fig. 14.1: Maculopopular drug rash—generalised itchy erythematous maculopapular rash

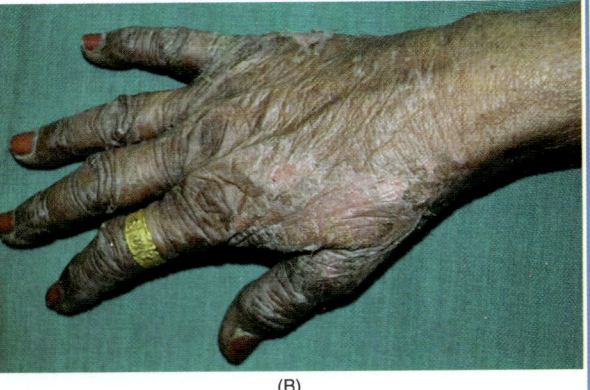

(A)

(B)

Fig. 14.2A and B: Drug induced photoallergy—diffuse erythema and scaling over face and hand

Chapter
14

Drug Eruptions including
Erythema Multiforme and its Variants

eruption and erythema multiforme) frequently need a short course of systemic steroids for rapid resolution. Topical therapy for drug eruptions includes soothing calamine lotion and steroid creams.

Stevens Johnson syndrome and toxic epidermal necrolysis are life-threatening medical emergencies and their therapy resembles that of extensive superficial burns. Admission to an acute care unit, warm surroundings, restoring water and electrolyte balance (input/output records and serum electrolytes to be monitored), and parenteral nutrition are the supportive measures. Administration of parenteral dexamethasone 0.2–0.4 mg/kg/day for short duration is of value in preventing progression. Recent additions to successful therapy have been oral cyclosporine 3–5 mg/kg/day and intravenous immunoglobulin 2 g/kg in divided doses over 3–5 days.

Summary: Drug eruptions are uncommon in children. They appear usually within a few days or hours of beginning a new drug. They are pruritic. Antibacterials, nonsteroidal anti-inflammatory drugs (NSAIDs) and antiepileptics are the commonest causes of drug eruptions. Minor rashes subside on withdrawal of the concerned drug and application of topical steroids. Severe (blistering) or extensive (exfoliative dermatitis) rashes need systemic steroids tapered over 1–2 weeks. Stevens Johnson syndrome and toxic epidermal necrolysis are medical emergencies and the latter needs to be treated like 100% superficial burns. Oral cyclosporine and intravenous steroids or immunoglobulin (IVIg) are life saving in Stevens Johnson syndrome and toxic epidermal necrolysis.

FIXED DRUG ERUPTION

The peculiarity of this drug eruption is that if affects a particular body site repeatedly with every exposure to a particular drug, i.e. it is fixed to a particular site. This is a common drug eruption in India. Sulphonamides, NSAIDs, quinolones, tetracyclines, phenolphthalein, barbiturates and phenytoin are common causes (Fig. 14.7A).

Morphology

Initial lesion of fixed drug eruption is a circular or oval, erythematous patch or a barely elevated plaque that appears within 1–2 days of the intake of the offending agent (Fig. 14.3). Accompanying sensation of burning or stinging is common. Occasionally, vesicle or bulla may develop (Fig. 14.4). Within a few days the lesion starts darkening in the centre, the margins still showing signs of erythema. After a couple of weeks (usually with the withdrawal of the implicated drug) only a rounded patch of greyish black discolouration remains at the

commonly affects dorsae of hands and feet, palms and soles, lips, genitalia (Fig. 14.6), periorbital region, face and oral mucosa. However, it is not uncommon on trunk or proximal extremities.

Therapy

Please *see* therapy of drug eruptions.

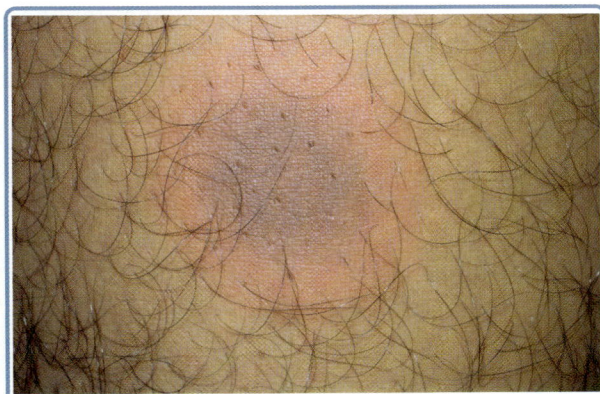

Fig. 14.3: Fixed drug eruption—a fresh lesion showing erythema and central pigmentation

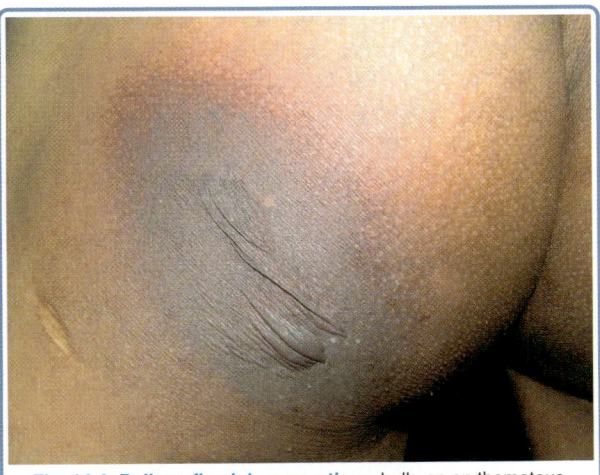

Fig. 14.4: Bullous fixed drug eruption—bulla on erythematous, hyperpigmented background

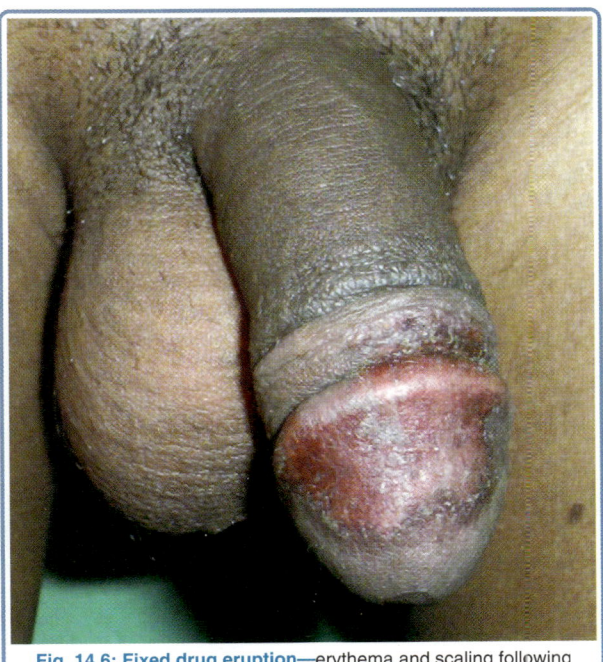

Fig. 14.6: Fixed drug eruption—erythema and scaling following ingestion of ibuprofen

site and this persists for 6 months to 2 years (Fig. 14.5). When challenged with the offending drug (knowingly unknowingly), the site turns erythematous again and later darker.

Distribution

Acral regions and mucocutaneous junctions are the favoured sites. Hence, fixed drug eruption

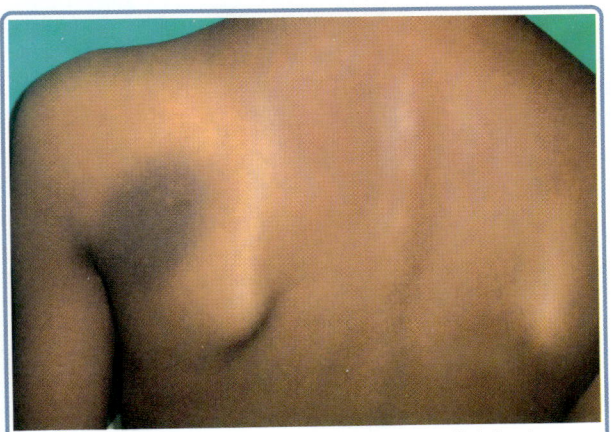

Fig. 14.5: Fixed drug eruption—persistent, ill defined hyperpigmented patch

Summary: Fixed drug eruption recurs at the same site after every exposure to the offending drug. Sulphonamides, NSAIDs and phenolphthalein are common causes. Initial lesions are one or many, dusky red, circular macules that soon turn greyish black in colour. The pigmentation takes many months to fade and hence, patients may present with only pigmented macules or patches that represent inactive lesions. Acral and mucocutaneous junctional regions are commonly affected. Treatment is avoidance of the suspected drug and topical steroids, when lesions are active.

Chapter 14

Erythema Multiforme, Stevens Johnson Syndrome and Toxic Epidermal Necrolysis

Erythema multiforme, Stevens Johnson syndrome and toxic epidermal necrolysis are best considered together because of striking clinicopathologic and aetiologic similarities. They probably represent morphologic and distributional variants of the same pathologic process. The inflammatory pattern of these disorders can be induced not only by drugs but also by infections.

Drug Eruptions including Erythema Multiforme and its Variants

ERYTHEMA MULTIFORME

Aetiology

Drugs commonly implicated are sulphonamides, NSAIDs (aspirin, pyrazolones, oxicams, acetic acid derivatives, etc.), tetracyclines, penicillins, phenytoin, barbiturates, quinolones, rifampicin, isonicotinythydrazide (INH), para-aminosalicylate sodium (PAS), thiacetazone, phenothiazines and nevirapine.

Common infections that are proposed to be causative include viral (herpes simplex), bacterial (streptococcal), mycobacterial (tuberculosis) and mycoplasmal. Recurrent herpes simplex is known to be associated with recurrent erythema multiforme (Fig. 14.7B).

Rare Causes for Erythema Multiforme

- Infections like infectious mononucleosis, syphilis, trichomoniasis and histoplasmosis.
- Systemic diseases like lymphomas, leukaemias, systemic lupus erythematosus and sarcoidosis.
- Physiologic states like pregnancy.
- Ingestants like food additives.
- Inhalants like organophosphorus compounds.

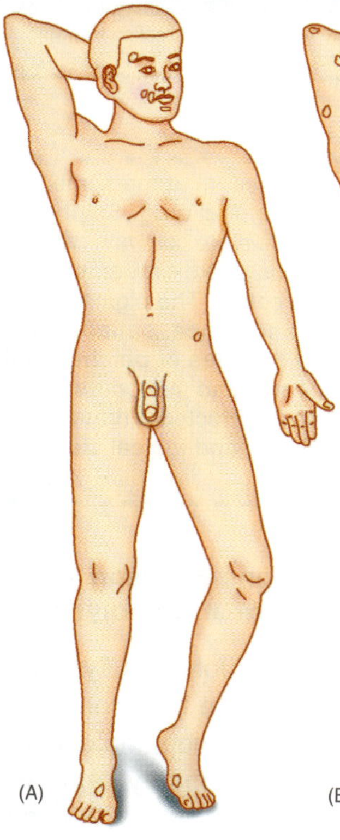

Erythema multiforme and Stevens Johnson syndrome are reported to be commoner in the human immunodeficiency virus (HIV) infected especially following sulphonamides or nevirapine. Despite this long list, the exact cause for erythema multiforme/Stevens Johnson syndrome frequently remains undetermined.

Patient Profile

Most patients are young adults. Children and elderly are involved uncommonly. Both sexes are affected equally. Mild constitutional disturbance is common.

Morphology

As implied in the name, lesions are multiform (varied morphology). Initial lesions are erythematous macules and patches that rapidly become elevated to form papules and plaques which develop a dark red centre. Within a few days, the lesions progress to typical target lesions (also called bull's eye lesion or iris lesion) that comprise three concentric zones, from outside in, erythema (bright red), oedema (pale) and the dark red or gray centre that represents either purpura or vesiculation (Figs 14.8, 14.9). Erosions surrounded by erythema characterise the mucosal affection.

Distribution

Mucocutaneous junctions (lips, glans penis), mucosae (oral, conjunctival), acrae (palms, soles, dorsa of hands and feet) and extremities are preferentially affected. Trunk is affected commonly, though the density of lesions is lesser. Widespread involvement with many bullous lesions with severe mucosal involvement is termed as erythema multiforme major.

Fig. 14.7A: Fixed drug eruption—hyperpigmented patches

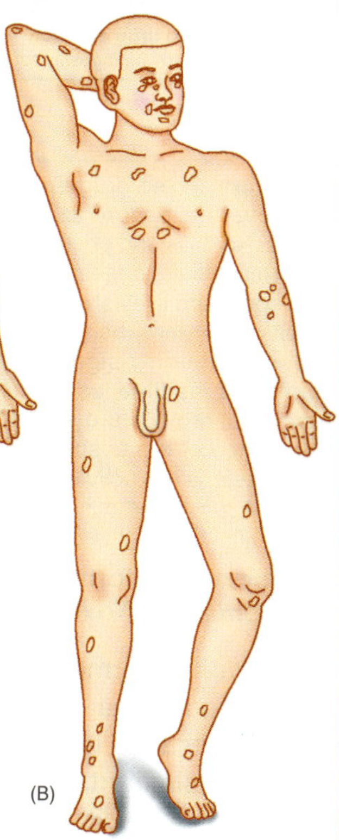

Fig. 14.7B: Erythema multiforme—erythematous papules, plaques, vesicles, target lesions

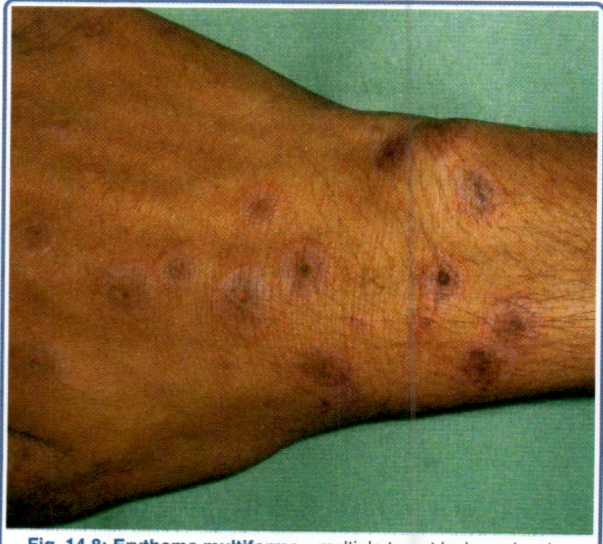

Fig. 14.8: Erythema multiforme—multiple target lesions showing three colour zones in each lesion

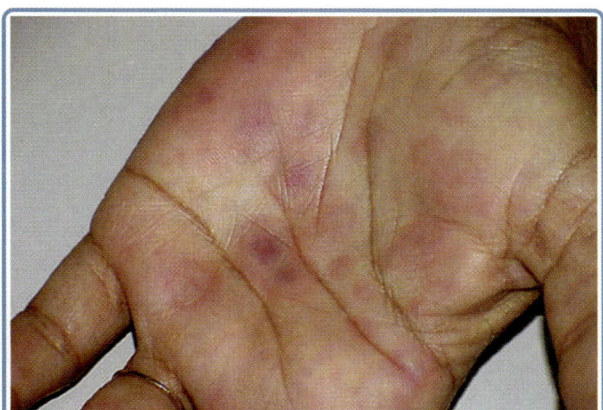

Fig. 14.9: Erythema multiforme—target lesions show three zones inside out-purpura, oedema and erythema

Diagnosis

In the presence of typical target lesions and sudden appearance of polymorphic lesions in characteristic distribution, biopsy is rarely needed to establish diagnosis.

Therapy

Please *see* therapy of drug eruptions.

Summary: Erythema multiforme is a hypersensitivity reaction to herpetic, streptococcal, mycobacterial or mycoplasmal infections or to drugs like sulphonamides, NSAIDs, antibiotics, antituberculous agents and anti-epileptics. Polymorphous rash includes the characteristic target lesions that comprise a dark centre, surrounded by pale and bright red zones of oedema and erythema respectively (Fig. 14.10). Acral regions and mucocutaneous junctions are preferred sites. Therapy is symptomatic (other than identifying and treating the cause) except in severe cases when systemic steroids may be used.

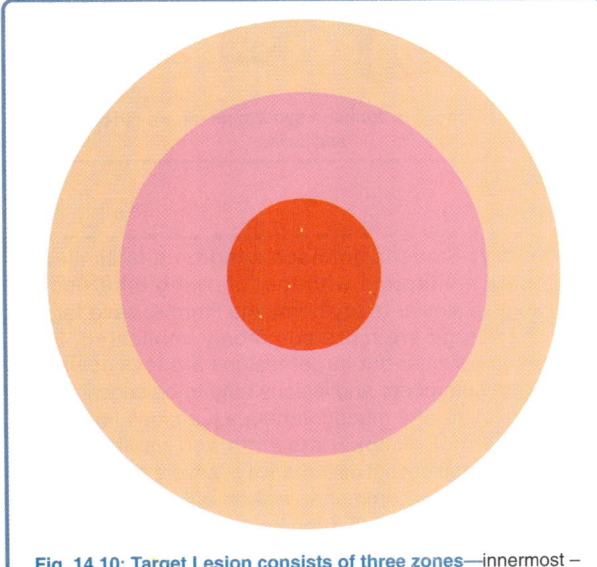

Fig. 14.10: Target Lesion consists of three zones—innermost – **dusky red**   middle – **pink**   outermost – **brighter red flare**

STEVENS JOHNSON SYNDROME

Patient Profile

Adolescents and young adults of both sexes are commonly affected. Children and elderly are affected less frequently. A mild prodrome of fever, malaise, body ache, and sore throat is frequently noted by the patient. Drugs given for these symptoms may sometimes be blamed unjustifiably as the rash is noticed 1–2 days after the other symptoms (Fig. 14.11).

Morphology

Typical target lesions are absent. Most lesions begin as tender dusky red patches of erythema that turn dark red to brown-black for most of the part of the lesion except the rim that remains erythematous (Figs 14.11 and 14.13). The centre often develops into a haemorrhagic vesicle in a few days and may get deroofed to leave behind an erosion. Mucosal lesions are similar to erythema multiforme but are more widespread and confluent. Painful erosions of lips are covered with thick, adherent, haemorrhagic crusts (Fig. 14.14). Severe erosions of oropharynx may be painful enough to prevent the movements of eating or talking.

Distribution

Mucocutaneous junctions, mucosae and per orificial regions are preferentially or exclusively involved. Other regions of the body may also be affected albeit to a lesser extent. Severe ocular involvement leads to keratitis, corneal ulceration and its resultant complications.

Diagnosis

Morphology and distribution are characteristic enough. Skin biopsy is diagnostic and shows

Chapter
14

Drug Eruptions including
Erythema Multiforme and its Variants

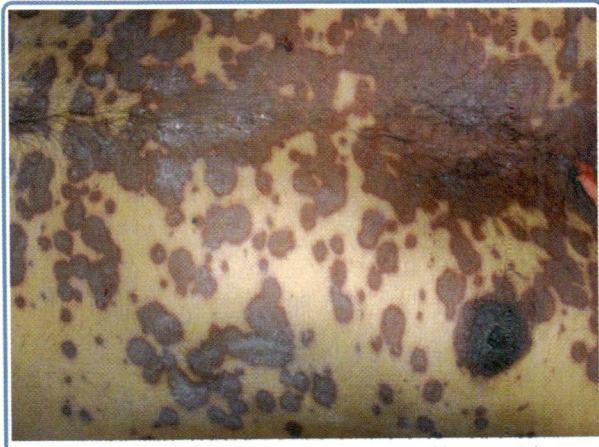

Fig. 14.11: Stevens Johnson syndrome—red brown patches resembling superficial burns

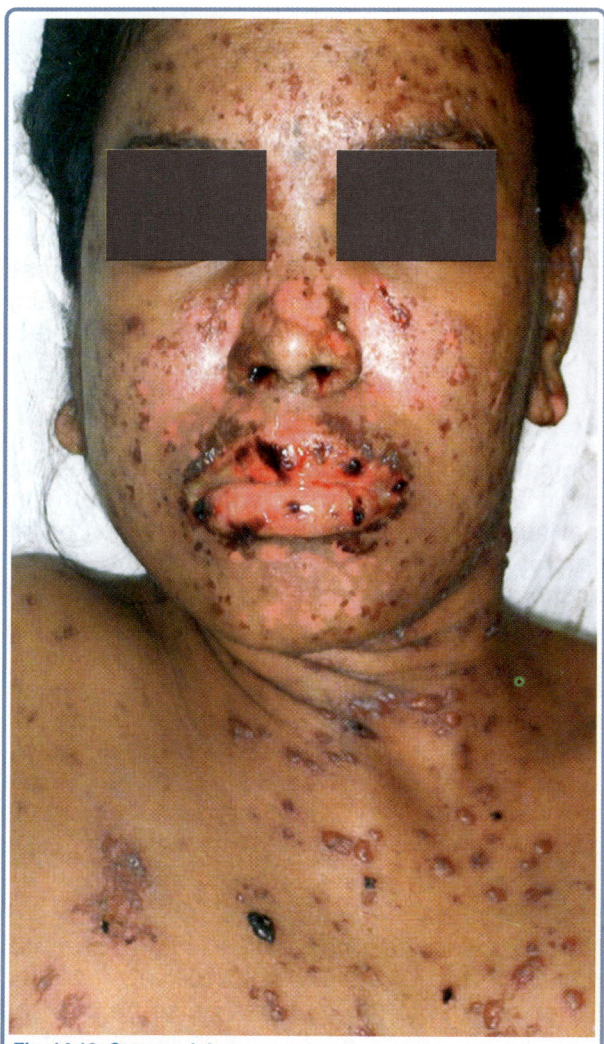

Fig. 14.12: Stevens Johnson syndrome—vesicles and bullae on the neck and chest. Erosions and haemorrhagic crusts on lips are characteristic

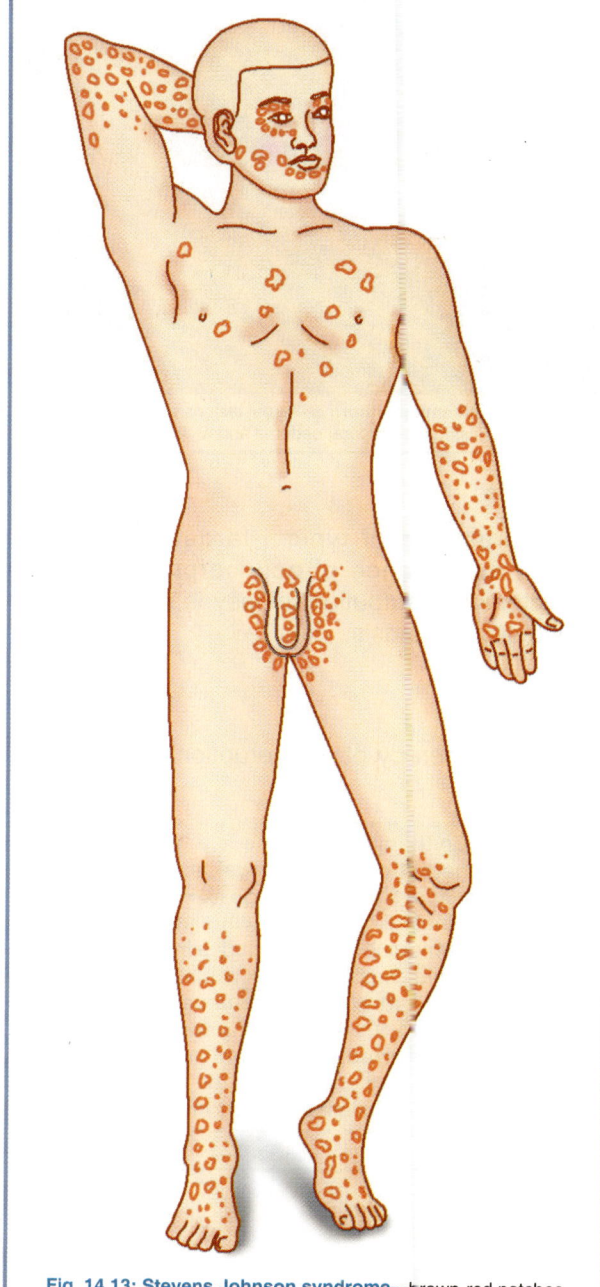

Fig. 14.13: Stevens Johnson syndrome—brown-red patches and bullae

confluent epidermal necrosis or interface change with necrotic keratinocytes.

Therapy

Please *see* under 'therapy of toxic epidermal necrolysis'.

Systemic Affection in Stevens Johnson Syndrome and Toxic Epidermal Necrolysis

This is common in patients who have more than 25% body area involvement or have toxic epidermal necrolysis. Extensive erosions of pharynx, oesophagus, and stomach hamper oral feeds or make the patient unable to tolerate a Ryle's tube. Pneumonitis, hepatitis, nephritis, leucopenia, and gastrointestinal bleeding may supervene. Patients with extensive body area involvement are prone to fluid and electrolyte imbalances. Toxaemia, aspiration pneumonia and septicaemia are other complications.

Summary: Stevens Johnson syndrome is similar to erythema multiforme with the following differences. Aetiology is similar to erythema multiforme, save for the fact that drugs are more commonly implicated. Skin lesions are similar but target lesions are less common, bullae are commoner and lesions tend to be concentrated over mucosae and mucocutaneous junctions leading to severe painful mucosal erosions and haemorrhagic crusting. Constitutional disturbance is severe and systemic complications are commoner. A short course of high dose systemic steroids (0.2–0.4 mg/kg/day of dexamethasone) along with supportive therapy in an acute care unit is needed.

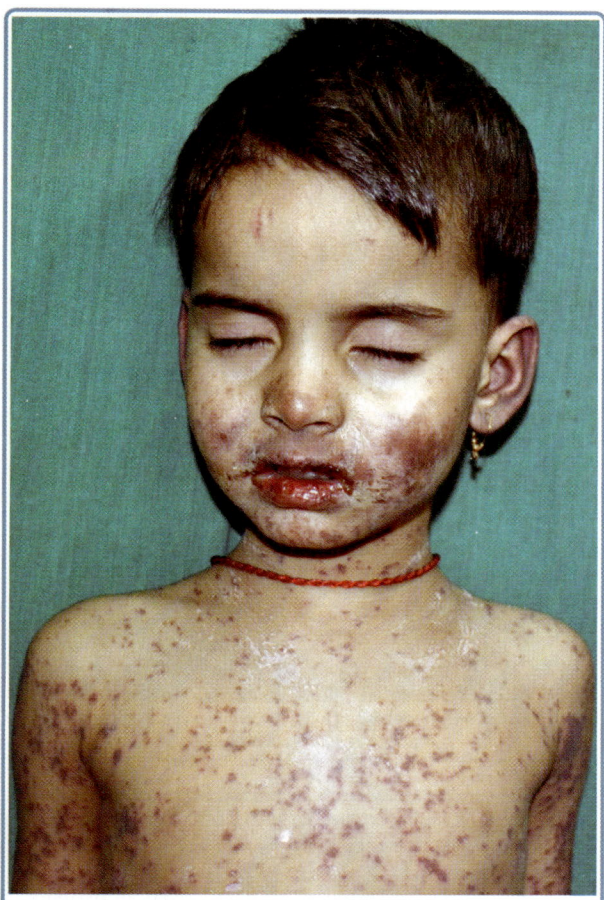

Fig. 14.14: Stevens Johnson syndrome—condition tends to be milder in children with better outcome

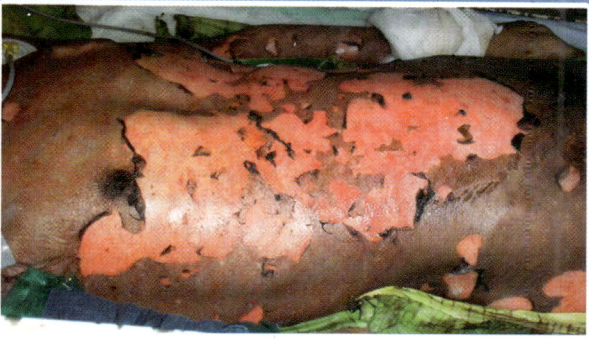

Fig. 14.15: Toxic epidermal necrolysis—separation of the necrotic epidermis in large sheets

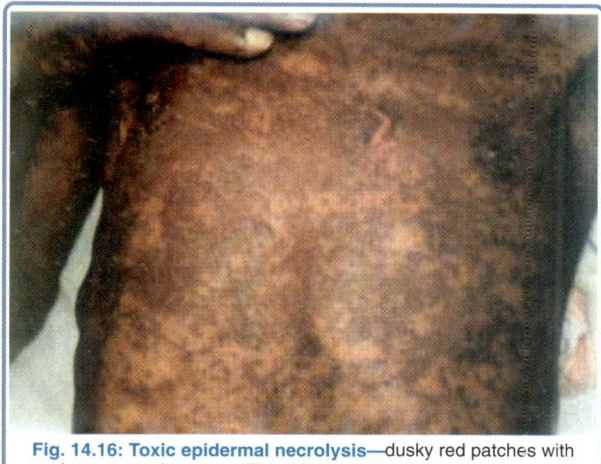

Fig. 14.16: Toxic epidermal necrolysis—dusky red patches with tendency to coalescence. The skin is fragile and erodes on trauma

TOXIC EPIDERMAL NECROLYSIS

This generalised skin affection carries about 50% mortality. Drugs implicated in its pathogenesis include NSAIDs (especially pyrazolones), sulphonamides, penicillins, phenytoin, barbiturates and allopurinol. As opposed to erythema multiforme, infections account for a minority of cases.

Patient Profile

Young adults are affected more commonly. Elderly individuals and children are affected less frequently.

Morphology and Distribution

Large patches of tender dusky erythema involve the whole body. Within 24–48 hours fluid begins to collect under the upper layer of the skin (epidermis) forming vesicles that coalesce and form bullae. As adjacent large flaccid bullae coalesce, their roof is shed as a sheet leaving behind large erosions which ooze serosanguinous fluid (Figs 14.15 and 14.16). Application of a rotational shearing force with thumb over erythematous or even apparently normal skin, preferably over a bony prominence, leads to peeling (Nikolsky's sign). Mucosal lesions are indistinguishable from Stevens Johnson syndrome. Severe palmoplantar affection is common.

Toxic epidermal necrolysis needs to be differentiated from staphylococcal scalded skin syndrome which is more common in infants, spares palms, soles and mucosae, and being caused by staphylococci, has to be treated with antibacterials like cloxacillin.

Therapy of Toxic Epidermal Necrolysis

Patients must be managed in an intensive care unit. A short course of high dose steroids early in the course of the disease may be beneficial (please *see* therapy of drug eruptions). Rest of the therapy is supportive, i.e. maintenance of nutrition, fluid and electrolyte intake, urinary catheterisation and management of any other complications as and when they arise. Avoidance of friction between skin and clothes or bed prevents extensive denudation. Ocular antibiotic and moistening preparations are useful for keratoconjunctivitis.

Summary: Although, aetiopathologically related to erythema multiforme, toxic epidermal necrolysis is a life-threatening disease due to necrosis of whole body epidermis and mucosal epithelia. Epidermis peels off in large sheets on a background of diffuse tender erythema and bullae all over the body. Mucosal lesions resemble Stevens Johnson syndrome. Nikolsky's sign is positive. Systemic complications are fluid, electrolyte and temperature imbalance and propensity for developing infections. Therapy is similar to that of 100% superficial burns.

DRUG HYPERSENSITIVITY REACTION

Drug hypersensitivity reaction presents with fever generalised skin eruption and internal organ involvement. The skin rash begins as an itchy, erythematous, maculopapular rash that soon becomes generalised and later may lead to erythroderma (Figs 14.17 and 14.18). Liver is the most common internal organ involved leading to hepatitis with or without jaundice. Lymphadeno-pathy and kidney involvement can also occur. The reaction usually starts after a few weeks following exposure to the suspected drug. Antiepileptics, dapsone and sulphonamides are common causes of this reaction. Peripheral blood examination may show eosinophilia and atypical lymphocytosis. Reaction subsides after weeks to months following withdrawal of the offending drug. Severe reactions need to be treated with systemic steroids.

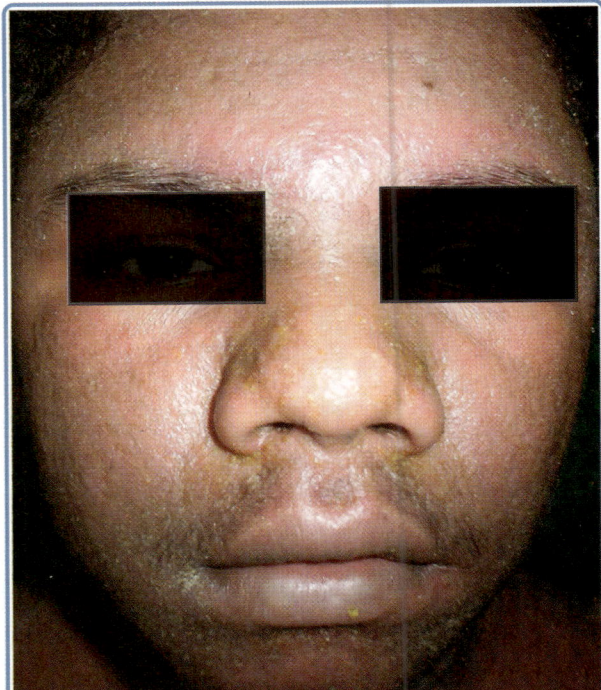

Fig. 14.18: Drug hypersensitivity reaction—erythema, oedema of face with scaling and crusting

body involvement (erythroderma). Rash resembles a viral exanthem (e.g. measles), but is more oedematous and is pruritic (Fig. 14.1).

Penicillins esp. ampicillin (particularly in patients with infectious mononucleosis), NSAIDs, antidiabetics, anti-hypertensives and nevirapine are common culprits.

Acneiform drug eruption: Lesions are monomorphic follicular papules resembling papular acne vulgaris but occur predominantly over the trunk (Fig. 14.19). Isonicotinylhydrazide (INH) and systemic steroids are commonly implicated.

Lichenoid drug eruption: Rash resembles lichen planus but lacks Wickham's striae. Rash is generalised and does not show preference for flexors and does not affect mucosae as with lichen planus.

Drug-induced photodermatitis: *See Chapter 15, Photosensitive Dermatoses.*

Other Drug-induced Rashes

See Table 14.1 for causes. These include:

Drug-induced urticaria: Morphology is that of urticaria. Urgent therapy may be necessary if accompanied by anaphylactoid syndrome. Please *see* management of acute urticaria on page 144.

Maculopapular drug eruption: Generalised erythematous macules and papules that coalesce and lead to full

---

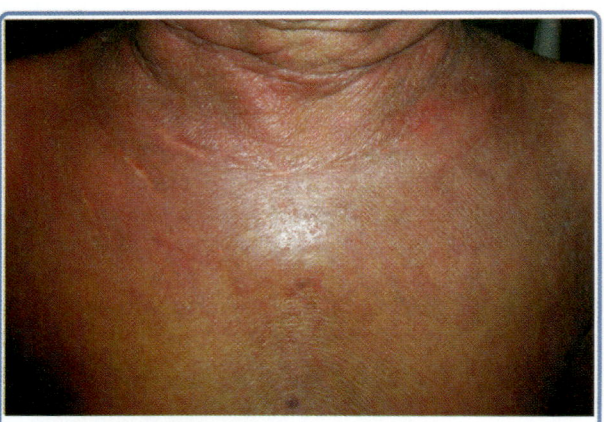

Fig. 14.17: Drug hypersensitivity reaction—generalised erythema and scaling

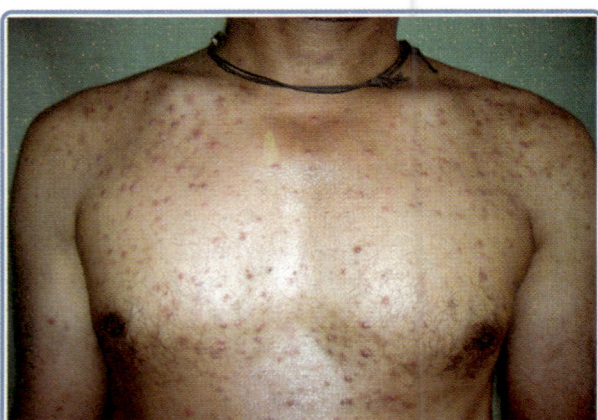

Fig. 14.19: Acneiform eruption—erythematous and skin colored papules in a patient on oral cortecosteroids

MCQs

1. Drug eruption is not a common side effect with which of the following drugs?
a. Ciprofloxacin
b. Carbamazepine
c. Azithromycin
d. Nevirapine

2. Drug eruption is a common side effect of which of the following drugs?
a. Cotrimoxazole
b. Erythromycin
c. Paracetamol
d. Digitalis

3. Which of the following drug reactions may be life threatening?
a. Fixed drug eruption
b. Maculopapular drug eruption
c. Angio-oedema
d. Lichenoid drug eruption

4. Which of the following drug eruption has high mortality rate?
a. Toxic epidermal necrolysis
b. Drug induced erythroderma
c. Drug induced urticaria
d. Stevens Johnson syndrome

5. Which of the following drugs is not a common cause of drug eruptions?
a. Ampicillin
b. Omeprazole
c. Sulphamethoxazole
d. Phenobarbitone

6. Which drug eruption is characterised by prominent post-inflammatory hyperpigmentation?
a. Erythema multiforme
b. Stevens Johnson syndrome
c. Fixed drug eruption
d. Maculopapular drug eruption

7. Which of the following drug eruptions may present as a bullous eruption?
a. Erythema multiforme
b. Lichenoid drug eruption
c. Urticaria
d. Photoallergic dermatitis

8. Which of the following drug eruptions is not associated with development of blisters?
a. Erythema multiforme
b. Fixed drug eruption
c. Toxic epidermal necrolysis
d. Urticaria

9. A 35-year-old male presented with burning, dusky red coloured, rounded patches over hands, feet and face since 3 days. The patient appeared comfortable but had been taking treatment for backache for the last few days. What is the most probable diagnosis for his skin rash?
a. Stevens Johnson syndrome
b. Photoallergic dermatitis
c. Urticaria
d. Fixed drug eruption

10. A 25-year-old female complained or recurrent reddening and persistent pigmentation of a 2 inch spot on the arm. She had been taking an over the counter preparation for headache off and on. The most likely diagnosis is:
a. Lichenoid drug eruption
b. Photoallergic dermatitis
c. Urticaria
d. Fixed drug eruption

11. Which of the following antiepileptics does not commonly cause a drug eruption?
a. Carbamazepine
b. Phenobarbitone
c. Phenytoin
d. Sodium valproate

12. Which of the following drugs does not commonly cause fixed drug eruption?
a. Sulphamethoxazole
b. Ibuprofen
c. Ciprofloxacin
d. Erythromycin

13. Which of the following drug eruptions is associated with prominent lip involvement?
a. Angio-oedema
b. Stevens Johnson syndrome
c. Fixed drug eruption
d. Maculopapular drug eruption

14. Which of the following drug eruptions is characterised by target lesions?
a. Stevens Johnson syndrome
b. Erythema multiforme
c. Toxic epidermal necrolysis
d. Fixed drug eruption

15. A drug eruption which resembles measles is called:
a. Morbilliform drug eruption
b. Erythema multiforme
c. Stevens Johnson syndrome
d. Rubeola

16. **A drug eruption with prominent affection of mucosae is:**
    a. Stevens Johnson syndrome
    b. Urticaria
    c. Maculopapular drug eruption
    d. Photoallergic dermatitis

17. **A drug eruption which affects sun-exposed areas of the body is:**
    a. Erythema multiforme
    b. Stevens Johnson syndrome
    c. Drug induced exfoliative dermatitis
    d. Photoallergic dermatitis

18. **Nonsteroidal anti-inflammatory drugs (NSAIDs) that is least likely to cause drug eruption is:**
    a. Indomethacin
    b. Ibuprofen
    c. Paracetamol
    d. Naproxen

19. **Antibacterial drug that is least likely to cause drug eruption is:**
    a. Penicillin
    b. Tetracycline
    c. Chloramphenicol
    d. Cephalosporin

20. **Antibacterial drug that is least likely to cause drug eruption is:**
    a. Ciprofloxacin
    b. Erythromycin
    c. Rifampicin
    d. Cotrimoxazole

21. **A drug that is not known to have caused toxic epidermal necrolysis is:**
    a. Allopurinol
    b. Carbamazepine
    c. Cotrimoxazole
    d. Ketoconazole

22. **Maculopapular drug eruption is distinguished from a viral exanthem based on:**
    a. Pruritic nature
    b. Associated peripheral eosinophilia
    c. Associated lymphadenopathy
    d. All of the above

23. **A 23-year-old woman presented to the casualty department with fever and tender erythema of the skin of one day duration. Within 2 days of admission, his skin became darker all over and started forming large flaccid haemorrhagic bullae. What is the probable diagnosis?**
    a. Pemphigus vulgaris
    b. Staphylococcal scalded skin syndrome
    c. Toxic shock syndrome
    d. Toxic epidermal necrolysis

24. **Target lesions of erythema multiforme are commonly seen over:**
    a. Lips
    b. Palms
    c. Oral mucosa
    d. Genital mucosa

25. **Maculopapular rash due to ampicillin occurs more frequently in the setting of:**
    a. Chickenpox
    b. Infective hepatitis
    c. Infectious mononucleosis
    d. Primary HIV infection

26. **Post-inflammatory hyperpigmentation due to fixed drug eruption lasts for**
    a. 15 days
    b. 1 month
    c. 3 months
    d. More than 6 months

27. **A drug that is known to improve prognosis of Stevens Johnson syndrome when given within the first couple of days of the skin rash is:**
    a. Oral steroids
    b. Intravenous immunoglobulin G
    c. Intravenous steroids
    d. Intravenous antihistamines

28. **Mortality rate of toxic epidermal necrolysis is:**
    a. Less than 5%
    b. More than 5%
    c. More than 25%
    d. Nearly 50%

29. **Hives are characteristic lesions of this drug eruption:**
    a. Maculopapular drug eruption
    b. Erythema multiforme
    c. Urticaria
    d. Fixed drug eruption

30. **All cause erythema multiforme *except*:**
    a. Herpes simplex infection
    b. Drugs
    c. Mycoplasma infection
    d. Human papilloma virus infection

31. **Most common cause of erythema multiforme is:**
    a. Herpes simplex infection
    b. Diabetes mellitus
    c. Pitiriyasis rosea
    d. Erysipelas

32. **Target or iris lesion is seen in:**
    a. Urticaria
    b. Erythema multiforme
    c. Erythema nodosum
    d. Lichen planus

Chapter
14

Drug Eruptions including
Erythema Multiforme and its Variants

33. A 60-year-old patient presented with numerous bullous lesions all over body for the last 3 days. Each bulla is surrounded by erythematous haloes. There were multiple target lesions. The patient had oral erosions. The most likely diagnosis is:
    a. Chickenpox
    b. Herpes simplex
    c. Herpes zoster
    d. Stevens Johnson syndrome

34. Nikolsky sign is positive in all *except*:
    a. Pemphigus
    b. Bullous pemphigoid
    c. Toxic epidermal necrolysis
    d. Staphylococcal scalded skin syndrome

35. Diagnostic lesion of erythema multiforme is:
    a. Wheal
    b. Purpura
    c. Target lesion
    d. Umbilicated papule

Chapter
14

Drug Eruptions including
Erythema Multiforme and its Variants

ANSWERS

1-c,	2-a,	3-c,	4-a,	5-b,	6-c,	7-a,	8-d,	9-d,	10-d,
11-d,	12-d,	13-a,	14-b,	15-a,	16-a,	17-d,	18-c,	19-c,	20-b,
21-d,	22-d,	23-d,	24-b,	25-c,	26-d,	27-b,	28-d,	29-c,	30-d,
31-a,	32-b,	33-d,	34-b,	35-c					

Photosensitive Dermatoses

Sunlight is the main source of energy for humans. However, at times it plays as villain for persons who develop photodermatitis. According to the ability of the normal skin to tan and to get sunburnt, it is classified into five types (Fitzpatrick skin types).

Type I : Always burns; never tans

Type II : Usually burns; then tans

Type III : May burn; tans well

Type IV : Rarely burns; always tans well

Type V : Very rarely burns; always tans well; brown-skin

Type VI : Very rarely burns; always tans well; black skin

Such classification helps us in advising patients about how much sun exposure is allowed for them and which sun protection methods, they should use.

PHOTODERMATITIS (PHOTOSENSITIVE DERMATITIS)

A state of heightened sensitivity of the skin to ultraviolet and, at times, visible spectrum of light is termed as photosensitivity. Such sensitivity may manifest as photodermatitis (Fig. 15.1).

Distribution of Lesions

This is common to all photosensitive disorders as only the sun exposed areas are affected. Face, ears, 'V' area of the chest (Fig. 15.2), back and sides of the neck (Fig. 15.3), forearms and dorsa of hands are some of the commonly affected sites. Upper eyelids, submental and postauricular regions and covered body parts are usually spared. However, sites differ in patient according to her/his clothes and circumstances (occupational and home) in which such exposure occurs.

Photodermatitis may occur due to:

- Phototoxicity, i.e. a predisposition to develop an eruption simulating sunburn or

- Photoallergy, i.e. a delayed type of hyper-sensitivity simulating 'eczema'

- Besides these, photodermatitis may also occur as:

  - A component of multi-system diseases like:

    - Pellagra (niacin deficiency)

    - Systemic lupus erythematosus

    - Porphyrias except acute intermittent porphyria (AIP)

- Tendency to sunburn is a constant accompaniment of skin devoid of melanin as in:

  - Oculocutaneous albinism

  - Vitiligo

  - White skin of Caucasians (Type I and II skin)

  - Phenylketonuria

- Exacerbation of skin lesions with sunlight is known with:

  - Rosacea

  - Lichen planus (actinic type)

  - Seborrhoeic dermatitis

  - Pemphigus and other bullous disorders

- Photosensitivity due to unknown cause—Polymorphous light eruption

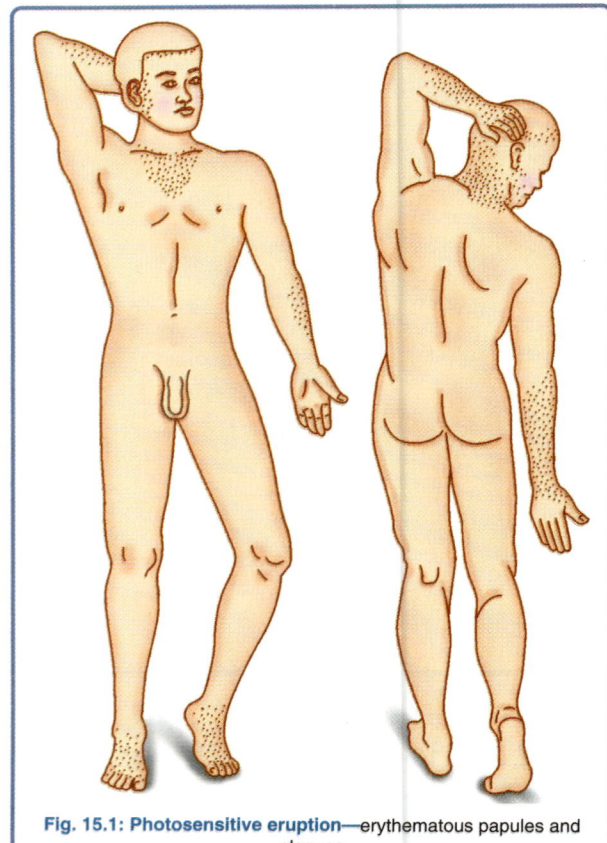

Fig. 15.1: Photosensitive eruption—erythematous papules and plaques

Phototoxicity

This is a sunburn-like response of the skin on ordinary exposure to sunlight or artificial light. This non-immunologically mediated heightened sensitivity of skin may follow first exposure to topical application of or systemic administration of phototoxic chemicals. Examples of such agents are:

- Topical agents—psoralens, certain perfumes and dyes, certain plants and their extracts (that contain psoralens or similar compounds) and,
- Systemic agent—psoralens, tetracyclines, phenothiazines, sulphonylurea and furosemide.
- The affected skin, usually of face and extensor forearms shows bright red erythema that quickly turn red-brown to give a sun-baked appearance. In severe cases oedema and vesiculation may occur. Lesions resolve with scaling and pigmentation.

Plants Causing Photosensitive Reactions in India
Parthenium hysterophorus
Psoralea corylifolia (Babchi)
Chrysanthemum
Cinnamon
Citrus fruits
Garlic
Latex
Eucalyptus
Sunflowers, cosmos, marigold and asters
Vegetables like lettuce, chicory and artichokes
Herbal medicines like feverfew (*Tanacetrim parthenium*), pot marigold (calendula)

Photoallergy

This is an immunologically mediated hypersensitivity to ordinary or less than ordinary amounts of light. Lesions are pruritic maculo-papules or papulovesicles with a tendency to coalesce resembling eczema over sun-exposed sites. They follow repeated exposures to topical or systemic agents that include exposures topical—antibacterials like hexachlorophene, salicylanilides, perfumes, plants like parthenium (Fig. 15.2), or ragweed and systemic—phenothiazines, sulphonylureas, furosemide, thiazides, some nonsteroidal anti-inflammatory drugs and oestrogens. Photoallergic dermatitis due to parthenium is common in India. Due to airborne nature of this allergen, relatively sun-protected areas like upper eyelids and flexures are also involved in these cases (Fig. 15.3). Also contact dermatitis to parthenium, page 118.

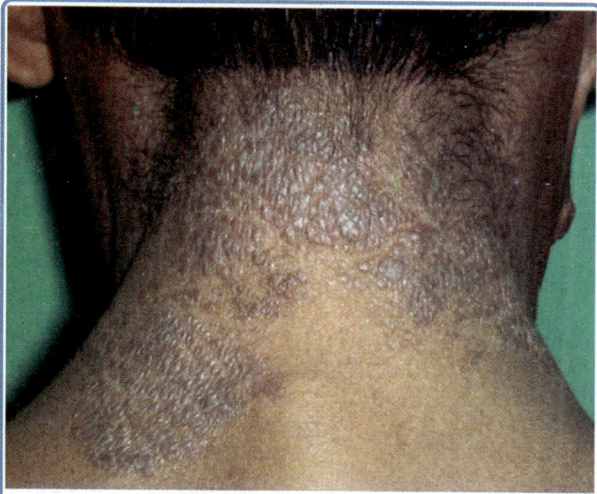

Fig. 15.2: Photoallergic dermatitis—erythematous lichenoid papules over exposed area of neck

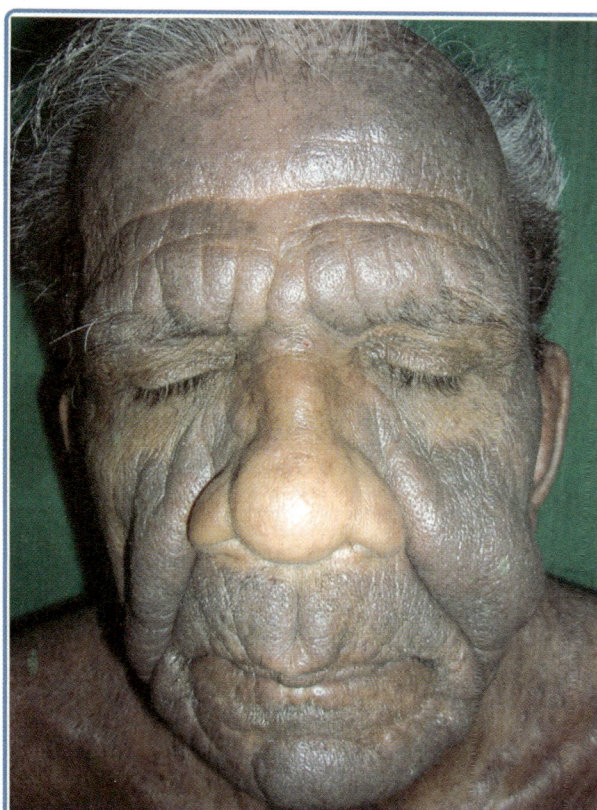

Fig. 15.3: Persistent photoallergic dermatitis to parthenium—hyperpigmentation and thickening of skin. Note involvement of upper eyelids due to airborne nature of the allergen

Polymorphous Light Eruption

Polymorphous light eruption is a diagnosis to be reached by exclusion (Figs 15.4–15.7). Hence, only when all other causes of photosensitivity are ruled out, should it be considered. Airborne contact dermatitis to parthenium also needs to be ruled out. Polymorphous light eruption usually occurs in adults of both sexes. Lesions may be small or

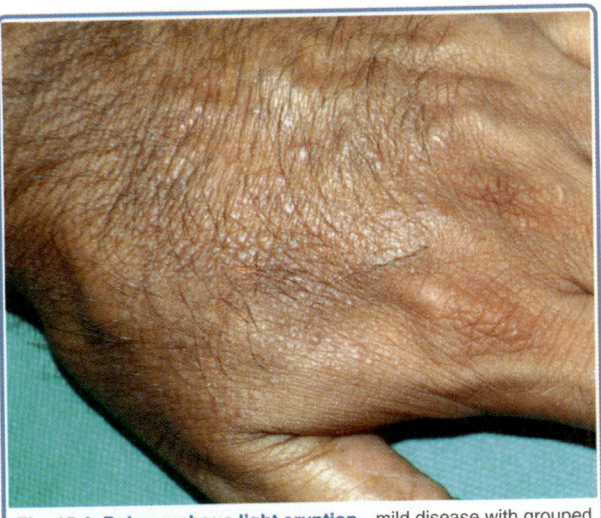

Fig. 15.4: Polymorphous light eruption—mild disease with grouped itchy papules over exposed areas is common

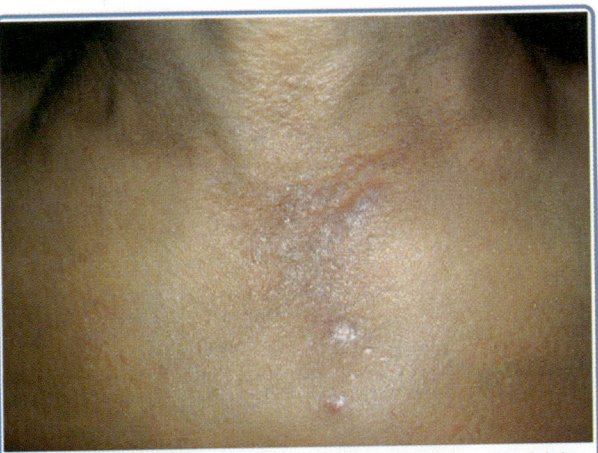

Fig. 15.5: Polymorphous light eruption—skin coloured to slightly hyperpigmented papules and plaque on 'V' area of chest

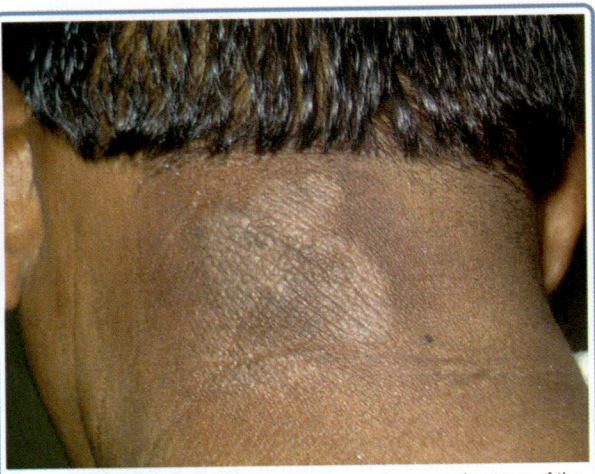

Fig. 15.6: Polymorphous light eruption—plaque on the nape of the neck

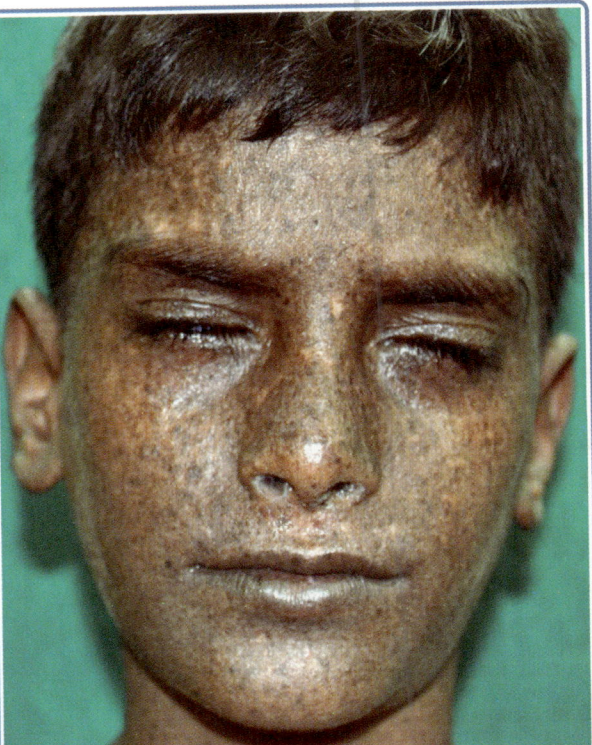

Fig. 15.7: Xeroderma pigmentosum—numerous freckle like lesions, keratoses over face with photophobia. Evoultion into Squamous cell carcinoma may occur over years

Summary: Photosensitive disorders include phototoxicity (induced by systemic or topical agents), photoallergy (systemic or topical agents), tendency to photosensitivity due to reduced melanin (albinism, vitiligo) or to systemic disease pellagra, systemic lupus erythematosus (SLE), porphyria and photosensitivity of unknown cause (polymorphous light eruption).

Distribution of these diseases is restricted to sun-exposed parts of face, neck, chest, hands, forearms and feet. Phototoxicity is a sunburn-like response that occurs following local use of psoralens or certain perfumes. Photoallergy is an immunologically mediated eczematous response to topical (antibacterials, parthenium) or systemic (phenothiazines, sulphonylureas) agents. Polymorphous light eruption is diagnosed by exclusion of other photo-dermatoses.

MANAGEMENT OF PHOTOSENSITIVE DISORDERS

Identifying an aetiologic agent is tough but rewarding, Hence, all patients should be carefully questioned about possible contactants or ingestants. Topical steroids hasten healing. However, eliminating the cause and photoprotection are essential for lasting benefit.

Photoprotection

Reducing sunlight exposure by remaining indoors during the late morning and afternoon hours,

large papules, papulovesicles that may either resemble prurigo or eczema or they may be plaques. Erythematous or hypopigmented scaly patches over the face or forearms are common.

carrying an umbrella, wearing a broad brimmed sun-cap or hat, full sleeved, high collar clothes or covering adequately with a saree need to be integrated into lifestyles.

Topical sunscreens are agents which when applied to the skin, shield it from the effects of ultraviolet light. Opaque sunscreens like zinc cream, calamine cream or titanium dioxide are cosmetically unacceptable but highly effective. Para-aminobenzoic acid (PABA) and its esters block ultraviolet B (UV-B) spectrum. Salicylates, cinnamates and benzophenones block both UV-A and B spectrum. Sunscreens should be applied 30 minutes before expected sun exposure and may need to be reapplied following excessive sweating, swimming and washing. Their effect usually wears off over 2–3 hours.

Hydroxy-chloroquine and chloroquine are the only commonly used systemic agents that have a photoprotective effect. However, because of their potential for ocular toxicity, their use should be restricted to unresponsive cases. They are administered in doses of 200 mg 1 or 2 times a day for up to 1–3 weeks. Pre and intratherapy monitoring for ocular toxicity is recommended.

Other orally active agents that have a photo-protective effect include beta carotene and urocanic acid. Psoralen and ultraviolet-A (PUVA) therapy, administered in gradually increasing doses, para-doxically increases skin tolerance to sunlight.

Summary: Topical steroids induce remission in mild cases, but identification and avoidance of a contactant or an ingestant responsible for the rash is crucial for cure. Avoiding sunlight, adequate photocover with umbrella, clothes or sunscreens (zinc cream, PABA and its esters) is essential. Moderate to severe cases of polymorphous light eruption need a short course of hydroxy-chloroquine therapy (200 mg BD) if necessary, with ophthalmic monitoring.

Chapter

15

Photosensitive Dermatoses

MCQs

1. **Photoallergy is a type of allergy towards:**
   a. Sunlight and chemicals
   b. Photography chemicals
   c. Camera flashlight
   d. Sunlight

2. **Photoallergy may be induced by:**
   a. Macrolides
   b. Paracetamol
   c. Metformin
   d. Quinolines

3. **Polymorphous light eruption does not affect:**
   a. Forehead
   b. Paranasal area
   c. Preauricular area
   d. Postauricular area

4. **Photoallergy can be induced by:**
   a. Soaps
   b. Sunscreens
   c. Fragrances
   d. All of these

5. **To be effective, chemical sunscreens need to be applied at least _____ before exposure to sunlight.**
   a. 0 minutes
   b. 2 minutes
   c. 5 minutes
   d. 30 minutes

6. **A metabolic disorder associated with photosensitivity is:**
   a. Amyloidosis
   b. Mucopolysaccharidosis
   c. Xanthomatosis
   d. Porphyria

7. **Polymorphous light eruption lesions may be all *except*:**
   a. Papules
   b. Plaques
   c. Vesicles
   d. Pustules

8. **A plant which causes photoallergy is:**
   a. China grass
   b. Elephant grass
   c. Congress grass
   d. India grass

9. **This plant is the commonest cause of air borne contact dermatitis in India, it is:**
   a. Parthenium
   b. Chrysanthemum
   c. Rhus
   d. Celery

10. **Which of the following drugs does not cause photoallergic rash?**
    a. Ciprofloxacin
    b. Glibenclamide
    c. Cotrimoxazole
    d. Colchicine

11. **Photoallergic rash which is mediated by Coombs and Gell hypersensitivity, is:**
    a. Type I
    b. Type II
    c. Type III
    d. Type IV

12. **Oral drug of choice for the treatment of polymorphous light eruption is:**
    a. Hydroquinone
    b. Chloroquine
    c. Clioquinol
    d. Hydroxychloroquine

13. **The effect of most of the sunscreens lasts for:**
    a. 3 hours
    b. 6 hours
    c. 8 hours
    d. 12 hours

14. **Paradoxical sun-protective effect is seen with:**
    a. Chloroquine
    b. Hydroxychloroquine
    c. Psoralens
    d. Beta carotene

15. **Fitzpatrick type IV skin:**
    a. Always tans; never burns
    b. Always tans; rarely burns
    c. Sometimes tans; sometimes burns
    d. Always burns; rarely tans

16. **Most of the Indians have Fitzpatrick skin type:**
    a. I or II
    b. II or III
    c. III or IV
    d. IV or V

17. **To be effective, physical sunscreens need to be applied at least _____ before exposure to sunlight.**
    a. 1 minute
    b. 5 minutes
    c. 20 minutes
    d. 30 minutes

18. **The morphology of a photoallergic rash resembles:**
    a. Urticaria
    b. Pellagra
    c. Eczema
    d. Porphyria

19. **Phototoxic dermatitis is mediated by Coombs and Gell hypersensitivity:**
    a. Type I
    b. Type II
    c. Type IV
    d. None of these

20. **Area spared by photoallergic dermatitis is:**
    a. Upper eyelids
    b. Lower eyelids
    c. Ears
    d. Nose

21. **A 23-year-old lady developed erythematous, non-pruritic macular lesions over bridge of the nose and cheeks following exposure to sunlight. The probable diagnosis is:**
    a. Systemic lupus erthematosus
    b. Acne rosacea
    c. Melasma
    d. Photodermatitis

22. **A 45-year-old farmer has itchy erythematous papular rash on the face, neck, 'V' area of chest, dorsa of hands and forearms for 3 years. Rash increases in summer and improves in winter. The likely diagnosis is:**
    a. Pellagra
    b. Photoallergic dermatitis
    c. Lichen planus
    d. Psoriasis

23. **Photosensitivity is a feature of:**
    a. Porphyria cutanea tarda
    b. Psoriasis
    c. Pemphigoid
    d. Pompholyx

24. **Which of the following is not photosensitive?**
    a. Porphyria
    b. Discoid lupus erythematosus
    c. Systemic lupus erythematosus
    d. Lichen planus

25. **Photosensitive butterfly rash with nephritis, arthritis and psychosis are features of:**
    a. Systemic lupus erythematosus
    b. Lyme's disease
    c. Porphyria
    d. Psoriasis

26. **Test to confirm photoallergic dermatitis is:**
    a. Skin biopsy
    b. Serum IgE levels
    c. Photopatch test
    d. Intradermal prick test

Chapter 15

Photosensitive Dermatoses

ANSWERS

1-a,	2-d,	3-d,	4-d,	5-d,	6-d,	7-d,	8-c,	9-a,	10-d,
11-d,	12-d,	13-a,	14-b,	15-b,	16-d,	17-a,	18-c,	19-d,	20-a,
21-a,	22-b,	23-a,	24-d,	25-c,	26-c				

Alopecia

Visible hair is the end product of cornification of cells of a skin appendage called the hair follicle. The structure of a hair follicle is like a cup that gives rise to, supports, and shapes the hair shaft. Ordinarily, there are about 1,00,000 hair on the scalp. Out of these, about 100 are lost every day. This is because the follicles continually pass through the 3 phase cycle of anagen (growth phase), catagen (phase of decay) and telogen (resting phase). When telogen ends, anagen begins, forming a new hair shaft that pushes the old resting shaft out of the follicle.

DIFFERENTIAL DIAGNOSIS OF ALOPECIA

Loss of previously existing scalp hair is termed as alopecia. It may be permanent (scarring or cicatricial) wherein the follicles are not permanently damaged. Examination of the bald area with a lens reveals follicular openings without hair shafts in cases of non-scarring alopecia. Follicular openings are absent in areas of scarring alopecia.

Non-scarring alopecias are divided into those accompanied by signs of inflammation (inflammatory) and those without them (non-inflammatory). Erythema, oedema, pustules and scaling are noted in the inflammatory non-scarring alopecias caused by tinea capitis (some cases) and superficial bacterial infections of the scalp like folliculitis.

Non-inflammatory non-scarring alopecias can be divided into localised and generalised. Such localised loss of hair is seen in alopecia areata and traumatic alopecia. Generalised non-inflammatory non-scarring alopecia is the commonest form of hair loss encountered in medical practice. Androgenetic alopecia, telogen effluvium, drug induced alopecias and alopecias due to systemic diseases like thyroid disease and systemic lupus erythematosus fall under this category.

Summary: Out of about 1,00,000 scalp hair, close to 100 are lost every day. Hair are formed by hair follicles which continually pass through growth (anagen), catabolic (catagen) and rest (telogen) phases in a cyclical manner.

Loss of hair is termed alopecia. When follicles are destroyed (as judged by absence of follicular openings) the hair loss is said to be scarring and this is irreversible. Scarring alopecia occurs due to deep bacterial, viral or fungal infections, discoid lupus erythematosus and scleroderma. Non-scarring alopecia may be inflammatory (tinea capitis) or non-inflammatory which can be localised (alopecia areata) or generalised (androgenetic alopecia, telogen effluvium).

SCARRING ALOPECIA (CICATRICIAL ALOPECIA)

Hair loss accompanied by loss of hair follicles (as evidenced by absence of follicular openings) is termed as scarring alopecia (Figs 16.1 and 16.2A and B). Most of these conditions are associated with deep inflammations that destroy follicles. Common causes of scarring alopecia include:

I. Infections

a. Bacterial infections (pyoderma including chronic folliculitis, carbuncle, and abscesses).

b. Fungal infections (inflammatory tinea capitis kerion, favus).

c. Viral infections (herpes zoster)

d. Parasitic infections (maggots)

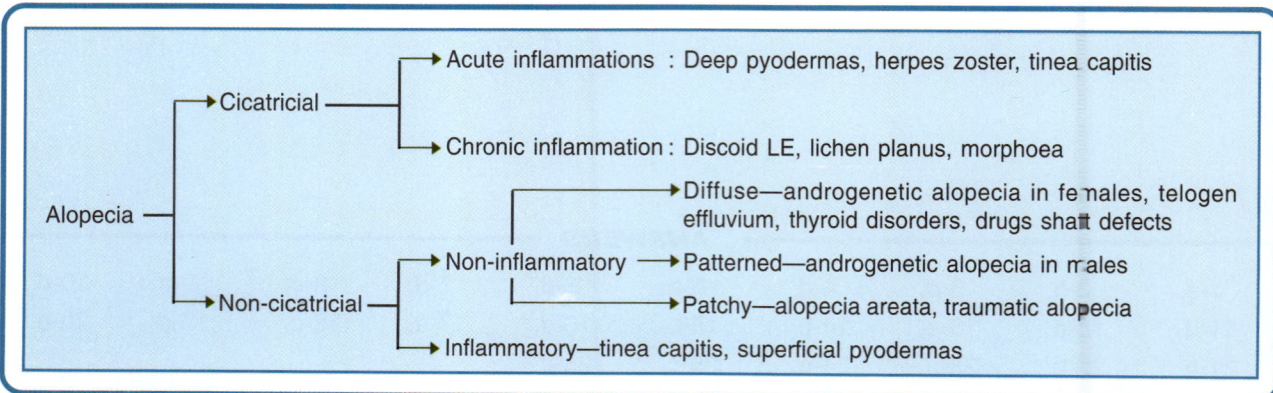

Alopecia —
- Cicatricial —
  - Acute inflammations : Deep pyodermas, herpes zoster, tinea capitis
  - Chronic inflammation : Discoid LE, lichen planus, morphoea
- Non-cicatricial —
  - Non-inflammatory —
    - Diffuse—androgenetic alopecia in females, telogen effluvium, thyroid disorders, drugs shaft defects
    - Patterned—androgenetic alopecia in males
    - Patchy—alopecia areata, traumatic alopecia
  - Inflammatory—tinea capitis, superficial pyodermas

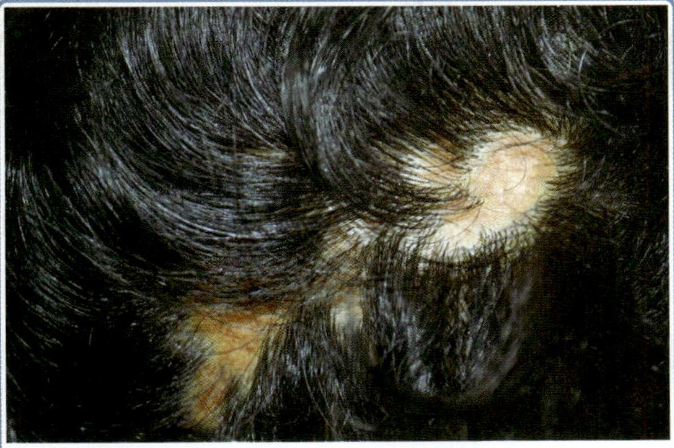

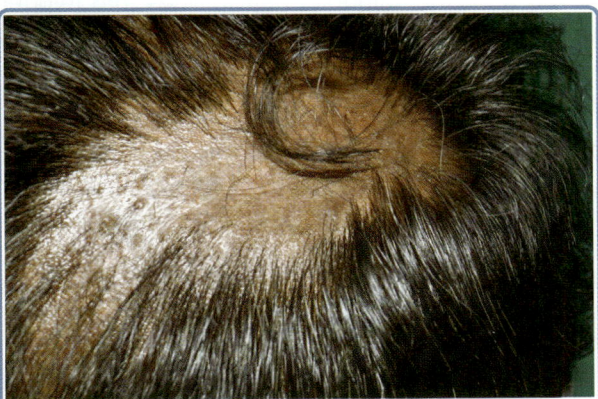

Fig. 16.1: Cicatricial alopecia—multiple shiny depressed patches without follicular openings

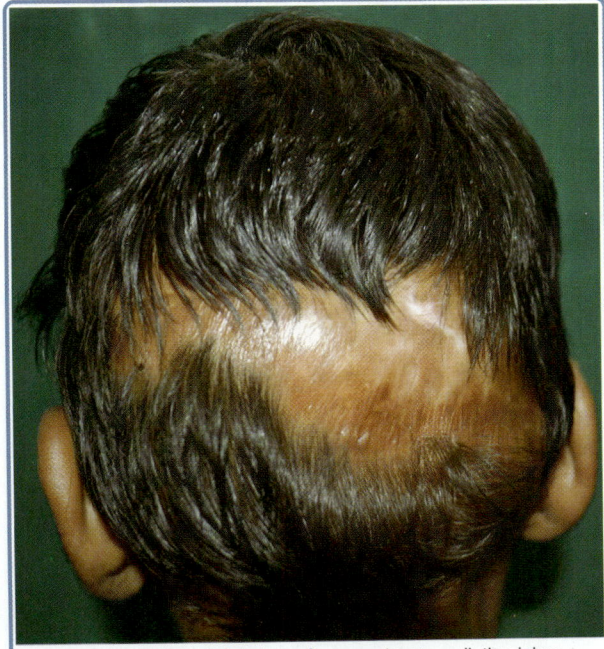

Fig. 16.2A: Patch of cicatricial alopecia with lichenoid follicular papules at the margins seen in lichen planopilars

Fig. 16.2B: Cicatricial alopecia secondary to radiation injury

II. Trauma

a. Thermal trauma (burns or cold injury due to cryotherapy)

b. Chemical trauma (acid burns or application of caustics like phenol or salicylic acid)

c. Mechanical trauma (lacerated wounds)

d. Radiation trauma (following radiotherapy)

III. Inflammatory causes

a. Autoimmune diseases (discoid lupus erythematosus, lichen planus, and orphoea)

b. Pseudopelade (unknown cause)

c. Metabolic (porphyria)

IV. Genetic causes

Dystrophic epidermolysis bullosa.

History and examination play a crucial part in reaching a diagnosis. Sometimes, biopsy is necessary to find out the cause of scarring alopecia. However, when a biopsy is done from an old patch of scarring alopecia, histopathologic signs of the original disease leading to the scarring may no longer be seen.

Treatment consists of arresting the progression of disease by identifying the cause and treating it. Since no regrowth of hair can occur once follicles are lost, surgery is one of the means of cosmetic correction. This can be done by simply excising the patch of scarring alopecia followed by primary closure. Alternatively, hair transplant can be done at the site using punches or by other methods. Artificial hairs have added a new avenue for treatment of such cases. Hair patch (weaving) provides a way of cosmetic camouflage.

DIFFUSE ALOPECIA

Diffuse loss of hair is one of the commonest complaints in dermatology. Since no bald patch is visible, it is common for the doctor to under-estimate the severity of the complaint. No signs are obvious except in the very severe cases where slight sparsity of hair ('diffuse thinning') is visible.

Causes of diffuse hair loss include:

- Androgenetic alopecia
- Telogen effluvium
- Thyroid disorders
- Drugs like colchicine, antithyroid drugs, cytotoxic and immunosuppressant drugs, high dose vitamin A and oral retinoids
- Iron deficiency anaemia, protein energy malnutrition
- Diffuse alopecia areata

Chapter
16

Alopecia

- Senile alopecia
- Hair shaft disorders, many of which are genetic diseases

The commonest cause of diffuse hair loss in women is female pattern alopecia (androgenetic alopecia in women) and this is detailed under androgenetic alopecia later in this chapter. Another common and reversible cause of alopecia is telogen effluvium which is detailed below. While androgenetic alopecia affects women with family history of alopecia, telogen effluvium follows some stressful precipitating event a few months earlier. Positive history of thyroid disease, nutritional deficiency or drug ingestion is helpful in identifying the cause of diffuse hair loss. While senile alopecia affects the elderly beyond the age of 60 years, hair shaft disorders present during childhood. Alopecia areata is rarely diffuse but can be diagnosed by a skin biopsy.

TELOGEN EFFLUVIUM

Literally, this term means shedding of telogen hair. Hair matrix, during the anagen (growth) phase, is one of the fastest multiplying tissues of the body. Hence, in times of stress, probably in order to conserve resources, many (but not all) follicles are precipitated suddenly into telogen. Since most telogen hair are shed only when a new anagen hair pushes the old hair out, it takes about 2–3 months (average duration of telogen) for the hair fall to be noticed.

The internal stressful stimuli that can induce telogen effluvium include febrile episodes especially persistent high fever (malaria, typhoid, tuberculosis, etc.), surgery, major trauma, difficult labour, emotional stress, cyable diets, etc.

Ordinarily, about 10% of the 1,00,000 scalp follicles are in telogen. In telogen effluvium this proportion goes up to about 20%. However, since most of the hair are still in anagen, visible thinning of scalp is unusual. Reassurance that the hair are going to regrow spontaneously is most important.

Summary: Sudden precipitation of anagen follicles into telogen by major stresses (e.g. persistent high fever, difficult labour, major trauma) leads to loss of these telogen hair (about 20% of scalp hair) 2–4 months after the stressful event. Hair grow back spontaneously.

ANAGEN EFFLUVIUM

Hair Shaft Disorders

Hair loss may uncommonly result from breakage of hair shafts. This may happen due to genetic defects in hair shaft strength (e.g. in some aminoacidurias) or due to external trauma. Repetitive trauma due to frequent use of a strong shampoo, due to rapid drying of hair with a hair drier or due to use of a rough comb are some of the traumatic events. However, in such cases, hair loss is not severe enough to cause patches of baldness. Cessation of trauma leads to gradual regrowth of hair.

PATCHY HAIR LOSS

ALOPECIA AREATA

An autoimmune disorder, alopecia areata manifests as patchy loss of hair due to sudden precipitation of a group of contiguous hair follicles into telogen (resting phase).

Patient Profile

Although common in young adults, about 20% patients are children. Most patients do not have an associated condition (common type). A small minority of cases show association with other autoimmune diseases (autoimmune type), atopy (atopic type) and hypertension in parents (prehypertensive type).

Morphology

Loss of hair in well define rounded patches is typical (Figs 16.3 and 16.4). The bald skin is hairless, smooth and lacks any sign of inflammation. However, careful examination with a lens reveals openings of follicles, indicating that this is a non-scarring alopecia. Spreading margins bear broken stubs of hair that taper towards the skin surface, are easily pluckable and when plucked, show a rounded bulb (exclamation mark hair).

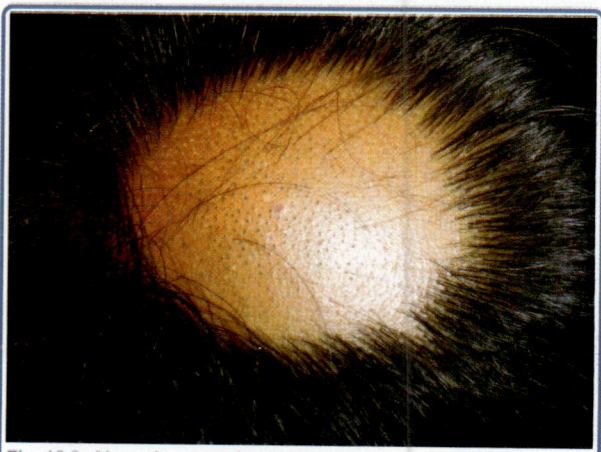

Fig. 16.3: Alopecia areata (early lesion)—oval patch of non-cicatricial alopecia. Note preservation of follicular openings and presence of broken hair at the periphery

Chapter 16

Alopecia

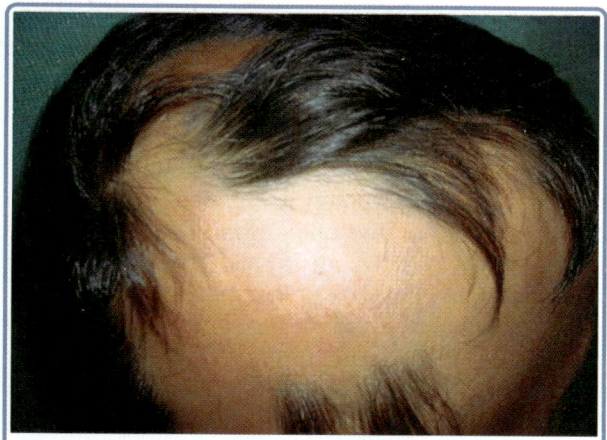

Fig. 16.4: Alopecia areata—large patches of compete non-scarring and non-inflammatory alopecia

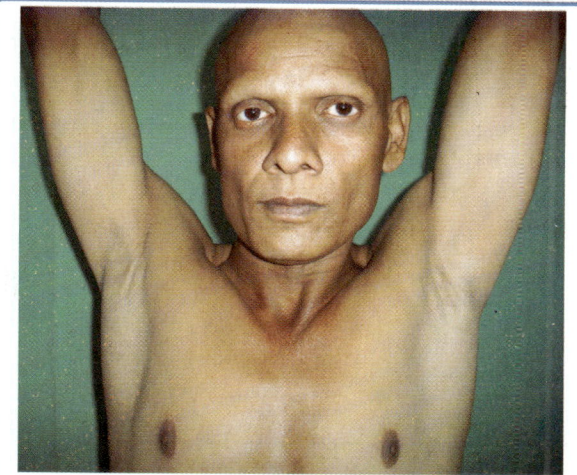

Fig. 16.6: Alopecia universalis—generalised loss of hair on the scalp, eyebrows, eyelashes and axilla

Distribution

Scalp is affected most often, alone or in combination with other regions. Beard, mustache, eyebrows, eyelashes, axillae, pubis or extremities are some of the other sites. Involvement of the whole scalp leading to complete baldness is termed as **alopecia totalis** (Fig. 16.5). When hair are lost over the whole body it is termed as **alopecia universalis** (Fig. 16.6). Both these conditions have poor prognosis.

Diagnosis

Clinical findings of non-scarring, non-inflammatory alopecia in localised patches are characteristic. Differential diagnosis includes trichotillomania, tinea capitis and pseudopelade. Skin biopsy shows perifollicular infiltrates of lymphocytes around the hair roots.

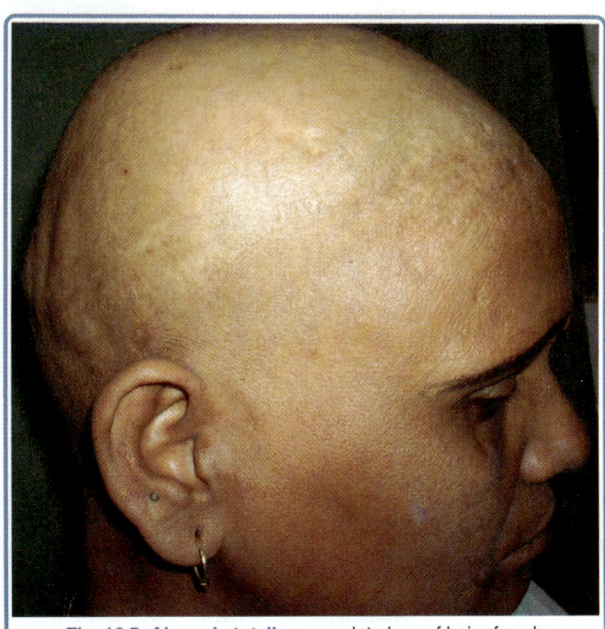

Fig. 16.5: Alopecia totalis—complete loss of hair of scalp

Therapy

Spontaneous regrowth of hair is seen in 60–75% cases and occurs as a rule in patients with one or two patches of short duration (less than 6 months). However, since most patients are anxious about the hair loss, primary line of therapy may begin immediately. Potent **topical steroids** (clobetasol or betamethasone) or **intralesional steroids** (hydrocortisone or triamcinolone) induce regrowth in about 60% cases. **Topical tacrolimus** 0.1% lotion is claimed to give results, albeit slowly but without the side effects of local steroids. **Topical minoxidil** solution, 2–5%, applied twice daily stimulates regrowth in a fair proportion and can also be used as a first line therapy (Table 16.1).

Topical or systemic psoralen and ultraviolet-A (PUVA) therapy is successful in a proportion of unresponsive cases. Induction of contact allergic dermatitis to diphenylcyclopropenone (DPCP) leads to hair regrowth in some recalcitrant cases. Topical irritants like phenol, trichloracetic acid, salicylic acid, etc., were used in the past in an attempt to stimulate hair growth. However, due to the risk of inducing scarring alopecia by causing deep ulceration, these agents should be used with caution.

Systemic steroids are not generally indicated in alopecia areata because of their serious side effects and a very high relapse rate on tapering of steroids. Their only justified use may be to prevent the spread of a rapidly evolving alopecia areata threatening to become total. Even in those uncommon cases, alternative immunosuppressive agents should be started simultaneously and steroids withdrawn as soon as possible.

In unresponsive cases of alopecia areata or totalis careful counselling is needed. Cosmetic camouflage options like hair weaving or hair wig may be considered.

Chapter
16

Alopecia

TABLE 16.1: Treatment modalities in alopecia areata	
Topical agents	• Corticosteroids with or without occlusion • Topical tacrolimus 0.1% lotion • Topical minoxidil 2–5% • Topical PUVA therapy • Topical irritants like phenol, salicyclic acid and anthralin • Topical contact sensitisers like diphenylcyclopropenone (DPCP)
Intralesional	Corticosteroids
Systemic agents	• Corticosteroids (oral minipulse therapy or intramuscular injections) • Cyclosporine • Azathioprine • Systemic PUVA
Cosmetic camouflage	• Tattooing • Hair pieces or Hair weaving • Wigs

Summary: Alopecia areata is an autoimmune disease of hair follicles that affects young adults. It is occasionally associated with atopy and other autoimmune disease. Well defined patches of non-scarring, non-inflammatory hair loss are characteristic. Any part of scalp or body (e.g. beard, mustache) may be affected. Affection of all scalp hair (alopecia totalis) and all body hair (alopecia universalis) carry bad prognosis. More than 50% cases regrow spontaneously. However, as most patients are worried about the condition, topical or intralesional steroid or topical minoxidil are the first line of therapy. Unresponsive cases can be managed with topical or systemic PUVA or topical DPCP. Systemic steroids are best avoided.

Chapter 16

Alopecia

TRAUMATIC ALOPECIA

Hair loss due to mechanical stresses on hair shaft is termed as traumatic alopecia. It may occur due to traction, pulling, plucking or pressure.

Traction Alopecia

Persistent abnormal traction on the hair may lead to their breakage resulting in alopecia. A common example of these occurs in girls or women who tie their hair bands very tightly. The alopecia is seen either as a recession of the hairline at the scalp margin where the pull is the maximum or as small ill-defined patches at the margins with short broken hair. It may be sometimes seen in males who grow and tie their hair of scalp or beard. Alteration of hair styling with relief of the traction solves the problem.

Trichotillomania (Hair Pulling Tick)

Trichotillomania is a habit tic, usually seen in children or young women who, consciously or subconsciously, twist and pull at their hair producing a patch of hair loss. This presents typically as one or a few localised patches of incomplete non-scarring, non-inflammatory alopecia over accessible areas of scalp (Fig. 16.7). The patient is usually a child between 5–10 years of age and the patches show broken stubs of hair. Close questioning usually reveals a habit tic involving handling (twisting and pulling) of scalp hair. KOH mount of hair does not show any fungi thus differentiating it from tinea capitis. Skin biopsy differentiates it from alopecia areata. Stoppage of trauma invariably leads to regrowth.

Pressure Alopecia

This non-inflammatory, non-scarring and completely reversible patchy alopecia is seen at sites exposed to persistent pressure. Occipital areas are commonly affected in young infants in this way. Comatose patients may occasionally develop this type of hair loss.

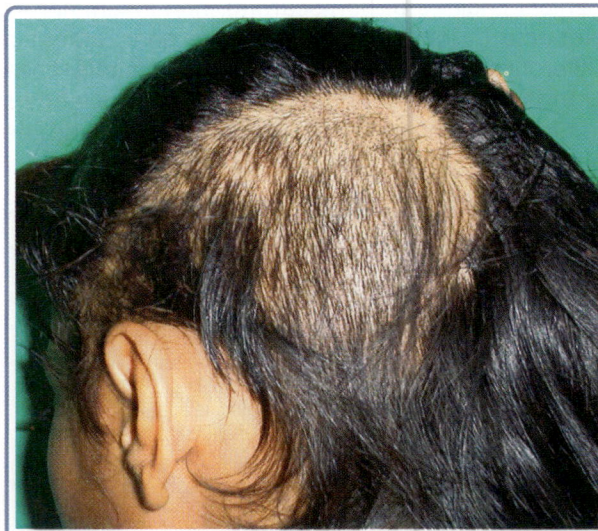

Fig. 16.7: Trichotillomania—patch of incomplete non-inflammatory alopecia with irregularly broken stubs of hair

ANDROGENETIC ALOPECIA (ANDROGENIC ALOPECIA, COMMON BALDNESS, PATTERN ALOPECIA BALDNESS)

This is the commonest cause of alopecia. Androgens and an appropriate genetic background are prerequisites for developing this alopecia. It is transmitted as an autosomal dominant trait. Alopecia becomes manifest under these conditions at an appropriate age. Thus, scalp hair are normal in childhood. Excess hair loss is initially noticed in second or third decade of life and may gradually progress to cause pattern baldness.

Male Pattern Alopecia

Initial sign is thinning of hair shafts and later, increase in the number of villus (short, fine) hair. Afterward, the majority of hair in the region turn into vellus hair, only a few thick terminal hair being left. Finally, the scalp looks smooth and bald with only fine vellus hair that may be visualised only by a lens.

First sign of male pattern baldness is seen during the early twenties as recession of temporal hair line and then in the late twenties, the frontal hair line (Fig. 16.8). During the early thirties, thinning of hair over vertex becomes evident. As the condition progresses, there is further frontal and temporal recession and a patch of baldness on the vertex (Fig. 16.9). Later, the vertical, frontal and temporal areas of baldness coalesce leaving only the parietal and occipital hair intact (Figs 16.10 and

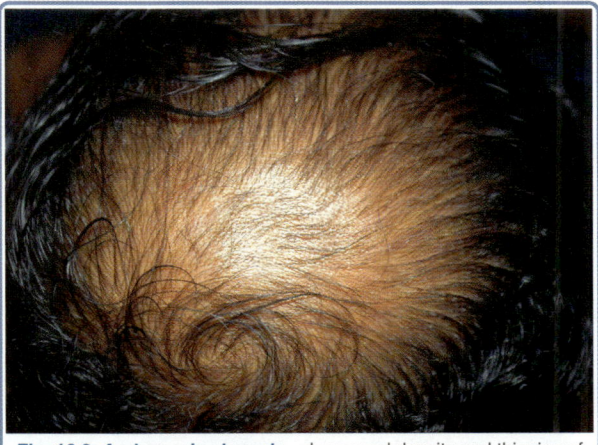

Fig. 16.9: Androgenic alopecia—decreased density and thinning of hair shafts involving the vertex

16.11). Finally, even the parietal and then occipital hair may be lost leading to complete baldness. In most individuals, the condition does not progress fully.

Female Pattern Alopecia

In genetically predisposed women, androgenetic alopecia presents as partial diffuse hair loss beginning during the twenties or thirties. However, this rarely leads to bald patches. When the onset is early, the patient may be evaluated for polycystic ovaries or metabolic syndrome.

Therapy

Therapy for androgenetic alopecia remains suboptimal. Topical minoxidil, 5% solution, to be applied twice a day (once daily in women), after hair washing, stops further hair fall and improves hair thickness. It gives cosmetically acceptable results only in patients who have a majority of hair of a thickness intermediate between vellus and terminal hair. The result take 6–12 months and is maintained only if minoxidil is continued. Besides, minoxidil requires monitoring of response and side effects by an expert. Increased hair loss is a common complaint during the initial months of minoxidil therapy. Hypertrichosis is an infrequent

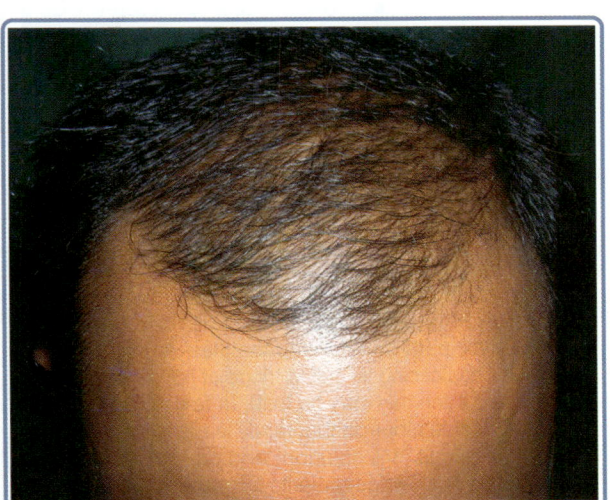

Fig. 16.8: Androgenic alopecia—decreased density, length and thickness of hairs with recession of hairline in temporal and frontal region

Chapter 16

Alopecia

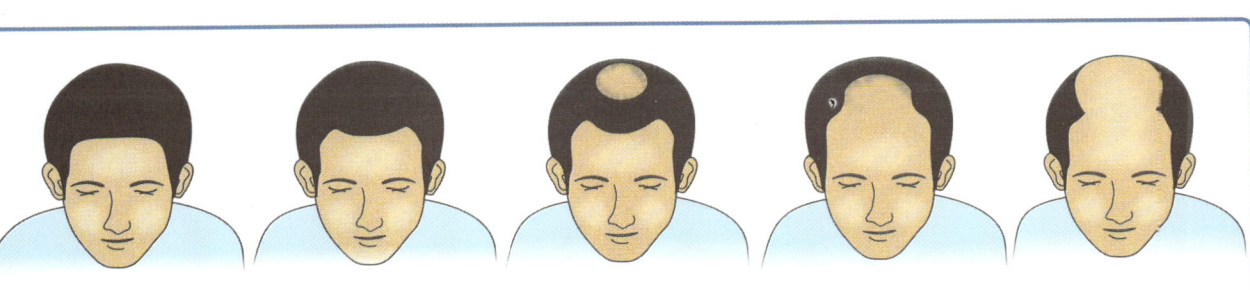

Fig. 16.10: Progression of androgenetic alopecia in men

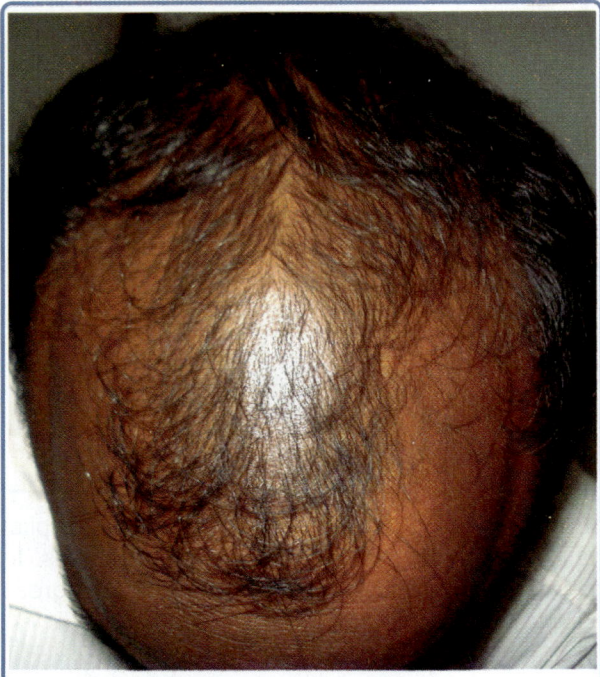

Fig. 16.11: Androgenic alopecia (advanced)—coalescence of vertical, frontal and temporal areas of baldness

TABLE 16.2: Treatment of androgenetic alopecia	
Topical agents	• 5% topical minoxidil alone or in combination with tretinoin 0.025% and azelaic acid 5%
Adjuvant therapy (optional)	• Intradermal platelet rich plasma injection • Dermaroller • Topical agents containing capixyl, arginine • Wigs/Hair piece • Low level laser light therapy
Systemic agents	• Anti-androgens (finasteride/ dutasteride in males, cyproterone acetate, drosperinone, spironolactone in females) • Oral contraceptive pills
Cosmetic camouflage	• Hair weaving • Hair fibre powder • Wigs
Surgical	• Follicular unit transplantation (FUT—donor strip graft) • Follicular unit extraction (FUE) • Mini and micro punch grafting • Rotation flaps • Scalp reduction • Artificial hair fibre implants

side effect of topical minoxidil in women. Hence, sometimes 2% solution is preferred for women.

Finasteride, a 5-alpha reductase inhibitor, is useful in a dose of 1 mg/day orally for men and 2.5 mg/day for women. Oral antiandrogens are contraindicated in men but may be used cyclically in females in combination with 35 mcg of ethinyl oestradiol. Oral medications are contraindicated in women who are planning pregnancy. Side effects should be explained to the patient and watched for, during the therapy. Surgical options for motivated men include hair transplant and scalp reduction. The older technique of transplanting small punch grafts from the occipital to frontal/temporal regions has been given up due to the embarrassing 'crop-like' appearance. Newer techniques involve dissecting out follicular units of two or three hair follicles or even single hair follicle and transplanting them into tiny slits onto the recipient areas. The surgery is time consuming and somewhat expensive but the results are satisfying.

Summary: This autosomal dominant trait needs androgens for its expression. The hair gradually become thinner and finally are lost. In males, it progresses in characteristic pattern (forehead-temples-vertex, gradually all regions coalescing till only a fringe of hair is left over the occiput and even this may be lost). In females, it presents as partial diffuse alopecia that rarely leads to bald patches. Topical minoxidil (5% solution) and oral finasteride give good results in selected patients but need to be continued to maintain the improvement. Surgical options like hair transplant and scalp reduction are available for motivated patients.

MCQs

1. The approximate number of scalp hair in a healthy young adult is:
   a. Ten million
   b. One million
   c. One hundred thousand
   d. Ten thousand

2. The average number of hair lost in one day in a young healthy adult is:
   a. 10 per day   b. 25 per day
   c. 50 per day   d. 100 per day

3. The phases of normal hair cycle are all *except*:
   a. Anagen   b. Nanogen
   c. Telogen   d. Catagen

4. The phase of hair cycle in which the hair follicle degenerates is called:
   a. Anagen   b. Nanogen
   c. Telogen   d. Catagen

5. The type of hair seen over the healthy adult scalp is:
   a. Terminal   b. Intermediate
   c. Vellus   d. Lanugo

6. The growth phase of the hair cycle is called:
   a. Anagen   b. Nanogen
   c. Telogen   d. Catagen

7. The approximate percentage of telogen hair in a young healthy adult is:
   a. 0–1%   b. 1–2%
   c. 2–5%   d. 10%

8. The approximate percentage of anagen hair in a young healthy adult is:
   a. 50%   b. 75–80%
   c. 85–90%   d. 90–95%

9. The approximate average duration of anagen in a healthy young adult male is:
   a. 3 months   b. 9 months
   c. 3 years   d. 10 years

10. The approximate average duration of telogen in a healthy young adult is:
    a. 1 month   b. 3 months
    c. 9 months   d. 3 years

11. The average rate of growth of scalp hair in a young healthy adult is:
    a. 1 mm every day
    b. 1 mm every 3 days
    c. 1 mm every 7 days
    d. 1 mm every 10 days

12. The outermost layer of the hair shaft is called the:
    a. Cuticle   b. Outer root sheath
    c. Infundibulum   d. Isthmus

13. The part of the follicle that makes the hair shaft is called:
    a. Infundibulum   b. Isthmus
    c. Stem   d. Bulb

14. Which of the following is a common cause of diffuse alopecia?
    a. Alopecia areata   b. Tinea capitis
    c. Trichotillomania   d. Telogen effluvium

15. Which of the following is a cause of localised alopecia?
    a. Telogen effluvium
    b. Anagen effluvium
    c. Female pattern alopecia
    d. Follicular lichen planus

16. Which of the following is a cause of inflammatory alopecia?
    a. Alopecia areata   b. Telogen effluvium
    c. Trichotillomania   d. Kerion

17. Which of the following is a cause of non-inflammatory alopecia?
    a. Alopecia areata
    b. Tinea capitis
    c. Herpes zoster
    d. Discoid lupus erythematosus

18. Which of the following alopecias do not show broken stubs of hair?
    a. Thyroid alopecia   b. Trichotillomania
    c. Tinea capitis   d. Alopecia areata

19. Which of the following scalp diseases is caused by a fungus?
    a. Kerion   b. Tinea amiantacea
    c. Trichotillomania   d. Scalp folliculitis

Chapter
16

Alopecia

20. **A feature which is missing in cicatricial alopecia is:**
    a. Follicular openings   b. Atrophy
    c. Wrinkling   d. Scarring

21. **Which of the following conditions may lead to cicatricial alopecia?**
    a. Alopecia areata
    b. Androgenic alopecia
    c. Telogen effluvium
    d. Tinea capitis

22. **The outcome of cicatricial alopecia is:**
    a. Hair never regrow
    b. Hair may regrow but fall out again
    c. Hair usually regrow
    d. Hair always regrow

23. **This is a cause of patterned alopecia:**
    a. Androgenic alopecia
    b. Telogen effluvium
    c. Anagen effluvium
    d. Drug induced alopecia

24. **Drug which does not commonly causes alopecia is:**
    a. Oral retinoid acid   b. Amoxycillin
    c. Colchicine   d. Azathioprine

25. **Causes of telogen effluvium include all except:**
    a. High grade fever
    b. Major surgery
    c. Unusual mental stress
    d. Oral enalapril

26. **Anagen effluvium may be caused by all except:**
    a. Vitamin A   b. Colchicine
    c. Azathioprine   d. Hydroxyurea

27. **Internal diseases which may not cause hair loss include:**
    a. Hypothyroidism
    b. Hyperthyroidism
    c. Hypertension
    d. Iron deficiency anaemia

28. **The type of hair seen at the periphery of a patch of alopecia areata is:**
    a. Vellus hair
    b. Terminal hair
    c. Exclamation mark
    d. Intermediate hair

29. **Which of the following show scaling within a patch of alopecia?**
    a. Trichotillomania
    b. Alopecia areata
    c. Tinea capitis
    d. Androgenic alopecia

30. **Which of the following is an infective cause of alopecia?**
    a. Dandruff   b. Tinea capitis
    c. Tinea versicolor   d. Lichen planus

31. **Chance of regrowth in alopecia areata worsens with:**
    a. Increase in area of bald patches
    b. Affection of total scalp
    c. Long duration of disease
    d. All of the above

32. **The modality of first line treatment for single patch alopecia areata is:**
    a. Topical steroids
    b. Topical PUVA therapy
    c. Oral steroids
    d. Topical anthralin

33. **The aetiology of alopecia areata is:**
    a. Fungal infection
    b. Viral infection
    c. Autoimmune process
    d. Hormonal cause

34. **Androgenic alopecia is transmitted as _____ trait.**
    a. Autosomal dominant
    b. Autosomal recessive
    c. Multifactorial
    d. X-linked recessive

35. **Trichotillomania refers to:**
    a. Hair pulling tic
    b. A type of mania
    c. A type of schizophrenia
    d. Psychologic affection in alopecia areata

36. **Hair follicle roots in trichotillomania are usually:**
    a. Damaged   b. Intact
    c. Lost   d. Inflamed

37. **First line therapy of androgenic alopecia is:**
    a. Topical steroids
    b. Topical minoxidil
    c. Topical finasteride
    d. Topical oestrogen

Chapter
16

Alopecia

38. Finasteride acts in androgenic alopecia by its action on:
a. Testosterone
b. 5 alpha reductase inhibitor
c. 5 alpha reductase
d. Oestrogen receptors

39. The recommended dose of finasteride in male pattern alopecia is:
a. 0.5 mg daily   b. 1 mg daily
c. 2.5 mg daily   d. 5 mg daily

40. Surgical technique of hair restoration used in androgenic alopecia is called:
a. Hair transplantation
b. Scalp reduction
c. Follicular unit transplantation
d. All of the above

41. Cosmetic camouflage technique for patterned alopecia is:
a. Hair wig   b. Hair weaving
c. Artificial hair   d. All of these

42. The commonest cause of diffuse alopecia in women is:
a. Telogen effluvium
b. Thyroid disease
c. Androgenic alopecia
d. All of the above

43. In telogen effluvium, the percentage of hair in telogen phase is:
a. 10   b. 20
c. 30   d. 40

44. The following requires skin biopsy for confirmation of diagnosis:
a. Telogen effluvium
b. Androgenic alopecia
c. Lichen planopilaris
d. Tinea capitis

45. The following are types of alopecia areata *except*:
a. Classical   b. Prehypertensive
c. Atopic   d. Childhood

46. Poor prognostic sign in alopecia areata is:
a. Loss of hair over the beard
b. Loss of hair over moustache
c. Alopecia universalis
d. None of the above

47. The following is a common initial side effect of minoxidil therapy for androgenic alopecia:
a. Vomiting
b. Increased hair loss
c. Strabismus
d. Dermatitis

Chapter
16

Alopecia

ANSWERS

1-c,	2-d,	3-b,	4-c,	5-a,	6-a,	7-d,	8-c,	9-d,	10-b,
11-b,	12-a,	13-d,	14-d,	15-d,	16-d,	17-a,	18-a,	19-a,	20-a,
21-d,	22-a,	23-a,	24-b,	25-d,	26-a,	27-c,	28-c,	29-c,	30-b,
31-d,	32-a,	33-c,	34-a,	35-a,	36-b,	37-b,	38-b,	39-b,	40-d,
41-d,	42-c,	43-b,	44-c,	45-d,	46-c,	47-b			

CHAPTER 17

Disorders of Nail

Nails are being increasingly recognised as cosmetically important skin appendages. However, they serve many useful day-to-day functions in protecting the fingertips and improving our manual abilities. Healthy nails are pink, translucent, smooth and have a little luster. Their affection may manifest as change in thickness (excessively thick or thin nails), separation of nail plate from nail bed (onycholysis), change in surface texture (pits, ridges, irregularity or dystrophy or excessive shininess), or change in structural strength (excessive fragility). Sometimes, the nail bed may be affected leading to collection of keratotic debris under the nail plate (subungual hyperkeratosis).

Common conditions that affect the nail include psoriasis, lichen planus, dermatophyte infection and traumatic nail dystrophy. Occasionally, systemic diseases affect the nails in a specific way to be able to serve as markers (clubbing in cardiopulmonary diseases or white nails in hepatic disease).

NAIL PSORIASIS

About 30–80% of patients suffering from skin psoriasis show nail changes. These include irregular pitting (Figs 17.1 and 17.2) and transverse ridging of nail plate, subungual hyperkeratosis and yellowish-gray discolouration of the nail plate. In severe cases onycholysis and dystrophy of nails can occur. Tinea unguium is the main differential diagnosis.

Patients who are treated with systemic agents for skin or joint psoriasis, viz. methotrexate or

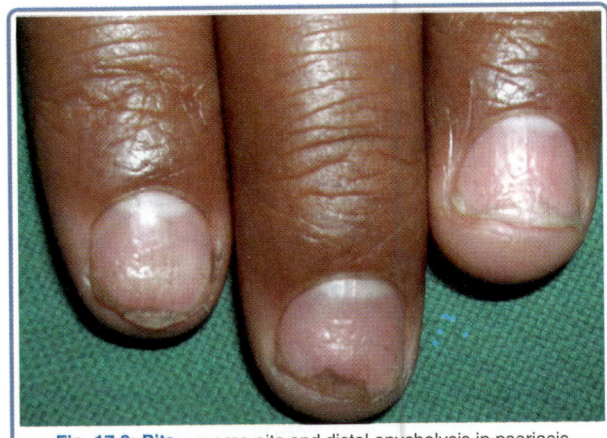
Fig. 17.2: Pits—coarse pits and distal onycholysis in psoriasis

retinoids, show simultaneous improvement in nail psoriasis. Treatment of isolated nail psoriasis is difficult as systemic agents are best avoided for a predominantly cosmetic problem. Topical application of highly potent steroids (under occlusion) or 5-fluorouracil or tazarotene show marginal benefit. Intralesional injections of steroids into the nail matrix can be tried.

NAIL LICHEN PLANUS

Nail involvement can be seen in 10% cases of lichen planus. Sometimes nail involvement can occur without any evidence of skin lesions. Nail changes in lichen planus include pterygium (wing like extension of proximal nail fold over the nail bed) (Figs 17.3 and 17.4), thinning of nail plates, longitudinal ridging and grooving of nail plates and

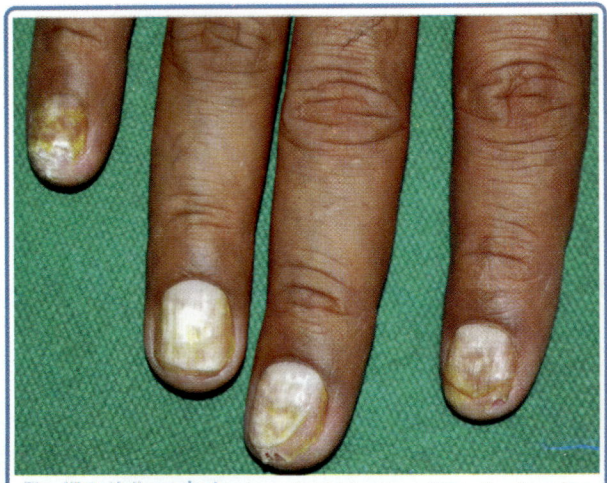
Fig. 17.1: Nail psoriasis—irregular thickening, pitting, discolouration of the nail plate with subungual hyperkeratosis

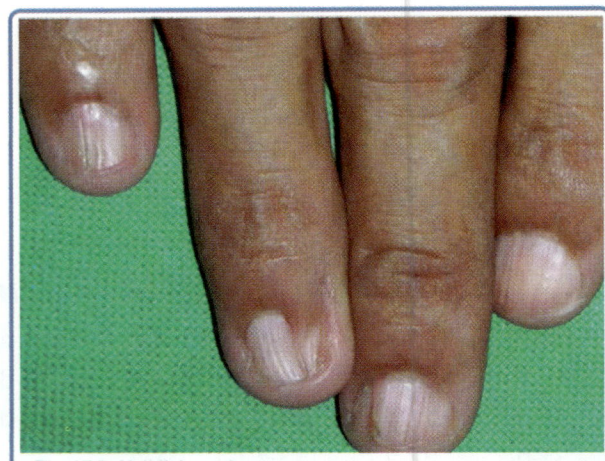
Fig. 17.3: Nail lichen planus—band-like extension of proximal nail fold over nail bed (pterygium of ring finger). Other nails show longitudinal ridging

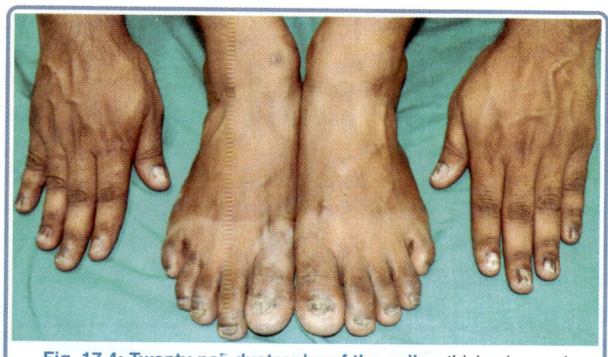

Fig. 17.4: Twenty nail dystrophy of the nails—thickening and discolouration of all twenty nails

eventually permanent loss of nails. In a few cases involvement of all the nails of hands and feet (twenty nail dystrophy) can occur. As in nail psoriasis, systemic treatment of skin or mucosal lichen planus may benefit nail lichen planus; however, treatment of isolated nail lichen planus is difficult. Intralesional steroid injections have been tried with variable success.

TINEA UNGUIUM (ONYCHOMYCOSIS)

This refers to infection of the nail plate by dermatophytes or other fungi. Affected nails show discolouration, thickening (Figs 17.5 and 17.6), fragility, loss of luster, dystrophy and subungual hyperkeratosis (Figs 17.7 and 17.8). Diagnosis is

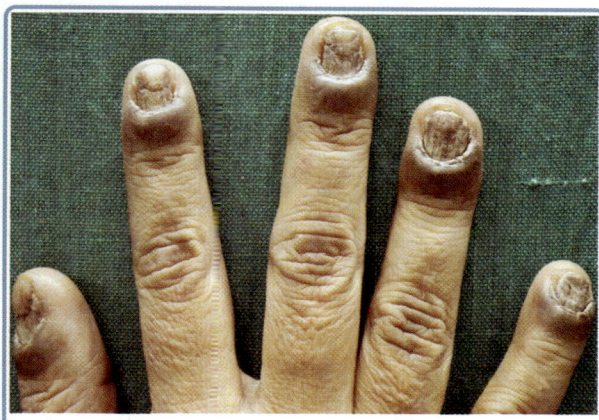

Fig. 17.5: Chronic paronychia with secondary nail dystrophy

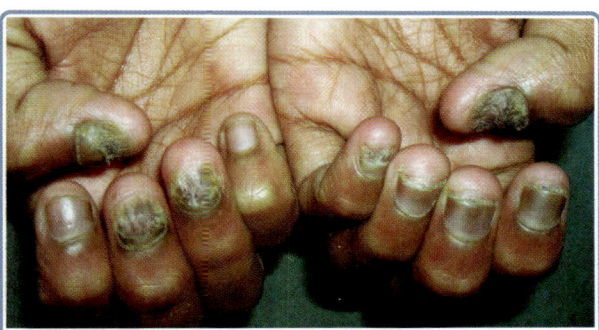

Fig. 17.6: Onychomycosis—dystrophy and discolouration of nail plates. Some of the nail plates are thick and fragile

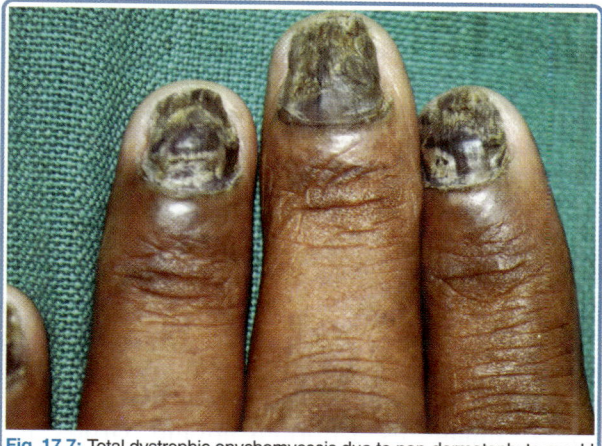

Fig. 17.7: Total dystrophic onychomycosis due to non-dermatophyte mould

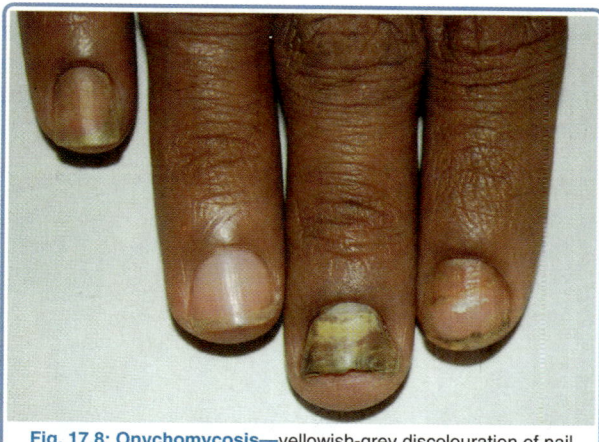

Fig. 17.8: Onychomycosis—yellowish-grey discolouration of nail plates and separation from the nail bed (onycholysis)

confirmed by scraping of keratotic debris under the nail plate or nail plate clippings to demonstrate fungal elements on KOH mount or on periodic acid-schiff (PAS) stain.

ONYCHOLYSIS

This refers to separation of nail plate from the nail bed. It can occur due to trauma, psoriasis, Reiter's disease and bacterial or fungal infections involving the nail. Excessive filling, chemical overexposure in manicures or nail tip application can also cause onycholysis. Some drugs like tetracycline, minocycline, psoralens can induce onycholysis.

NAILS IN SYSTEMIC DISEASES

Clubbing of nails is a well known association of cardiovascular and pulmonary diseases. Koilonychia, i.e. spoon shaped nail on platynychia (Hat nails) are seen in iron deficiency anaemia and Plummer Vinson syndrome. Dilated and tortuous nail fold capillaries are a well recognised feature of collagen vascular diseases like systemic sclerosis, rheumatoid arthritis or lupus erythematosus. Pterygium, seen typically in nail lichen planus, may also be seen in peripheral vascular disease and systemic sclerosis. Subungual haemorrhage or splinter haemorrhage may be associated with psoriasis and subacute bacterial endocarditis.

NAIL PLATE DISCOLOURATION

Melanonychia is occurrence of longitudinal black or brown lines on nail plates (Fig. 17.9) and can be seen in Addison's disease and vitamin B$_{12}$ deficiency. It may also occur in dark skinned individuals or in some families as a normal finding. Drugs like zidovudine, minocycline, antimalarials and cancer chemotherapeutic agents like cyclophosphamide, can induce hyperpigmented streak, may be the earliest sign of a subungual melanoma. However, similar streaks may be caused by benign melanocytic nevi.

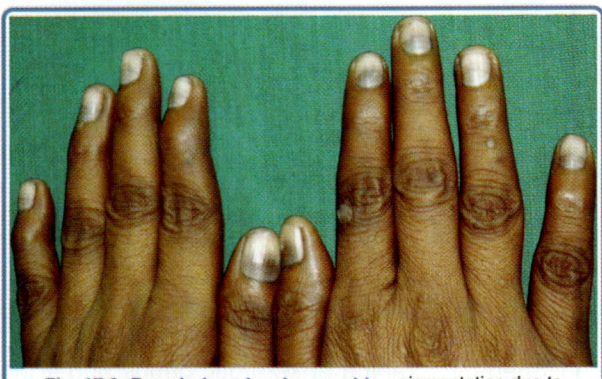

Fig. 17.9: Drug induced melanonychia—pigmentation due to adriamycin

Leuconychia refers to white discolouration of a nail plate. It can be spotty (unknown cause) or patchy (onychomycosis) or may involve the whole of the nail (onychomycosis) or may affect all the nails (hepatic disease). Green discolouration of nail plate is seen in persons involved with wet work due to overgrowth of pseudomonas under the nails (green nail syndrome). Yellow discolouration can occur due to increased bilirubin levels but may also result from psoriasis, or fungal infection. Blue discolouration of lunulae (azure lunulae) is seen in Wilson's disease.

TABLE 17.1: Nails in systemic diseases	
Clubbing	Cardiovascular and pulmonary diseases
Koilonychia (spoon shaped nail)	Iron deficiency anaemia
Platynychia (flat nail)	Plummer Vinson syndrome
Beaus lines	Malnutrition, drugs, cancer, trauma
	Myocardial infarction, liver disease, severe infections
Mee's lines	Arsenic poisoning
	Sickle cell anaemia
	Myocardial infarction
Pterygium	Nail lichen planus
	Peripheral vascular disease
	Sarcoidosis
Subungual/Splinter haemorrhage	Psoriasis
	Hypertension
	Subacute bacterial endocarditis

MCQs

1. **The nail plate is made of:**
   - a. Calcium
   - b. Keratin
   - c. Cartilage
   - d. Desmosomes

2. **The nail plate is made mainly by the:**
   - a. Nail bed
   - b. Nail matrix
   - c. Nail folds
   - d. Cuticle

3. **The finger nails grow on an average in a day by:**
   - a. 0.1 mm
   - b. 0.5 mm
   - c. 1 mm
   - d. 2 mm

4. **The rate of nail growth is reduced by:**
   - a. Peripheral vascular disease
   - b. Increasing age
   - c. Injury to the nail
   - d. All of the above

5. **The potential space between the nail fold and nail plate is sealed by:**
   - a. Use of adhesives
   - b. Lunula
   - c. Cuticle
   - d. Hyponychium

6. **Beau's lines have been described following:**
   - a. Consumption of NSAIDs
   - b. Injury to a nail unit
   - c. Myocardial infarction
   - d. Lichen planus of the nail

7. **Pterygium of nail occurs in:**
   - a. Psoriasis
   - b. Diabetes mellitus
   - c. Renal disease
   - d. Lichen planus

8. **Coarse pits over nail plate are common in:**
   - a. Psoriasis
   - b. Diabetes mellitus
   - c. Renal disease
   - d. Lichen planus

9. **White nails are seen in:**
   - a. Psoriasis
   - b. Hepatic disease
   - c. Renal disease
   - d. Lichen planus

10. **Clubbing of nails may be a feature of:**
    - a. Heart disease
    - b. Lung carcinoma
    - c. Hepatic disease
    - d. All of the above

11. **In clubbing of nails, the altered angle is between the nail plate and the:**
    - a. Nail bed
    - b. Nail matrix
    - c. Lateral nail fold
    - d. Proximal nail fold

12. **Onycholysis refers to:**
    - a. Loss of nail plate
    - b. Loss of nail unit
    - c. Separation of nail plate from nail bed
    - d. Dissolution of keratinocytes making up the nail plate

13. **Tinea unguium usually begins under the:**
    - a. Nail bed
    - b. Proximal nail fold
    - c. Lateral nail fold
    - d. Lunula

14. **A frequent sign of tinea unguium is:**
    - a. Nail plate discolouration
    - b. Nail plate thickening
    - c. Nail plate fragility
    - d. All of the above

15. **Diagnosis of tinea unguium is confirmed by:**
    - a. KOH mount
    - b. Nail clipping culture
    - c. Nail biopsy
    - d. Any one of the above

16. **The drug of choice for treatment of onycho-mycosis is:**
    - a. Griseofulvin
    - b. Itraconazole
    - c. Ketoconazole
    - d. Terbinafine

17. **Nail psoriasis is often associated with:**
    - a. Proximal interphalangeal (PIP) joint arthropathy
    - b. Scalp psoriasis
    - c. Distal interphalangeal (DIP) joint arthropathy
    - d. Large joint (oligoarticular) affection

18. **Lunula refers to visible part of:**
    - a. Nail bed
    - b. Nail matrix
    - c. Hyponychium
    - d. Terminal nail plate

19. **Beau's lines of the nails are:**
    - a. Transverse lines
    - b. Longitudinal lines
    - c. Transverse ridges
    - d. Longitudinal ridge

20. **The nail finding associated with iron deficiency anaemia is:**
    - a. Beau's lines
    - b. Clubbing
    - c. Platynychia
    - d. Oil spots

Chapter
17

Disorders of Nail

21. **Nail fold capillaries are a marker of:**
    a. Systemic sclerosis
    b. Psoriasis
    c. Hereditary haemorrhagic telangiectasia
    d. Angiofibromas

22. **A single new melanotic streak in an adult may precede development of:**
    a. Addison's disease
    b. Congenital melanocytic nevus of the nail fold
    c. Malignant melanoma
    d. HIV infection

23. **Drug induced onycholysis may be caused by:**
    a. Isotretinoin
    b. Omeprazole
    c. Hydroxychloroquine
    d. Minocycline

24. **Inverse pterygium is seen in:**
    a. Psoriasis
    b. Systemic sclerosis
    c. Lichen planus
    d. Onychomycosis

25. **Blue lunula is seen in:**
    a. Methotrexate toxicity
    b. Wilson's disease
    c. Tinea unguium
    d. Chronic hand dermatitis

26. **Fine pits are seen in all *except*:**
    a. Lichen planus
    b. Alopecia areata
    c. Psoriasis
    d. Atopic dermatitis

27. **All of the following are associated with nail changes *except*:**
    a. Psoriasis
    b. Lichen planus
    c. Darier's disease
    d. None of the above

28. **Diffuse nail pigmentation is seen in:**
    a. Iron deficiency anaemia
    b. Vitamin B_{12} deficiency
    c. Pellagra
    d. Vitamin C deficiency

ANSWERS

1-b,	2-b,	3-a,	4-d,	5-c,	6-c,	7-d,	8-a,	9-b,	10-d,
11-d,	12-c,	13-c,	14-d,	15-d,	16-b,	17-c,	18-b,	19-c,	20-c,
21-a,	22-c,	23-d,	24-b,	25-b,	26-c,	27-d,	28-b		

Skin and Internal Diseases

Appearance of skin is closely related to the state of internal systems of our body. Imbalanced function of any of the systems manifests as skin disease of one type or the other.

SKIN MANIFESTATIONS OF INTERNAL DISEASES

Skin is said to be a mirror of health of the internal systems of the body. Some examples of internal diseases that manifest on the skin are mentioned here with the skin lesions enumerated in parenthesis.

- **Brain and spinal cord diseases**
  - Tuberous sclerosis (adenoma sebaceum, ash leaf macules)
  - Neurofibromatosis (café au lait spots neurofibromas)
  - Sturge Weber syndrome (port wine stain)

- **Cardiovascular system**
  - Bacterial endocarditis (splinter haemorrhages)
  - Coronary artery disease due to hyperlipidaemias (xanthomas)
  - Rheumatic fever (erythema marginatum, subcutaneous nodules)

- **Endocrine diseases**
  - Diabetes mellitus (carbuncle, unresponsive or recurrent candidiasis/furunculosis/dermatophytosis and necrobiosis lipoidica)
  - Myxoedema (thickened, dry skin of face and extremities, alopecia)
  - Hyperthyroidism (alopecia, pretibial myxoedema)
  - Cushing's syndrome (striae, easy bruisability, acne, hirsutism, moon face and buffalo hump)
  - Addison's disease (hyperpigmentation of exposed regions, bony prominences and mucosae)
  - Adrenal hyperplasia and virilising adrenal and ovarian humors (hirsutism, acne and baldness)

- **Gastrointestingal diseases**
  - Cirrhosis of liver (spider angioma, palmar erythema, loss of axillary and pubic hair, gynaecomastia)
  - Peutz Jeghers syndrome (lentigines)
  - Hereditary haemorrhagic telangiectasia (telangiectasia)

- **Haematologic disorders**
  - Thrombocytopenia (purpura)
  - Disseminated intravascular coagulation (peripheral gangrene)
  - Lymphoma (pruritus, erythroderma)

- **Joint diseases**
  - Reiter's disease (keratoderma blenorrhagica, urethritis and conjunctivitis)
  - Gout (gouty tophi)
  - Rheumatoid arthritis (rheumatoid nodules)

- **Renal disorders**
  - Pruritus and dry scaly skin occurs in renal failure due to any cause.

- **Autoimmune diseases**
  - Systemic lupus erythematosus (butterfly erythema, discoid lesions)
  - Systemic sclerosis (generalised sclerosis, Raynaud's phenomenon)
  - Dermatomyositis (heliotrope erythema of eyelids)
  - Behcet's syndrome (aphthous ulcers, genital ulcers)

- **Deficiency disorders**
  - Pellagra (photosensitivity, glossitis and stomatitis)
  - Vitamin A deficiency (phrynoderma)

- **Metabolic diseases**
  - Hyperlipidaemia (xanthomas)
  - Porphyria (photosensitivity)
  - Amyloidosis (eyelid purpura, nodules)

- **Internal malignancy**
  - ❑ Carcinoma (metastasis)
  - ❑ Carcinoid syndrome (flushing)
  - ❑ Virilising tumours (hirsutism)

- **Infections**
  - ❑ Urticaria, erythema multiforme and erythema nodosum can be induced by a variety of infections

- **Unknown cause**
  - ❑ Sarcoidosis (papulonodules)

> **Summary:** In addition to the various body systems like the cardiovascular, central nervous system (CNS), renal, haematologic, joints, endocrine, gastrointestinal systems, the skin examination provides valuable clues to the diagnosis of underlying malignancies, nutritional deficiencies, metabolic diseases, infections and autoimmune diseases like systemic lupus erythematosus.

Following conditions affect internal systems as well as the skin and, being relatively common or important, will be dealt with more detail in the following sections. They are:

- **Collagen vascular diseases:** These multi-system autoimmune diseases affected many body systems including the skin.
- **Vesiculobullous disorders of the skin:** They are autoimmune diseases of the skin that may lead to systemic complications.
- **Nutritional deficiencies:** These affect many systems including the skin.
- Others like erythema nodosum, erythroderma (exfoliative dermatitis), hirsutism and acanthosis nigricans are also discussed. Many more like erythema multiforme or chickenpox are placed in other chapters.

CUTANEOUS CHANGES IN ENDOCRINE DISORDERS

Skin may be affected in a variety of ways in the numerous endocrine disturbances. Commonest endocrine disease resulting in skin changes is diabetes mellitus. Thyroid, adrenal, ovarian and pituitary diseases are also not uncommon causes of skin problems.

Thyroid

Disorders of thyroid function affect the skin in several ways. Hypothyroidism may be associated with generalised thickening of skin due to mucin deposition (myxoedema). Diffuse swelling and thickening of facial skin, hands, forearms, feet and legs are the most obvious clinical features of myxoedema. The thickened facial skin may develop deep furrows leading to leonine facies. Skin of the limbs becomes dry, leading to acquired ichthyosis and at times xerotic eczema. Diffuse hair loss may be associated.

Skin in hyperthyroidism appears soft, smooth and erythematous. Diffuse hair loss is sometimes a presenting symptom of thyroid disease both hypothyroidism and hyperthyroidism. A small proportion of patients with hyperthyroidism develop asymptomatic, infiltrated nodules and plaques over legs due to mucin deposits (pretibial myxoedema). This may occur even when the thyroid function has returned to normal (Table 18.1).

TABLE 18.1: Skin manifestations of thyroid disease	
Hypothyroidism	Myxoedema over face, neck, hands and feet
	Acquired ichthyosis and palmoplantar keratoderma
	Xerotic eczema
	Diffuse hair loss
	Easy bruising
Hyperthyroidism	Soft smooth moist skin
	Flushing and telangiectasias
	Diffuse hyperpigmentation
	Hair become fine and friable with diffuse hair loss, alopecia areata
	Nails-soft and brittle with koilonychia
	Pretibial myxoedema
Other autoimmune diseases like alopecia areata, lichen planus can be associated with autoimmune thyroid disease	

Diabetes

Skin signs of diabetes include diverse infections that may be fungal or bacterial. Fungal infections include superficial infections like candidiasis or widespread dermatophytosis or deep infections like zygomycosis or cryptococcosis. Bacterial infections seen with diabetes include pyodermas like carbuncle or cellulitis and others like erythrasma.

Candidiasis in diabetics affects the genitals (candidal balanitis or vulvovaginitis) or less commonly the angle of the mouth (angular cheilitis) or the nail folds (paronychia). Candidal balanitis presents as pruritic erythema of glans with whitish cheesy discharge and radial fissures. Deep fungal infections are life threatening and therefore important to detect and treat in time. Zygomycosis presents as nasal stuffiness and sero-sanguinous discharge with swelling of nasal bridge. The infection is commonly neglected in its early stages and then spreads to orbit or skull with disastrous results. Treatment with amphotericin B and itraconazole is not always successful.

Non-infective associations include necrobiosis lipoidica diabeticorum, granuloma annnulare, acanthosis nigricans, scleroedema, lipodystrophy, diabetic dermopathy (shin spots) or diabetic bullosis. Necrobiosis lipoidica occurs as asymptomatic erythematous, yellowish coloured plaques over skin. The skin overlying the plaques shows atrophy or ulceration. Diabetic dermopathy refers to the common occurrence in diabetics of brownish coloured atrophic macules over shins (Table 18.2).

TABLE 18.2: Cutaneous manifestations of diabetes mellitus		
Infective	: Bacterial	: Carbuncle
		Furunculosis
		Cellulitis
		Erythrasma
	Fungal	: Candidal balanitis
		Candidal cheilitis
		Dermatophytoses
		Cryptococcosis
Non-infective	: Necrobiosis lipoidica diabeticorum	
	Diabetic dermopathy	
	Diabetic bullosis	
	Granuloma annulare	
	Scleroedema	
	Acanthosis nigricans	
	Lipodystrophy	

Necrobiosis Lipoidica Diabeticorum

These asymptomatic atrophic and granulomatous plaques over shins are associated with diabetes mellitus. They are not as common in Indians as in the white skinned persons. The lesions begin as asymptomatic plaques and may ulcerate at times. The lesions are indolent and tend to develop atrophy when persistent.

Cushing's Syndrome

This may occur due to adrenal or pituitary hyperfunction due to adenomas or hyperplasia. More commonly, iatrogenic Cushing's syndrome occurs due to systemic steroids. Skin in such cases is thinned with prominent veins and dilated venules (telangiectasia). The body fat is redistributed leading to truncal obesity, moon facies, buffalo hump and loss of fat from limbs. Striae tend to be wider and more numerous. Ecchymoses, skin fragility, acanthosis nigricans and hirsutism are other skin findings (Table 18.3).

TABLE 18.3: Skin manifestations of Cushing's syndrome	
Fat redistribution	Striae
Moon facies	Skin fragility
Buffalo hump	Purpura/Ecchymosis
Truncal obesity	Hirsutism (infrequent)
Thin limbs	Acanthosis nigricans (infrequent)

Ovarian Disease

Most common ovarian abnormality manifesting on the skin is polycystic ovarian disease (PCOD) leading to hirsutism, acne, and acanthosis nigricans accompanied by obesity, menstrual irregularities, anovulation and increased lutenizing hormone (LH) to follicle stimulating hormone (FSH) ratio. Less commonly ovarian tumours secreting androgens are associated with skin manifestations like hirsutism, recalcitrant acne, androgenic alopecia and seborrhoea.

Skin Changes in Polycystic Ovary Syndrome (PCOS)
- Hirsutism
- Acne
- Acanthosis nigricans
- Acrochordons (skin tags)
- Seborrhoea (oily skin)
- Hyperpigmentation
- Female pattern hair loss

Acanthosis nigricans

It manifests as hyperpigmented, velvety plaques in the flexor areas like neck folds (Fig. 18.12), axillae (Fig. 18.11) and inguinal region. It is considered to be a marker of insulin resistant diabetes mellitus but may also occur in families or with internal malignancies (Fig. 18.1). For more details please *refer* page 209.

Chapter 18

Skin and Internal Diseases

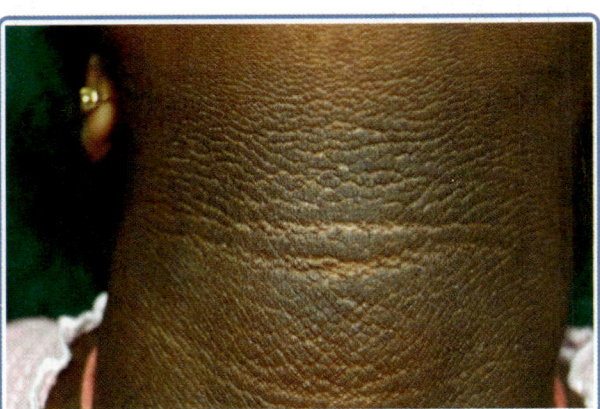

Fig. 18.1: Acanthosis nigricans—velvety hyperpigmented plaque over neck. Common associations include Diabetes mellitus, obesity and PCOD

Hirsutism

It refers to development of male pattern of distribution of hairs in a female, i.e. on upper lips, chin or beard region (Fig. 18.10). Hirsutism may be associated with ovarian tumours, PCOD, adrenal tumours and congenital adrenal hyperplasia. Treatment includes correction of the associated hormonal abnormality. Cosmetic correction may be done by various methods of hair removal like depilatories, waxing, shaving or hair reduction through use of intense pulse light, diode or long pulse neodymium-doped yttrium aluminum garnet (NdYAG laser). Topical application of eflornithine cream may also bring some improvement in appearance.

Hirsutism Aetiology

Constitutional

Ovarian tumours

Polycystic ovarian syndrome

Adrenal tumours

Congenital adrenal hyperplasia

Cushing's disease

Pituitary Disorders

Acromegaly or Gigantism lead to enlarged hands and feet, thickening of lips, tongue and skin over the forehead. Hypertrophy of the nose and chin is common and supraorbital ridges become more prominent. Cutis verticis gyarata, i.e. excessive thickened and folded scalp skin can occur. There can be hyperhidrosis, hypertrichosis and hyperpigmentation or even acanthosis nigricans.

AMYLOIDOSIS

The skin may be affected as one of the organs in the rare primary or myeloma associated multisystem

amyloidosis or may occur more commonly as localised cutaneous amyloidosis.

Systemic Amyloidosis

In this rare condition, lesions occur as skin coloured or erythematous papules, nodules or diffuse infiltration over face or other areas (Fig. 18.2). The lesions may become purpuric or vesicular. The purpura is seen especially over eyelids after Valsalva manoeuvre. The tongue is thickened (macroglossia), and the lips may be infiltrated. Biopsy of skin lesions reveals deposition of amyloid in the dermis and subcutaneous fat. Biopsy for demonstration of amyloid material may be done from the mucosae (rectal or oral) in case the skin lesions are absent. Associated multiple organ affection and clinical or subclinical myeloma makes the prognosis of this condition poor.

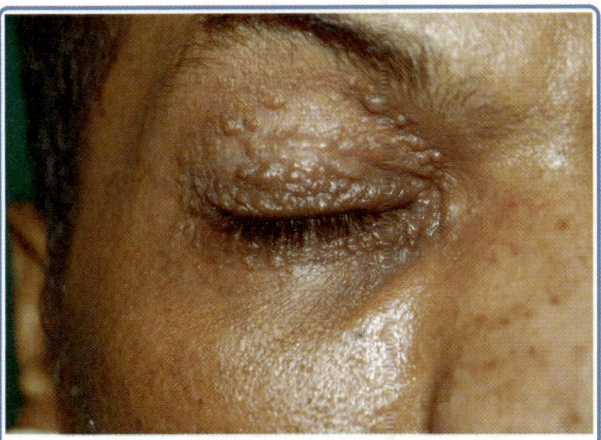

Fig. 18.2: Systemic amyloidosis—infiltrated papulonodules over upper eyelid in primary systemic amyloidosis

Localised Cutaneous Amyloidosis

This relatively common form of cutaneous amyloidosis may occur as hyperpigmented macules (macular amyloidosis) (Fig. 18.3) that when severe may progress to hyperpigmented and keratotic papular lesions (lichen amyloidosis) (Figs 18.4 and 18.5). The lesions are pruritic, grouped grayish-black coloured macules or papules of size 2–3 mm each. They are arranged close to each other in an orderly rippled pattern so that from a distance they appear as patches or plaques. Common sites are shins, forearms and upper back. Treatment consists of avoidance of friction (in the form of scratching or use of a bathing brush) and application of topical steroids. Improvement is extremely slow.

XANTHOMAS (YELLOW TUMOURS)

These yellow coloured lesions are caused by deposition of different types of fat into the skin.

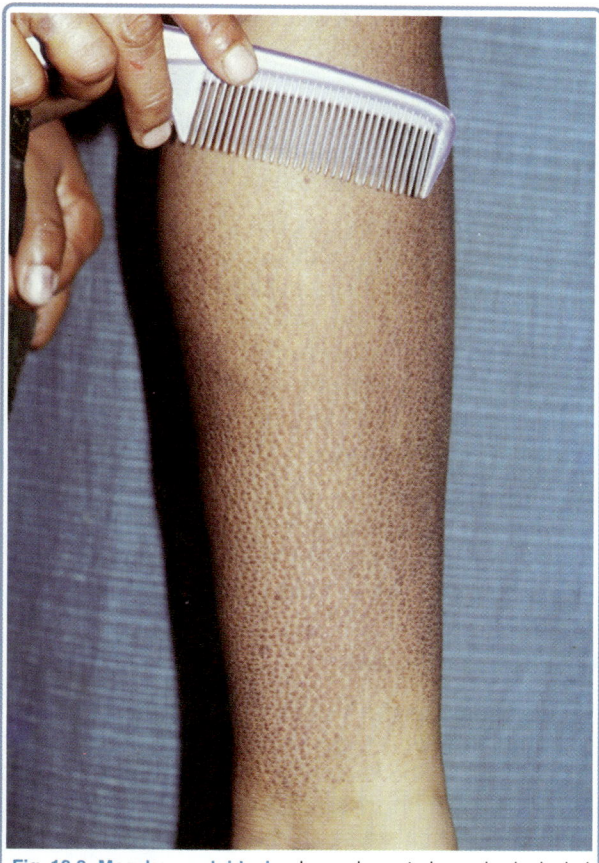

Fig. 18.3: Macular amyloidosis—hyperpigmented macules in rippled pattern as a result of repeated scratching with a comb

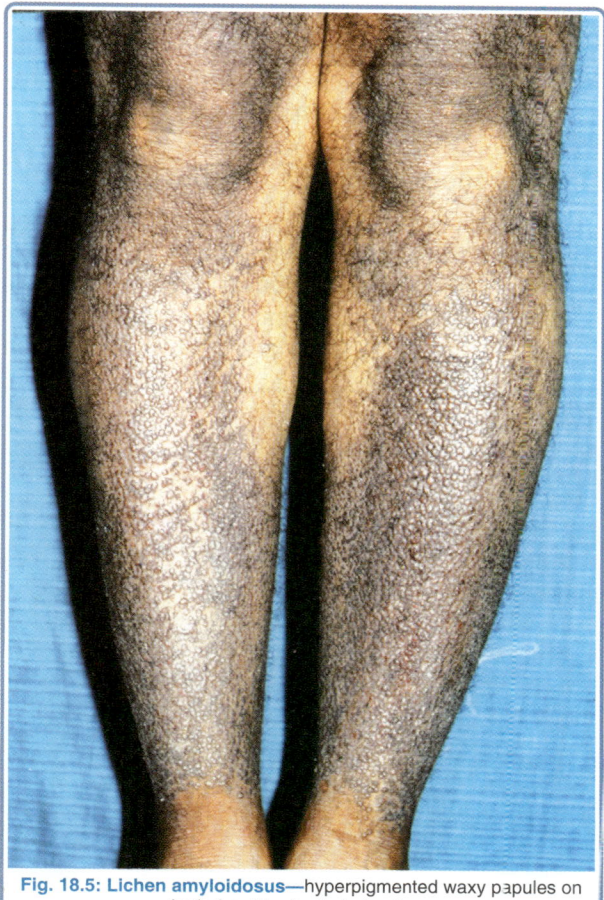

Fig. 18.5: Lichen amyloidosus—hyperpigmented waxy papules on both the shins in rippled pattern

They may be classified into xanthelasma, eruptive xanthomas, tuberous xanthomas, tendinous xanthomas and planar xanthomas.

I. Xanthelasma

Involve the upper and lower eyelids as soft yellowish flat papules and plaques (Fig. 18.6). They are the commonest type of xanthomas seen and appear frequently as an isolated finding in the absence of any hyperlipidaemia. They usually appear in fourth decade and are more common in females than in males. Less

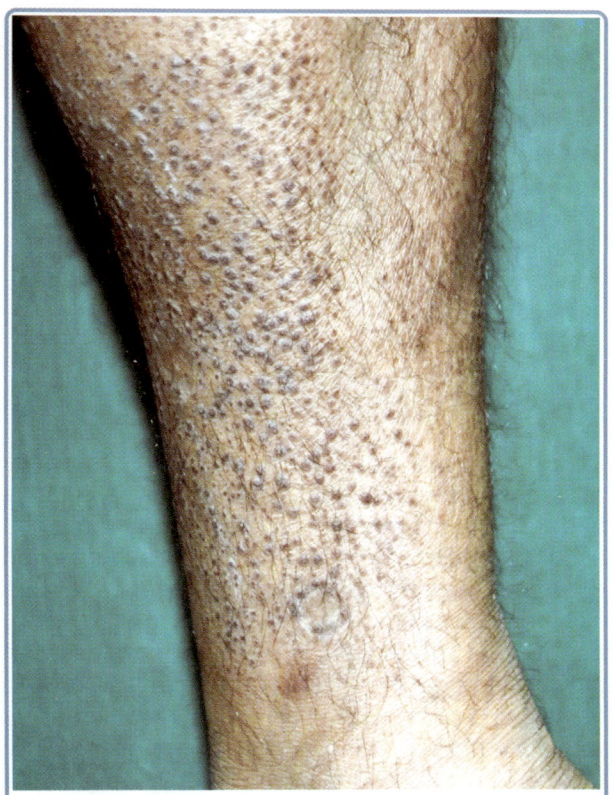

Fig. 18.4: Lichen amyloidosus—hyperpigmented uniform sized discrete keratotic papules. Bilateral affection of legs is common

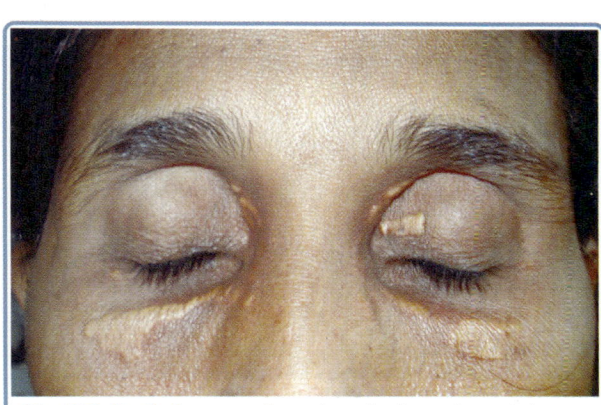

Fig, 18.6: Xanthelasma—yellow coloured soft papules and plaques

frequently they may occur in association with hyperlipidaemia esp. hypercholesterolaemia. Xanthelesma have been linked to atherosclerosis and ischaemic heart disease.

II. Tuberous xanthomas

Firm, painless, red-yellow nodules that develop around the pressure areas such as the knees (Figs 18.7A and B), elbows (Fig. 18.8), heels and buttocks. Nodules can join together to form knobby masses. They are usually associated

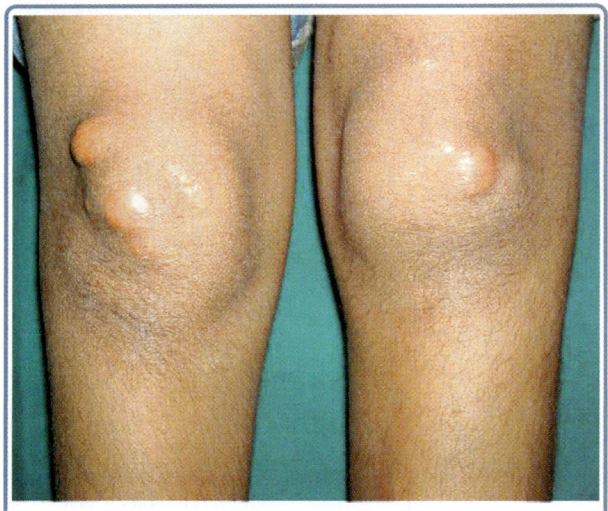

(A)

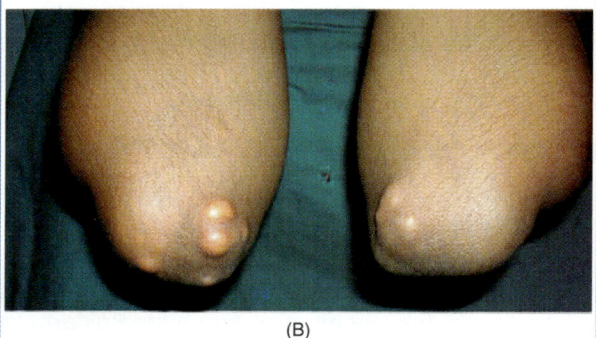

(B)

Fig. 18.7A and B: Tuberous xanthomas—yellowish, firm to hard nodules over bilateral knees and elbows are indicative of hyper-cholesterolaemia

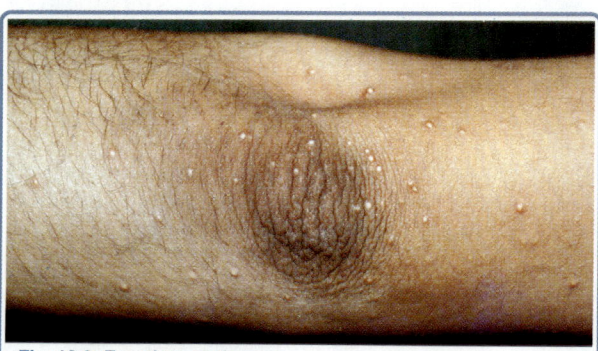

Fig. 18.8: Eruptive xanthomas—erythematous papules with yellow centre over extensors of body are seen in hypertriglyceridaemia

with hypercholesterolaemia and increased low-density lipoprotein (LDL) levels (Frederickson's type II).

III. Eruptive xanthoma (due to hypertriglyceridaemia)

They appear as crops of small yellowish papules, usually multiple in number. Eruptive xanthomas can be associated with pancreatitis. These lesions can be seen in patients with hypertriglyceridaemia with or without diabetes mellitus (Frederickson's type I, IV and V).

IV. Teinous xanthomas

These commonly occur in association with tuberous xanthomas with type II hyperlipidaemias (increases cholesterol and LDL) and are seen as firm nodules in tendons and ligaments.

V. Plain xanthomas

Lesions are flat papules or patches that can occur anywhere on the body. Lesions on the creases of the palms are indicative of a specific pattern of increased lipids in blood called Frederickson's type III dysbetalipoproteinaemia.

Management of xanthomas is that of the associated hyperlipidaemias. This includes dietary modifications to and use of lipid lowering drugs like statins, fenofibrates, cholestyramine, or nicotinic acid. Eruptive xanthomas associated with hypertriglyceridaemia are more amenable to dietary correction and can resolve completely while other types do not resolve completely with treatment. Management of associated systemic disorders like nephrotic syndrome or diabetes mellitus have a favourable effect on the xanthomas. Large tuberous masses may need to be excised.

PORPHYRIAS

Porphyrias are genetic or acquired disorders related to the haem metabolism. Porphyria cutanea tarda (PCT) is the most common type and may be associated with HIV infection, hepatitis C infection or use of hepatotoxic drugs or agents. Drugs like barbiturates, carbamazepine, griseofulvin, oestrogens, rifampicin, and sulphonamides can precipitate porphyrias. PCT is characterised by skin fragility and blisters on such exposure which heals with scarring (Fig. 18.9) and milia formation. Other features include hypertrichosis and hyperpigmentation of face. Diagnosis is made by detecting porphyrins in the urine.

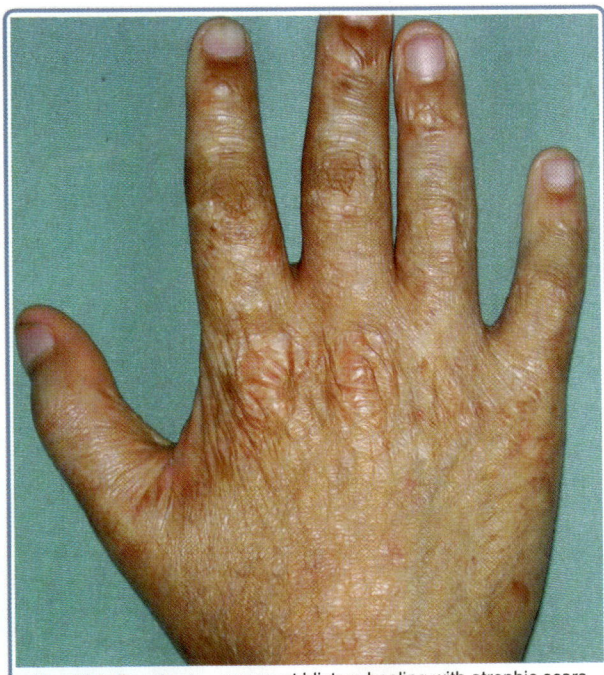

Fig. 18.9: Porphyria—recurrent blisters healing with atrophic scars

Acute intermittent porphyria has no associated skin lesions.

Congenital erythropoietic porphyria is the severe form of porphyria characterised by severe photosensitivity at birth or early infancy, red coloured urine and teeth (erythrodontia), mutilation of face and hands. Splenomegaly and anaemia are systemic associations with poor prognosis.

Management of porphyrias includes avoidance of sun exposure, alcohol and precipitating drugs. Phlebotomy, antimalarials and splenectomy are used for severe forms.

ERYTHEMA NODOSUM

This is a pattern of hypersensitivity response of the skin to various infections or drugs. However, many a times, no aetiology factor can be identified.

Aetiology

The different aetiologic factors implicated are:

- **Infections**

Bacterial	: Streptococcal upper respiratory tract infection (URTI), Yersinia, Brucella infections and Tularaemia. Cat Scratch Disease
Mycobacterial	: Tuberculosis
Chlamydial	: Lymphogranuloma venereum
Spirochaetal	: Leptospirosis
Fungal	: Histoplasmosis
Protozoan	: Toxoplasmosis

- **Drugs:** Sulphonamides, oestrogens, aspirin and iodides
- **Internal diseases:** Sarcoidosis, Behcet's disease, Crohn's disease
- **Malignancies:** Lymphoma and leukaemia

Clinical implication: Common investigations for detecting an underlying cause in the absence of any specific pointer include a careful drug history, complete blood count, X-ray chest, Mantoux test and throat swab/antistreptolysin O (ASO) titre.

Patient Profile

Young women are preferentially affected. Adult males and children are affected occasionally.

Morphology

Typical lesions are tender, reddish, barely elevated, deep seated nodules and plaques 1–10 cm in diameter. The initial yellowish red nodule turns deep red by the end of the first week, this is turn becomes bluish red, before subsiding with brownish hyperpigmentation over 3–6 weeks. Nodules do not ulcerate.

Distribution

Classically both shins are affected (Figs 18.10–18.12). Occasionally thighs, arms, buttocks, back or forearms may be involved.

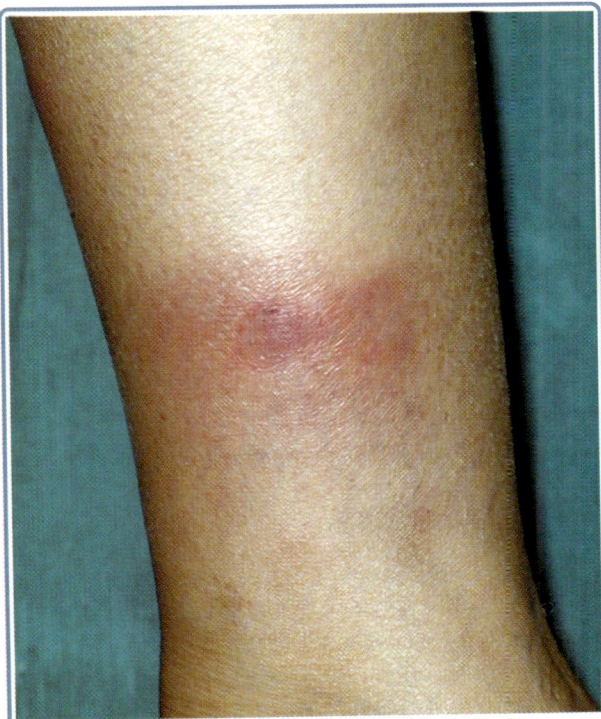

Fig. 18.10: Erythema nodosum—deep seated erythematous tender nodules and plaques over both legs are typical of erythema nodosum

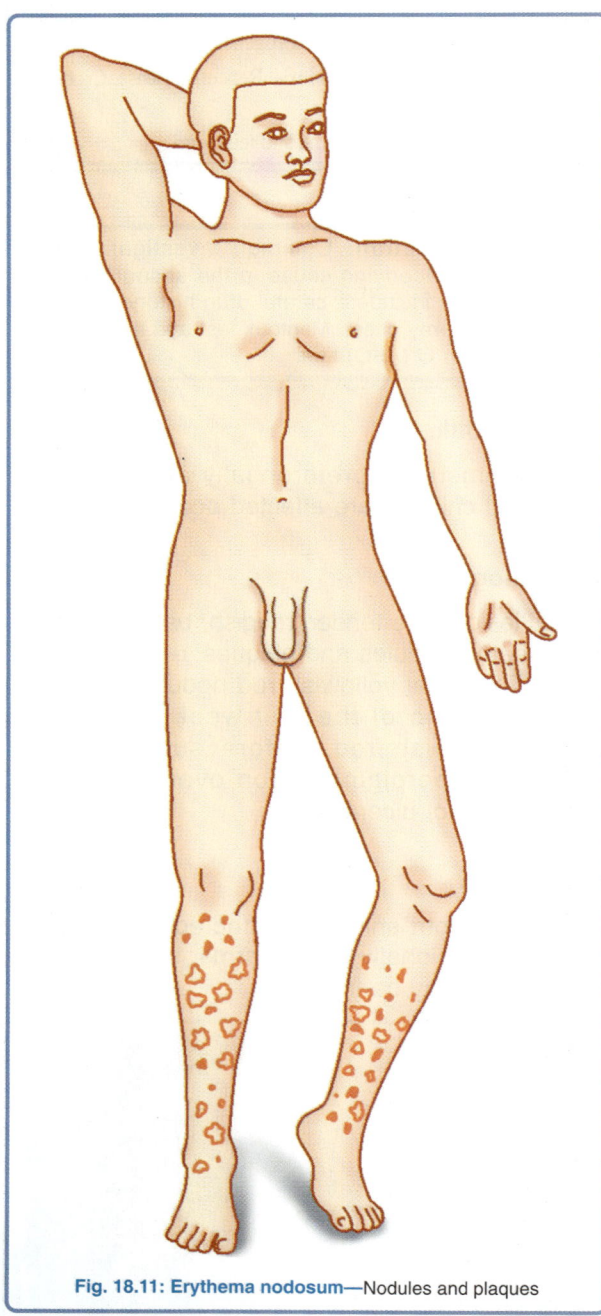

Fig. 18.11: Erythema nodosum—Nodules and plaques

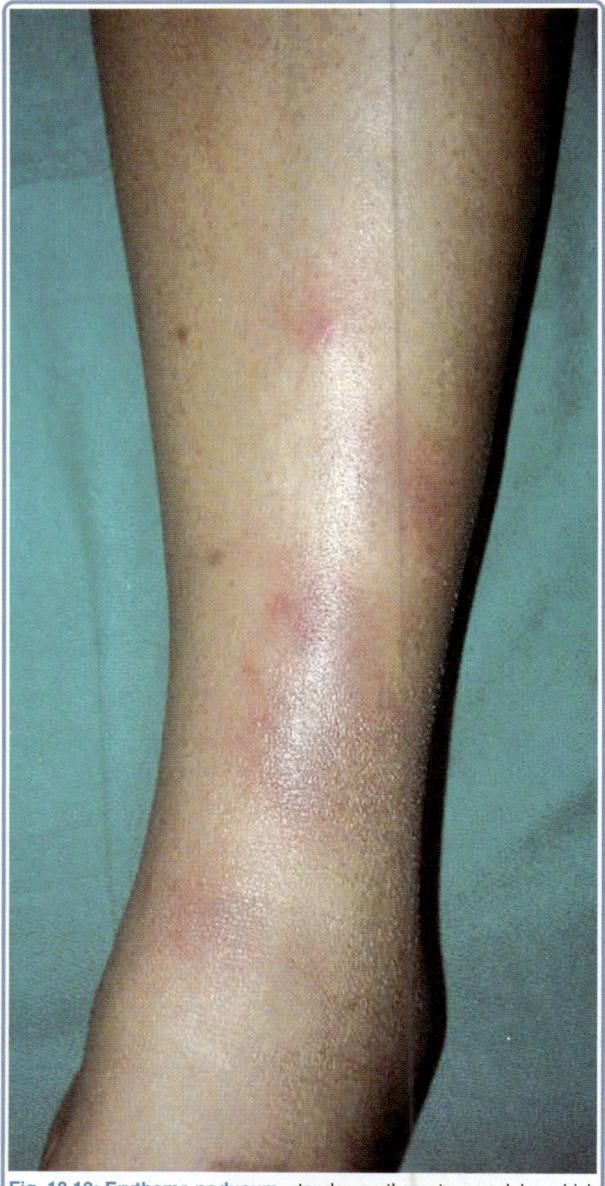

Fig. 18.12: Erythema nodusum—tender, erythematous nodules which are better palpated than seen

Other Systems

Fever, malaise, arthralgia, oedema of feet and body ache may accompany the skin lesions.

Therapy

If an underlying cause is detected, treat it. If none is found, therapy is only symptomatic since the disease is usually self-limiting. Ordinarily, it takes 3–6 weeks for the lesions to resolve by themselves. Nonsteroidal anti-inflammatory drugs (NSAIDs) like ibuprofen are helpful in relieving pain in the nodules and joints.

Summary: Symmetrical, tender, erythematous nodules over shins of young women accompany fever and arthralgia. Tuberculosis, streptococcal infections and drugs are commonly implicated. Lesions subside over 3–6 weeks without ulceration NSAIDs relieve the pain.

ERYTHRODERMA (EXFOLIATIVE DERMATITIS)

Erythema and scaling involving most or all of the body surface area is termed as exfoliative dermatitis or erythroderma (Figs 18.13 and 18.14). It develops either de novo (primary, idiopathic or due to unknown cause) or as a progression of a pre-existing skin disease (secondary erythroderma due to a known cause).

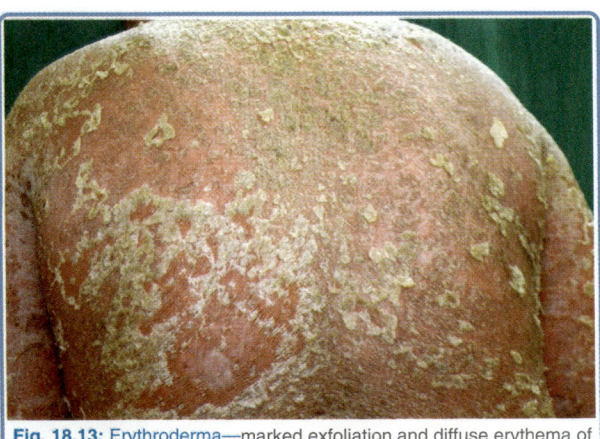

Fig. 18.13: Erythroderma—marked exfoliation and diffuse erythema of skin all over the body

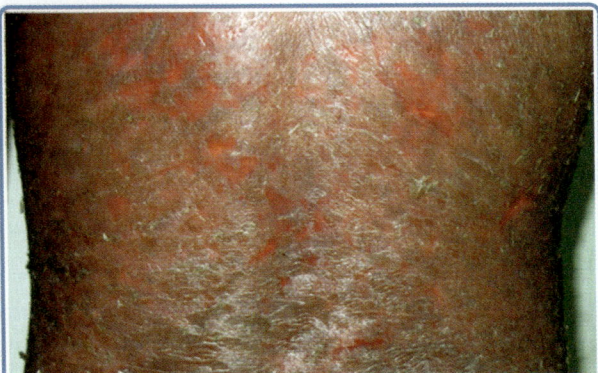

Fig. 18.14: Erythroderma—generalised erythema and scaling. Differentiating various causes requires careful examination and investigations including biopsy

Aetiology

- **Pre-existing skin diseases:** Skin diseases that lead to secondary erythroderma by virtue of extension of skin lesions all over the body are:

  - Psoriasis: Accounts for about 40% cases.

  - Eczema/Dermatitis group: Accounts for about 20%, and includes seborrhoeic dermatitis, allergic contact dermatitis and atopic dermatitis.

  - Miscellaneous: Account for about 10% cases like ichthyoses, pemphigus, toxic epidermal necrolysis, staphylococcal scalded skin syndrome, Norwegian scabies and lymphoma.

- **Drug-induced erythroderma:** Accounts for 10–15% cases and is caused by sulphonamides, dapsone, NSAIDs, antiepileptics, penicillins, etc.

- **Internal malignancy and lymphomas.**

- **Unidentified cause:** In a small proportion, no cause may be found.

Clinical Features

Apart from the diffuse and generalised erythema, oedema and scaling that constitute erythroderma, additional features that suggest a pre-existing skin disease may be present. These could vary from Auspitz sign and nail pitting for psoriasis or greasy scales in seborrhoeic distribution for seborrhoeic dermatitis to fragile vesicles and a positive Nikolsky's sign in pemphigus.

Erythroderma can end fatally, especially in the elderly, if not managed urgently and appropriately. This is because of the numerous medical complications that result from a serious compromise in skin function, increased peripheral blood flow and loss of protein and essential elements from skin.

Systemic Disturbances in Erythroderma

Persistent generalised dilation of peripheral vessels and loss of protein, vitamins and essential elements in scales has a profound effect on all systems.

Cardiovascular: Generalised peripheral vasodilation may lead to high output cardiac failure.

Gastrointestinal: Protein losing enteropathy develops due to intestinal villous atrophy.

Fluid/Electrolyte/Temperature: Due to hypoproteinemia, shift of fluid from intra to extravascular compartment results in oedema feet as well as oliguria and even anuria. Electrolyte imbalance is common. Hypothermia and concealed pyrexia are serious complications.

Renal: Oliguria, hyponatraemia and hyperkalaemia.

Lymphadenopathy: Generalised.

Management

Although, therapy would differ according to the pre-existing skin disease that led to erythroderma, the initial emergency care of all patients must ensure.

- Omit and avoid suspected drug(s).
- Warm clothing and monitoring core temperature.
- Monitor input/output, maintain fluid and electrolyte balance.
- High protein diet.
- Systemic steroids, oral or parenteral, equivalent of 1–2 mg/kg of prednisolone to be tapered gradually after 1–2 weeks.
- Topical applications of soothing ointment like white soft paraffin soften and separate scales. Topical steroids, applied in limited quantities, relieve pruritus and reduce erythema.
- Investigations to monitor fluid and electrolyte balance, serum proteins and renal function are repeated at intervals till the skin lesions subside and other systems regain normalcy.

Summary: Erythroderma indicates erythema and scaling of the whole body surface. It may result from aggravation of a pre-existing disease like psoriasis, contact allergic deratitis or seborrhoeic dermatitis or may be induced by drugs like sulphonamides or NSAIDs. Features of the original skin condition may be identifiable clinically or on biopsy. Systemic problems due to persistent erythroderma include hypoproteinaemia, cardiac failure, fluid, electrolyte and temperature imbalance and lymphadenopathy. Treatment is that of the pre-existing disease, if any. Offending drugs must be omitted. Supportive measures include high protein diet, warm clothing, maintaining fluid and electrolyte balance and topical application of soothing ointments. Systemic steroids are useful to expedite resolution.

HIRSUTISM

Growth of coarse hair in a male distribution, occurring in females and prepubertal children is termed as hirsutism.

Aetiology

High levels of circulating androgens or increased sensitivity of hair follicles to androgenic stimulation is causative.

Raised Androgens

Functional tumours or hyperplasias of the pituitary, adrenals and ovaries are responsible for some cases. However, many cases have only hyperplastic corpus luteum or ovarian follicles or may have increased peripheral production of androgens by excess adipocytes (obesity). Drugs, like androgens, anabolic steroids and less frequently, glucocorticoids, adrenocorticotropic hormone (ACTH) and progestagens, are responsible for some cases.

Raised End Organ (Hair Follicle) Sensitivity

This is responsible for many cases of 'idiopathic hirsutism' as these cases do not have a correctable hormonal imbalance. Genetic predisposition is present.

Morphology

Hair become thicker, darker and sometimes grow longer than usual. When the hair are not grossly coarse, it is important to be sure that there is either a significant change in the hair morphology or is associated with other features of virilisation. Comparison with other female members of the family is frequently useful.

Distribution

Upper lips and chin (Fig. 18.15) are involved in mild cases. Other regions like the submandibular, lower abdomen, thighs, are involved in severe cases.

Other Features of Virilization

These include change of voice quality, clitoromegaly, thick skin with coarse body hair, severe acne, hair loss in male type distribution, loss of female body outline due to well developed muscles and male type fat distribution (masculinisation). Patients frequently have amenorrhoea.

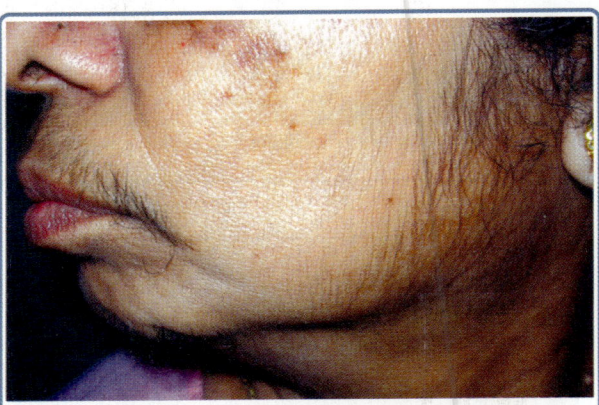

Fig. 18.15: Hirsutism—coarse hair growth resembling adult male

Investigations

Screening investigations for any androgen secreting tumour are urinary 17-ketosteroids and serum testosterone (total and free, if possible), serum dehydroepiandrosterone (DHEA) and ultrasonography of abdomen. Detailed investigations including dynamic tests are better left to endocrinologists.

Therapy

Although, patient's concern is cosmetic, it is important to rule out adenomas and carcinomas that can be surgically treated. Ovarian hyperplastic disorders with androgen excess can be treated with cyclical pills containing oestrogens or oestrogens with antiandrogens like cyproterone acetate. Symptomatic therapy of hirsutism includes waxing, plucking, bleaching and electrolysis. In electrolysis, the hair root is destroyed by electrical current passed with the help of a thin, long needle inserted through the follicular pore. The procedure is, however, tedious and significant proportion of hair may grow back. Epilatory lasers have the advantage of producing rapid results. Diode laser and long pulse Nd:YAG laser are preferred for hair removal. Transient inflammation and pigmentation are common but minor side effects. Due to a high rate of regrowth the term 'laser hair removal' is replaced by 'laser hair reduction.'

Summary: Hirsutism is growth of coarse hair in male distribution occurring in a female. Causes include androgen excess due to tumours or hyperplasias, increased follicular sensitivity to androgens or drugs like anabolic steroids. Other features of virilisation like clitoromegaly, husky voice and masculine body may be associated. Screening investigations include urinary 17-ketosteroids, serum testosterone and DHEA, and ultrasonography (USG) of abdomen. Plucking, waxing, bleaching and electrolysis provide a choice of therapeutic procedures. Epilatory lasers produce rapid results but are expensive. Oral antiandrogens with or without oestrogens are used in cases with ovarian hyperplasias. Ovarian tumours must be removed.

ACANTHOSIS NIGRICANS

This peculiar but benign condition of the skin is frequently a manifestation of an internal disorder.

Patient Profile

Young adults, male or female, are affected. Obesity is the commonest association. Endocrine disorders (polycystic ovarian disease, hypothyroidism, acromegaly, Cushing's syndrome and Insulin dependent diabetes mellitus) are frequently associated. Occasionally, the condition is familial and rarely it may be a manifestation of hidden internal malignancy. Drugs like oestrogens, corticosteroids, nicotinic acid can also induce acanthosis nigricans.

Morphology

Ill defined, brown-black plaques with a soft, velvety, papillated surface are typical. Skin tags may be associated. Initial stage is characterised by grey-brown, indistinct patches that develop central gentle papillations.

Hair become thicker, darker and sometimes grow longer than usual. When the hair are not grossly coarse, it is important to be sure that there is either a significant change in the hair morphology or is associated with other features of virilisation. Comparison with other female members of the family is frequently useful.

Distribution

Flexural regions are involved. Hence, axillae (Fig. 18.16) groins, neck (Fig. 18.17), popliteal and antecubital fossae are usually involved. Other flexures, palms, soles, mucosae and bony prominences are affected in severe cases. Due to cosmetic reasons face pigmentation is a frequent presenting symptom.

Therapy

Treatment of causative factor like obesity and endocrine disorders is crucial.

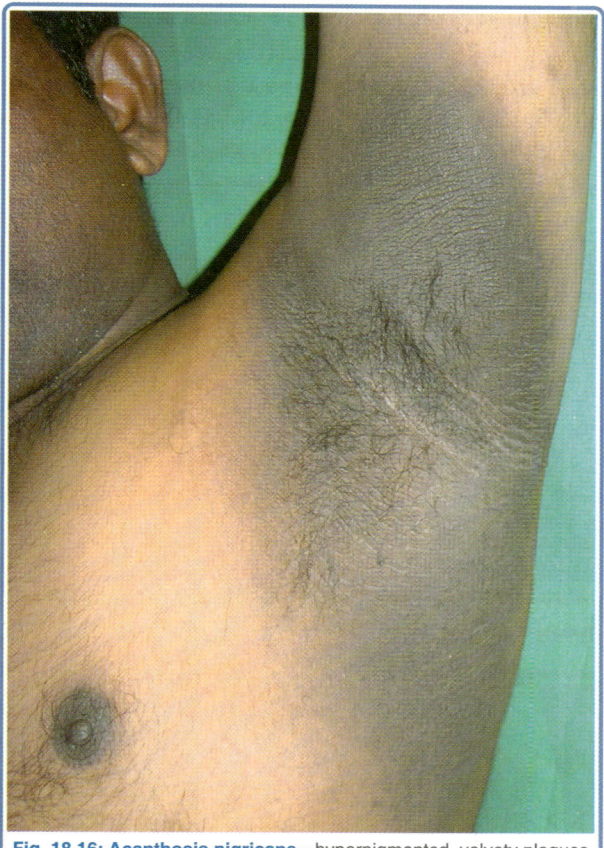

Fig. 18.16: Acanthosis nigricans—hyperpigmented, velvety plaques

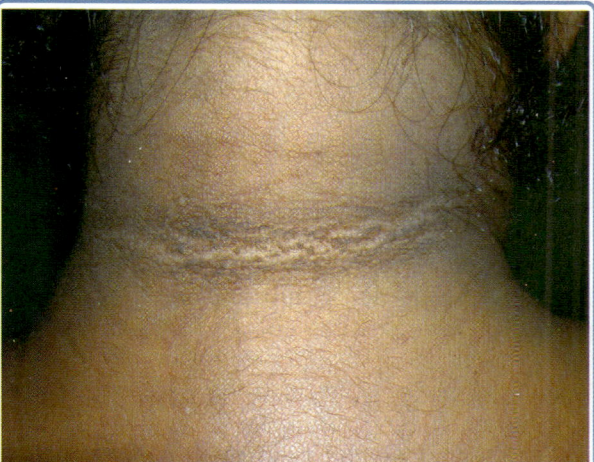

Fig. 18.17: Acanthosis nigricans—hyperpigmented velvety plaque in neck fold

LANGERHANS CELL HISTIOCYTOSIS

(Synonym: Histiocytosis X)

This proliferative disorder of Langerhans cell histiocytes involves not just the skin but also reticuloendothelial system and bones (skull and ends of long bones) (Fig. 17.19). Letterer-Siwe disease is the disseminated form of Langerhans cell histiocytosis (LCH), which presents as scaly

Chapter

18

Skin and Internal Diseases

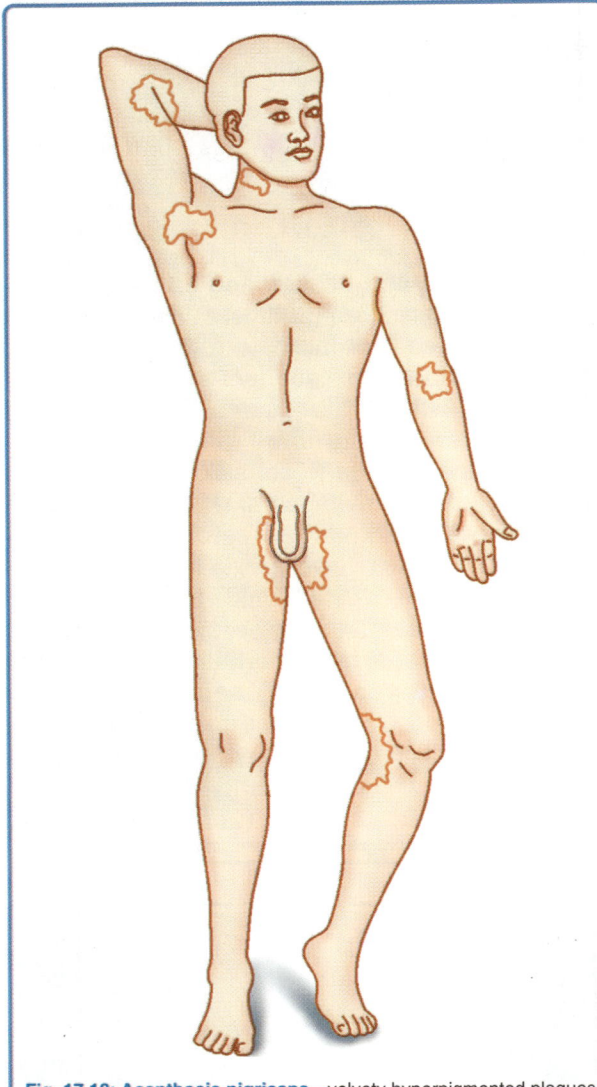

Fig. 17.18: Acanthosis nigricans—velvety hyperpigmented plaques

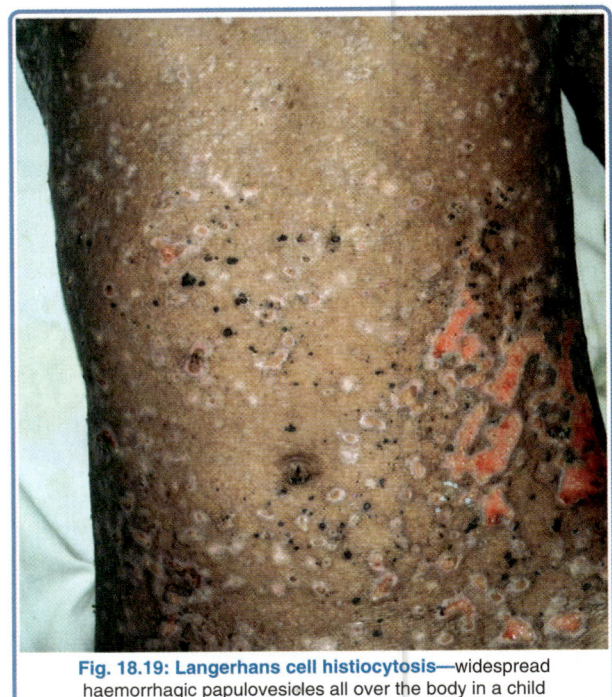

Fig. 18.19: Langerhans cell histiocytosis—widespread haemorrhagic papulovesicles all over the body in a child

crused papules in seborrhoeic areas, anaemia and thrombocytopenia. Hepatosplenomegaly and pulmonary infiltrates can occur and the condition is the localise form of LCH which manifests as a lesion in a bone, typically in the jaw bone leading to loose or 'floating' teeth. Hand Schuller Christian disease represents the middle part of the spectrum of LCH and is characterised by a triad of osteolytic lesions in skull bone, diabetes insipidus and exophthalmos. The prognosis is better than that in Letterer-Siwe disease but systemic involvement may occur.

Diagnosis is made on the basis of typical clinical features, skin biopsy findings, bone marrow examination and electron microscopic examination to demonstrate 'tennis racquet' shaped Birbeck granules. For solitary or few lesions in skin or bone, excision or curettage can be done. Extensive and systemic involvement may respond to chemotherapeutic agents.

NUTRITIONAL DEFICIENCIES

Vitamin A Deficiency

Vitamin A deficiency leads to dry skin and phrynoderma.

Phrynoderma

This follicular papular eruption, seen usually in prepubertal children from developing countries, is thought to be due to a deficiency of vitamin A. However, another school of though considers essential fatty acid deficiency as the cause. Ocular changes of vitamin A deficiency may be associated.

Morphology

Skin coloured conical follicular papules with or without a topping of dark coloured keratotic plugs characterise this disease (Figs 18.20 and 18.21). Lesions are grouped in areas of maximal affection but scattered in other regions.

Distribution

Initial lesions occurs over knees, lower anterolateral thighs, elbows, and posterolateral arms. Extensors of extremities, buttocks, back and face are involved later.

Therapy

Correction of dietary imbalance is important for avoiding relapses. Sources of vitamin A are eggs,

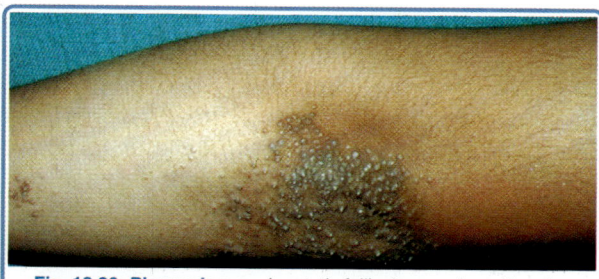
Fig. 18.20: Phrynoderma—keratotic follicular papules with spiny projections over elbow in a child

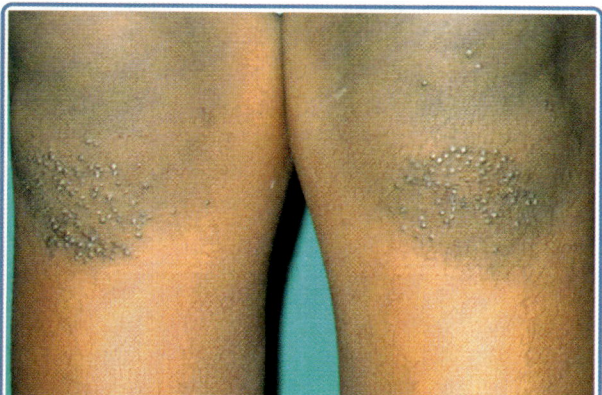
Fig. 18.21: Phrynoderma—bilaterally symmetrical grouped rough follicular papules

meat, mango, papaya, beet, carrots and green leafy vegetables. Daily requirement of vitamin A is 1000–4000 IU. Safflower and sunflower oil are rich in essential fatty acids.

Single large oral dose of vitamin A rarely clears phrynoderma. Oral vitamin A 5000–10000 IU per day (or 50000 IU per week) for many weeks leads to gradual flattening of lesions. Topical retinoic acid 0.05% or salicylic acid 3% are useful adjuvants.

Summary: Phrynoderma is due to vitamin A/essential fatty acid deficiency. Grouped, keratotic, skin coloured, conical, follicular papules over extensors of limbs are typical. Raising intake of vitamin A containing foods (eggs, meat, carrots, beet, papaya and green leafy vegetables) and oral supplementation (50000 IU once a week or 5000 IU daily improve lesions).

Vitamin B Complex

Many vitamin deficiencies from this group are commonly present in combination, thus some clinical features may overlap.

Riboflavin deficiency

Riboflavin is necessary for integrity of epithelia. It is also needed for activation of pyridoxine. Daily requirement is 2 mg, whereas therapeutic doses are 10–30 mg orally. Milk, eggs, liver and green leafy vegetables are rich in riboflavin.

Earliest change is angular cheilitis which refers to erythema and erosions of the angles of mouth. Lips may be red, scaly and fissured. Tongue is smooth and magenta red with prominent fungiform papillae. Later, conjunctivitis and keratitis may occur.

Skin changes over the face resemble seborrhoeic dermatitis. Diffuse erythema and yellowish powdery scaling of face with accentuation in areas of seborrhoeic dermatitis is seen. Similar erythema, and at times erosions, may affect the scrotal or vulval skin.

Pyridoxine deficiency

It is also involved with maintaining epithelia and its deficiency induces clinical features similar to those due to riboflavin deficiency. Pyridoxine is also necessary for synthesis of niacin and hence its deficiency may occasionally induce pellagra. Daily requirement is about 2 mg, the dietary sources being meat, liver, green vegetables and whole cereals and therapeutic doses 10–30 mg per day.

Summary: Actions of riboflavin and pyridoxine are closely related and interdependent. Hence, combined deficiency is a rule. Changes are early and prominent on face an include angular cheilitis, seborrhoeic dermatitis-like rash and a smooth magenta red tongue. Eggs, meat, liver, cereals and green vegetables are sources of riboflavin and pyridoxine. Oral therapeutic doses are 10–30 mg daily.

Pellagra (niacin deficiency)

Deficiency of niacin (nicotinic acid) leads to a multisystem disorder that affects primarily the skin, gastrointestinal tract and the brain (Fig. 18.22). Niacin is needed for synthesis of nicotinamide and thence for all hydrogen exchange—body metabolism dependent on nicotinamid adenine dinucleotide phosphate (NADP) and NADPH (reduced NADP). If left untreated, the outcome may be fatal. (Hence, it is said to be characterised by the 4 Ds viz. dermatitis, diarrhoea, dementia and death.)

Pellagra may also follow malabsorption disorders. Pellagra like state may result from metabolic diversion of tryptophan for other uses (carcinoid syndrome), deficient with niacin synthesis (INH induced). Thyrotoxicosis, pregnancy, persistent fever and high carbohydrate intake raise niacin requirement and may precipitate pellagra.

Chapter **18**

Skin and Internal Diseases

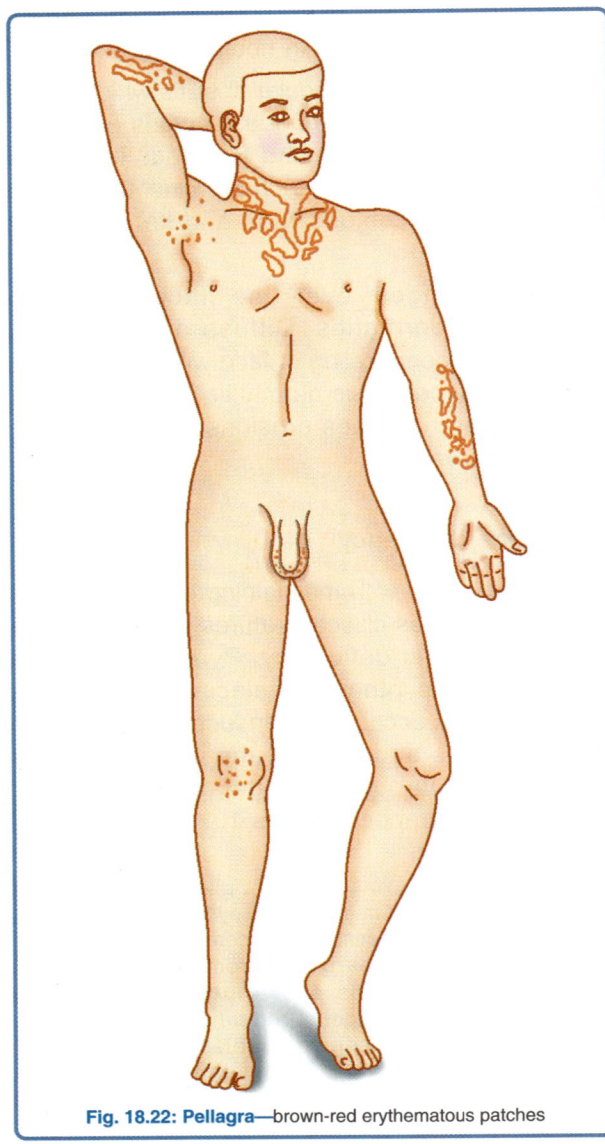

Fig. 18.22: Pellagra—brown-red erythematous patches

sharply restricted to sun-exposed regions. When severe, vesicles or blisters may occur. Persistent lesions turn brown and later, brownish black plaques, topped with scales, appear. Neck, upper chest, forearms, dorsa of hands and face are involved commonly (Fig. 18.23). Sharp delineation of lesions over the 'V' of the chest and around the neck has been termed Casal's necklace (Figs 18.24 and 18.25).

Similar ill defined patches occur over the pressure sites and body folds. Hence, elbows, knees, buttocks, trochanteric prominences, malleoli, axillae, groins, perineum and scrotum are affected commonly.

All mucosae turn red. Tongue is smooth (papillae flattened) and dark red. Fissuring and ulceration may occur later. Buccal, labial, palatal, conjunctival, vaginal and anal mucosae show erythema.

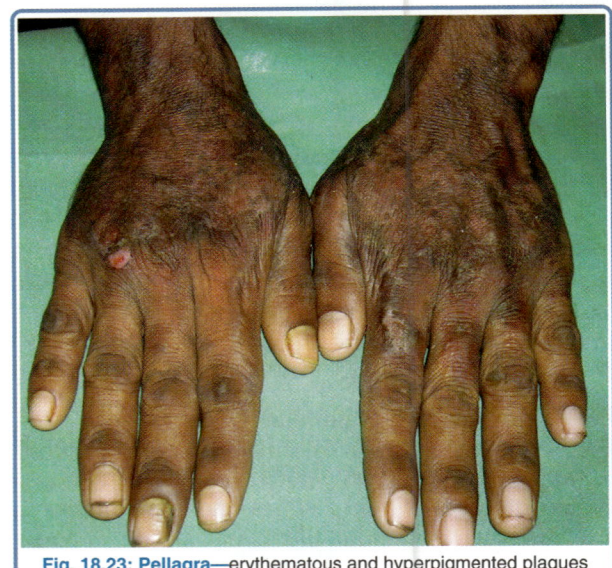

Fig. 18.23: Pellagra—erythematous and hyperpigmented plaques giving burnt out appearance

Normal daily requirement of niacin is 10 mg. Niacin is synthesised in the body from tryptophan. Hence, diet low in tryptophan, low proein diet, leads to pellagra.

Patient profile

Pellagra usually affects adult males. Chronic alcoholics, who have a higher requirement of niacin and lower intestinal absorption, develop pellagra in absence of adequate protein supplementation. Jowar contains excess leucine that retards the absorption of tryptophan whereas maize is poor in tryptophan. Therefore, a staple diet of jowar or maize predisposes to pellagra.

Morphology and distribution

Morphology of skin lesions resembles sunburn. They begin as burning erythematous patches

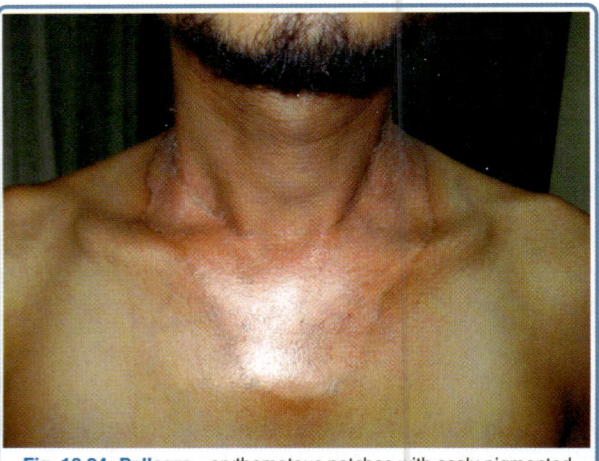

Fig. 18.24: Pellagra—erythematous patches with scaly pigmented border—Casal's necklace

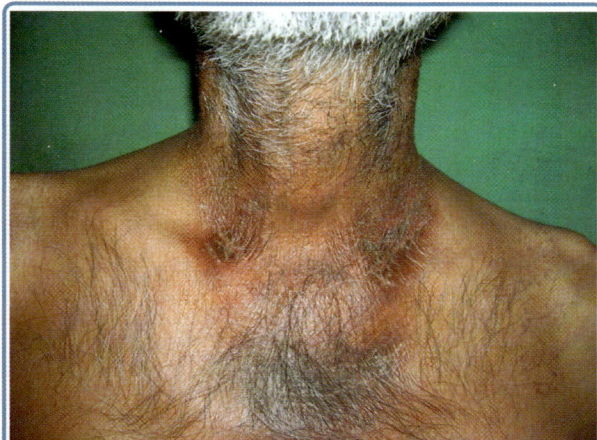

Fig. 18.25: Pellagra—hyperpigmented, brownish erythematous patches resembling sunburn

Earliest symptoms of pellagra are lethargy and a feeling of tiredness. Generalised inflmmmation of the gastrointestinal mucosa manifests as diarrhoea, nausea, vomiting and dyspepsia. Left untreated, encephalopathy reflects as poor memory, depression, psychosis, apathy, altered consciousness, coma and death.

Therapy

Pellagra responds rapidly to oral nicotinamide 50–100 mg tid. Diarrhoea is first to respond. CNS changes next and skin last, taking about 2 weeks to heal. Nicotinic acid, 100 mg tid, is equally effective but induces hypotension and flushing in some patients.

Inclusion of meat, eggs, pulses, cereals and nuts in diet or niacin supplementation (10–20 mg/day) prevents relapse.

Summary: Pellagra is due to niacin deficiency that affects NADP synthesis. Tryptophan is the dietary source of niacin and is present in eggs, meat, pulses, cereals and nuts. Alcoholism and a staple diet of jowar and maize predispose to pellagra sunburn-like lesions involving face, 'V' of neck, dorsa of hands and forearms are characteristic. Tongue is smooth and dark red and other mucosae are inflamed. Diarrhoea, behavioural changes, dementia and coma are the systemic changes that are serious but reversible with therapy. Nicotinamide 50 mg tid for many weeks and dietary correction are curative.

Vitamin Deficiencies that Rarely Present with Skin Complaints

Thiamine

Skin changes are not characteristic. Along with oedema of feet and legs, skin over the legs becomes stretched, dry, scaly and at times fissured. Trophic changes of acral skin are seen in dry beriberi.

Pantothenic acid

Skin manifestations are uncommon except for the burning feet syndrome (Gopalan syndrome) which responds slowly to 200 mg/day of oral pantothenic acid.

Folic Acid and Cyanocobalamin

These deficiencies are commonly associated. Hyperpigmentation of the skin and mucosae is observed in some patients. Stimulation of melanin synthesis is hypothesised as the mechanism.

Hyperpigmentation typically affects the knuckles, dorsa of interphalangeal joints, dorsa of hands and feet, palmar creases, forearms, lips, oral mucosa and face.

Vit. C: Skin in infantile scurvy shows petechiae, ecchymoses and haematomas. Bleeding from gums in seen in older infants. Classic adult scurvy has petechial haemorrhages in perifollicular location with the central hair twisted like a corkscrew. Other evidences of mucocutaneous bleeding are common (esp. from gums). Therapeutic doses are 100 mg per day.

Vit. E: Vitamin E deficiency is uncommon. Scaling, papular lesions and dryness are reported.

Vit. K: Cutaneous haemorrhages can occur in severe vitamin K deficiency seen usually in premature babies.

It commonly affects vegetarians or those who have gastrointestinal absorption problems. Serum vitamin B_{12} levels are low.

It responds to oral or intramuscular vitamin B_{12} but has a tendency to relapse. Hence, maintenance and supplements are commonly needed.

Chapter 18

Skin and Internal Diseases

MCQs

1. **Which of the following is true for skin in hypothyroidism?**
   a. Skin feels moist
   b. Skin thinning occurs
   c. Diffuse hair loss is common
   d. Fungal infections are common

2. **Infections associated with diabetes mellitus include all *except*:**
   a. Carbuncle
   b. Candidiasis
   c. Herpes simplex
   d. Mucormycosis

3. **Acanthosis nigricans affects all of these sites *except*:**
   a. Axillae
   b. Neck
   c. Lower back
   d. Face

4. **Acanthosis nigricans is associated with all of the following *except*:**
   a. Diabetes mellitus
   b. Polycystic ovarian disease
   c. Obestiy
   d. Systemic lupus erythematosus

5. **A 27-year-old overweight diabetic male complained of increasing pigmentation over neck. The lesions were not pruritic but had velvety appearance. The most probable diagnosis is:**
   a. Acanthosis nigricans
   b. Casal necklace
   c. Atopic dermatitis
   d. Lichen simplex chronicus

6. **Thyroid disease which is not associated with this skin manifestation is:**
   a. Myxoedema
   b. Pretibial myxoedema
   c. Scleroderma
   d. Hair loss

7. **This is not a manifestation of Cushing's syndrome:**
   a. Striae
   b. Purpura
   c. Skin thinning
   d. Generalised hyperpigmentation

8. **Photosensitivity is a component of these systemic diseases *except*:**
   a. Porphyria
   b. Lupus erythematosus
   c. Albinism
   d. Amyloidosis

9. **A 45-year-old diabetic presented with extremely painful nodule on the nape of the neck. On enquiry he was feeling feverish since one day. The most probable diagnosis is:**
   a. Carbuncle
   b. Furuncle
   c. Tuberculous lymphadenitis
   d. Lymphoma

10. **This is not a cutaneous manifestation of lymphoma:**
    a. Pruritus
    b. Ichthyosis
    c. Pityriasis rosea
    d. Herpes zoster

11. **The type of porphyria which does not show any photosensitivity is:**
    a. Porphyria cutanea tarda
    b. Acute intermittent porphyria
    c. Congenital erythropoietic porphyria
    d. Erythropoietic protoporphyria

12. **Cutaneous feature of polycystic ovarian disease does not include:**
    a. Hirsutism
    b. Ichthyosis
    c. Acanthosis nigricans
    d. Acne

13. **This is not a cause of hirsutism:**
    a. Congenital adrenal hyperplasia
    b. Ovarian tumours
    c. Adrenal tumours
    d. Testicular tumours

14. **The specific sign of lupus erythematosus is:**
    a. Discoid lesions
    b. Alopecia
    c. Vasculitis
    d. Fingertip ulcers

15. **Butterfly rash affects:**
    a. Bilateral periocular area
    b. Forehead and ears
    c. Cheeks and nose
    d. Chest and limbs

16. **The oral ulceration in systemic lupus erythematosus typically affects the:**
    a. Buccal mucosa
    b. Tongue
    c. Palate
    d. Lower lip

17. **Which of the following is not a sign of systemic lupus erythematosus?**
    a. Hair fall
    b. Hidebound skin
    c. Butterfly rash
    d. Discoid lesions

18. **This is troublesome for patients with systemic sclerosis:**
    a. Photosensitivity
    b. Dry skin
    c. Raynaud's phenomenon
    d. Oral ulceration

19. **Photosensitivity is a sign of:**
    a. Rheumatoid arthritis
    b. Psoriasis
    c. Lupus erythematosus
    d. Systemic sclerosis

20. **Localised scleroderma is characterised by:**
    a. Yellowish discolouration of skin
    b. Induration
    c. Calcium deposit in the skin
    d. Bony deposit in the skin

21. **The skin sign of Addison's disease is:**
    a. Acanthosis nigricans
    b. Generalised hyperpigmentation
    c. Striae
    d. Purpura

22. **Patients with dermatomyositis characteristically have:**
    a. Eyelid oedema
    b. Lip oedema
    c. Hand oedema
    d. Feet oedema

23. **Behcet's disease is characterised by ulceration of:**
    a. Leg
    b. Genital
    c. Stomach
    d. Eye

24. **The characteristic skin lesion of Rieter's disease is called as:**
    a. Keratoderma climactericum
    b. Palmoplantar keratoderma
    c. Keratoderma blenorrhagicum
    d. Palmoplantar pustulosis

25. **Genital lesions in Rieter's disease are:**
    a. Plasma cell balanitis
    b. Circinate balanitis
    c. Candidal balanitis
    d. Erosive balanitis

26. **The distribution of rash in acute cutaneous lupus erythematosus is on:**
    a. Exposed regions
    b. Flexures
    c. Hair skin
    d. Sun-exposed areas

27. **This may be a cutaneous sign of internal malignancy:**
    a. Hypopigmented macules
    b. Acanthosis nigricans
    c. Saw tooth acanthosis
    d. Tinea capitis

28. **A sign of primary systemic amyloidosis is:**
    a. Pigmented purpura
    b. Palpable purpura
    c. Gun metal purpura
    d. Palpebral purpura

29. **Macroglossia is a sign of this multisystem disorder:**
    a. Systemic lupus erythematosus
    b. Diabetes mellitus
    c. Hyperthyroidism
    d. Systemic amyloidosis

30. **Skin lesions in Letterer Siwe disease resemble:**
    a. Psoriasis
    b. Xanthoma
    c. Lichen planus
    d. Seborrhoeic dermatitis

31. **Skin lesions in phrynoderma are:**
    a. Flat topped papules
    b. Dome shaped smooth papules
    c. Conical rough papules
    d. Rounded papules

32. **The typical skin sites of affection in riboflavin deficiency are:**
    a. Sun exposed areas
    b. Frictional sites
    c. Seborrhoeic areas
    d. Exposed areas

33. **This is not a predisposing factor for pellagra:**
    a. Alcohol abuse
    b. Excessive smoking
    c. Malabsorption disorders
    d. Staple diet of jowar

34. **Normal daily requirement of niacin is:**
    a. 1 mg
    b. 10 mg
    c. 100 mg
    d. 1 g

35. **Classical site of affection of erythema nodosum is:**
    a. Face
    b. Feet
    c. Forearms
    d. Shins

Chapter
18

Skin and Internal Diseases

36. **Butterfly rash in lupus erythematosus needs to be distinguished from:**
    a. Erythema multiforme
    b. Rosacea
    c. Pityriasis rosea
    d. Erythema nodosum

37. **The most common form of xanthomas seen in clinical practice are called:**
    a. Eruptive xanthoma
    b. Tuberous xanthoma
    c. Xanthelasma
    d. Planar xanthoma

38. **The type of xanthomas carried risk of cardiac events is:**
    a. Eruptive xanthoma
    b. Tuberous xanthoma
    c. Xanthelasma
    d. Xanthoma disseminatum

39. **The type of xanthoma that is linked to hypertriglyceridaemia is:**
    a. Tuberous xanthoma
    b. Eruptive xanthoma
    c. Tendinous xanthoma
    d. Planar xanthoma

40. **The skin sign which is associated with diabetes mellitus is:**
    a. Ichthyosis
    b. Herpes simplex
    c. Necrobiosis lipoidica
    d. Erythema marginatum

41. **Acrodermatitis enteropathica occurs due to deficiency of:**
    a. Zinc
    b. Iron
    c. Copper
    d. Vitamin A

42. **Flaky paint appearance of skin is seen in:**
    a. Dermatitis
    b. Pellagra
    c. Marasmus
    d. Kwashiorkar

43. **Casal's necklace is seen in:**
    a. Lichen planus
    b. Pellagra
    c. Pernicious anaemia
    d. SLE

44. **'Pinch' purpura is diagnostic of:**
    a. systemic primary amyloidosis
    b. secondary systemic amyloidosis
    c. idiopathic thrombocytopenic purpura
    d. drug induced purpura

45. **Which of these statements is false of lesions of erythema nodosum?**
    a. They are considered as hypersensitivity reaction
    b. Skin overlying lesions is red, smooth and shiny
    c. They are usually non-tender
    d. They can be associated with tuberculosis

46. **Erythema nodosum is seen in all of the following *except*:**
    a. Streptococcal infections
    b. Tuberculosis
    c. Lymphogranuloma venereum
    d. Donovanosis

47. **Exfoliative erythroderma is seen in all of the following *except*:**
    a. Drug hypersensitivity
    b. Pitriyasis rubra pilaris
    c. Pitriyasis rosea
    d. Psoriasis

48. **Erythroderma is:**
    a. Erythema of the dermis
    b. Erythema of the skin
    c. Erythema and scaling affecting most of the body surface area (BSA)
    d. Erythema and scaling affecting all of the BSA

ANSWERS

1-c,	2-c,	3-c,	4-d,	5-a,	6-c,	7-d,	8-d,	9-a,	10-c,
11-b,	12-b,	13-d,	14-a,	15-c,	16-c,	17-b,	18-c,	19-c,	20-b,
21-b,	22-a,	23-b,	24-c,	25-b,	26-d,	27-b,	28-d,	29-d,	30-d,
31-c,	32-c,	33-b,	34-b,	35-d,	36-b,	37-c,	38-c,	39-b,	40-c,
41-a,	42-d,	43-b,	44-a,	45-c,	46-d,	47-c,	48-c		

Collagen Vascular Diseases

SKIN MANIFESTATIONS OF COLLAGEN VASCULAR DISEASES

Collagen vascular diseases (sometimes referred to as collagen diseases or connective tissue diseases) are a group of multi-system autoimmune diseases that affect connective tissue, among other tissues. They include lupus erythematosus, scleroderma, dermatomyositis, rheumatoid arthritis, rheumatic fever and Sjogren's syndrome.

Lupus Erythematosus

Lupus erythematosus (LE) may present as a multi-system disorder with affection of the skin, mucosae and internal organs (systemic LE) or be restricted to the skin and mucosae (chronic cutaneous LE). Please *see* the following section on systemic LE for details of skin lesions. In chronic cutaneous LE only discoid lesions occur over sunexposed regions of face and scalp without any other systemic affection.

Scleroderma

Once again, this may be a multisystem disease (systemic sclerosis) with generalised/symmetric affection of the skin or it may be restricted to the skin (morphoea/localised scleroderma). Essential feature of scleroderma is cutaneous sclerosis, i.e. the skin is thickened, indurated and bound down (difficult to pick up). Skin lesions pass

through the stages of oedema, induration and atrophy (Figs 19.1–19.4).

Systemic sclerosis is seen as diffuse sclerosis of skin predominantly affecting the acral regions, i.e. hands (Fig. 19.5), feet, fingers, toes and face. Other systemic affections include:

- Raynaud's phenomenon with or without fingertip ulcers and scars
- Bibasilar pulmonary fibrosis leads to dyspnoea
- Gastrointestinal dysmotility manifests as difficulty in deglutition, gastrooesophageal

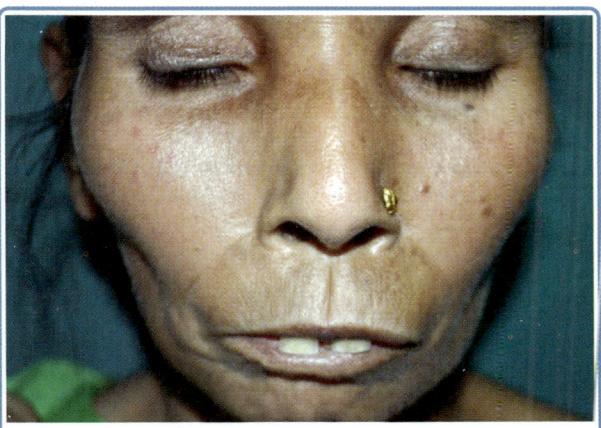

Fig. 19.2: Systemic sclerosis—mask like face due to tightening of skin

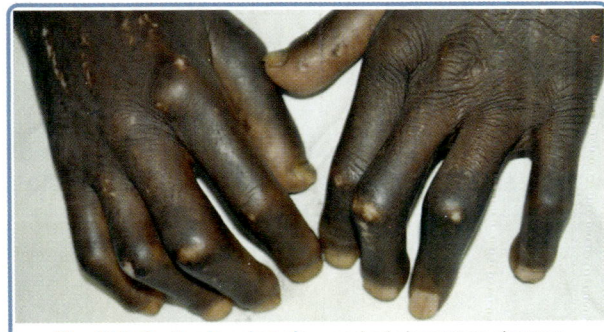

Fig. 19.3: Systemic sclerosis—marked pigmentary changes, thickening and hardening of skin of both hands with flexion contracture

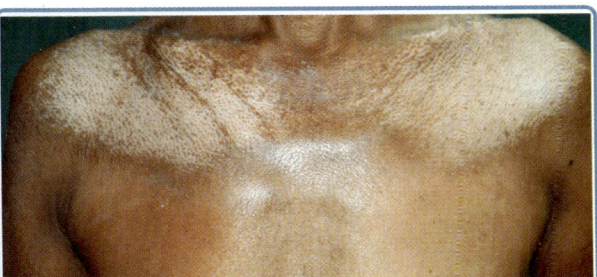

Fig. 19.4: Systemic sclerosis—salt and pepper pigmentation with generalised hide bound skin

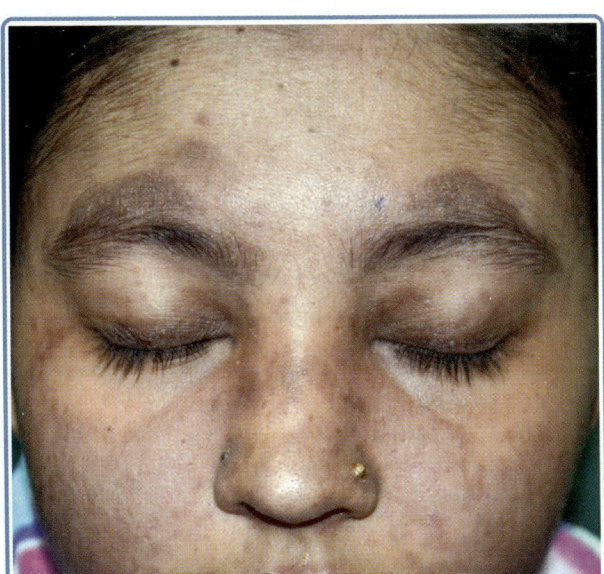

Fig. 19.1: Systemic lupus erythematosus—butterfly erythema affecting cheeks, nose, forehead and eyelids

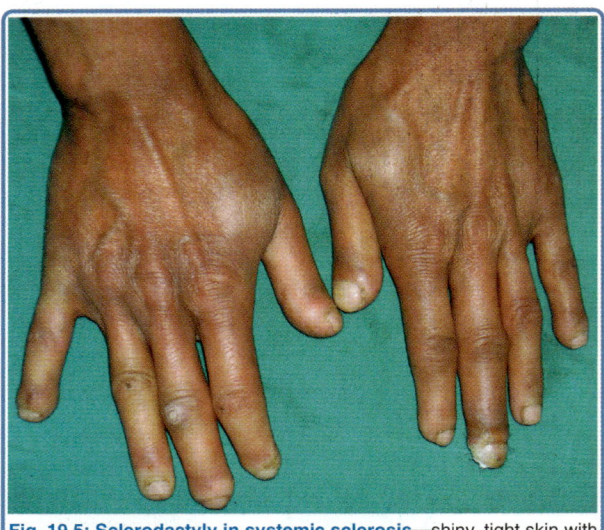

Fig. 19.5: Sclerodactyly in systemic sclerosis—shiny, tight skin with resorption of the fingers and calcinosis over dorsum of right middle finger

reflux, alternating diarrhoea and constipation, and pain in abdomen

- Glomerular sclerosis leads to hypertension

> Calcinosis cutis, Raynaud's phenomenon, oesophageal dysmotility, cutaneous sclerosis and skin telangiectasia occur together in the CREST syndrome, which has limited systemic affecton and better prognosis.
>
> Serious systemic affection occurs in diffuse systemic sclerosis wherein sclerosis is not restricted to the face, head and feet but extends to proximal extremities or trunk.

Localised scleroderma (morphoea) presents as a rounded or linear indurated dyspigmented plaque with or without atrophy. Affected skin is sclerosed (Fig. 19.6).

Dermatomyositis

Inflammation of proximal limb muscles manifests as weakness and tenderness of limb girdle muscles.

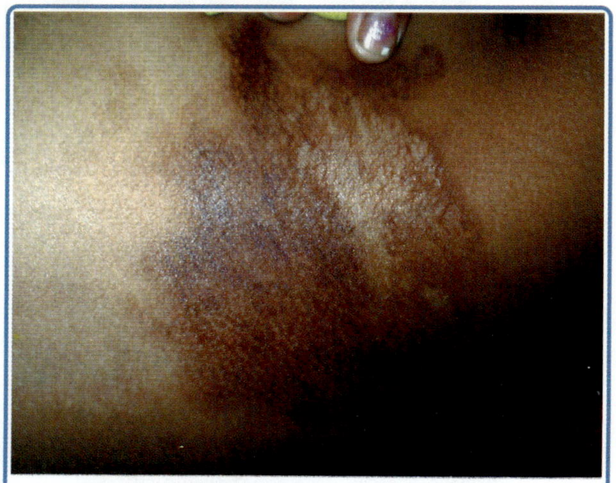

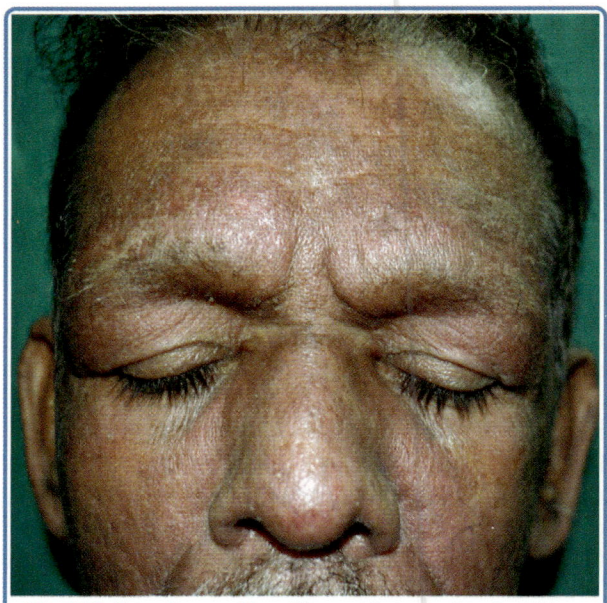

Fig. 19.6: Localised scleroderma (morphoea)—hyperpigmented indurated plaque with atrophy of skin

Common complaints are inability to get up from squatting position or to comb hair. These features of proximal muscle weakness are associated with facial erythema, violaceous lid oedema (heliotrope rash) and lichenoid papules over dorsa of interphalangeal (IP) joints (Gottron's papules) in dermatomyositis (Figs 19.7–19.9).

Fig. 19.7: Dermatomyositis—diffuse erythema and scaling of face particularly accentuated over upper eyelids

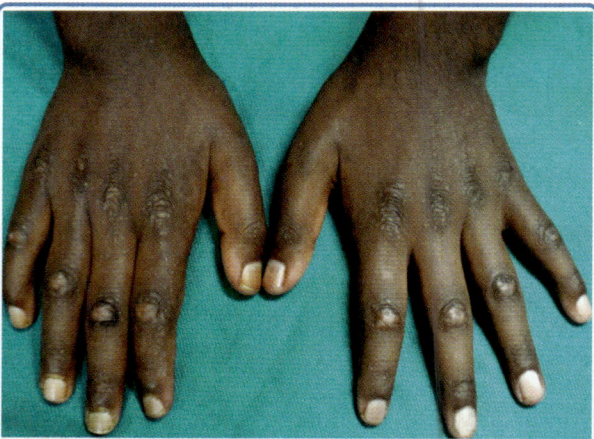

Fig. 19.8: Gottron papules—lichenoid papules over extensors of interphalangeal and metacarpophalangeal joints are characteristic of dermatomyositis

> **Rheumatoid Arthritis**
>
> Rheumatoid nodules are asymptomatic stable, skin coloured, deep seated nodules varying in size from 1–3 cm and occurring over extensors of metacarpophalangeal (MP) joints, elbows, knees or malleoli.
>
> **Rheumatic fever**
>
> In contrast to rheumatoid nodules, subcutaneous nodules

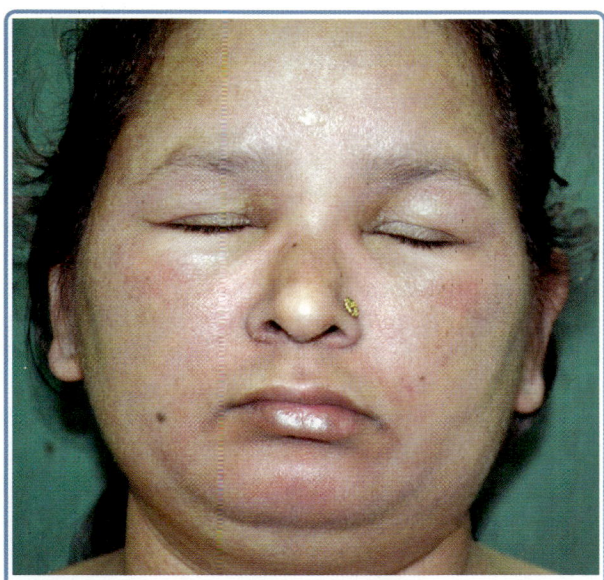

Fig. 19.9: Dermatomyositis—facial erythema and oedema

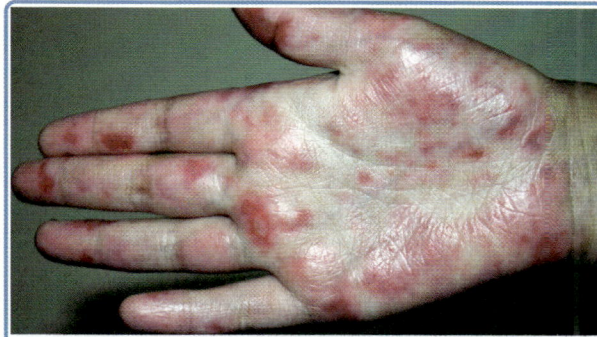

Fig. 19.10: Systemic lupus erythromatosus—tender palmar erythema in acute cutaneous lupus erythromatosus

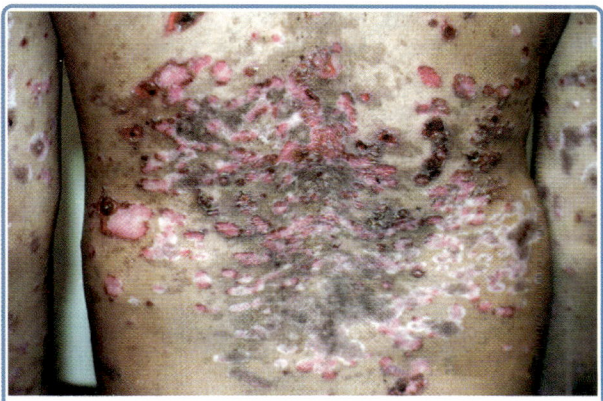

Fig. 19.11: Systemic lupus erythromatosus—disseminated discoid lupus erythromatosus

in rheumatic fever are transient, smaller (0.5–1 cm), occur over extensors of extremities and can be best felt against bony surfaces. Erythema marginatum rheumaticum is a transient erythema that spreads rapidly in a gyrate fashion.

Sjogren's syndrome

Skin may also be dry in this disorder which primarily affects the mucosae. Dryness of conjunctiva is demonstrated by Schirmer's test.

Summary: Lupus erythematosus manifests on skin as discoid lesions, butterfly rash, oral ulcers, photosensitivity, alopecia and Raynaud's phenomenon. Localised scleroderma is seen as an indurated dyspigmented plaque with atrophy. Skin findings in systemic sclerosis include diffuse or acral skin sclerosis, Raynaud's phenomenon, telangiectasia, dyspigmentation, cutaneous calcinosis and fingertip ulcers and scars. Violaceous lid oedema and lichenoid papules on hands are manifestations of dermatomyositis. Subcutaneous nodules can be seen in rheumatoid arthritis as well as in rheumatic fever. Erythema marginatum is a feature of rheumatic fever.

SKIN MANIFESTATIONS OF SYSTEMIC LUPUS ERYTHEMATOSUS

A variety of cutaneous lesions are observed in systemic lupus erythematosus (CSLE). Conventionally, they are divided into:

- **Specific**—Those, being specific for the disease, have a diagnostic value (Figs 19.10 and 19.11).

  - ❑ **Discoid lesions (discoid lupus erythematosus)**—they are seen as erythematous, indurated, rounded plaques with depigmented, atrophic centres and hyperpigmented margins (Fig. 19.12). Active lesions have a central adherent scale that has minute tacs on its undersurface (carpet tac sign). Malar regions, nose, ears, forehead, scalp and postauricular area are affected commonly (Fig. 19.13).

  - ❑ **Facial erythema (butterfly rash)**—bright red erythema involves the malar regions and nose symmetrically in a 'butterfly' distribution (Fig. 19.1 and 19.14). The rash has a tendency to wax and wane with disease activity.

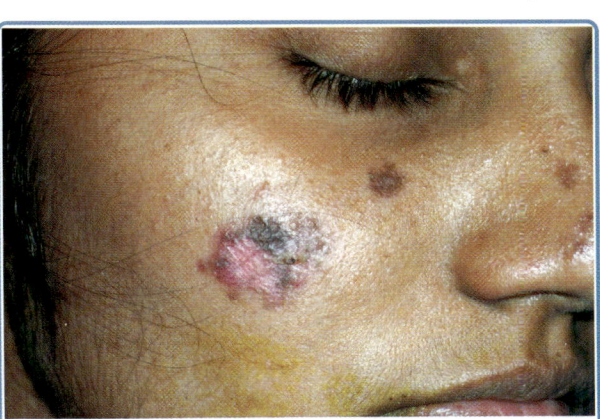

Fig. 19.12: Discoid lupus erythematosus—erythematous hyperpigmented plaque with scaling and atrophy

Chapter

19

Collagen Vascular Diseases

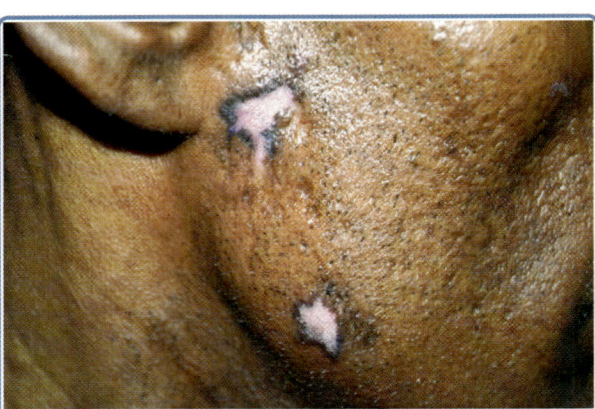

Fig. 19.13: Discoid lupus erythromatosus—discoid plaques with central atrophy and depigmentation in chronic cutaneous lupus erythromatosus

- **Non-specific**—non-specific cutaneous findings in SLE include:

  - **Photosensitivity:** Burning and itching on exposure to sunlight is followed by an erythematous maculopapular rash.

  - **Oral and nasopharyngeal ulceration:** Erosions and superficial ulceration of these mucosae (esp. hard palate) are common and keep step with the disease activity.

  - **Raynaud's phenomenon:** Exposure to cold elicits a vasospastic response, passing through the stages of pallor, cyanosis and rubor and is accompanied by pain.

  - **Alopecia:** Diffuse non-scarring alopecia that is in phase with disease activity is typical of SLE. Patchy scarring alopecia, related to discoid lesions, may occur in addition.

  - **Telangiectasiae:** Punctate macular and papular telangiectasiae over face, exposed regions, palms and soles are typical of SLE. Additionally, linear telangiectasiae may be seen over the face and proximal nail folds.

  - **Purpura:** This may be seen in SLE as a result of either thrombocytopenia or due to vasculitis (Fig. 19.10).

  - Thrombophlebitis

  - Peripheral gangrene and non-healing ulcers

> **Summary:** Specific cutaneous findings of systemic lupus erythematosus (seen only in lupus erythematosus) include discoid lesions and butterfly rash. Discoid lesions are erythematous plaques with central depigmentation, atrophy, follicular plugging and adherent scaling and affect the face and scalp. Butterfly rash is erythema that affects the malar regions. Non-specific lesions include photosensitivity, oral ulceration, Raynaud's phenomenon, alopecia and telangiectasia.

BUTTERFLY RASH

Symmetric bright red erythema and oedema in the malar region, cheeks and bridge of the nose is termed as butterfly erythema and is characteristic of acute cutaneous lupus erythematosus (Fig. 19.14). This manifestation of lupus erythematosus, unlike the discoid lesions, is invariably associated with systemic involvement in lupus erythematosus (systemic lupus erythematosus) and hence carries serious clinical implications. The condition is common in young women.

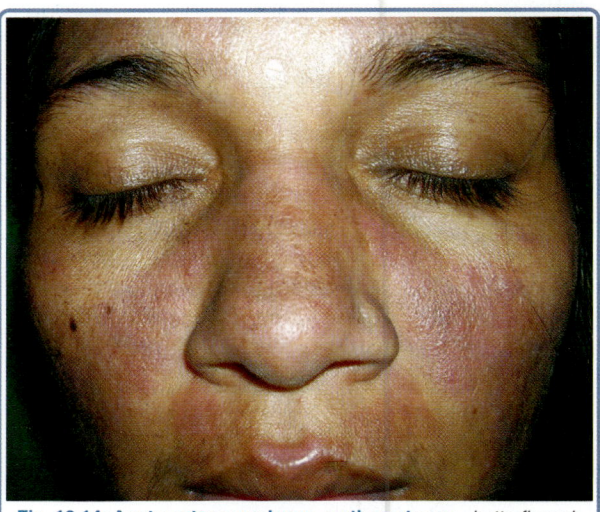

Fig. 19.14: Acute cutaneous lupus erythematosus—butterfly rash

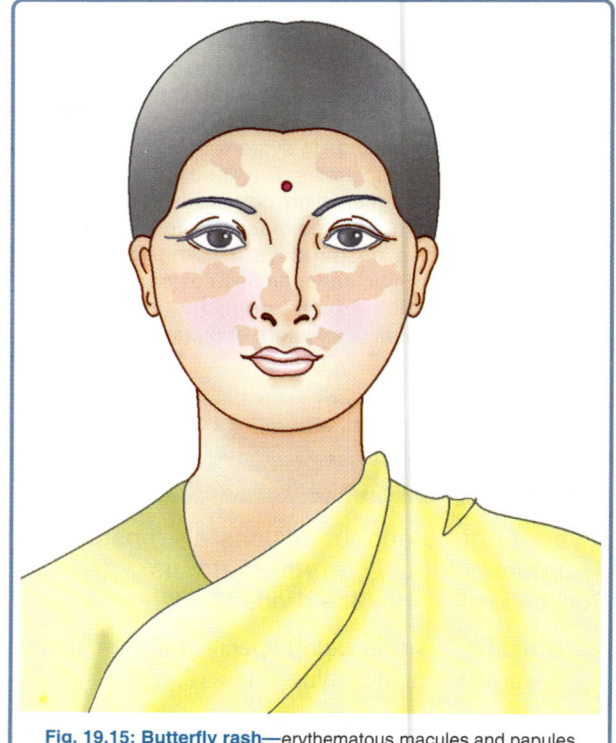

Fig. 19.15: Butterfly rash—erythematous macules and papules

A history of photosensitivity is commonly present. The intensity of erythema is usually in phase with the severity of the disease. In severe cases, the erythema may involve other parts of face, ears, neck, upper chest, forearms, hands, palms and soles. Occasionally, lesions may vesiculate. Healing occurs with or without scaling.

Other Skin Lesions of Lupus Erythematosus

Discoid lesions, photosensitivity, alopecia, Raynaud's phenomenon, oral and nasopharyngeal ulceration, telangiectasia and purpura are other skin lesions to be sought in such patients.

Other Systems

Lymphadenitis, nephritis, arthritis, pleuritis, pneumonitis, pericarditis, myocarditis, endocarditis, hepatitis, peritonitis, anaemia, thrombocytopenia, lymphopenia, behavioural changes and convulsions are some of the systemic changes that may accompany the butterfly erythema.

Investigations

Blood counts show anaemia, lymphopenia and thrombocytopenia. Erythrocyte sedimentation rate (ESR) is raised and significant proteinuria is common. Antinuclear antibody (ANA) is positive in most cases. Anti-DNA antibody, anti-Ro antibody are other helpful tests. A skin biopsy is also helpful.

Therapy

Therapy is that of SLE and depends primarily on the presence of systemic involvement. Active disease can be managed with hydroxychloroquine or chloroquine (if mild) or systemic steroids (if severe). Fulminant disease can be brought under control with pulse therapy of intravenous steroids and immunosuppressants (e.g. azathioprine).

Differential Diagnosis of Butterfly Rash

Other causes of facial erythema and oedema include:

- *Physiological* flushing of face during menopause, pregnancy and febrile episodes.
- *Acute Contact Dermatitis*—Asymmetric involvement with frequent vesiculation. History of contactant can be elicited.
- *Seborrhoeic Dermatitis*—Erythema covered with yellowish greasy scales preferentially affects eyebrows, eyelashes, nasolabial and paranasal folds and is associated with itching.

- *Photosensitivity*—Other features of lupus erythematosus are absent. History of contact or ingestion of photosensitiser is present.
- *Pellagra*—Rash resembles sunburn, i.e. has a brownish tint. History of predisposing factors can be elicited.
- *Dermatomyositis*—Purplish colour of rash with oedema of eyelids is distinctive. Manifestations of proximal muscle weakness are present.

Summary: Erythema involving butterfly region of face (cheeks and nasal bridge) suggests acute skin lesion of systemic lupus erythematosus. Other findings of lupus erythematosus in the skin (discoid lesions, photosensitivity, oral ulcers, alopecia, Raynaud's phenomenon, etc.) and other systems (serositis, renal, CNS, haematologic, cardiac, hepatic etc.) should be sought. Blood examination may show pancytopenia, ESR is elevated and there is proteinuria. ANA is positive. Other causes of facial erythema include other photodermatoses, flushing due to physiologic causes like fever, contact allergic dermatitis and dermatomyositis.

VASCULITIS

Vasculitis are a group of diseases that cause their manifestations through vessel occlusion due to an autoimmune inflammatory process. They affect multiple systems and skin, being the easily seen and accessible organ for biopsy, is an important affected system. Various types of skin lesions seen in this group of diseases include palpable purpura (Henoch Schoenlein purpura) (Figs 19.16 and 19.17), vesicles (Fig. 19.18), bullae, ulcers, and nodules (periarteritis nodosa) (Fig. 19.19). Commonly affected regions are ankles, feet, legs, buttocks, elbows and knees. Diagnosis requires skin biopsy and treatment includes steroids and immunomodulatory agents.

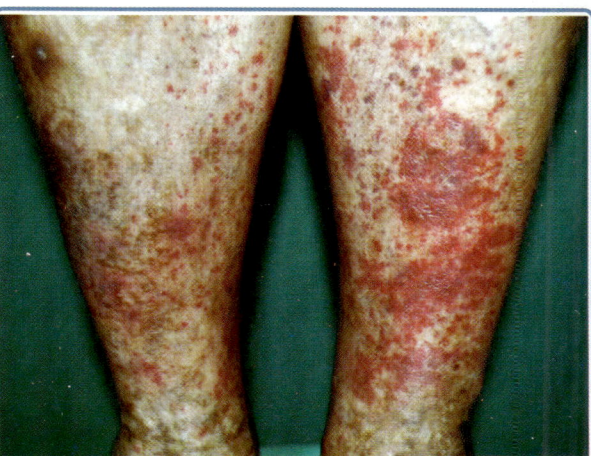

Fig. 19.16: Vasculitis—bilateral palpable purpura over legs, a sign of small vessel vasculitis

Chapter 19

Collagen Vascular Diseases

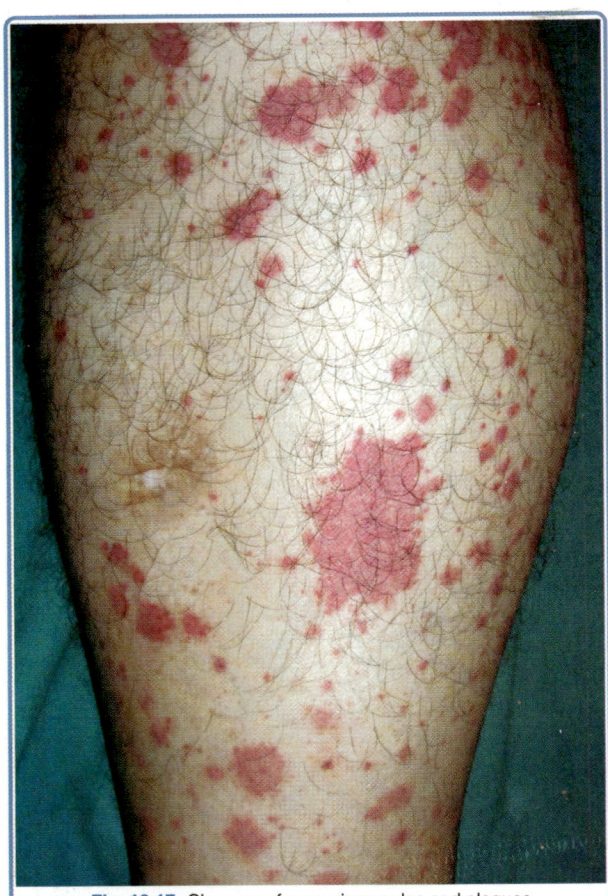

Fig. 19.17: Close up of purpuric papules and plaques (palpable purpura) due to small vessel vasculitis

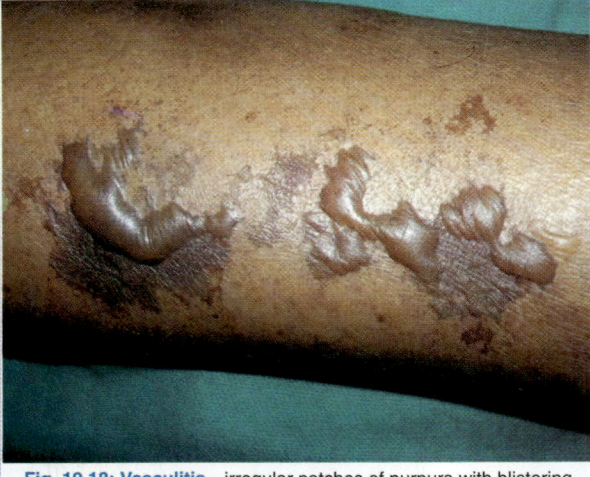

Fig. 19.18: Vasculitis—irregular patches of purpura with blistering

SARCOIDOSIS

Sarcoidosis is a multisystem granulomatous disease of unknown aetiology. Skin is frequently

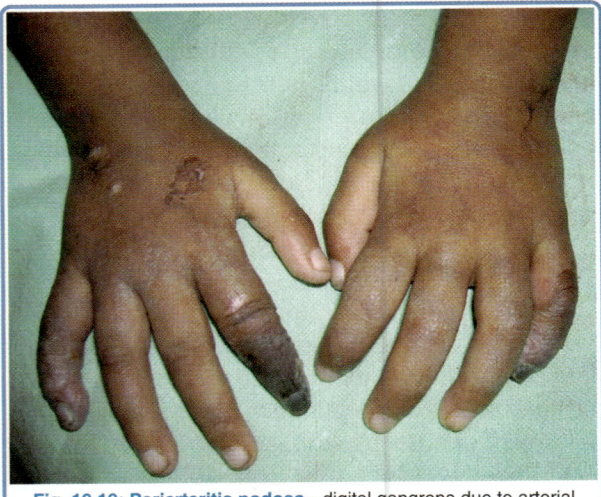

Fig. 19.19: Periarteritis nodosa—digital gangrene due to arterial occlusion

affected in sarcoidosis. The skin lesions may be in the form of asymptomatic skin coloured (Fig. 19.20) or erythematous papules, plaques or nodules and may affect the face, extremities or the back. Mucosal dryness with salivary gland enlargment is common. Since sarcoidosis is a diagnosis by exclusion it is important to rule out infectious granulomas (e.g. leprosy, tuberculosis, leishmaniasis) by biopsy and other relevant tests. Mantoux test is negative in sarcoidosis and Kveim test is positive. Serum calcium and serum angiotensin converting enzyme (ACE) levels are raised. Other tests include X-ray or computed tomography (CT) scan of chest for mediastial lymphadenopathy and pulmonary involvement. Skin biopsy shows sarcoidal (naked) granulomas with fibrinoid necrosis.

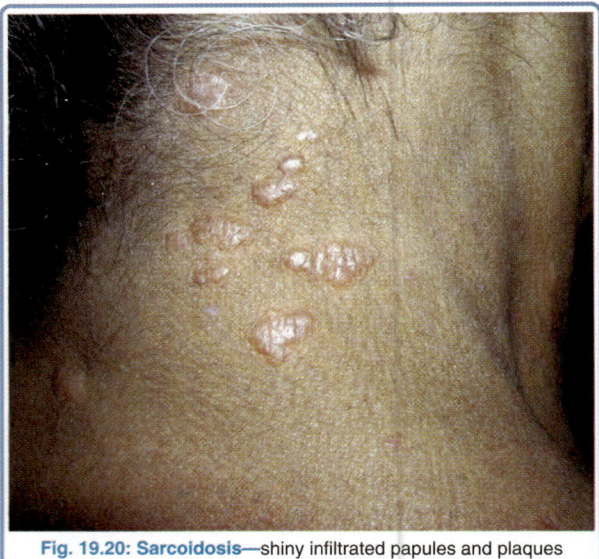

Fig. 19.20: Sarcoidosis—shiny infiltrated papules and plaques

MCQs

1. **This is not an autoimmune disorder:**
   a. Pemphigus vulgaris   b. Psoriasis
   c. Lichen planus   d. Acne vulgaris

2. **A 40-year-old woman presented with 8 months history of erythema and swelling of periorbital region and papules and plaques on the dorsolateral aspect of the forearm with ragged cuticles. The most likely diagnosis is:**
   a. Systemic lupus erythematosus
   b. Dermatomyositis
   c. Systemic sclerosis
   d. Mixed connective tissue disorder

3. **Gottronus papules are:**
   a. Erythematous papules on cheek
   b. Erythema seen over elbows and knees
   c. Periorbital lesions
   d. Violaceous papules over knuckles

4. **Gottron's papules seen in dermatomyositis are:**
   a. Vesicular   b. Psoriatic
   c. Lichenoid   d. Pustular

5. **All are dermatological manifestations of dermatomyositis except:**
   a. Gottron's papules
   b. Mechanics hands

   c. Periungual telangiectasias
   d. Salmon patch

6. **All are cutaneous manifestations of systemic sclerosis except:**
   a. Sclerodactyly
   b. Heliotrope rash
   c. Telangiectasias
   d. Oesophageal dysmotility

7. **A 28-year-old female presented with history of colour change of fingers from pallor to cyanosis on exposure to cold. This condition is mostly associated with:**
   a. Scleroderma   b. Leukaemia
   c. Lung infection   d. Diabetes mellitus

8. **A 42-year-female has palpable purpura with rash over buttocks, pain in abdomen and arthropathy. The most likely diagnosis is:**
   a. Sweet's syndrome
   b. Henoch Schonlein purpura
   c. Purpura fulminans
   d. Meningococcaemia

9. **Immunoglobulin A deposits on skin biopsy are seen with:**
   a. Henoch Schonlein purpura
   b. Giant cell arteritis
   c. Microscopic polyangiitis
   d. Wegener's granulomatosis

Chapter 19

Collagen Vascular Diseases

ANSWERS

1-d,   2-b,   3-d,   4-c,   5-d,   6-b,   7-a,   8-b,   9-a

CHAPTER 20

Chronic Vesicobullous Disorders

These are a group of antibody mediated auto-immune disorders that are characterised by formation of recurrent vesicles or bullae. They include pemphigus vulgaris, pemphigus foliaceous, bullous pemphigoid and dermatitis herpetiformis. Despite clinical similarities, they must be distinguished from one another as management guidelines are different for each disease (Table 20.1).

BULLOUS PEMPHIGOID

Middle aged and elderly patients with this condition show a propensity to form subepidermal bullae. The lesions start as urticarial plaques that develop vesicles and bullae on surface. The tense large bullae on a background of erythema and oedema rupture to form erosions (Figs 20.1–20.4) which, as against pemphigus, have a tendnency to heal spontaneously. However, new lesions continue to appear. Initially, lesions appear over flexors of trunk and extremities but soon become generalised. Mucosae are spared. The patient is in discomfort due to severe burning in lesions and itching. The

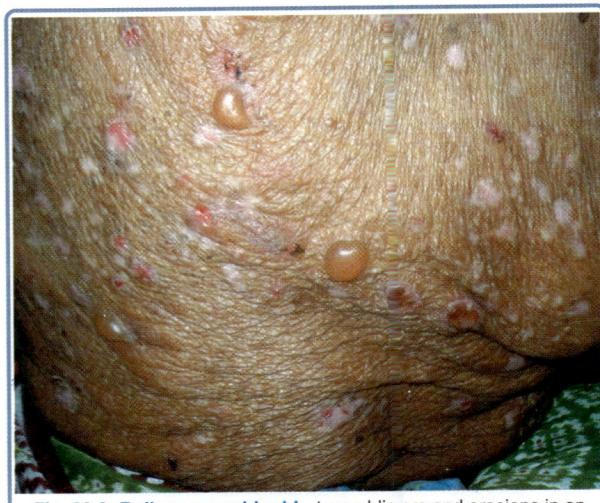
Fig. 20.2: Bullous pemphigold—tense blisters and erosions in an elderly woman

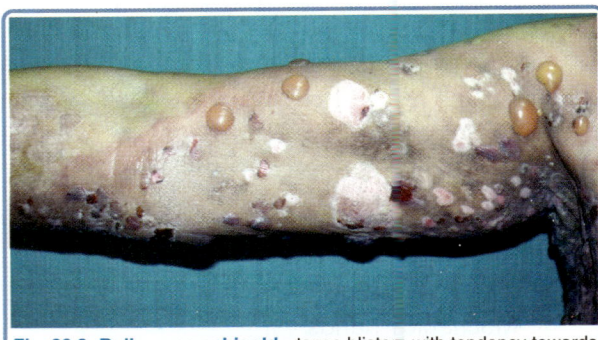
Fig. 20.3: Bullous pemphigold—tense blisters with tendency towards self-healing

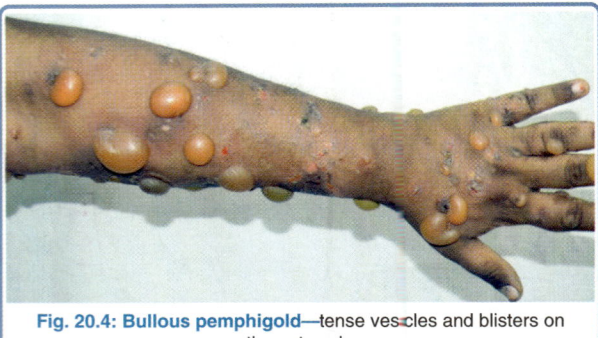
Fig. 20.4: Bullous pemphigold—tense vesicles and blisters on erythematous base

lesions heal on treatment without scarring but with post-inflammatory pigmentation.

DERMATITIS HERPETIFORMIS

Young adults are affected with this disorder in which vesicles or bullae are formed subepidermally.

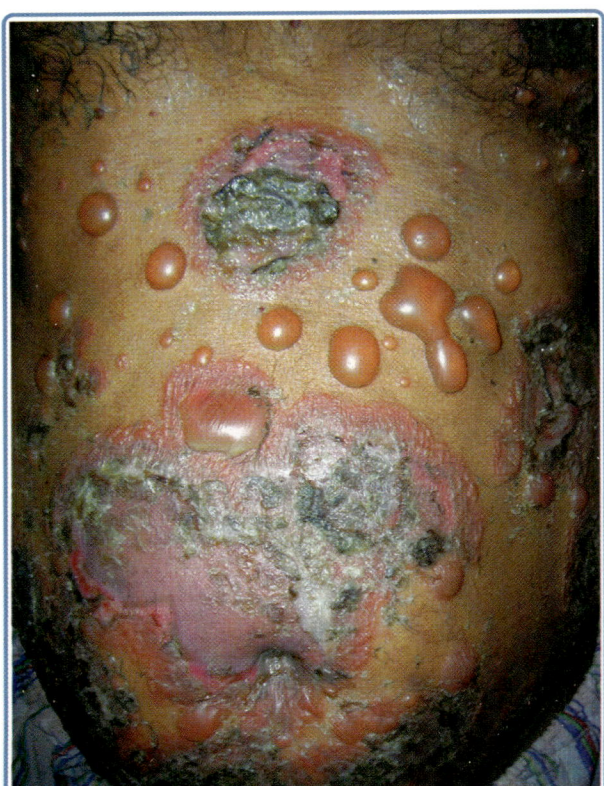
Fig. 20.1: Bullous pemphigold—widespread large tense blisters and erosions

TABLE 20.1 : Differential diagnosis of widespread bullous and erosive lesions

	Pemphigus vulgaris	Pemphigus foliaceus	Bullous pemphigoid	SJS/TEN	SSSS
Usual age (years)	20–40	20–40	40–60	20–40	1–2
Systemic symptoms	+	+	–	+++	++
Average curation	Weeks–months	Weeks–months	Months–years	days	days
Mucosal affection	++	–	–	+++	–
Skin sites	Face, scalp, upper trunk, flexures and periungual	Face, scalp, exposed and seborrhoeic	Flexures, proximal extremities and trunk	Acral, periorificial trunk if extensive	Trunk spares acral and periorificial
Bullae	Large, flaccid	Small, flaccid	Large, tense	Large, tense	Large, flaccid
Roof of bulla	Thick	Thin	Thick	Thick, comes of in thick sheets	Thin, peels off in thin scales
Skin around bullae	Normal	Normal	Red and oedematous	Red	Normal
Crusts	Thick, malodorous	Thin, malodorous	Thin, serosanguinous	Thick, haemorrhagic	Thin, seropurulent
Erosions	Deep and large	Superficial and small	Deep and large	Deep and large	Superficial and large
Target lesions	–	–	–	+	–
Self-healing of individual bullae	–	+	+	+	+
Nikolsky sign	+	++	–	+	++
Tzanck smear	Many acantholytic cells	Few acantholytic cells	Eosinophils	Necrotic epidermal cells	Elongated keratinocytes
Biopsy	Suprabasal acantholysis	Upper spinous acantholysis with eosinophils	Subepidermal blister necrotic epithelium	Subepidermal cleft no Inflammation	Subcorneal cleft
Direct :					
Immunofluorescence on skin biopsy	Intercellular IgG (Fish net)	Intercellular IgG (Fish net)	IgG at DE junction (linear)	–	–
Indirect :					
Immunofluorescence on blood	Intercellular IgG	Intercellular IgG	IgG at DE junction (linear)	–	–
ELISA on serum	Desmoglein III antibodies	Desmoglein I antibodies	Antibodies against BP 180, BP 230	–	–

N. B. : SJS = Stevens Johnson syndrome **TEN =** Toxic epidermal necrolysis **SSSS =** Staphylococcal scalded skin syndrome

Chapter
20

Chronic Vesicobullous Disorders

Lesions begin as extremely pruritus erythematous or oedematous papules and then vesiculate or blister. Extensors of extremities and trunk are affected. Gluten in wheat grain exacerbates the lesions and avoidance of wheat in diet improves lesions. Due to extreme pruritus lesions get excoriated and intact vesicles are difficult to find. Hence, presentation may vary from eczematous patches or prurigo-like lesions or blisters or urticarial wheals over extensors of limbs and trunk.

PEMPHIGUS VULGARIS AND FOLIACEUS

These disorders are due to lysis of the binding spines (desomosomes) that hold together the cells of the epidermis. Such keratinocytes, called acantholytic cells, are found within the bullae of these patients. This results in formation of flaccid, intraepidermal bullae and consequently erosions due to their rupture (Figs 20.7–20.11). Young and

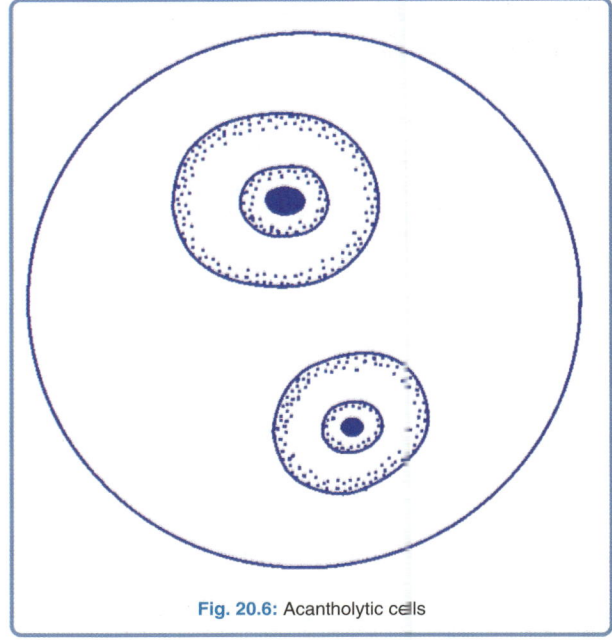
Fig. 20.6: Acantholytic cells

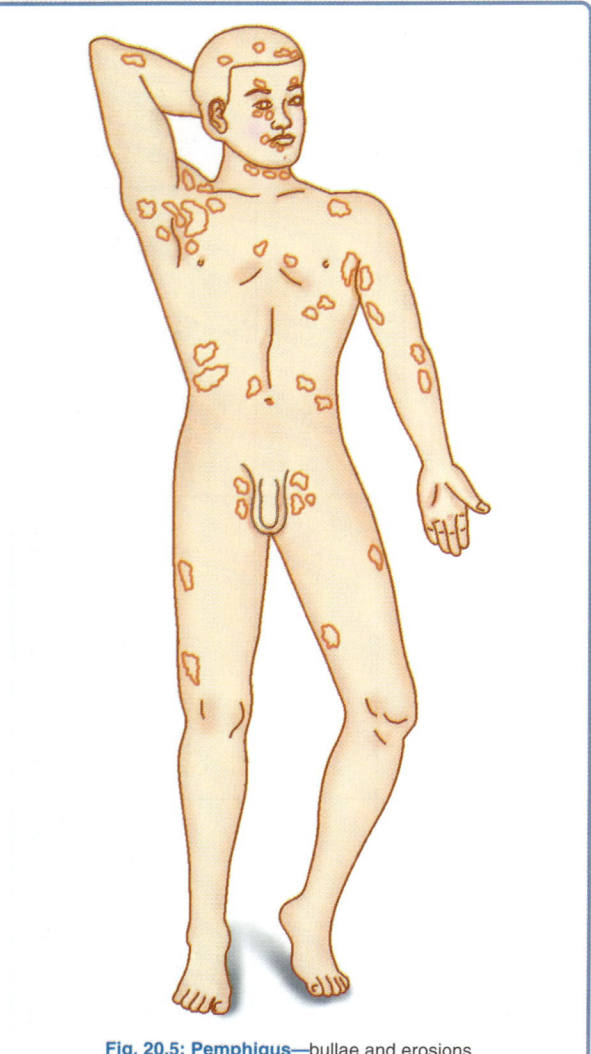
Fig. 20.5: Pemphigus—bullae and erosions

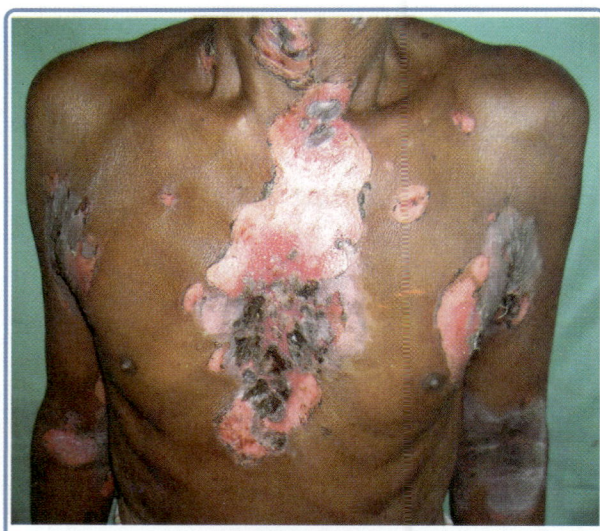
Fig. 20.7: Pemphigus vulgaris—widespread large erosions without any surrounding inflammation

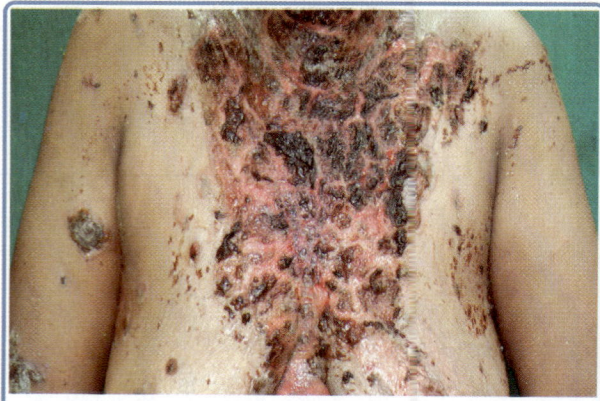
Fig. 20.8: Pemphigus vulgaris—extensive crusted erosions with fragile satellite vesicles

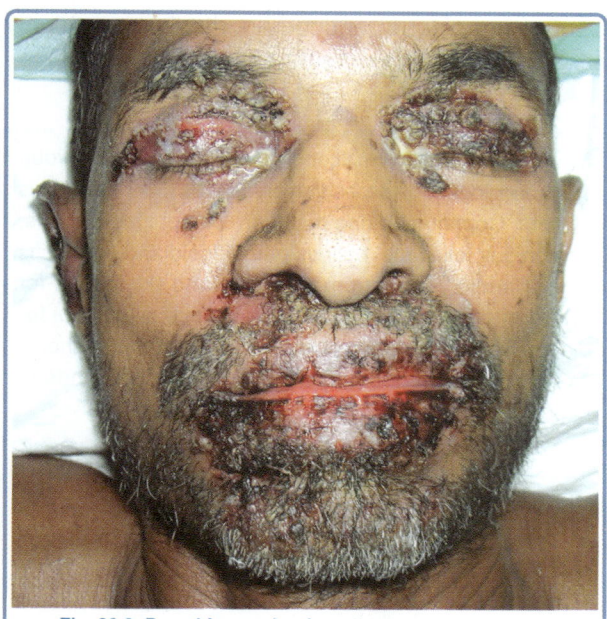

Fig. 20.9: Pemphigus vulgaris—affection of mucosae and periorificial areas is common

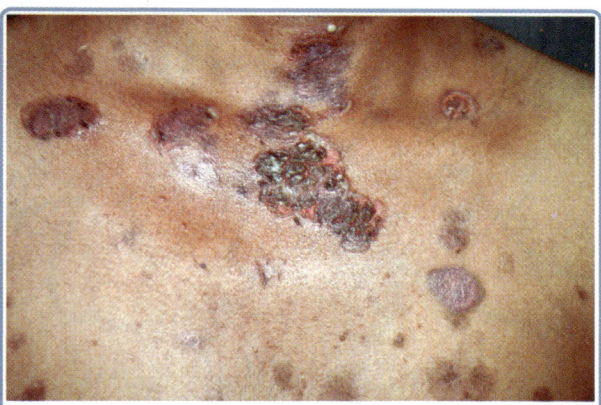

Fig. 20.10: Pemphigus vulgaris—partial resolution of lesions due to inadequate treatment

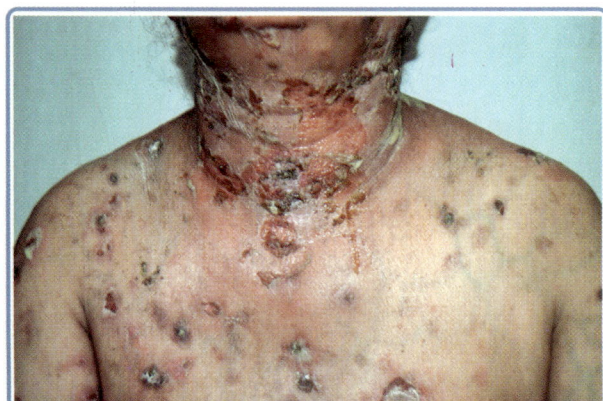

Fig. 20.11: Pemphigus foliaceus—numerous superficial blisters and erosions with secondary impetiginisation

middle aged adults are affected and extensive oozing erosions may lead to fluid, electrolyte and protein loss. Pemphigus vulgaris affects mucosae; oral mucosal (Fig. 20.12) affection leads to pain

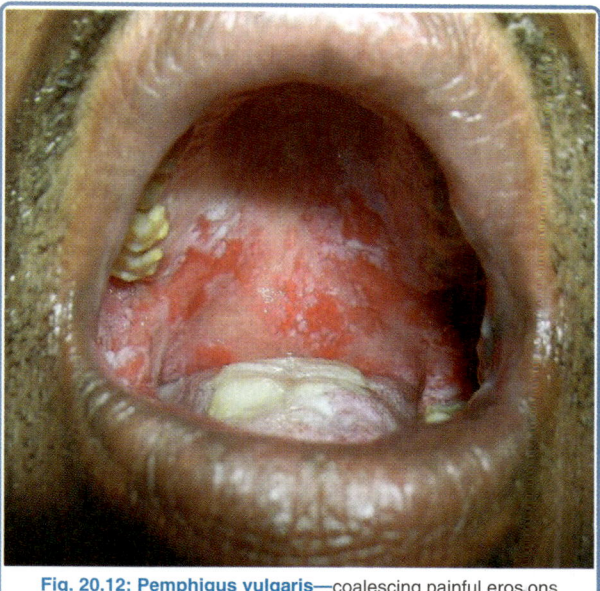

Fig. 20.12: Pemphigus vulgaris—coalescing painful erosions

and burning while eating or talking. Inability to take solid food adds to the electrolyte imbalance and hypoproteinaemia. Untreated extensive disease leads to debility, septicaemia and death.

Pemphigus vulgaris commonly begins as persistent painful oral erosions affecting buccal mucosa, gums and inner lips frequently mimicking oral aphthae or lichen planus. Diagnostic tests are detailed in Table 20.1. Scalp boils and a few scattered vesicles follow over several weeks or months. Lesions grow into flaccid and fragile blisters that tend to get infected and refuse to heal by themselves. Upon treatment lesions heal slowly without scarring with post-inflammatory pigmentation. In active disease even normal looking skin gets eroded on application of shearing force with thumb.

Pemphigus foliaceus differs from pemphigus vulgaris by the superficial nature of the erosions and sparing of the mucosae. The vesicles in pemphigus foliaceus are thin roofed, rupture easily and consequently are difficult to find. Left untreated, pemphigus foliaceus becomes extensive, leading to erythroderma and may even be fatal.

INVESTIGATIONS AND THERAPY OF VESICOBULLOUS DISORDERS

Smear from erosions or bulla fluid reveals acantholytic cells in pemphigus. Skin biopsy is diagnostic in most patients with these vesicobullous diseases. Immunofluorescence staining of the perilesional skin biopsy confirms the diagnosis.

Chapter
20

Chronic Vesicobullous Disorders

Serum antibodies against a component of desmosomes-desmoglein-III in pemphigus vulgaris and against dermaglein-I in pemphigus foliaceus are responsible for the disease. The antibody titre is useful for disease diagnosis and monitoring. All these disorders (except dermatitis herpetiformis) respond to high dose systemic steroid therapy with an extended tapering over many months or even years. Dermatitis herpetiformis responds to dapsone, 100–200 mg/day. Immunosuppressives like azathioprine are used as adjuncts to steroid therapy. Pulse therapy with steroids is claimed to have reduced side effects of steroid therapy. Anti CD-20 monoclonal antibody— rituximab is highly effective in minimising side effects of other drugs.

Summary: Chronic vesticobullous disorders are a group of immunological diseases that present as mucocutaneous blisters. Common among these are pemphigus vulgaris, pemphigus foliaceus, bullous pemphigoid and dermatitis herpetiformis. Smear from bulla floor and skin biopsy for histopathology and immunofluorescence are useful for diagnosis. Systemic steroids are the treatment of choice except for dermatitis herpetiformis which responds to dapsone.

MCQs

1. A 30-year-old female presented with persistent painful oral lesions with acantholytic cells. The most likely diagnosis is:

   a. Pemphigus vulgaris
   b. Dermatitis herpetiformis
   c. Epidermolysis bullosa
   d. Bullous pemphigoid

2. An 85-year-old woman has relapsing skin blisters on thigh and trunk with negative nikolsky sign. What is the probable cause?

   a. Pemphigus vulgaris
   b. Pemphigoid
   c. Lichen planus
   d. Dermatitis herpetiformis

3. Vesicles and bullae are seen in all of the following *except*:

   a. Pemphigus vulgaris
   b. Bullous pemphigoid
   c. Dermatitis herpetiformis
   d. Secondary syphilis

4. Linear IgG deposit is along the dermo-epidermal junction are seen in skin biopsy in:

   a. Dermatitis herpetiformis
   b. Bullous pemphigoid
   c. Pemphigus vulgaris
   d. None of the above

5. Gluten free diet is helpful in:

   a. Dermatitis herpetiformis
   b. Bullous pemphigoid
   c. Pemphigus vulgaris
   d. None of the above

6. Which of the following diseases is potentially fatal?

   a. Dermatitis herpetiformis
   b. Bullous pemphigoid
   c. Pemphigus vulgaris
   d. None of the above

Chapter
20

Chronic Vesicobullous Disorders

--- ANSWERS ---

| 1-a, | 2-b, | 3-d, | 4-b, | 5-a, | 6-c |

Cutaneous Neoplasms, Cysts and Hyperplasias

Malignant neoplasms of the skin, though uncommon, must be studied as they are potentially fatal and yet completely curable when diagnosed early. They include squamous cell carcinoma, basal cell carcinoma and melanoma. On the other hand, benign neoplasms of the skin and cutaneous cysts are common and the majority are of only cosmetic import.

MALIGNANT NEOPLASMS

SQUAMOUS CELL CARCINOMA

This malignant neoplasm has the potential to lead to death by metastasis or local spread if left untreated. Affection of mucosae and mucocutaneous junctions is much more common in the brown skinned Indians than in the whites who develop these tumours on sun-exposed skin.

Patient Profile

Spices, spirits, syphilis, sharp tooth, smoking or other carcinogens, chewing tobacco or other of irritants in gutka and some types of pan masala and submucous fibrosis are the predisposing factors for oral cavity squamous cell carcinoma. The syndrome of acquired immune deficiency is associated with carcinoma of other mucosae and mucocutaneous junctions. Several varieties of human papilloma virus infections have been identified as a risk factor for cervical, penile, vulval, vaginal and anal carcinomas. Excessive exposure to sunlight leads to carcinoma of sun-exposed regions of skin in whites and albinos. Squamous cell carcinomas occasionally develop within scars follwoing burns (Fig. 21.1). Although, senility is a risk factor, many patients are middle aged adults. Persistent exposure to severe heat is responsible in some (Kangri cancer) cases. Some cases follow persistent skin inflammations like edges of non-healing ulcers, untreated hypertrophic or ulceration lichen planus or discoid lupus.

Morphology

Two morphologic types are seen. Exophytic type is seen as a pink, firm to hard, papillomatous nodule (Figs 21.2–21.4) with moist, eroded or ulcerated surface covered with serosanguinous discharge. Endophytic variety is seen as an indurated, pink

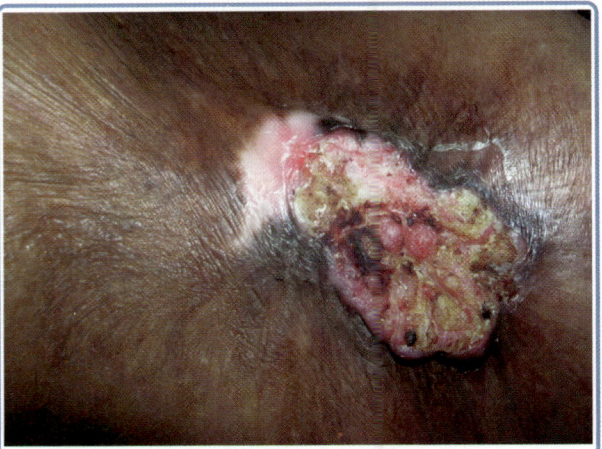

Fig. 21.1: Marjolin's ulcer—sqamous cell carcinoma arising in an old burns scar

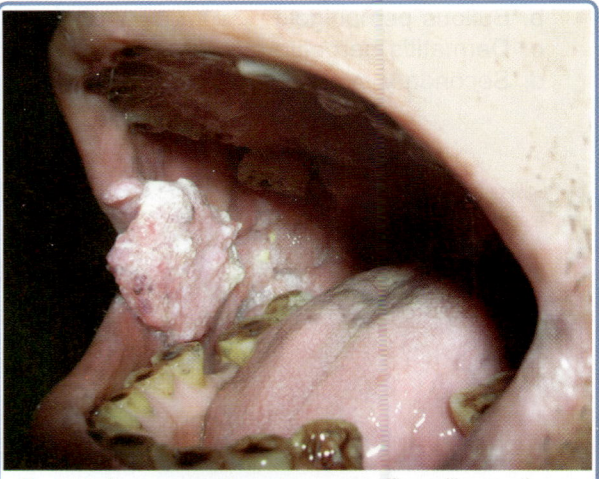

Fig. 21.2: Squamous cell carcinoma—cauliflower like growth over buccal mucosa in a tobacco chewer

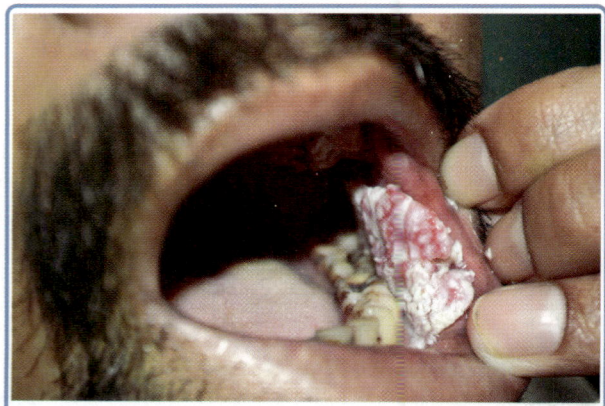

Fig. 21.3 : Squamous cell carcinoma—well circumscribed plaque with ulcerogranulomatous surface. Differentation from verrucous leucoplakia requires biopsy

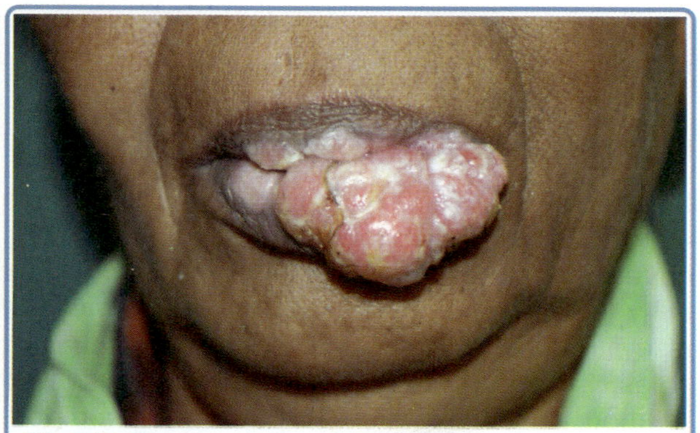

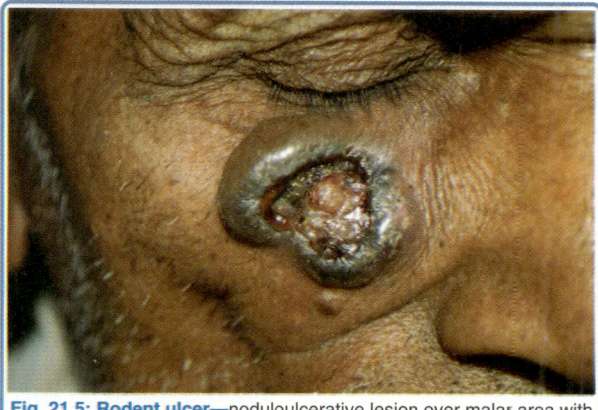

Fig. 21.4: **Squamous cell carcinoma** of verrucous carcinoma type

plaque with ulcerated or eroded surface. The ulcer discharges serosanguinous fluid has everted edges and bleeds on manipulation. A combination of both types may also be present. The ulcer refuses to heal with conservative therapy. Regional lymph nodes may be enlarged and hard due to lymphatic spread and if left untreated, may even ulcerate. Metastases to skin or other orgns are uncommon but can occur if the condition is allowed to progress. The lesions progress slowly over many months or years and are painless.

Distribution

Common sites seen in Indian patients are the mucosae (buccal, gingiva, cervical and anal) and mucocutaneous junction like penis, lips, tongue, perianal and vulval regions. In albinos, if proper care for avoiding sun exposure is not taken, and in fair skinned Indians exposed to excessive sunlight squamous cell carcinomas develop over sun exposed regions by adulthood. Squamous cell carcinoma also develops in the edge of a non-healing ulcer of any cause, if the ulcer persists for several years.

Diagnosis

Keeping a high index of suspicion clinically and choosing the right area for biopsy are very important. Biopsy is the gold standard in diagnosis. It may need to be done from multiple suspicious sites or may sometimes need to be repeated. Four quadrant biopsy is usually done for a non-healing ulcer to rule out squamous cell carcinoma (SCC).

Therapy

Complete excision (with 1 cm margin) is the treatment of choice. In case of lymph node involvement or metastasis, or if the tumour is inoperable, local radiation and chemotherapy may be used as palliative therapies.

BASAL CELL CARCINOMA (RODENT ULCER)

This locally malignant neoplasm rarely metastasises and may lead to local destruction of tissues (Figs 21.5 and 21.6).

Patient Profile

Sunlight and senility are the most important risk factors for basal cell carcinomas.

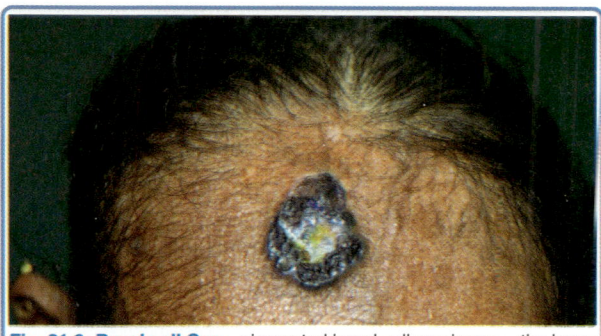

Fig. 21.5: **Rodent ulcer**—noduloulcerative lesion over malar area with rolled out edges

Fig. 21.6: **Basal cell Cap**—pigmented basal cell carcinoma—the lower edge is rolled out

Morphology

A typical lesion begins as a slow growing, asymptomatic, smooth surfaced, skin coloured or hyperpigmented papulonodule that after many months tends to ulcerate in the centre (Fig. 21.7). It left untreated, the ulcer enlarges, deepens and has an indurated base and rolled out, beaded edges (Fig. 21.8). Over several years, the spreading ulcer may distort and destroy the structures in its path. Hence the name, 'rodent ulcer'. Nose, eye, ear, skull bones and even brain are some of the structures that may thus be affected in severe cases. Many lesions begin as hyperpigmented plaques with beaded borders before they ulcerate. Variations in morphology include pigmented, superficial spreading and cicatrising forms. Most of the basal cell carcinomas in Indians are pigmented and noduloulcerative.

Chapter
21

Cutaneous Neoplasms, Cysts and Hyperplasias

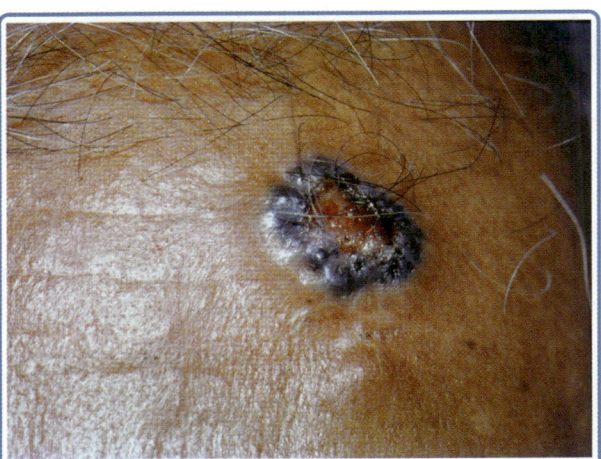

Fig. 21.7: Basal cell carcinoma—hyperpigmented nodule with central ulceration. Note beading of margin

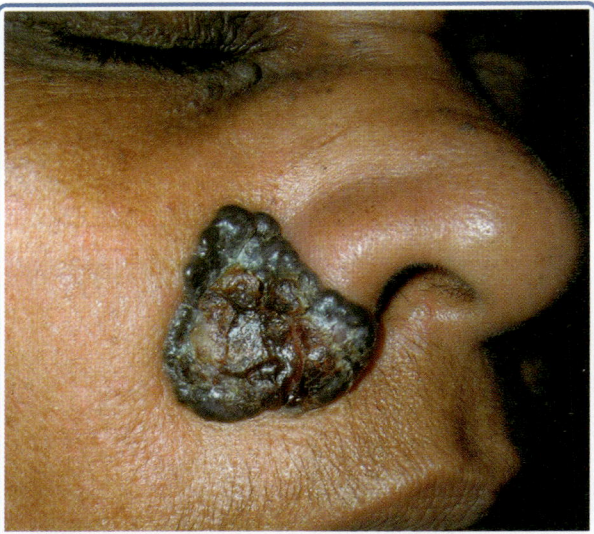

Fig. 21.8: Pigmented basal cell carcinoma—ulcerated nodule with beaded margins. Such pigmented lesions resemble nodular melanoma

Distribution

Sun exposed regions of the face (forehead, malar regions, nose and upper lip) are typical sites. In albinos and whites the lesions may be multiple and widespread.

Therapy

Simple excision (with a margin of 2–5 mm) is the treatment of choice. Recurring lesions may need Moh's chemosurgery and inoperable lesions, radiotherapy.

MELANOMA

This malignant tumour composed of melanocytes may arise in the skin or other tissues harbouring melanocytes, like the mucocutaneous junctions, mucosae including the conjunctiva, iris, choroid and substantia nigra.

Patient Profile

Melanomas are much more common in the middle aged and elderly white skinned population who have a history of repeated sunburns during their early years. In the brown skinned Indians, they are rare but occur at a younger age, affect palms or soles, fingers or toes and genitalia and have no relation to sun exposure except in the albinos. Melanomas occasionally arise in giant (larger than 15 cm) congenital hairy melanocytic nevi. Very rarely, they may arise within the common variety of small acquired melanocytic nevi.

Morphology

All cutaneous melanomas probably begin as brown to black coloured macules/patches (melanoma *in situ*) at which stage they are restricted to the epithelium. The irregular shape, large (more than 1 cm) size, poor definition and variegated colour of such macules/patches are clues to an evolving melanoma.

Over many months or years, such macules or patches become thicker or elevated at one point and evolve into pigmented papules or nodules which indicates dermal involvement. Once dermal involvement occurs, the chances of satellite, lymph node or distant organ metastasis are fairly high. Further progression of nodules leads to their ulceration (Fig. 21.9), bleeding and satellite or lymph node metastasis.

> **Clinical implication:** Although rare, melanoma still occurs in Indians and deaths due to metastases of cutaneous melanoma are wholly preventable by completely excising the macules or patches at an early stage. Once the lesions become elevated, the prognosis worsens.

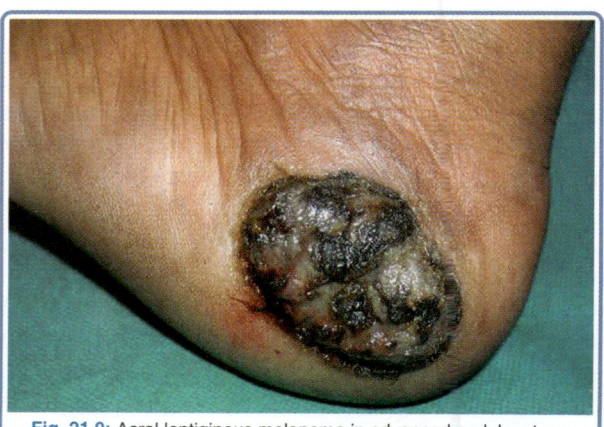

Fig. 21.9: Acral lentiginous melanoma in advanced nodular stage

Distribution

Sun-exposed regions like face are affected in the white skinned. Among Indians, palmoplantar skin and sub, and periungual areas are affected more commonly (acral lentiginous melanoma).

Diagnosis

Skin biopsy is a must for diagnosis. An excision biopsy is advocated.

Therapy

Complete excision of the skin lesion, with a free margin of at least 1 cm, is the only reliable therapy. Other options, which are applicable to local, regional or metastatic disease, include wider excision, lymph node resection, chemotherapy and immunotherapy. However, once metastases have occurred prognosis for life is grave (5-year survival about 10%).

Summary: Melanoma is the malignant tumour of melanocytes. Sun-exposed regions are involved in whites whereas palms and soles are affected in Indians. It begins as a pigmented macule that grows slowly over months or years and then evolves into a papule or nodule on its surface indicating dermal involvement. Metastatic nodules signify poor prognosis. In the absence of metastasis, complete surgical excision, with a free margin of 1 cm is usually curative.

PARANEOPLASTIC SYNDROMES

Skin may be involved in internal malignancy by many mechanisms.

i. Continuity or Contiguity due to extension from underlying organs like in breast cancer
ii. Spread through lymphatics and skin overlying lymph node metastasis
iii. Spread through blood borne metastasis (Fig. 21.10)
iv. Paraneoplastic dermatosis: Occurrence of a skin disease in association with internal malignancy but without the infiltration of malignant cells into the affected skin is termed as paraneoplastic dermatosis (Fig. 21.11).

Paraneoplastic dermatoses include conditions that occur due to some hormone secreting neoplasm like Cushing's syndrome induced by adrenocorticotropic hormone (ACTH) producng bronchogenic carcinoma or acanthosis nigricans due to a carcinoma secreting insulin like growth factor or hirsutism caused by an androgen secreting ovarian neoplasm.

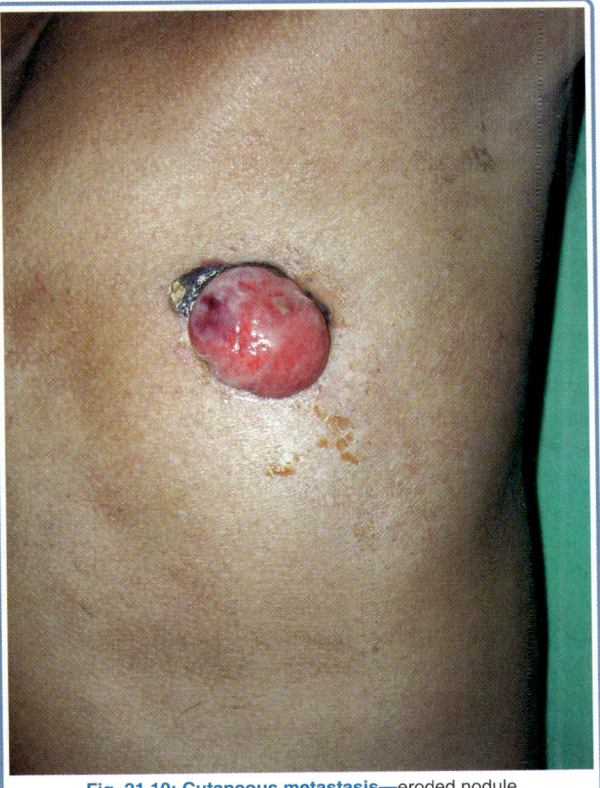

Fig. 21.10: Cutaneous metastasis—eroded nodule

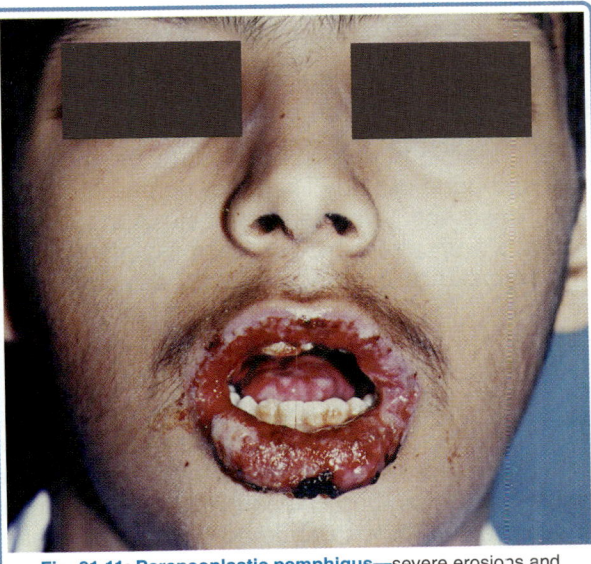

Fig. 21.11: Paraneoplastic pemphigus—severe erosions and ulcerations involving the lips and tongue

Erythema gyratum repens is another para-neopastic disorder characterised by concentric scaly erythematous circles on the trunk. Erythema multiforme and erythema nodosum may also be rarely associated with internal malignancy.

Certain autoimmune dermatoses like para-neoplastic pemphigus, dermatomyositis cr bullous pemphigoid may be the presenting feature of internal malignancies.

Chapter 21

Cutaneous Neoplasms, Cysts and Hyperplasias

Rare genodermatoses like ataxia telangiectasia or dyskeratosis congenita are also associated with internal malignancies like lymphoma or squamous cell carcinoma respectively. While some other genodermatoses like albinism and xeroderma pigmentosm make the skin prone to squamous cell carcinoma.

PREMALIGNANT LESIONS

Bowen's Disease

This is a premalignant condition which presents as well demarcated scaly, keratotic or crusted plaques resembling eczema or psoriasis. When it occurs on uncircumcised glans penis it is known as erythroplasia of Queyrat. Erosions or Reddish patches are seen in erythroplasia of Queyrat. Both the clinical entities are common in the elderly. Histological findings show atypical keratinocytes with mitotic figures involving full thickness of epidermis giving a disorderly 'wind blown' appearance. Sqamous cell carcinoma may develop in untreated and long standing lesions. Medical modalities of treatment include application of 5% imiquimod cream 3 times in a week or 5-fluorouracil cream (5-FU). Irritation, burning and ulceration are common side effects with 5-FU. Other modalities like cryotherapy and surgical excision can be tried.

Solar Keratosis (Actinic Keratosis)

As the name indicates, it occurs on the sun-exposed parts of body like face, dorsae of hands, ears, nose and bald areas of scalp in the elderly. Patients with albinism, xeroderma pigmentosum and fair skin are more prone to develop solar keratoses. Papules or plaques with scaly, crusted surface are common. Other changes due to sun damage are also seen (Fig. 21.12).

Involvement of the lip is known as actinic cheiltis. Microscopic features include parakeratosis and atypical keratinocytes in lower part of the epidermis. Squamous cell carcinoma may develop in such lesions if left untreated. Imiquimod cream 5% is an effective topical treatment for actinic keratoses. However, chance of recurrence is high. 5-fluorouracil has comparabe efficacy but is more irritant. Other modalities include protection from sun exposure, surgical excision, curettage and electro-cauterisation and photodynamic therapy.

Leucoplakia

It is seen as a well to ill defined white coloured plaques associated with the same high risk factors as for squamous cell carcinoma in the mouth. If

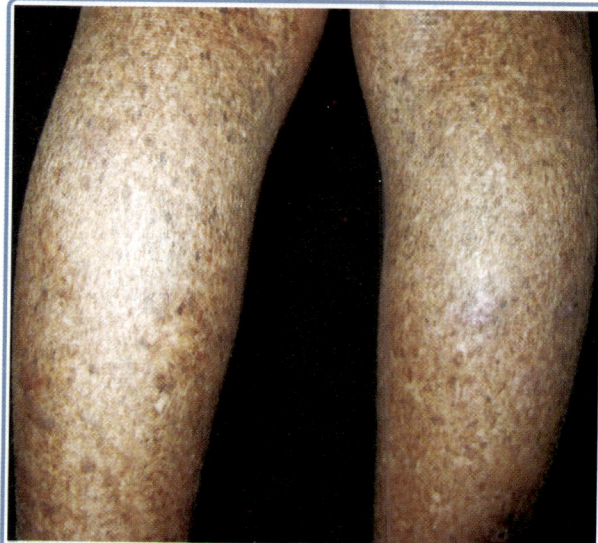

Fig. 21.12: Hyperpigmented macules and premalignant keratoses in a patient with xeroderma pigmentosum

exposure to the high risk factors is continued it has a tendency to progress to squamous cell carcinoma. Biopsy is important to establish the diagnosis. Changes of grade I leucoplakia may revert with avoidance of high risk activity. More advanced cases will have to be treated with ablative therapy like cryotherapy, electrocautery or laser ablation. Surgical excision may be needed for less responsive cases (Fig. 21.13).

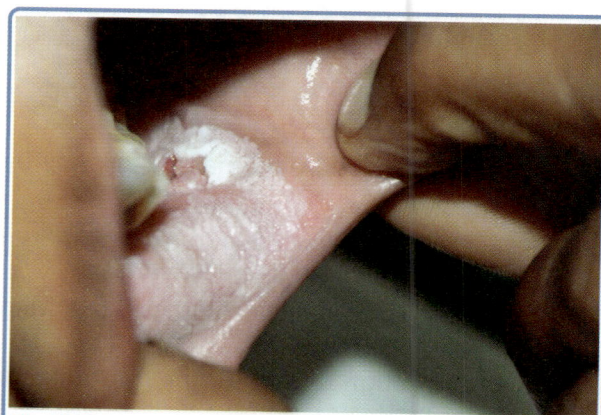

Fig. 21.13: Leucoplakia—well circumscribed white plaque with ebbing tide appearance of surface

BENIGN NEOPLASM

SEBORRHOEIC KERATOSIS

These are probably the commonest of the skin tumours.

Patient Profile

Genetic predisposition and increasing age are the risk factors. Lesions begin appearing in the second or third decade though they are notice in the third or fourth decade.

Morphology

They are seen as brown to black coloured papules or plaques of sizes varying from 1 mm to 3 cm (Fig. 21.14). The papules may be small, pedunculated and soft or may be larger, flat and rough surfaced. Larger lesions show a greasy scale that covers dilated follicular openings occluded with black plugs (Fig. 21.15).

Distribution

Face, neck and upper trunk are common sites. Lower eyelids, malar regions, sides of neck, chest and upper back are particularly involved. Lower trunk and proximal extremities may also be affected.

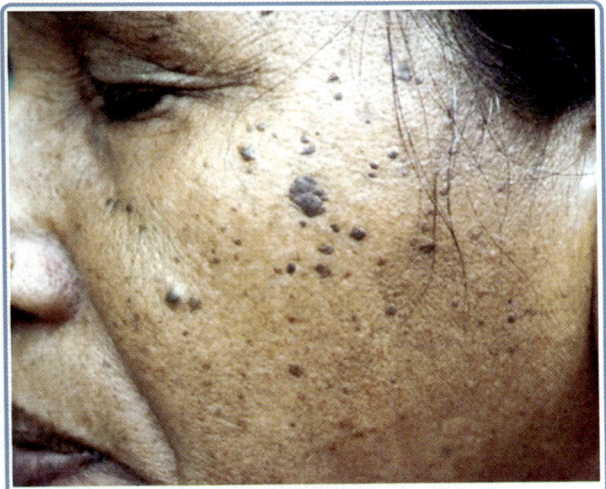

Fig. 21.14: Seborrheic keratoses—multiple hyperpigmented papules and plaques over face

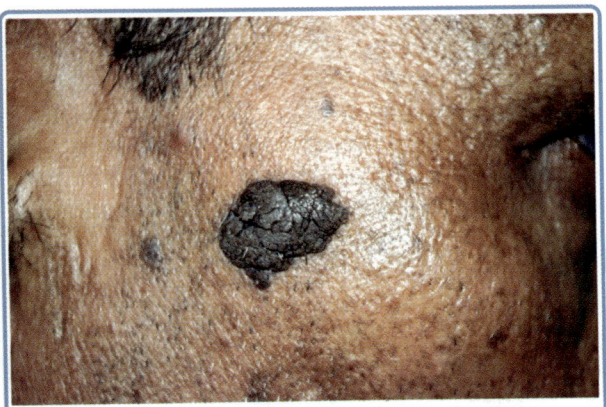

Fig. 21.15: Seborrheic keratosis—close up view shows hyperkeratotic cerebriform surface with follicular plugs

Treatment

Destruction with electrocautery or cryotherapy is the therapy of choice. Radiofrequency or carbon dioxide laser give better cosmetic results. Large lesions need surgical excision.

SOLAR LENTIGO (SENILE LENTIGO, LIVER SPOT)

These are brown coloured, well defined macular lesions, varying in size from a few mm to a few cm that develop on sun exposed sites. They are seen usually in the elderly but may begin in adulthood. Face, dorsa of hands and bald area of scalp are commonest sites affected. Individual macules may coalesce to form a larger patch. Some lesions may become elevated and keratotic with time and evolve into a seborrhoeic keratosis. Treatment includes preventive measures like avoidance of sun exposure and application of a sunscreen. Topical retinoids can be effective for smaller lesions while larger ones may need treatment with chemical peels or switched neodymium-doped yttrium aluminum garnet (NdYAG) laser.

FRECKLES

Freckles are multiple, light brown coloured and small macules, which occur over the sun-exposed parts of the body, commonly on the central part of face. They are common in persons with fair complexion and are usually familial. Lighter colour of hair and brown, gray or blue iris colour are common associations. Freckles are more prominent in summer but face considerably or disappear in winter. Treatment is not a must as they subside on their own, if sun exposure is avoided but can recur on such exposure. Patients who are concerned about their appearance may be treated with either chemical peel or Q switched NdYAG laser.

MELANOCYTIC NEVI

These extremely common skin lesions are benign neoplasm comprising melanocytes. They may be divided into congenital and acquired types. Their basic clinical characteristics are enumerated below.

Congenital (Figs 21.16–21.19)
- Present at birth
- Larger (>1 cm)
- Black or Bluish-black
- Usually hairy
- Small chance of melanoma developing in giant nevi.

Acquired (Fig. 21.20)
- Appear during first, second or third decades of life

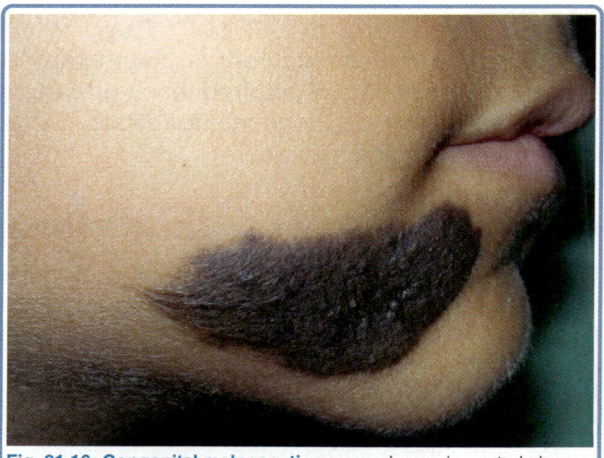

Fig. 21.16: Congenital melanocytic nevus—hyperpigmented plaques with coarse hairs

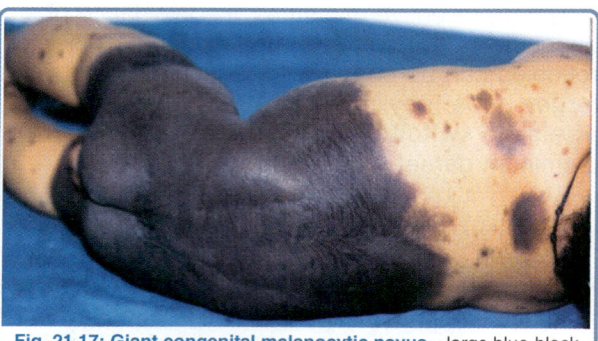

Fig. 21.17: Giant congenital melanocytic nevus—large blue-black hairy plaque in bathing trunk distribution

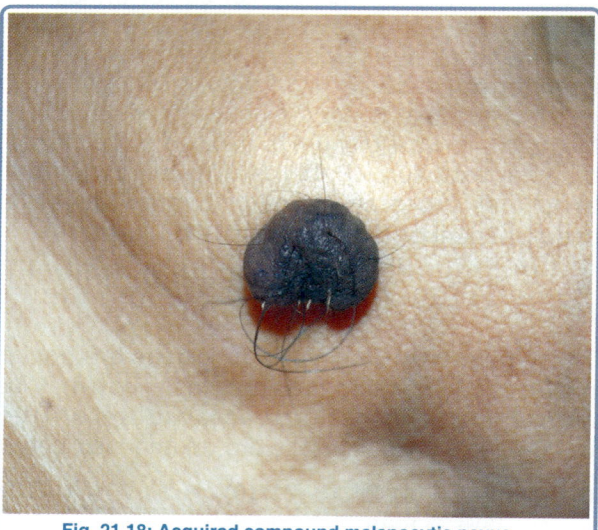

Fig. 21.18: Acquired compound melanocytic nevus—hyperpigmented nodule with coarse hair

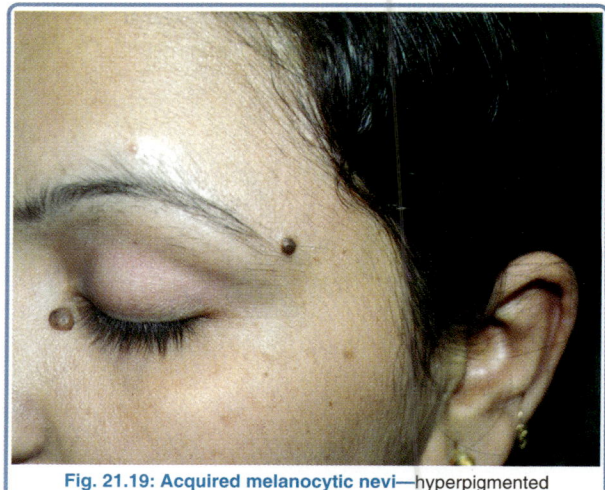

Fig. 21.19: Acquired melanocytic nevi—hyperpigmented papulonodules with occasional terminal hair

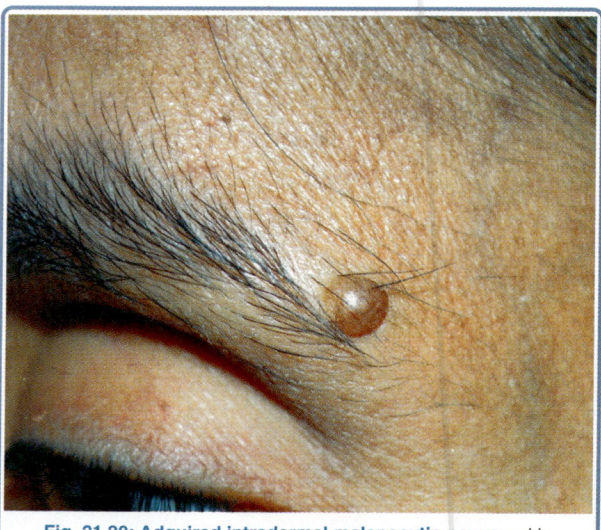

Fig. 21.20: Adquired intradermal melanocytic nevus—skin coloured nodule

- Smaller (<1 cm)
- Brown-black or Skin coloured
- Sometimes hair
- Development of melanoma is very rare

Melanocytic nevi may further be classified based on histopathology into junctional, compound and intradermal types. Junctional nevi appear jet-black in colour while intradermal nevi are born or skin coloured.

Management

Since melanoma rarely develops within acquired melanocytic nevi, they should be left untreated unless (a) they appear during the fourth decade or later and, (b) show persistent enlargement, ulceration, bleeding or irregular pigmentation. Large congenital melanocytic nevi may be removed in stages to avoid the risk of melanoma.

SKIN TAGS

These are asymptomatic lesions seen more commonly in overweight individuals. Lesions are usually multiple and may be associated with acanthosis nigricans. It may be a pedunculated, soft, skin coloured papule seen over flexural regions like axillae, neck, groins, or inner thighs. It grows slowly over months or years to form a soft, pedunculated, papillomatous, skin coloured nodule of up to 2–3 cm diameter. Smaller lesions may be removed by electrocautery or cryosurgery. Radiofrequency or carbon dioxide laser give better cosmetic results. Large lesions need excision (Fig. 21.21).

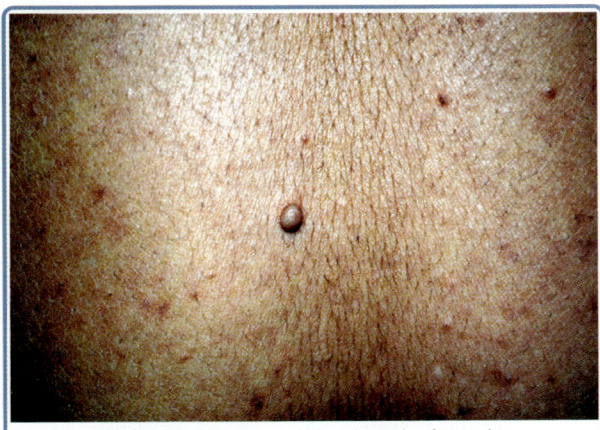

Fig. 21.21: **Skin tags**—skin coloured soft papules

HAEMANGIOMAS

These are vascular neoplasms (strawberry haemangioma) or malformations that may have either a capillary (port wine stain), venular (cavernous haemangioma) or arterial (arteriovenous malformation) component or may be mixed.

Port Wine Stain

These are flat capillary malformations that are difficult to blanch and remain largely unchanged since birth. Sharply defined, irregular, bright or dark red, or bluish red patch of several inches diameter is typical (Fig. 21.22). Most commonly noticed on the face, it follows a segmental pattern of involvement. In Sturge-Weber syndrome, port wine stain is seen over the face, above the level of outer canthus. Glaucoma may be associated. Port wine stains do not regress but are amenable to pulse dye laser therapy.

Strawberry Haemangioa

An elevated capillary haemangioma, is seen as a bright red, circular or oval, plaque or nodule that is compressible (Figs 21.23–21.26). The lesion is frequently noticed at or soon after birth and grows at a rapid pace, during the first 6 months during which time it may ulcerate. After the first year of life, it stops growing and is static for some time

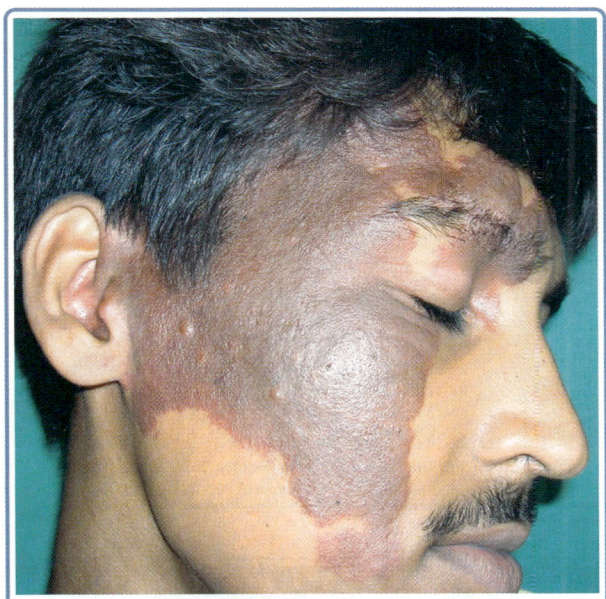

Fig. 21.22: **Portwine stain**—a large red coloured unilateral, slightly elevated plaque on the face since birth

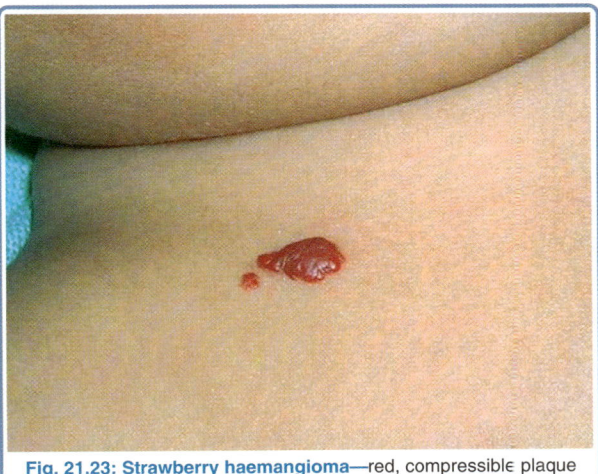

Fig. 21.23: **Strawberry haemangioma**—red, compressible plaque since birth

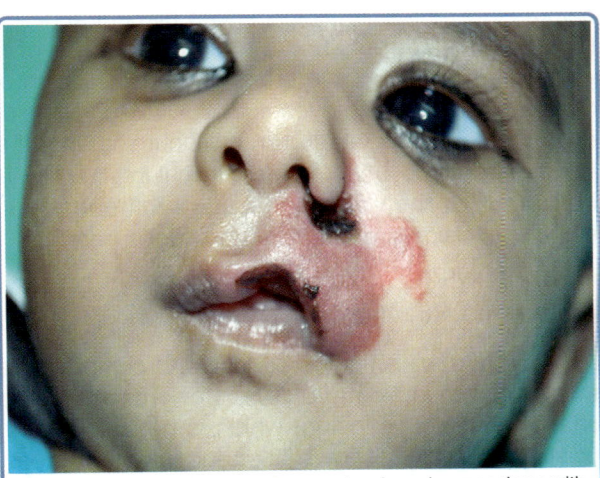

Fig. 21.24: **Infantile haemangioma**—strawberry haemangioma with ulceration

Chapter **21**

Cutaneous Neoplasms, Cysts and Hyperplasias

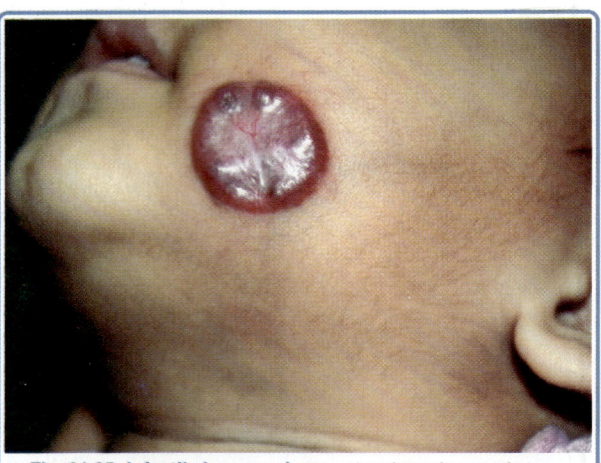

Fig. 21.25: Infantile haemangioma—starwberry hemangioma—Central whitening is suggestve of resolving phase

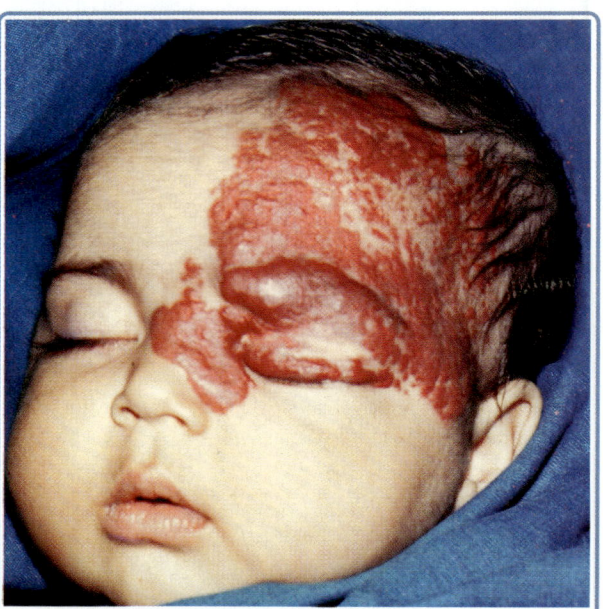

Fig. 21.26: Strawberry haemangioma—red compressible plaque since birth interfering with vision

before slow regression is evidenced by central pallor. Most lesions regress completely by the age of 5 years without appreciable scarring. Early institution of oral propranolol may prevent full evolution of lesion or even result in complete healing without scarring. If a lesion persists beyond 7 years surgical intervention is indicated. Carbon dioxide laser, cryotherapy and surgical excision are therapies to choose from.

Cavernous Haemangioma

An ill defined, bluish coloured, soft and compressible swelling that may have a bag of worms feel is characteristic. The lesion, which is noticed at birth or soon thereafter, shows little tendency to regress. Surgical intervention (sclerotherapy or excision) is indicated.

SENILE ANGIOMA (CHERRY ANGIOMA)

These are small, bright red coloured, asymptomatic papules and macules which occur in the middle aged and elderly. Trunk and proximal extremities are common sites followed by face. Bleeding can occur following trauma. Usually no treatment is required, but if cosmetically displeasing then can be removed by radiofrequency or carbon dioxide laser (Fig. 21.27).

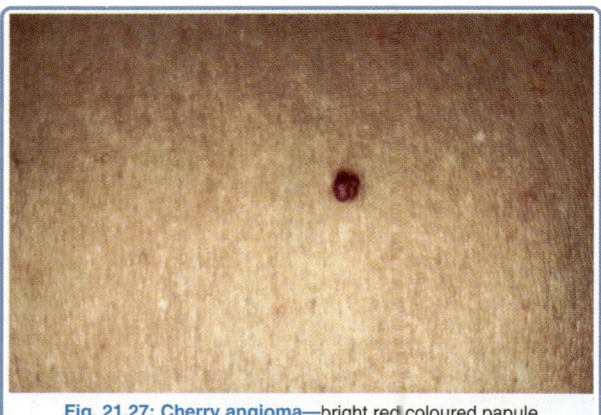

Fig. 21.27: Cherry angioma—bright red coloured papule

SYRINGOMA

These benign neoplasms of sweat ducts occur as multiple papules over the lower eyelids of middle aged females (Fig. 21.28). The condition is familial and the lesions are asymptomatic, skin coloured,

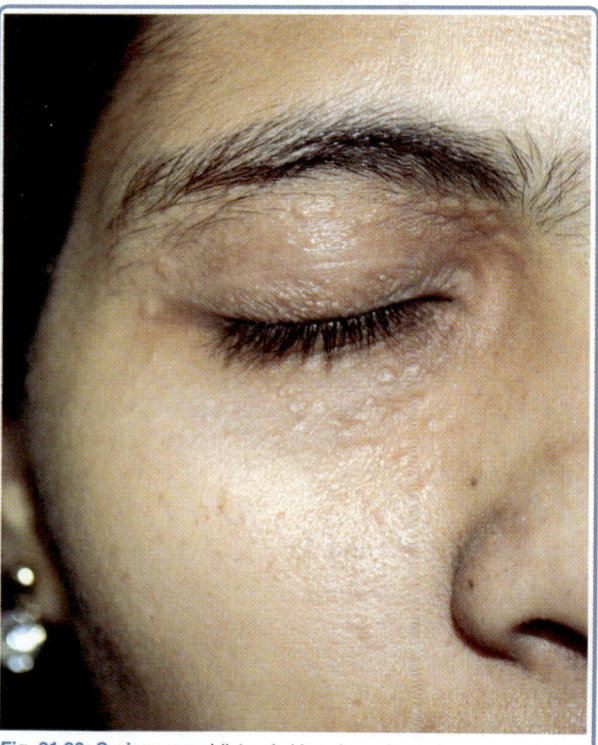

Fig. 21.28: Syringoma—bilateral skin coloured papules over eyelids in young/middle-aged ladies

or slightly yellowish multiple tiny papules of size 1–3 mm. No effective treatment is available though ablative treatment like radiofrequency or carbon dioxide laser can be tried.

EPIDERMAL NEVUS

This is a developmental malformation that presents as skin or dark coloured verrucous, keratotic papules and plaques arranged in linear fashion (Figs 21.29–21.31). The lesions are frequently noticed at birth as flat or slightly elevated hyperpigmented macules or patches. During childhood or adolescence, they may increase in size or become papillomatous gaining their characteristic appearance. They remain stable once they have achieved their full size. Treatment includes excision and skin grafting if small in size, or ablation with radiofrequency or carbon dioxide laser.

CYSTS

Cysts are defined as sac like structures lined by epithelium. Cysts are usually soft and compressible but sometimes may feel firm or hard if internal contents have undergone inspissation or calcification. The clinical term 'sebaceous cyst' is used loosely to designate epidermal or pilar cysts or a steatocystoma. One or A few cysts are best dealt with by surgical excision.

Epidermoid (Infundibular) Cyst

These are the commonest cysts that occur in the skin and show central or eccentric comedone like punctum (Figs 21.32 and 21.33). Epidermal cysts are slightly blue gray or yellowish in colour, have a cystic feel and may show the sign of fluctuation. Pressure over the cyst may cause expression of putty material through the punctum or may lead to change of shape of the hemispherical nodule (moulding). Trauma or Manipulation, may make the cyst to rupture inside the skin leading to erythema and tenderness of the surrounding skin. Sometimes secondary infection may occur leading to abscess formation.

Pilar Cyst

These commonly occur on the scalp and have a tendency to calcification or even ossification. They

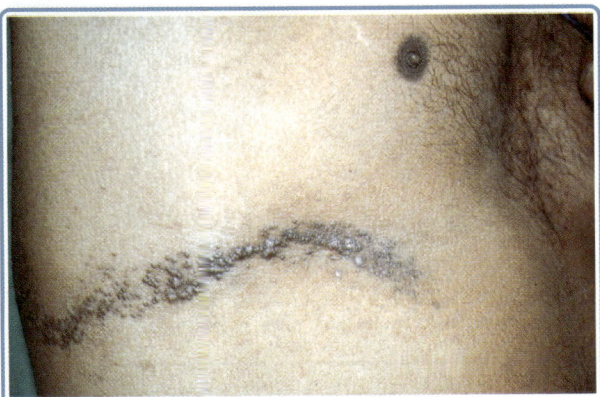

Fig. 21.29: Epidermal nevus—unilateral verrucous papules and plaques following linear pattern

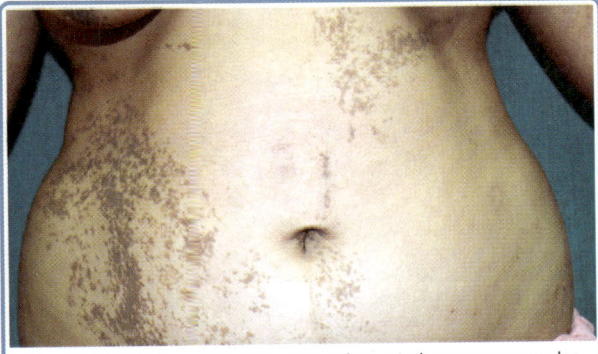

Fig. 21.30: Epidermal nevus—hyperpigmented verrucous papules involving multiple dermatomes

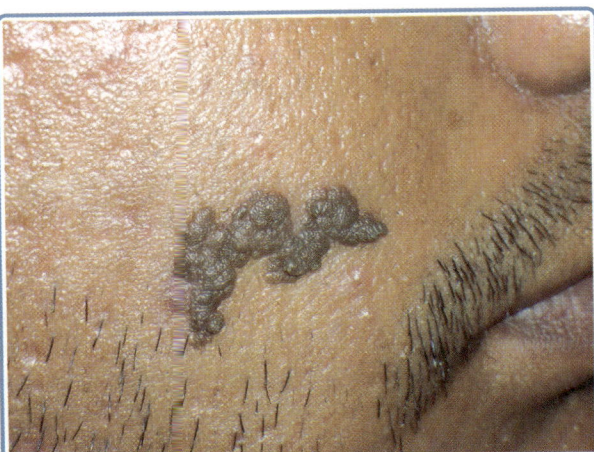

Fig. 21.31: Verrucous epidermal nevus—hyperpigmented verrucous plaque

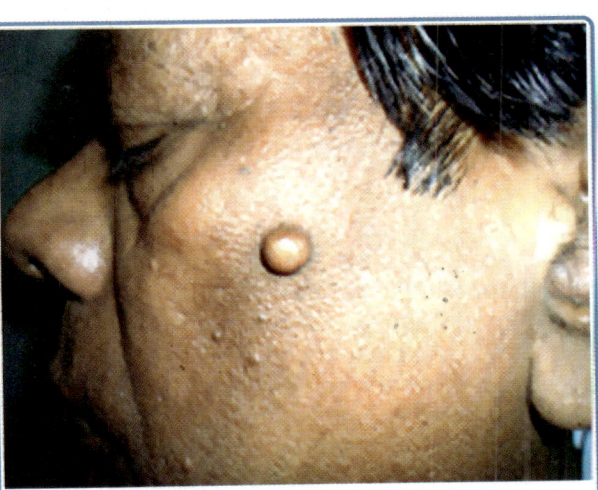

Fig. 21.32: Sebaceous cyst—single sessile nodule of yellowish colour

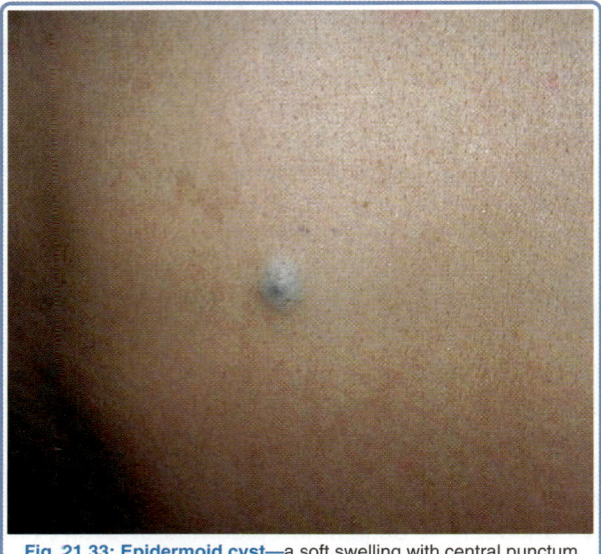

Fig. 21.33: Epidermoid cyst—a soft swelling with central punctum

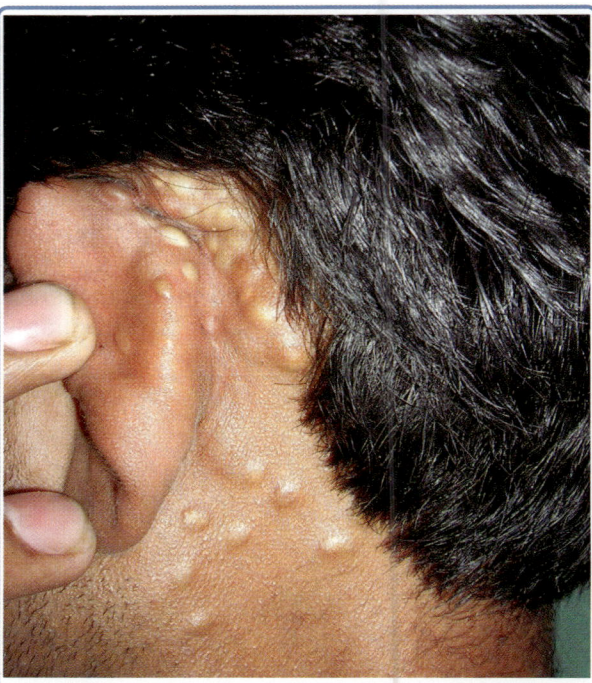

Fig. 21.34: Steatocystoma multiplex—yellowish deep seated cystic nodules

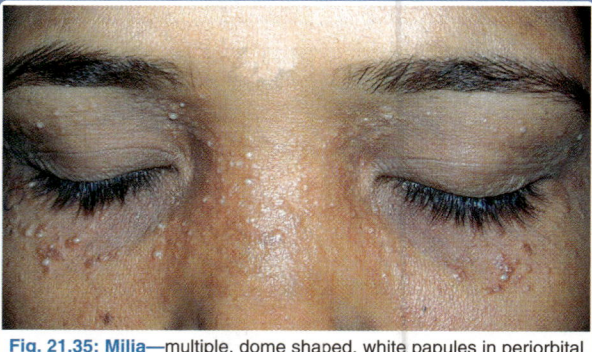

Fig. 21.35: Milia—multiple, dome shaped, white papules in periorbital area

appear similar to epidermoid cysts clinically and the term sebaceous cysts is clinically used collectively describe them. Histopathologically, lining of epidermoid cyst resemble the epidermis while that of pilar cyst resembles the isthmic portion of the hair follicle.

Steatocystomas

These are asymptomatic cutaneous cysts which occur as multiple skin to yellowish coloured cystic nodules in young adults. The cysts occur due to an autosomal dominantly transmitted genetic trait. They are commonly seen over the upper part of chest. (Fig. 21.34) back, and on the scrotum. Surgical excision is effective but may be cumbersome.

Dermoid Cysts

These are developmental defects that occur along the embryonic closure lines. Common sites include face over lateral end of the eyebrows, nasal root and midline on the forehead. Contents of dermoid cysts are varied from putty matter to hair or even teeth.

Milia

These are tiny keratin cysts which occur over the face around the lower eyelids. They have sized of 1–3 mm and appear as whitish to pearly papules (Fig. 21.35). A kernel of rice like white material can be extracted when they are pricked with a sterile needle. They are commonly seen on upper cheeks, nose and chin in newborn babies and disappear spontaneously after a few days. Milia can develop over scars or following healing of lesions as seen in vesiculobullous diseases like porphyria cutanea tarda and dystrophic epidermolysis bullosa. Extraction with the help of a needle is effective treatment. Topical retinoids are useful when lesions are numerous.

CUTANEOUS HYPERPLASIAS

KELOID

Keloid results from an excessive reparative response on the part of the skin to common clinical (e.g. following traumatic wounds) and subclinical (so called 'spontaneous' occurrence) injuries. Multiple lesions are common and a person with one lesion is likely to develop another after similar injury or upon excision of the first lesion.

Patient Profile

Adolescents and young adults are affected commonly. Keloids are more common in males but can occur in both sexes and all ages. Black races are particularly prone.

Morphology

Skin coloured, pruritic, irregularly shaped but well demarcated firm plaques that have pseudopod like extensions at the growing margins are characteristic. Early lesions are nodules, which in some locations (e.g. earlobes) (Fig. 21.36) may become pedunculated. Lesions enlarge gradually over several months or even years, after which they remain quiescent.

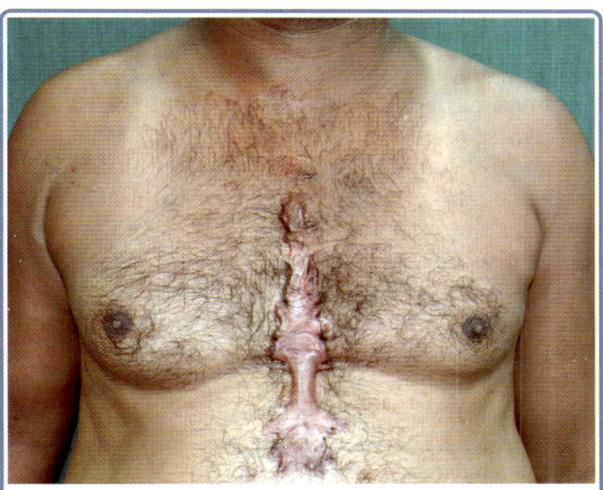

Fig. 21.37a: Keloid—claw-like extensions from the central plaque. Lesions followed open heart surgery

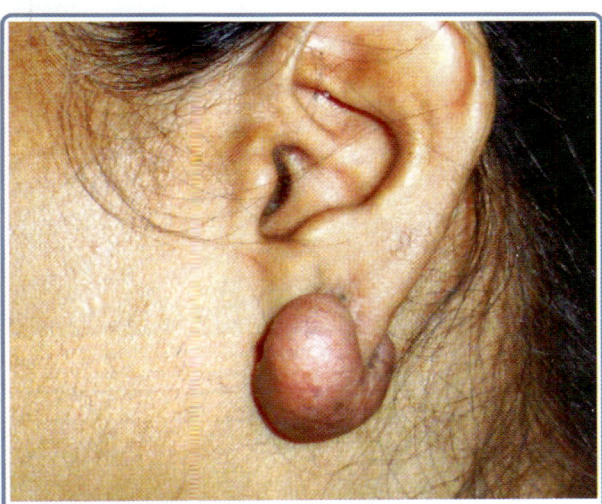

Fig. 21.36: Keloid—firm nodule on ear lobe following ear piercing

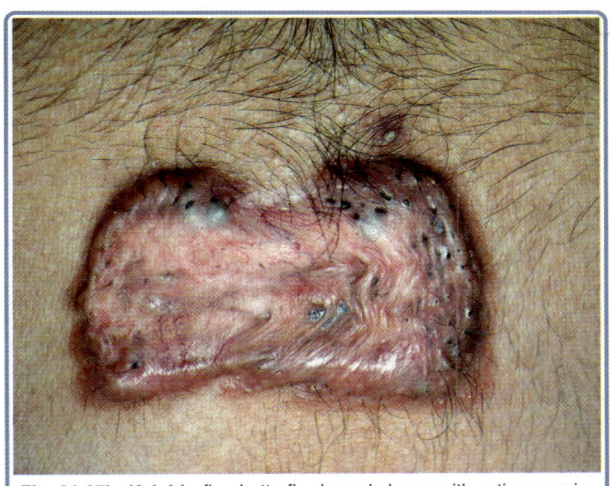

Fig. 21.37b: Keloid—firm butterfly shaped plaque with active margin. Presternal area is commonly affected

Distribution

Common sites of trauma (vaccination scars on shoulders, ear piercing, tattoos and lower legs) are prone to develop the lesions. Spontaneous lesions are common over the pre-sternal region (Fig. 21.37a and b), upper chest, shoulders, upper back and upper arms. Prior skin wounds (infected ulcers, burns scars and surgical wounds under tension) and diseases (scrofuloderma, acne vulgaris epecially nodulocystic type) may heal with scars in which keloids may develop.

Differential Diagnosis

As against hypertrophic scars keloids are pruritic, have irregular pseudopod like outline, continue to grow in size even after 6 months, become pedunculated, show keloidal collagen on biopsy and recur after surgical excisions. In the early stages it may be difficult to differentiate the two conditions (Table 21.1).

TABLE 21.1: Differential diagnosis of keloid and hypertrophic scar

	Hypertrophic scar	Keloid
Previous trauma	+	+
Growth in size for	< 6 months	usually > 6 months
Recurrence after excision	–	+
Symptoms pruritic or tender	Nil	Usually
Claw-like extensions at the border	Absent	Present
Biopsy	No keloidal collagen	Keloidal collagen +

Chapter **21**

Cutaneous Neoplasms, Cysts and Hyperplasias

Therapy

Therapy of keloids is not satisfactory. Intralesional injections of triamcinolone acetonide 10–20 mg/mL on several occasions may stop growth and soften the lesion. Persistent pressure with elastic bands has similar effect. Local cryotherapy or radiotherapy have a salutary effect on keloid growth. Surgical excision or laser ablation are fraught with the risk of recurrence. However, when surgery is followed up with intralesional steroid injection or pressure therapy or radiotherapy of the excision scar the chances of recurrence are considerably reduced.

Palmoplantar Keratoderma

Thickening of palms and soles (keratoderma) can be acquired or congenital (Fig. 21.38). Acquired causes include occupational keratoderm (due to the friction of manual labour), psoriasis or keratoderm blenorrhagicum of Reiter's disease. Hereditary palmoplantar keratodermas present as diffuse thickening of the skin of palms and soles. Some cases may be associated with other genetic diseases like Darier disease while others, rarely, may have internal organ affection like carcinoma of oesophagus. Thus, palmoplantar keratoderma serves as a marker for internal disease in such patients.

Morphology and Distribution

Palms and soles are visibly thickened and roughened. In severe cases the thickened stratum corneum cracks leading to painful fissures that are especially common over the sides of soles. Fissures may hamper foot and hand function.

Therapy

Treatment includes topical application of emollients like white soft paraffin or urea or keratolytic agents like salicylic acid. Systemic treatment includes oral retinoids like isotretinoin.

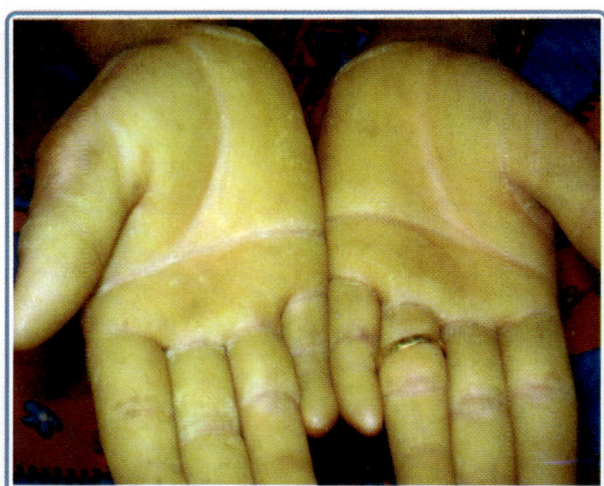

Fig. 21.38: Palmar keratoderma—diffuse yellowish discolouration and marked hyperkeratosis of palms

PYOGENIC GRANULOMA

These are fleshy, red coloured nodules (Fig. 21.39a and b) which bleed on touch or minor trauma. Pyogenic granulomas occur at trauma prone sites and on mucosa. Fingers, scalp, face, gingiva and lips are commonly affected. During pregnancy they occur on the gums and then known as epulis gravidarum. Complications like erosion, ulceration and bleeding can occur following trauma. The cause of pyogenic granuloma is unknown. Histologically lobules of capillary proliferation are seen. Management includes surgical excision, cryotherapy or chemical cauterisation with phenol or silver nitrate. Pyogenic granulomas have a tendency to recurrence after excision.

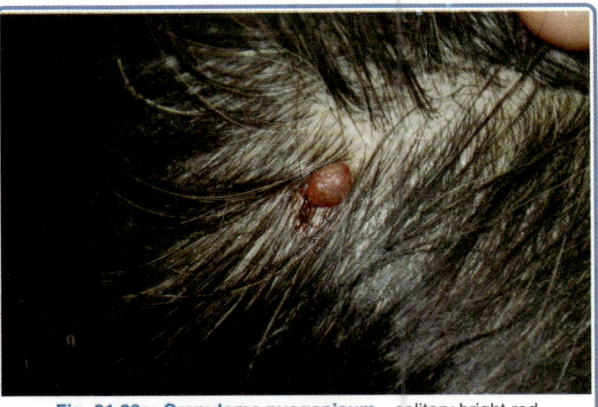

Fig. 21.39a: Granuloma pyogenicum—solitary bright red compressible nodule with bleeding surface

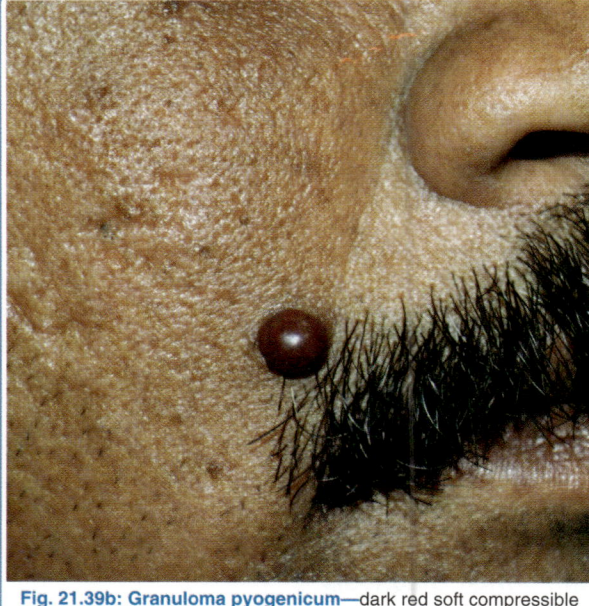

Fig. 21.39b: Granuloma pyogenicum—dark red soft compressible nodule

CLAVUS (CORN)

Corns result from abnormal distribution pressure leading to excessive concentration of pressure at one point.

Patient Profile

Corns are rarely seen in bare foot walkers. Abnormal pressure distribution due to ill fitting footwear or deformities of the foot or abnormal gait, is causative.

Morphology

Seen as a painful thickening of the skin, corns have rounded outlines and show loss of dermatoglyphic lines in the centre of the lesion. The lesion turns white on moistening and is tender when pressure is applied perpendicular to the skin surface. Shaving the superficial dead keratin layer with a blade exposes the conical white core made of soft keratin. The tip of the cone is pointed internally whereas the base is formed by the skin surface.

Distribution

Most commonly they occur over the pressure bearing points of the foot. Bases of the first and fourth metatarsals and heel are the common sites. Other pressure bearing points, normal or abnormal, may also be affected.

Differential Diagnosis

As against a corn, a callus has prominent dermatoglyphic lines over surface, is not as sharply demarcated and does not display the central core on paring the top layer. A palmar or plantar wart, like a corn, also shows loss of dermatoglyphic lines. However it is more painful on horizontal pressure, when pressed between fingers, than on vertical pressure on the centre of the lesion. Besides, removal of the top layer, by paring with a blade, reveals black points in a wart as against the soft keratin core of a corn.

Treatment

Identification and correction of predisposing factors is necessary to prevent recurrence. If correction is difficult, pressure distribution can be ensured by use of a soft lining for footwear. Resolution of painful lesions can be hastened by application of up to 40% salicylic acid under occlusion ('corn caps') for 24–48 hours and following it up with shaving of the softened dead keratin by using a sterile blade. The procedure can be repeated till the soft white core is removed. No anaesthesia is needed if the removal is done in steps. Application of 20% salicylic acid lotion is effective with smaller lesions.

Callus (Callosity)

Callus is a localised thickening of the stratum corneum as a result of repeated rubbing.

Patient Profile

Callosities are common in manual labourers and bare foot walkers. Sites of callositis may serve as a clue to one's occupation. Callosities on soles may result from ill fitting shoes or due to hard points in the insole. Callosities are protective in their early stages. Once they become too thick they result in abnormal concentration of pressure which makes them painful. In patients with leprosy, who lack pain sensation over the feet, such concentration of pressure leads to skin necrosis and trophic ulcer.

Morphology

Callus is seen as an ill defined skin coloured plaque. When examined closely, the surface shows prominent dermatoglyphic lines and on touching it, the surface is rough. For differentiation of callosity from corn and warts, *see* page 89 and 242.

Therapy

Topical salicyclic acid in suitable concentration (5–25%) is effective.

PYOGENIC GRANULOMA

This hyperplasia of vascular tissue is localised to sites of injuries or cuts or follow pyogenic infections of the skin. Vascular areas prone to trauma like fingertips or nailfolds or scalp or body folds or bony prominences are prone to develop such lesions. The condition is common in adolescents and young adults.

Morphology

Soft friable, bright red nodules that are sessile or pedunculated and have a wet surface that oozes serosanguinous or purulent discharge at above sites. They are tender, soft, at times, compressible and their base is not indurated.

Treatment

Control of bacterial infection, silver nitrate application and if needed cryo or electrocautery.

Chapter
21

Cutaneous Neoplasms, Cysts and Hyperplasias

MCQ

1. **This is not a predisposing factor for oral squamous cell carcinoma:**
   a. Gutka abuse
   b. Alcohol abuse
   c. Smoking
   d. Persistent candidiasis

2. **This is not a predisposing factor for oral squamous cell carcinoma:**
   a. Sharp tooth
   b. HIV infection
   c. Leucoplakia
   d. Submucous fibrosis

3. **This is not a predisposing factor for cutaneous squamous cell carcinoma:**
   a. Excessive exposure to sunlight
   b. Old age
   c. Excess exposure to ultraviolet radiation
   d. Dark coloured skin

4. **This is not a predisposing factor for cutaneous squamous cell carcinoma:**
   a. White skin
   b. Persistent heat
   c. Recurrent bacterial infections
   d. Old burns scar

5. **This is not a predisposing factor for oral squamous cell carcinoma:**
   a. Leprosy
   b. Syphilis
   c. Lichen planus
   d. Arsenic ingestion

6. **Edges of an ulcer of squamous cell carcinoma are:**
   a. Everted
   b. Punched out
   c. Rolled out
   d. Sloping

7. **This is not a clue to squaous cell carcinoma:**
   a. Long standing non-healing ulcer
   b Bloody discharge
   c. Irregular pigmentation
   d. Rapidly enlarging lesion

8. **Cutaneous squamous cell carcinoma does not usually spread by:**
   a. Continuity
   b. Contiguity
   c. Lymphatic spread
   d. Blood borne metastases

9. **Edges of an ulcer of basal cell carcinoma are:**
   a. Everted
   b. Punched out
   c. Rolled out
   d. Sloping

10. **The type of biopsy recommended for a non-healing ulcer is:**
    a. Punch biopsy
    b. Incision biopsy
    c. Excision biopsy
    d. Four quadrant biopsy

11. **The base of a squamous cell carcinoma is:**
    a. Broad
    b. Narrow
    c. Soft
    d. Indurated

12. **This is not a common site for squamous cell carcinoma in Indians:**
    a. Cheek
    b. Lower lip
    c. Mouth
    d. Penis

13. **This is a clue to basal cell carcinoma on face in Indian patients:**
    a. Pigmented plaque
    b. Persistent lesion
    c. Asymptomatic nodule on face
    d. Old acne scars

14. **Rodent ulcer is another name for:**
    a. Rat bite fever
    b. Rat bite
    c. Squamous cell carcinoma
    d. Basal cell carcinoma

15, **The type of melanoma which occurs in Indians is:**
    a. Superficial spreading melanoma
    b. Lentigo maligna
    c. Lentigo maligna melanoma
    d. Acral lentiginous melanoma

16. **The cutaneous malignancy with worst prognosis is:**
    a. Squamous cell carcinoma
    b. Melanoma
    c. Basal cell carcinoma
    d. Atypical fibroxanthoma

17. **In its early stage melanoma presents as:**
    a. Macule
    b. Papule
    c. Nodule
    d. Plaque

18. **Melanoma rarely occurs within:**
    a. Melanocytic nevus
    b. Burns scar
    c. Lichen planus
    d. Epidermal nevus

19. **The macular stage of acral melanoma lasts for:**
    a. Days
    b. Weeks
    c. Months
    d. Years

20. **Once a lesion of melanoma turns nodular:**
    a. Chance of lymphatic metastasis increases
    b. Chance of blood borne dissemination increases
    c. 5-year survival becomes poor
    d. All of the above

21. **Congenital melanocytic nevi, when large, run the risk of developing:**
    a. Keloid
    b. Cancer
    c. Scar
    d. Melanoma

22. **Commonest site of melanoma in Indians is:**
    a. Sole
    b. Face
    c. Back
    d. Neck

23. **This is a paraneoplastic skin condition:**
    a. Acanthosis nigricans
    b. Stevens Johnson Syndrome
    c. Bowen's disease
    d. Leucoplakia

24. **This lesion has a high chance of evolving into a squamous cell cacinoma:**
    a. Leucoplakia
    b. Bowen's disease
    c. Actinic keratosis
    d. Lichen planus

25. **Erythroplasia of Queyrat occurs over the:**
    a. Lip
    b. Buccal mucosa
    c. Tongue
    d. Penis

26. **This is a benign keratosis of the skin:**
    a. Actinic keratosis
    b. Arsenical keratosis
    c. Seborrhoeic keratosis
    d. Solar keratosis

27. **Another name for cutaneous squamous cell carcinoma in situ is:**
    a. Leucoplakia
    b. Bowen's disease
    c. Actinic keratosis
    d. Seborrhoeic keratosis

28. **Congenital melanocytic nevi can be differentiated from acquired melanocytic nevi except by their:**
    a. Age at onset
    b. Colour
    c. Size
    d. Amount of hair on surface

29. **The type of vascular lesion which does not change much after birth and does not regress is:**
    a. Strawberry haemangioma
    b. Spider angioma
    c. Port wine stains
    d. Cherry angioma

30. **Eye finding in Sturge Weber syndrome is:**
    a. Cataract
    b. Capillary angiomas
    c. Glaucoma
    d. Iridocyclitis

31. **Neurologic findings in Sturge Weber syndrome include:**
    a. Epilepsy
    b. Mental retardation
    c. Cerebral calcification
    d. All of the above

32. **Strawberry haemangioma regresses usually by this age:**
    a. 6 months
    b. 12 months
    c. 2 years
    d. 5 years

33. **Strawberry haemangiomas tend to grow initially till the age of:**
    a. 3 months
    b. 6 months
    c. 9 months
    d. 12 months

34. **Intervention for strawberry angioma includes:**
    a. Intralesional steroid injections
    b. Carbon Dioxide laser
    c. Cryotherapy
    d. Topic imiquimod

35. **A vascular lesion that is not elevated above the surface of skin is:**
    a. Strawberry haemangioma
    b. Spider angioma
    c. Port wine stains
    d. Cherry angioma

36. **Cavernous haemangiomas are of this colour:**
    a. Dull red
    b. Bright red
    c. Fiery red
    d. Bluish red

Chapter 21

Cutaneous Neoplasms, Cysts and Hyperplasias

37. Senile angiomas are of this colour:
a. Dull red
b. Bright red
c. Bluish red
d. Bluish green

38. Linear arrangement of pigmented papules since birth is usually a:
a. Epidermal nevus
b. Becker's nevus
c. Congenital melanocytic nevi
d. Cafe au lait macules

39. This is not a type of cutaneous cyst:
a. Pilar cyst
b. Epidermoid cyst
c. Milia
d. Cystic hygroma

40. Epidermal cysts have this in the centre:
a. Umbilication
b. Punctum
c. Projecting spine
d. Hair shaft jutting out

41. As against keloids, hypertrophic scars do not continue to grow beyond this period after injury:
a. 1 month
b. 3 months
c. 6 months
d. 1 year

42. A typical site of affection of keloids is:
a. Scalp
b. Back
c. Bony prominences
d. Chest

43. Keloids may follow:
a. Acne scars
b. Injury marks
c. Striae
d. All of the above

44. Keloids have a tendency to:
a. Heal
b. Recur
c. Local invasion
d. Disseminate

45. Presternal keloids are usually of this shape:
a. Oval
b. Butterfly shaped
c. Geographic
d. Annular

46. Common medical therapy for keloids includes:
a. Intralesional steroids
b Oral isotretinoin
c. Oral steroids
d. Topical isotretinoin

47. This is a common site for pyogenic granuloma:
a. Nail fold
b. Back
c. Neck
d. Shoulder

48. Corns do not occur in the:
a. Bare-foot walkers
b. Diabetics
c. Middle aged
d. People who wear shoes

49. These are prominent over a callus:
a. Keratin core
b. Blood vessels
c. Dermatoglyphic lines
d. Projecting spines

50. Commonest site for occurrence of corns is base of:
a. First metatarsal
b. Third metatarsal
c. Second metatarsal
d. Fifth metatarsal

51. All of the following sentences are true about melanoma *except*:
a. It is the most common tumour of the skin
b. Long term sunexposure is a risk factor
c. Metastatic nodules signify poor prognosis
d. Melanoma *in situ* has good prognosis

52. The most common mucocutaneous malignancy in India is:
a. Melanoma
b. Basal cell carcinoma
c. Squamous cell carcinoma
d. None

53. All of the following are paraneoplastic syndromes, *except*:
a. Erythema gyratum repens
b. Acanthosis nigricans
c. Paraneoplastic pemphigus
d. Cutaneous metastases

54. False regarding hypertrophic scars is:
a. They are pruritic
b. Limited to the site of injury
c. Donot recur
d. None of the above

55. **Post-traumatic vascular proliferation is:**
    a. Infantile haemangioma
    b. Keloid
    c. Pyogenic granuloma
    d. Scar

56. **Predisposing factors for skin cancer are:**
    a. Smoking
    b. UV light
    c. Chronic ulcer
    d. Infrared light

57. **Mycosis fungoides affects:**
    a. T cell
    c. NK cell
    b. B cell
    d. K cell

58. **Not true about skin tag:**
    a. Associated with seborrhoeic keratosis
    b. Pedunculated
    c. Most common site—skin and axilla
    d. Premalignant

ANSWERS

1-d,	2-b,	3-d,	4-c,	5-a,	6-a,	7-c,	8-d,	9-c,	10-d,
11-d,	12-a,	13-c,	14-d,	15-d,	16-b,	17-a,	18-c,	19-c,	20-d,
21-d,	22-a,	23-a,	24-b,	25-d,	26-c,	27-b,	28-c,	29-c,	30-c,
31-d,	32-d,	33-d,	34-a,	35-c,	36-d,	37-a,	38-a,	39-c,	40-b,
41-b,	42-d,	43-d,	44-b,	45-b,	46-a,	47-a,	48-a,	49-c,	50-c,
51-a,	52-c,	53-d,	54-a,	55-c,	56-b and c,	57-a,	58-d		

Genetic Diseases of the Skin

Genetic diseases predominantly affecting the skin are termed genodermatoses. Many of the geno-dermatoses show associated affection of other body systems (e.g. tuberous sclerosis or neurofibro-matosis). In such conditions, the skin lesions provide early pointers to the diagnosis of the genodermatosis. In tuberous sclerosis, screening newborns or infants for presence of ash leaf macules by a Wood's lamp may be used as a tool for early identification. In neurofibromatosis, screening newborns or infants for café au lait macules helps in early diagnosis of the condition. While most of the genodermatoses are not life-threatening there are exceptions like some forms of epidermolysis bullosa and ichthyosiform erythroderma.

EPIDERMOLYSIS BULLOSA

This is a genetic disorder in which bullae and erosions (Figs 22.1 and 22.2) occur following minor day-to-day trauma or friction. Presentation is at birth or in infancy. Feet, hands (Fig. 22.3), knees and elbows, and buttocks are commonly involved. The lesions heal without or with scarring which may be severe enough to cause deformities in some patients. At times the mucosae are affected.

No treatment is effective. General measures include avoidance of trauma and prevention of secondary infection with the use of topical

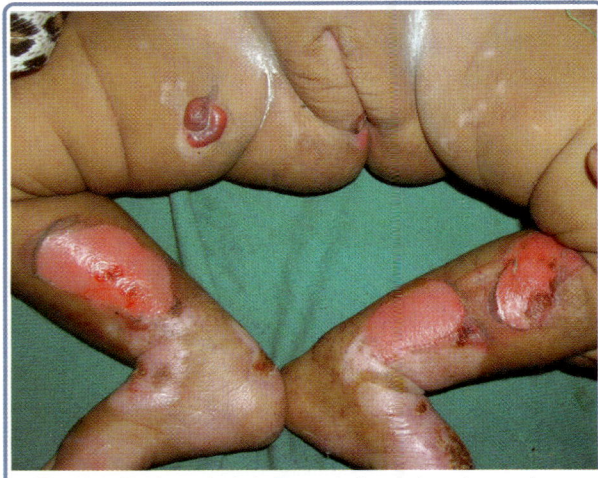

Fig. 22.2: Epidermolysis bullosa—bullae and erosions on lower extremities

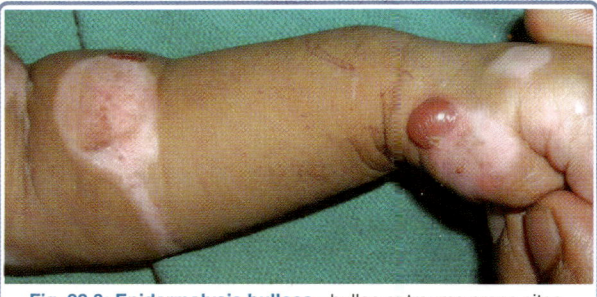

Fig. 22.3: Epidermolysis bullosa—bullae at trauma prone sites, healing with post-inflammatory depigmentation

antibiotics. Oral phenytoin and vitamin E have been used with inconsistent results.

PALMOPLANTAR KERATODERMA

Thickening of palms (Fig. 22.4) and soles (keratoderma) can be acquired or congenital. Acquired causes include occupational keratoderma (due to the friction of manual labour), psoriasis or keratoderma blenorrhagicum of Reiter's disease. Hereditary palmoplantar keratodermas present as diffuse thickening of the skin of palms and soles since birth or childhood. The affected skin feels rough or hard and shows prominent dermato-glyphic lines. Painful cracks (fissures) occur over the thickened skin. Some cases may be associated with other genetic diseases while others may have internal organ affection. Thus, palmoplantar kerato-derma serves as a marker for internal disease in such patients. Treatment includes topical application of emollients like white soft paraffin or urea or

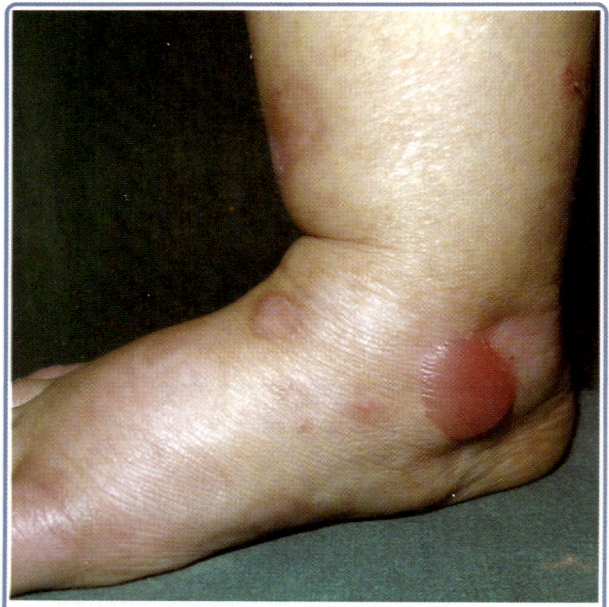

Fig. 22.1: Epidermolysis bullosa—bullae over trauma prone skin in a child

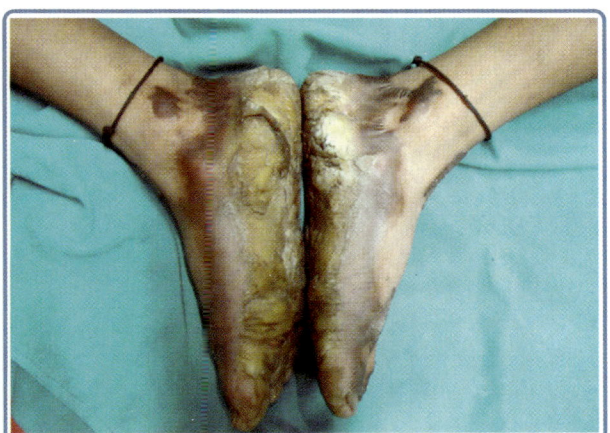

Fig. 22.4: Plantar keratoderma—marked thickening of palms and soles with fissuring in a child is usually due to hereditary palmoplantar keratoderma

keratolytic agents like salicyclic acid. Systemic treatment includes oral retinoids like isotretinoin.

DARIER'S DISEASE

This dominantly inherited genodermatosis is characterised by hyperpigmented, verrucous, scaly, crusted papules in seborrhoeic areas of the face, scalp and trunk (Fig. 22.5). Grayish dirty warty keratotic papules occur over scalp, retroauricular and nasolabial folds, and central part of chest. Pits and keratoses can occur on the palms and soles. Lesions show summer exacerbation with maceration and secondary infection producing a peculiar malodour. Nails show longitudinal striations and terminal nicking. Skin biopsy is diagnostic. Oral retinoids like isotretinoin induce a temporary remission or improvement. Oral and topical antibiotics can be used if there is secondary bacterial infection.

ICHTHYOSES

This, usually inherited, group of disorders is characterised by dry, scaly and rough skin. The scales somewhat resemble those of a fish (Greek, *ichthys*—fish). The scales result from either excess keratin production or increased adherence of corneocytes leading to inability to shed keratin material. Ichthyosis can be acquired or congenital.

> **Acquired ichthyosis may result from**
> - *Infections:* Leprosy, HIV infection.
> - *Drugs:* Cholesterol lowering agents, butyrophenones.
> - *Metabolic causes:* Malnutrition, essential fatty acid deficiency.
> - *Systemic causes:* Hypothyroidism, renal failure, antihidrosis due to neuropathies.
> - *Malignancies:* Hodgkin's lymphoma.

Ichthyosis vulgaris is the commonest and the mildest type of ichthyosis that is transmitted as an autosomal dominant trait. It presents after 3 months of age as fine brown-coloured scales with 'pasted on' appearance, distributed predominantly on the extensors of the extremities and trunk with sparing of flexors. Other associated manifestations are follicular papules and hyperkeratosis of palms and soles. Features of atopy are common in these patients. The condition may improve with increasing age.

Lamellar ichthyosis is inherited as an autosomal recessive condition and manifests as large, brown, thick, quadrangular scales at birth. At birth, a thick membrane of keratin may be present encasing the baby called collodion membrane. The scales are more prominent over the extensors but the flexors are not spared.

X-linked ichthyosis is inherited as an X-linked recessive trait; hence, only males are affected. Scales are dark, large and prominent on sides of the neck and extensors of the extremities (Fig. 22.6) and trunk. Other features include punctate corneal opacities and cryptorchidism.

Treatment includes maintaining the moisture of the skin with application of topical agents like liquid paraffin, white soft paraffin or coconut oil. Topical urea, salicylic acid, retinoids and propylene glycol are also useful. In severe cases oral retinoids like isotretinoin or acitretin are useful to give partial and temporary benefit.

NEUROFIBROMATOSIS (VON RECKLINGHAUSEN'S DISEASE)

This is an autosomal dominantly inherited disorder. Classical type 1 neurofibromatosis is most common and characterised by multiple neurofibromas, café au lait macules, axillary freckles and Lisch nodules

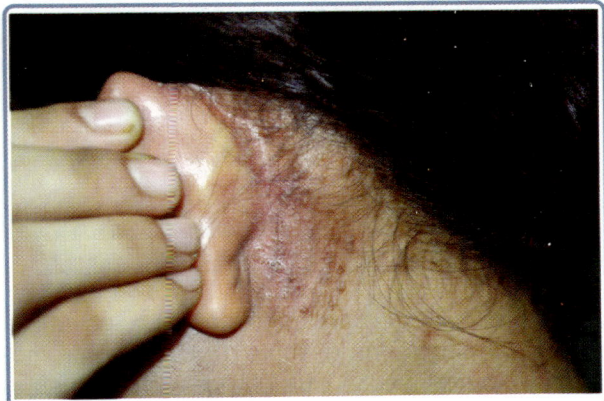

Fig. 22.5: Darier's disease—keratotic erythematous papules behind ears in distribution resembling seborrhoeic dermatitis is characteristic

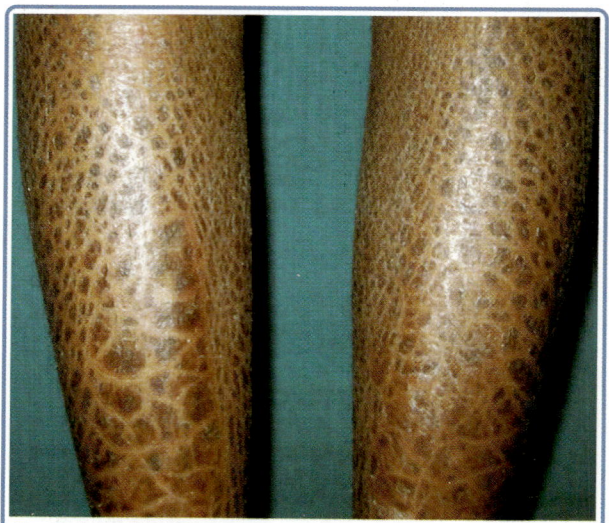

Fig. 22.6: Ichthyosis vulgaris—large fish-like scales with dry surface affecting extensors of extremities

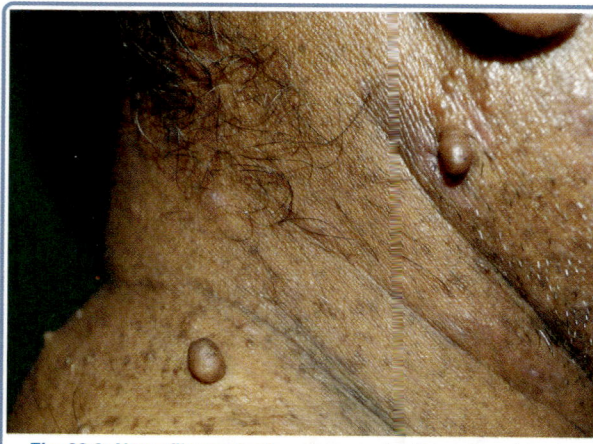

Fig. 22.8: Neurofibromatosis—close up of soft papulonodules in neurofibromatosis. Note background freckling

in the iris. Type 2 neurofibromatosis presents as bilateral acoustic neuromas. Cutaneous neurofibromas (Figs 22.7 and 22.8) are soft in consistency and can be pushed down into the skin through a dermal defect by light pressure using a finger and pop out when pressure is released (button hole sign). Crow's rule states that presence of 5 or more café au lait spots of size 5 cm diameter in an adult makes the possibility of neurofibromatosis quite high (Fig. 22.9). Crow's sign refers to the occurrence of small hyper-pigmented macules ('freckles') over axillae.

The neurofibromas may also be subcutaneous may follow the course of a nerve trunk or may be present along the nerve roots. Plexiform neurofibromas are large, soft and pendulous masses of neural tissue which have bag of worms like feel on palpation (Fig. 22.10). Neurofibromas along nerve roots may compress them against vertebrae and lead to compression signs. Neurofibromas can be

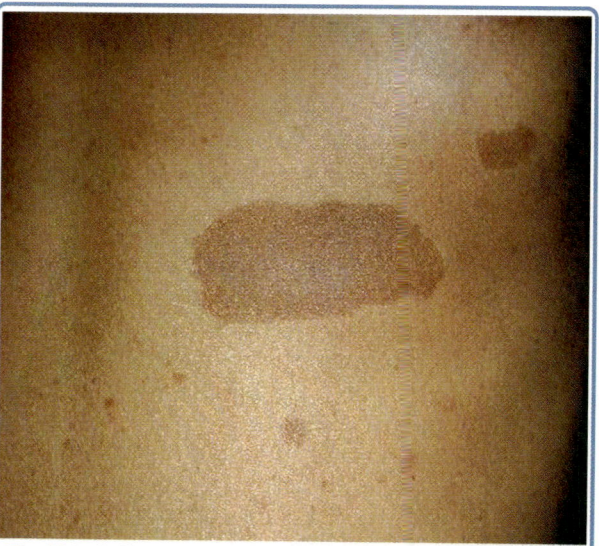

Fig. 22.9: Café au lait spots—well defined brown-coloured macules and patches

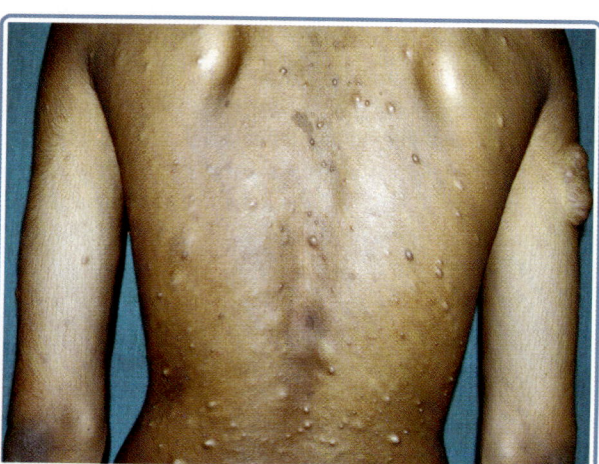

Fig. 22.7: Neurofibromatosis—multiple soft nodules of variable size and cafe au lait spots

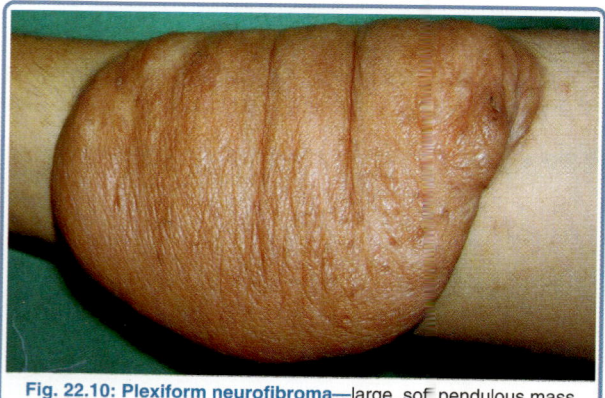

Fig. 22.10: Plexiform neurofibroma—large, soft pendulous mass

associated with multiple endocrine neoplasias like medullary carcinoma of thyroid or phaeochromocytoma. During the life time of a patient with neurofibromatosis there is a small chance of malignancy (neurofibrosarcoma) developing in a neurofibroma.

TUBEROUS SCLEROSIS

This is a neurocutaneous disorder with autosomal dominant inheritance. Tuberous sclerosis is also known by the acronym epiloia (epi—epilepsy, loi—low intelligence, a—adenoma sebaceum) a classic triad of this disorder. Adenoma sebaceum are the angiofibromas that occur as brown-coloured papules on the cheeks, nose and forehead (Fig. 22.11). Other skin manifestations include knobby, skin-coloured 'shagreen plaques' over lower back,

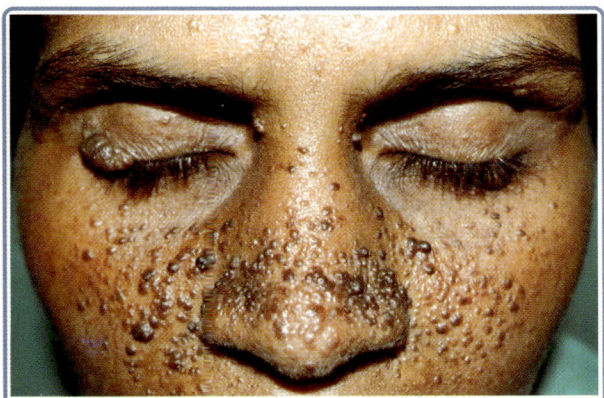

Fig. 22.11: Adenoma sebaceum in tuberous sclerosis—firm papules over central face in symmetrical distribution

Koenen's tumours (periungual fibromas) and ash leaf macules. Ash leaf macules are the earliest to develop being frequently detectable at birth under Wood's lamp. They are seen as oval hypopigmented macules over trunk (Figs 22.12–22.14) or extremities. Complications like astrocytomas or ependymomas of brain may occur; retinal phakomas and renal tumours can also develop later in life.

STURGE WEBER SYNDROME

This syndrome is characterised by a bright red-coloured capillary malformation (portwine stain) on the face in the area supplied by ophthalmic division of trigeminal nerve along with epilepsy and mental retardation. Vascular malformation of the

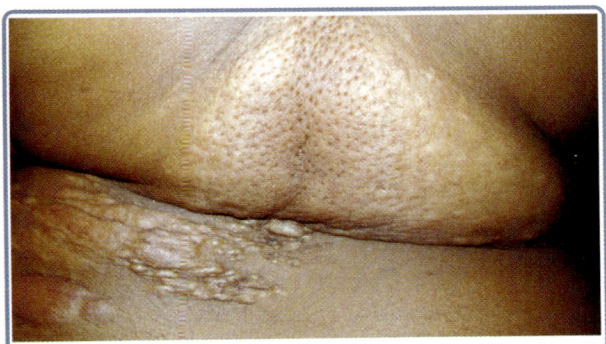

Fig. 22.12: Shagreen plaque in tuberous sclerosis—skin-coloured plaque of collagen nevi with peau d'orange appearance

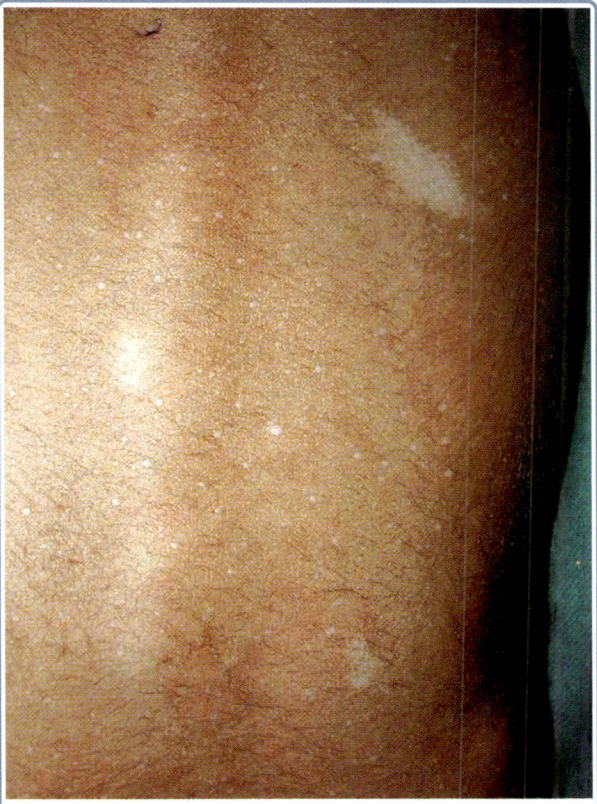

Fig. 22.13: Large ash leaf macules and multiple confetti-like smaller macules in tuberous sclerosis

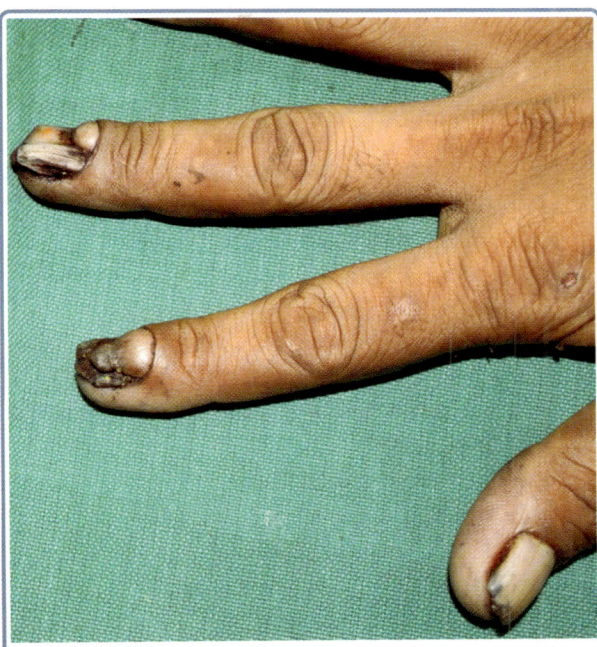

Fig. 22.14: Koenen's periungual firbomas in tuberous sclerosis

leptomeninges leads to epilepsy, mental retardation, hemiparesis and hemianosmia. Calcification along the arteries of cerebral cortex gives the appearance of double-contoured 'tram tracks'. Ocular abnormalities like glaucoma may also be present.

Chapter

22

Genetic Diseases of the Skin

MCQs

1. **An example of an autosomal dominantly transmitted skin disease is:**
   a. Albinism
   b. Neurofibromatosis
   c. Lamellar ichthyosis
   d. Xeroderma pigmentosum

2. **An example of an autosomal recessively transmitted skin disease is:**
   a. Darier's disease
   b. Tuberous sclerosis
   c. Ichthyosis vulgaris
   d. Albinism

3. **An example of life-threatening genetic skin disease is:**
   a. Tuberous sclerosis
   b. Ichthyosis vulgaris
   c. Neurofibromatosis
   d. Epidermolysis bullosa

4. **A genetic skin disease that leads to skin lesions at site of trauma is:**
   a. Tuberous sclerosis
   b. Palmoplantar keratoderma
   c. Neurofibromatosis
   d. Epidermolysis bullosa

5. **A skin disease characterised by dirty warty papules on the body is:**
   a. Darier's disease
   b. Tuberous sclerosis
   c. Neurofibromatosis
   d. Albinism

6. **Which of the following is true of epidermolysis bullosa?**
   a. It begins in childhood
   b. Big bullae are rarely seen
   c. Bullae occur over flexural regions
   d. Effective treatment is available

7. **Which of the following is false for Ichthyoses?**
   a. They are always genetically transmitted
   b. Skin lesions resemble fish scales
   c. Skin is dry and flaky
   d. Condition improves with application of emollients

8. **Which of the following is false for neuro-fibromatosis?**
   a. It is also known as Osler-Weber-Rendu syndrome
   b. Nodular nerve thickening is common
   c. Numerous café au lait spots are diagnostic
   d. Malignant tumours are uncommon in neuro-fibromatosis

9. **Which of the following is true for tuberous sclerosis?**
   a. Ash leaf macules are pinkish brown in colour
   b. Adenoma sebaceum lesions are present from birth
   c. Adenoma sebaceum lesions are seen all over the body
   d. Wood's lamp is useful for diagnosis

10. **Which of the following is true to Sturge-Weber syndrome?**
    a. Strawberry haemangioma over face is present
    b. Vascular malformation is present over face
    c. X-ray skull shows nodular calcification
    d. Epilepsy and mental retardation are uncommon associations

11. **Which of the following is false for Darier's disease?**
    a. Recessively inherited
    b. Skin biopsy is diagnostic
    c. Oral retinoids are helpful
    d. Lesions show summer exacerbation

12. **All of the following may cause acquired ichthyosis except:**
    a. Leprosy
    b. Lymphoma
    c. Malnutrition
    d. Parkinsonism

13. **Lisch nodules are seen in:**
    a. Von Recklinghausen's disease
    b. Lupus vulgaris
    c. Leprosy
    d. Lymphogranuloma venereum

14. **Café au lait spots are seen in:**
    a. Neurofibromatosis
    b. Gardner syndrome
    c. Cockayne syndrome
    d. Down syncrome

15. **A patient has multiple meningiomas, acoustic neuroma and hyper-pigmented skin lesions. The most likely diagnosis is:**
    a. Neurofibromatosis
    b. Tuberous sclerosis
    c. Von Hippel-Lindau disease
    d. Sturge-Weber syndrome

16. **Adenoma sebaceum is a feature of:**
    a. NF
    b. Tuberous sclerosis
    c. Xanthomatosis
    d. Incontinentia pigmenti

17. **All of the following are features of tuberous sclerosis *except*:**
    a. Koenen's tumour   b. Ash leaf macule
    c. Nevus depigmentosus d. Shagreen patch

18. **Koenen's tumour is seen in:**
    a. Tuberous sclerosis   b. NF
    c. Verruca vulgaris   d. SLE

Chapter 22

Genetic Diseases of the Skin

ANSWERS

1-b,	2-d,	3-d,	4-d,	5-a,	6-a,	7-a,	8-a,	9-d,	10-b,
11-a,	12-d,	13-a,	14-a,	15-a,	16-b,	17-c,	18-a		

Miscellaneous Disorders

DIFFERENTIAL DIAGNOSIS OF SUBCUTANEOUS NODULES

As is explicit in the term, subcutaneous nodules are the result of a pathological process that affects the subcutaneous fat (panniculus). Before considering the following conditions one must be sure that the nodules are not related to lymph nodes (lymphadenitis), tendons (ganglion), veins (thrombophlebitis) or nerves (leprosy or neurofibroma).

Broadly the processes affecting the panniculus can be divided as follows.

HYPERSENSITIVITY PHENOMENA

Inflammatory diseases of the panniculus are termed panniculitis. They include the following:

Erythema Induratum (Bazin's Disease)

Seen as ulcerating nodules over calves of young females with underlying tuberculosis.

Erythema Nodosum Leprosum

Seen over face and extremities as tender erythematous papulonodules and are due to a reaction to killing of lepra bacilli usually after therapy for lepromatous leprosy.

Erythema Nodosum

Seen over shins of young women as a symmetric eruption of tender reddish nodules and is a hypersensitivity response to streptococcal or tuberculous infections.

Periarteritis Nodosa

A multisystem leucocytoclastic vasculitis involving smaller arteries. Nodules are erythematous, purpuric and pulsatile.

INFECTIONS

Furuncles

One or many, tender, warm, erythematous nodules with central pointing are a result of staphylococcal infection of a deep-seated hair follicle.

Abscesses

Tender, warm, swellings with or without overlying erythema or softening are accompanied by bouts of fever with chills.

Cold Abscess

Non-tender, skin-coloured or reddish, slowly evolving, soft, cystic swelling that overlies a tuberculous focus (lymph node, joint, bone, etc.).

Nodulocystic Acne

Insidious cystic skin-coloured or erythematous nodules with comedones over face, neck or back of young males.

GRANULOMATOUS DISORDERS

Rheumatoid Nodules

Asymptomatic skin-coloured nodules over bony prominences of limbs in rheumatoid arthritis (Fig. 23.1).

Rheumatic Fever

Small, transient, asymptomatic nodules over extensors of limbs in children with rheumatic fever.

Sarcoidosis

Asymptomatic skin-coloured or erythematous nodules on trunk or limbs of patients with sarcoidosis. Upper or lower respiratory tract, bones, lymph nodes and liver are commonly involved.

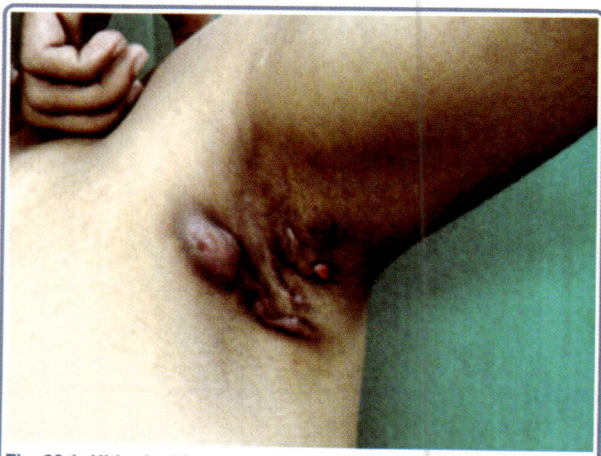

Fig. 23.1: Hidradenitis suppurativa—suppurative nodules, bridge-like scars and comedones in axillae and groins are the typical presentation

DEPOSITS

Gouty Tophi

Yellowish red nodules over ears and bony prominences of limbs later break down to discharge urate crystals. Joints are predominantly involved in gout.

Amyloidosis

Asymptomatic nodules over face with or without purpura, macroglossia, peripheral neuropathy and nephropathy occur here. Myeloma is associated.

TUMOURS

Neurofibroma

Soft, asymptomatic, skin-coloured nodules accompany café au lait spots in neurofibromatosis.

Fibroma

One or two, firm asymptomatic, skin-coloured nodules.

Lipoma

Single or multiple, soft, lobulated, skin-coloured swellings with pseudofluctuation and slipping of edge under the examining finger.

Metastasis

Single or multiple, firm, skin-coloured or reddish, smooth, rounded nodules situated over normal skin usually in elderly persons.

MISCELLANEOUS

Hematoma

Skin coloured or bluish, tender nodules that follow a history of blunt trauma.

Sebaceous Cysts

Skin-coloured or yellowish, smooth surfaced, rounded, swellings with cystic feel, with or without a punctum. Pressure may elicit foul smelling, thick, white discharge from the punctum.

> **Summary:** Subcutaneous nodules may result from hypersensitivity phenomena like erythema nodosum, infections like furuncles and abscess, granulomatous disorders like rheumatoid nodules, deposits like gouty tophi or tumours like neurofibromas.

DIFFERENTIAL DIAGNOSIS OF VESICULAR RASH

The numerous causes of vesicular skin rash include the following.

INFECTIONS

Chickenpox

Appearance of crops of red papules and papulovesicles on erythematous base over trunk, extremities and mucosae in the young.

Herpes Simplex

Grouped vesicle based in erythema affecting mucocutaneous junctions and adjacent skin and mucosa and accompanied by mild constitutional symptoms and regional lymphadenitis.

Herpes Zoster

Unilateral, grouped vesicles based on erythema affecting one or two nerve segments and accompanied by pain and paraesthesiae in the elderly or the immunocompromised.

Impetigo

Clustered thin-walled clear or cloudy vesicles over face of infants and young children are accompanied by erosions covered with thin honey-coloured crusts and a few pustules.

ECZEMAS

In this group, vesicular lesions are grouped and are based on erythema and oedema. With progression, the vesicles burst to form erosions, which ooze serous fluid. Distribution differs according to the type of eczema.

Atopic Dermatitis

Face and extremities are affected in infants.

Contact Dermatitis

Lesions are localised to the area of contact. Photo-contact dermatitis affects those areas of contact that are exposed to the sun. Airborne photocontact dermatitis affects exposed regions and flexures.

Autosensitisation Eczema

Sudden symmetric involvement of flexor aspects of the trunk, limbs and face.

Chapter 23

Miscellaneous Disorders

Id Eruption

Scattered papulovesicular lesions erupt simultaneously all over the body.

HYPERSENSITIVITY PHENOMENA

Erythema Multiforme

Vesicles accompany erythematous macules, papules, purpura and the diagnostic target lesions. Mucosae and palms/soles are preferentially affected.

Stevens-Johnson Syndrome

Severe mucosal erosions with painful haemorrhagic crusts of lips are associated with scattered or widespread purpura and erythema with vesiculation. Target lesions may occur and palms and soles are usually affected.

PHOTOSENSITIVE DERMATOSES

Drug-induced Photosensitivity

History of drug ingestion is present. Vesicles and erythema occur over sun-exposed regions.

Polymorphous Light Eruption

Papulovesicles over sun-exposed regions (face, neck, hands and forearms).

CHRONIC VESICOBULLOUS DERMATOSES

Dermatitis Herpetiformis

Papules and vesicles, in grouped configuration, over elbows, knees, scapulae, buttocks and extensors or limbs occur in this autoimmune disorder.

Pemphigus Foliaceus

Superficial vesicles, with a tendency to burst and form thin scale crusts, may involve the whole of the body.

Pemphigus Vulgaris

Although most cases show bullae and erosions, a few may present with scattered vesicles and occasional bullae in initial stages. Oral erosions are present.

Bullous Pemphigoid

Although a typical case shows large tense bullae, some cases present with vesicles on a background of large patches of burning erythema. Oral cavity is spared.

MISCELLANEOUS

Miliaria Crystallina

Tiny (few mm), thin roofed, clear coloured vesicles occur over extremities and trunk during summer or following fever.

Prurigo (Insect Bite Reaction)

Vesicular and papulovesicular lesions on exposed parts (extremities and face) in children suggest this diagnosis.

> **Summary:** Differential diagnosis of vesicular rash includes infections caused by the herpes viruses and staphylococcal impetigo, eczematous dermatoses like contact allergic dermatitis and id eruption, hypersensitivity dermatoses like erythema multiforme and Stevens-Johnson syndrome, photosensitive dermatoses like polymorphous light eruption, chronic vesicobullous disorders like dermatitis herpetiformis and pemphigus foliaceus and miscellaneous conditions like miliaria crystallina and prurigo mitis.

DIFFERENTIAL DIAGNOSIS OF RASH WITH FEVER

This common combination of symptoms can result from numerous causes. In most patients the rash and fever are due to the same cause except when drug rash occurs in a case with pyrexia due to other causes.

VIRAL INFECTIONS

Chickenpox

The condition affects older children and adolescents. Fever and constitutional symptoms are followed by crops of centripetal polymorphic rash consisting of scattered papules and vesicles, the red flare around the latter gives 'dew drop on rose petal' appearance (Fig. 23.2).

Measles

Preschool children are the commonest victims. Fever and constitutional symptoms are followed closely by Koplick spots on the buccal mucosa and a generalised erythematous maculopapular rash with a tendency to coalesce, scale and pigment as the lesions evolve.

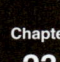

Chapter
23

Miscellaneous Disorders

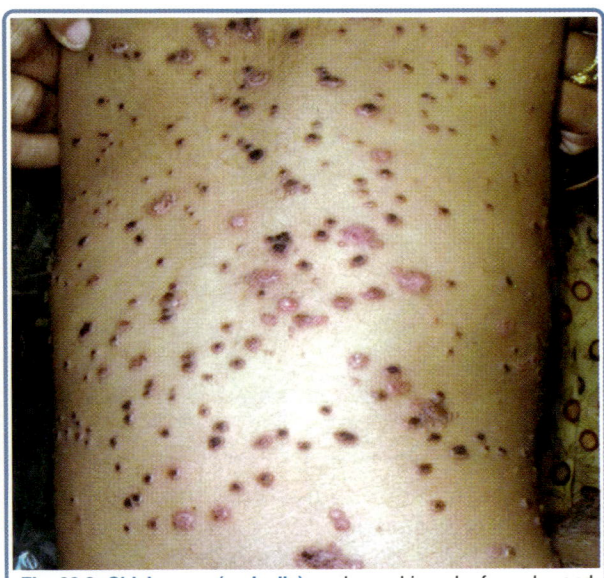

Fig. 23.2: Chickenpox (varicella)—polymorphic rash of papules and papulovesicles over trunk in various stages of evolution

Rubella

Older children, adolescents and young adults are affected. Fever, mild constitutional symptoms and lymphadenopathy are followed by an erythematous maculopapular rash that fades away within 3–5 days without pigmentation.

Primary HIV Infection

Young adults with a risk factor for HIV (which may need to be elicited with direct questioning) present with fever, constitutional symptoms and a generalised maculopapular rash that may coalesce and resemble measles.

Infectious Mononucleosis

Young adults are commonly affected. Fever and constitutional symptoms are followed by hepatitis (with or without icterus), lymphadenopathy and a generalised maculopapular rash. Ampicillin administered for the initial complaint of fever precipitates the rash. Paul-Bunnel test is positive.

Other Viral Infections

Coxsackie, echo, adenoviruses and hepatitis B can induce both fever and rash. Dengue haemorrhagic fever presents with a generalised purpuric rash that appears after several days of high fever.

NON-VIRAL INFECTIONS

Rickettsial Infections

Rocky Mountain spotted fever (fever, toxaemia and generalised erythematous, and purpuric rash).

Spirochaetal Infections

Commonest of these is secondary syphilis, the widespread papular or papulopustular rash of which is accompanied by fever, joint pains, malaise and lymphadenopathy. Uncommon example is leptospirosis (fever with rash over lower limbs).

Bacterial Infections

Type II lepra reactions may be a presenting manifestation of lepromatous leprosy. It presents with erythema nodosum leprosum lesions on face and limbs with fever and neuritis. Skin smears and a biopsy are necessary to confirm the diagnosis.

Meningococcaemia is accompanied by purpuric and pustular lesions. Uncommonly, typhoid may be accompanied by a bright red, macular (roseolar rash) rash on trunk at the height of fever. Bacterial endocarditis presents as fever with palmoplantar erythema, purpura and cutaneous infarcts.

HYPERSENSITIVITY PHENOMENA

Drug Eruptions

Maculopapular drug eruptions and drug-induced exfoliative dermatitis are sometimes accompanied by fever, which may either be due to the same drug or be due to the underlying condition for which the drug was given.

Erythema Multiforme, Stevens-Johnson Syndrome and Toxic Epidermal Necrolysis

Whether drug-induced or otherwise they are commonly associated with fever.

Erythema Nodosum

These painful nodules on legs are usually associated with fever.

AUTOIMMUNE DISEASES

Systemic Lupus Erythematosus

Butterfly erythema, photosensitivity and discoid lesions may occur with fever.

Dermatomyositis

Facial erythema with violaceous lid oedema accompanies fever and proximal muscle weakness.

Rheumatic Fever

Erythema marginatum and subcutaneous nodules are transient lesions associated with active rheumatic fever.

Chapter
23

Miscellaneous Disorders

Vasculitis of Small or Large Vessels of Varying Causes

This includes Henoch-Schönlein purpura, Wegener's granulomatosis, polyarteritis nodosa and rheumatoid vasculitis.

Juvenile Rheumatoid Arthritis

Active disease presents as fever with erythematous and urticarial rash.

MISCELLANEOUS

Malignancies

Lymphomas and leukemias may present with fever and a rash (leukemids).

Disseminated Intravascular Coagulation

Resulting usually from septicaemia, this causes fever, purpura, digital gangrene and cutaneous infarcts. Septicaemia can also cause pustules.

Opportunistic Infections

In the HIV era, opportunistic infections with a variety of organisms can induce fever and skin lesions. Examples include cryptococcosis, candidiasis, aspergillosis, cysticercosis, strongyloidosis and bacillary angiomatosis.

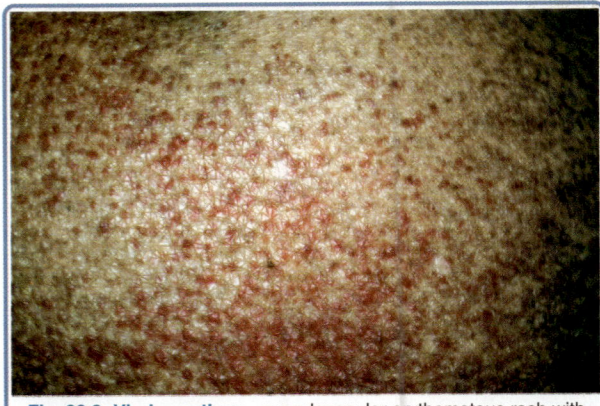

Fig. 23.3: Viral exanthem—maculopapular erythematous rash with purpura in some of the lesions

Although, maculopapular eruption is the most common presentation, an exanthem may also be vesicular, e.g. chickenpox. Although most exanthems are monomorphous or have just one or two types of skin lesions. Some conditions like chickenpox are characterised by three or more types of skin lesions (polymorphous, e.g. macules, papule and vesicles in chickenpox).

The commonest of the viral exanthems is measles. However, many other viruses can cause rash resembling measles [morbilliform rash]. These rashes are not easy to distinguish from maculopapular drug eruption. However, clinical features and investigations are helpful for making such a distinction (Table 23.1).

The rash of measles is preceded by an enanthem (Koplik spots). These are punctate

Summary: Common conditions that present with a combination of fever and skin rash are chickenpox, measles, rubella and other viral exanthems including primary HIV infection. Type II lepra reaction presents as fever with erythema nodosum leprosum. Occasionally, other infections like meningococcaemia, syphilis, typhoid and leptospirosis may present as fever wth rash. Drug eruptions, erythema multiforme, Stevens-Johnson syndrome and erythema nodosum are frequently associated with fever. Lupus erythematosus, dermatomyositis, rheumatic fever and vasculitis are some important autoimmune conditions presenting with this combination. Finally, malignancies and opportunistic infections in the HIV infected may also lead to fever and skin lesions.

EXANTHEMS

Any sudden widespread erythematous eruption on skin is termed an exanthem. Traditionally the term is used for describing viral rashes. However, other conditions resembling viral rashes (e.g. maculopapular drug eruption) also cause an exanthem (Fig. 23.3). Similar erythematous eruption on mucosae is termed an enanthem.

TABLE 23.1: Distinguishing viral exanthem and maculopapular drug rash

Parameter	Viral exanthema	Drug rash
Age	Common in young	Common in elderly
Associated fever	Common	Uncommon
Pruritus	Mild or absent	Moderate or severe
Drug history	May be absent	Present
Evolution of rash	Cephalocaudal	Begins on trunk
Constitutional s/s	Common	Less common
Enanthem	Common	Less common
Lymphadenopathy	Common	Uncommon
Blood counts	Lymphocytosis	Eosinophilia
Skin biopsy	Sparse lymphocytic infiltrate, vascular change	Moderate infiltrate of lymphocytes, eosinophils, necrotics, spongiosis, parakeratosis
Devolution	Subsides in 3–5 days	Subsides in 1–2 weeks after withdrawal of drug.

whitish spots that appear a couple of days before the exanthem when the child is febrile and therefore looking for them is helpful in early diagnosis of measles. The rash consists of ill-defined erythematous macules and slightly elevated papules that tend to coalesce. The rash tends to heal with scaling and pigmentation.

PRURIGO MITIS (PRURIGO SIMPLEX)

This is an allergic response to bites of common insects like mosquitoes and fleas (Fig. 23.4).

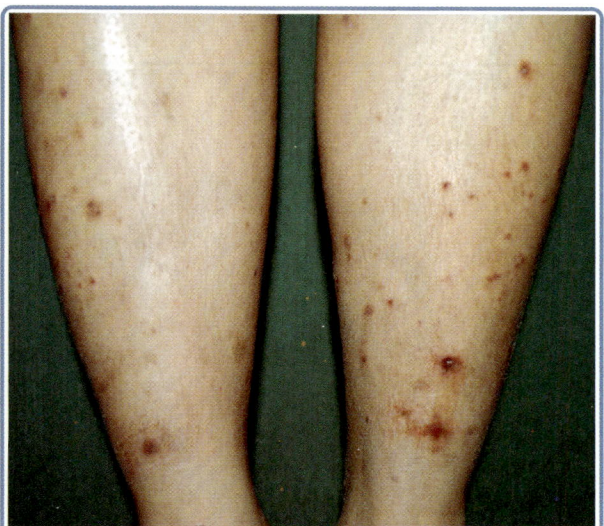

Fig. 23.4: Prurigo mitis—excoriated erythematous papules over legs

Patient Profile

The hypersensitivity affects preschool and young children, the severity of the response waning off as years pass with continued exposure to bites. Careful questioning of parents is necessary to elicit history of bites.

Morphology

Multiple pruritic erythematous, oedematous papules topped by tiny vesicles characterise the condition (Figs 23.5 and 23.6]. However, in most instances, the central vesicle is scratched off by the patient leaving behind a small serosanguineous crust.

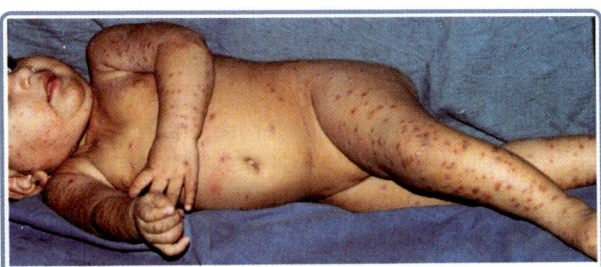

Fig. 23.5: Insect bite allergy—multiple, itchy papules on the extremities with relative sparing of covered parts

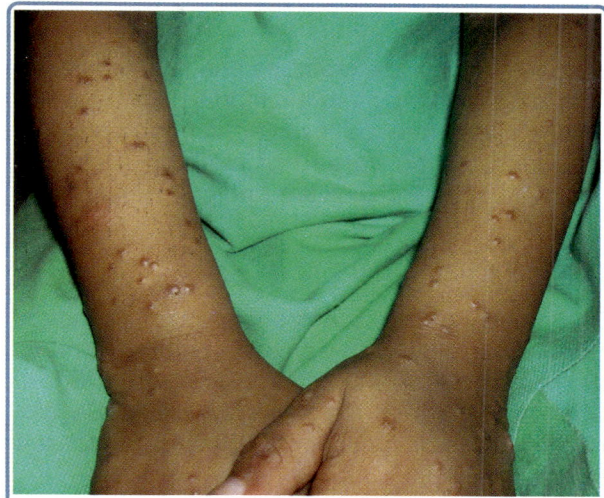

Fig. 23.6 : Prurigo mitis—multiple erythematous, oedematous papules on exposed areas

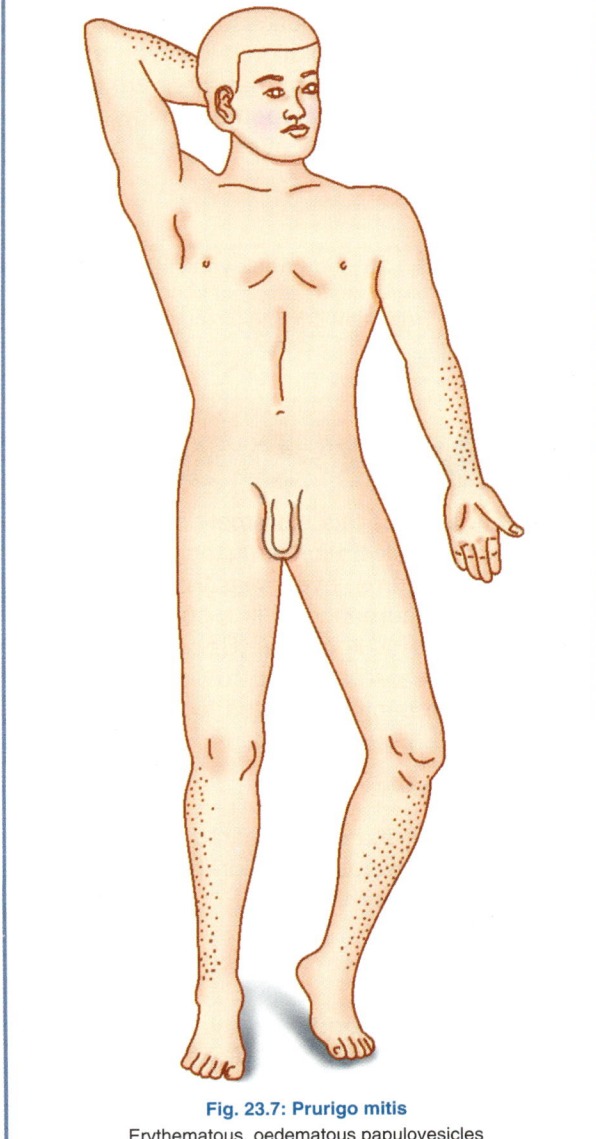

Fig. 23.7: Prurigo mitis
Erythematous, oedematous papulovesicles

Distribution

Exposed parts, viz. extremities and face are usually affected; extensors more than the flexors. However, other regions may be involved in young children, according to the pattern of clothing. Buttocks, genitals and inner thighs are rarely, if ever, involved.

Diagnosis

Differentiation from scabies is fequently required. Scabies affects web spaces, axillae, genitals, flexors of limbs, palms and soles in children, whereas these sites are spared in prurigo. Besides, mother and siblings commonly have symptoms or signs of scabies.

Therapy

Mild to moderate potency topical steroid like clobetasone butyrate or fluticasone applied for 5–7 days helps in rapid resolution. However, mosquito or flea control and repellant measures are crucial in avoiding a recurrence. Hypersensitivity gradually reduces and disappears over several months or years.

> **Summary:** Vesicular and papulovesicular lesions on exposed parts (extremities and face) in children suggest this diagnosis. Treatment comprises topical steroids and avoidance of mosquito/flea bites.

APHTHOUS ULCER

The exact cause of this extremely common variety of recurrent oral ulceration is unknown. Hypotheses proposed are trauma, hypersensitivity to drugs and immunologic disturbance. It is a component of the well defined oro-oculogenital (Behçet's syndrome) syndrome which, in addition to having a genetic basis, could probably be related to a viral infection.

Patient Profile

Although no age and sex is spared, the condition is common in young adults. Children and elderly are affected uncommonly.

Morphology

Single or a few, round or oval, 2–15 mm in diameter, rough edged, superficial or deep ulcers with a halo of erythema and oedema typify this condition (Figs 23.8 and 23.9). The ulcer is tender and its floor is covered with yellow slough. Large

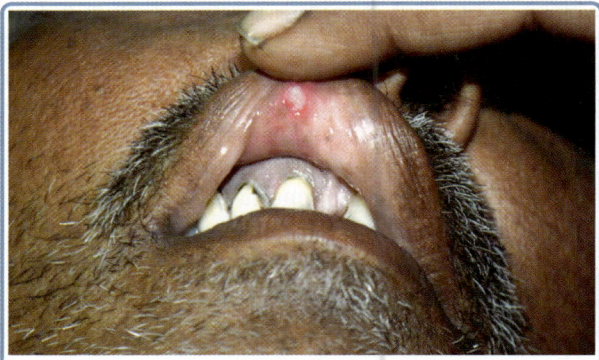

Fig. 23.8: Aphthous ulcer—small superficial ulcer covered with yellowish slough surrounded by erythematous halo

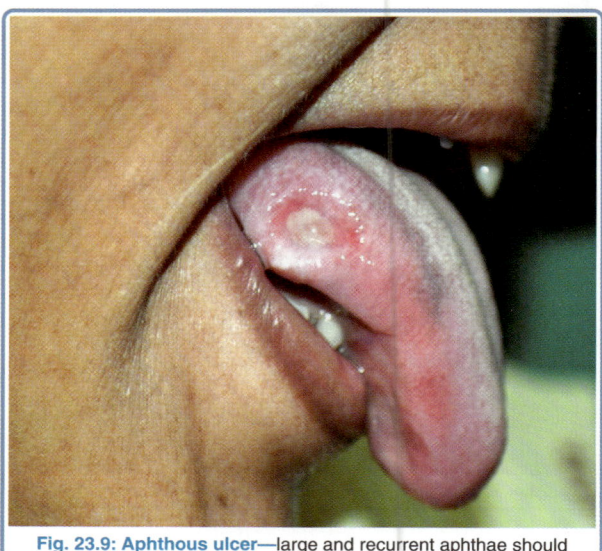

Fig. 23.9: Aphthous ulcer—large and recurrent aphthae should arouse suspicion of Behçet's disease

ones may have an indurated base, associated lymphadenopathy and heal with scars.

Distribution

Oral cavity is the commonest site. Inner aspects of lips, buccal mucosa, tongue and floor of the mouth are frequently affected. Gums, soft palate and hard palate are involved less commonly. Rarely, genital or perigenital lesions may occur, in which case. Behçet's syndrome should be considered.

Diagnosis

Differentiation from herpes simplex infections is required in case of multiple oral lesions. Presence of cutaneous papulovesicular lesions, coalescence of small superficial ulcers or erosions resulting in a polycyclic outline and a positive Tzanck smear for multinucleated cells favours herpes. Biopsy is helpful for ruling out herpetic infection. Drugs and immunodeficiency should be ruled out as causes in cases with recurrent lesions.

Therapy

Since aetiology is unknown and, the condition, self-limited within 5–10 days, therapy is symptomatic. Maintaining oral hygiene with antiseptic gargles, topical lignocaine before food and NSAIDs for large or painful lesions are helpful measures. Topical antibiotics and steroids as well as oral chloroquine and metronidazole have also been claimed to be useful.

Summary: Aphthae are a common cause of recurrent painful oral ulceration. Single or multiple, rounded ulcers with yellow slough over inner lips or cheeks characterise the disorder. Aetiology being unknown and the condition being self-limiting, the therapy is symptomatic.

MILIARIA (PRICKLY HEAT, HEAT RASH)

Miliaria is a common rash seen in hot and humid climates. It results from blockage of sweat pores (acrosyringia) by tiny keratin plugs. The blockage leads to either accumulation of fluid under the stratum corneum in clear-coloured vesicles (miliaria crystallina) or leakage of sweat within the epidermis and resultant superficial papulovesicular eruption (miliaria rubra) or secondary bacterial infection leading to papulopustular eruption (miliaria pustulosa) or bursting of duct in upper dermis and resultant dermal inflammation seen as persistent deep-seated papules (miliaria profunda).

Miliaria Crystallina

Sudden eruption of innumerable, asymptomatic, tiny (1–2 mm), superficial, clear vesicles that tend

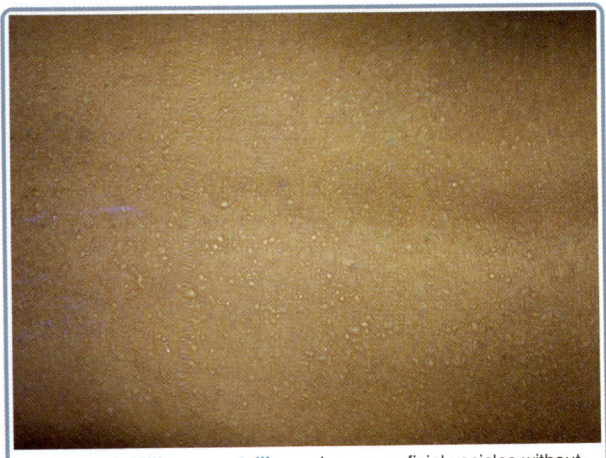

Fig. 23.10: Miliaria crystallina—clear, superficial vesicles without erythema

to coalesce is typical (Fig. 23.10). Lesions are commonly symmetric and widespread. Appearance following a febrile episode or in hot or humid environment is usual. Sometimes the vesicles may not be noticed until such time as they begin to heal with thin scaling.

Miliaria Rubra

Extremely pruritic, numerous, bright red-coloured, tiny (1–2 mm) papules based on erythema and involving large areas of trunk (Fig. 23.11) and extremities in symmetric fashion are typical. Some of the papular lesions may be topped by tiny vesicles. Extremes of heat and humidity, i.e. tropical climate, natural or man-made (ill-ventilated kitchens, basements, factories or boiler or furnace workers) are responsible.

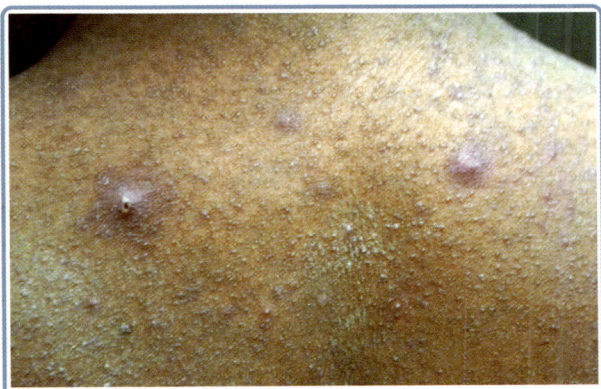

Fig. 23.11: Miliaria rubra—tiny erythematous papules and papulovesicles over covered parts. A few superimposed folliculitis lesions are also seen

Miliaria Pustulosa

Small pustules appear, topping the papular lesions of miliaria rubra. This is usually encountered in a severe case of miliaria rubra and may represent infection with gram-positive cocci.

Miliaria Profunda

This uncommon form follows long standing or recurrent miliaria rubra. Dull red- or skin-coloured papules, 2–4 mm in size, are seen over the trunk. Lesions may not itch and are slow to subside.

Therapy of all types of miliaria is based on providing cooler and drier environs and taking measures to soothe the skin, viz. apply talcum powder with antibacterial antipruritic and cooling agents and calamine lotion. Strong soaps and irritants should be avoided.

Chapter **23**

Miscellaneous Disorders

PRURITUS (ITCHING)

Definition

Pruritus or itching is an uncomfortable sensation that evokes an uncontrollable desire to scratch. Pruritus may be generalised or localised.

Generalised Pruritus

Generalised pruritus may occur:

- In absence of obvious skin lesions and dry skin (xerosis), scabies in the clean, pruritus of pregnancy, obstructive jaundice, renal failure, hypothyroidism, diabetes mellitus, lymphoma and polycythaemia.
- Associated with obvious skin lesions like scabies, pediculosis corporis, miliaria, drug eruptions, urticaria, widespread lichen planus, atopic dermatitis exfoliative dermatitis, dermatitis herpetiformis, etc.

Localised Pruritus

Localized pruritus may occur:

- In absence of obvious skin lesions: Neuro-dermatitis or seborrhoeic dermatitis to scalp or face wherein the severity of pruritus is frequently out of proportion to the visible lesions.
- Associated with obvious skin lesions like dermatophytosis, candidiasis, folliculitis, pediculosis capitis, insect bite allergy, lichen simplex chronicus, localised lichen planus, contact allergic dermatitis, photoallergic dermatitis, etc.

Treament of Pruritus

Successful therapy of pruritus depends on the physician's ability to pinpoint a cause and remove it. Oral H1 receptor blockers are popular antipruritic agents that temporarily relieve pruritus. H2 recceptor blockers and histamine release inhibitors are useful additives. Topical crotamiton and calamine lotion also alleviate pruritus.

Summary: Pruritus is a sensation that evokes a desire to scratch. It may be due to skin diseases like miliaria, scabies, pediculosis, dermatophytosis, candidiasis, insect bite allergy, urticaria, lichen planus, contact dermatitis, atopic dermatitis or seborrhoeic dermatitis. Systemic causes of pruritus include hypothyroidism, diabetes mellitus, obstructive jaundice, lymphoma and renal failure. Oral antihistaminics (H1 and H2), topical crotamiton and calamine lotion are useful in management which depends heavily on identification and treatment of underlying disorder.

GRANULOMA ANNULARE

As indicated by the name this granulomatous disorder presents as annular plaques that show a palisaded granuloma on biopsy. The condition is common in children and young adults and presents as asymptomatic, skin-coloured or slightly erythematous papules arranged in a ring. The papules frequently coalesce forming annular plaques. Extremities are commonly affected. In middle aged adults, the lesions are asociated with diabetes mellitus. The lesions subside spontaneously (frequently after a biopsy) after a variable period (Fig. 23.12).

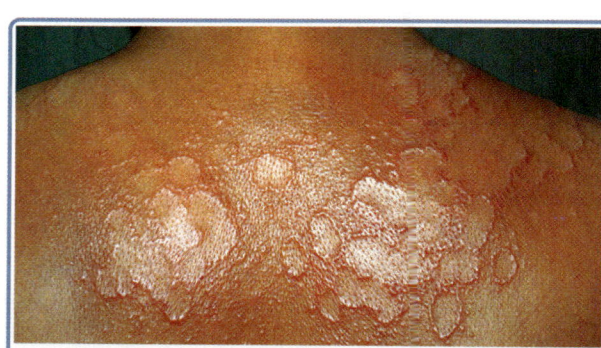

Fig. 23.12: Granuloma annulare—numerous infiltrated skin-coloured and erythematous papules arranged in annular and reticulate configuration

MCQs

1. **This is the commonest site of affection of erythema nodosum:**
   a. Face and limbs
   b. Shins
   c. Arms and thighs
   d. Hands and feet

2. **Erythema nodosum is characterised by:**
   a. Papulonodules
   b. Subcutaneous nodules
   c. Ulcerated nodules
   d. Crusted nodules

3. **Rheumatoic nodules are seen in:**
   a. Rheumatic diseases
   b. Rheumatic fever
   c. Rheumatoid arthritis
   d. Osteoarthritis

4. **Subcutaneous nodules are seen in all** *except*:
   a. Erythema multiforme
   b. Sarcoidosis
   c. Rheumatoid arthritis
   d. Rheumatic fever

5. **A 45-year-old man presented with firm nodule over ear rim that discharged powdery matter. He had past history of joint pains. The most probable diagnosis is:**
   a. Rheumatic fever
   b. Rheumatoid arthritis
   c. Gout
   d. Parathyroidism

6. **A 27-year-old male presented with severe constitutional symptoms and signs and tender papulonodules over face and limbs. The most likely diagnosis is:**
   a. Erythema nodosum leprosum
   b. Erythema nodosum
   c. Erythema multiforme
   d. Systemic lupus erythematosus

7. **The rash of dengue fever is described as:**
   a. Dew drop on rose petal
   b. Gun metal purpura
   c. Islands of white in a sea of red
   d. Mountain relief map

8. **Viral exanthem is distinguished from maculo-papular drug eruption on the basis of:**
   a. Lymph adenopathy
   b. Peripheral eosinophilia
   c. Pruritus
   d. All of the above

9. **Prurigo mitis affects these parts of the body:**
   a. Sun-exposed
   b. Covered
   c. Exposed
   d. Lower limbs

10. **Prurigo mitis affects this age group:**
    a. 6–12 months
    b. 1–5 years
    c. 6–10 years
    d. 11–20 years

11. **Prurigo simplex refers to hypersensitivity to:**
    a. Scabies mite
    b. Pollen grains
    c. Insect bite
    d. House dust mite

12. **Aphthous ulcers are known for their:**
    a. Self-healing nature
    b. Recurrence
    c. Painful nature
    d. Association with Reiter's disease

13. **Recurrent aphthous ulcers are sometimes a sign of:**
    a. Reiter's disease
    b. Behçet's disease
    c. Ritter's disease
    d. Sjögren's disease

14. **Which of the following diseases are known to be exacerbated in summer?**
    a. Xerotic eczema
    b. Ichthyosis
    c. Miliaria
    d. Psoriasis

15. **The commonest site of affection of miliaria is:**
    a. Trunk
    b. Upper limbs
    c. Face
    d. Lower limbs

16. **This is a form of iatrogenic miliaria:**
    a. Miliaria rubra
    b. Miliaria profunda
    c. Occlusion miliaria
    d. Miliaria pustulosa

17. **Miliaria results from blockage of:**
    a. Eccrine sweat gland openings
    b. Apocrine sweat gland openings
    c. Follicular openings
    d. Sebaceous gland openings

18. **This is a cause of pruritus without any skin lesions:**
    a. Dermatitis herpetiformis
    b. Urticaria
    c. Hypothyroidism
    d. Exfoliative dermatitis

Chapter 23

Miscellaneous Disorders

19. **This is a cause of pruritus with skin lesions:**
    a. Anal pruritus
    b. Obstructive jaundice
    c. Urticaria
    d. Lymphoma

20. **Ring-like arrangement of papules is seen in:**
    a. Secondary syphilis
    b. Granuloma annulare
    c. Tuberculoid leprosy
    d. All of the above

21. **Which of the following causes of pruritus is associated with insignificant skin lesions?**
    a. Dermatophytosis
    b. Insect bite allergy
    c. Scabies incognito
    d. Dermatitis herpetiformis

22. **Which of the following diseases are not pruritic?**
    a. Dermatitis herpetiformis
    b. Miliaria crystallina
    c. Lichen planus
    d. Atopic dermatitis

23. **Which of the following is are pruritic lesions?**
    a. Lichen planus
    c. Psoriasis
    b. Pemphigoid
    d. Both (a) and (b)

24. **A patient has recurrent oral ulcers with pain and erythematous halo around them. The most likely diagnosis is:**
    a. Aphthous ulcer   b. Herpes
    c. Chickenpox   d. Measles

ANSWERS

1-b,	2-b,	3-c,	4-a,	5-c,	6-a,	7-c,	8-d,	9-c,	10-c,
11-c,	12-b,	13-b,	14-c,	15-a,	16-c,	17-a,	18-c,	19-c,	20-d,
21-c,	22-b,	23-d,	24-a						

CHAPTER 24

Leprosy (Hansen's Disease)

Leprosy is a unique disease in many aspects. A brief summary of leprosy is listed in Table 24.1 on page 276.

Mycobacterium leprae, the causative organism of leprosy, inspite of being one of the earliest described (1872) pathogenic bacteria in humans, has not yet been grown in the laboratory. It can be grown in foot pads of mice, to a limited extent, and can cause disseminated infection in 9-banded armadillos (South American Anteaters).

M. leprae multiplies very slowly, doubling time being 14 days, compared to minutes or hours for most bacteria. The latter feature is responsible for the unusually long incubation period (2–10 years) and extremely slow evolution of the disease.

Importance of Host Immunity

Majority of the people in a leprosy endemic area, like India, are exposed to the infection but do not develop the disease. Hence, such healthy infected persons show serum antibodies to leprosy antigens (e.g. PGL-1) and have positive lepromin test. In short, whether a person is likely to develop leprosy is a function of host immunity.

Similarly, the type of leprosy that a person develops is also dependent on host immunity. Individuals with very poor immunity evolve into the lepromatous form and those with very good immunity (but not good enough to resist infection altogether) evolve into the tuberculoid form. Patients with intermediate immunity develop the borderline varieties.

EPIDEMIOLOGY OF LEPROSY

Mode of Transmission

Contrary to popular belief, leprosy is not transmitted by skin to skin contact but by droplet infection. Nasal droplets of patients with lepromatous leprosy contain thousands of bacilli (Fig. 24.1). However, most patients with leprosy have negative nasal smears and are therefore non-infectious.

Incubation Period

Usually, 3–5 years.

Prevalence

Of the total number of estimated leprosy cases in the world in the year 2000 (7,00,000) about 5,00,000 are in India. The prevalence of leprosy in India is between 0.5–1 per 1000 persons. The rate is higher (3–5/1000) in states like West Bengal, Odisha, Bihar, intermediate [1/1000] in Maharashtra, Tamil Nadu, Andhra Pradesh and low [0.1/1000] in Punjab, Haryana and Rajasthan. Mumbai has a higher rate of about 2 per 1000. For current figures of leprosy prevalence refer the note on 'elimination of leprosy' at the end of this chapter.

Patient Profile

Males are more commonly affected. Most patients are young or middle aged adults. It is relatively uncommon in children and the elderly.

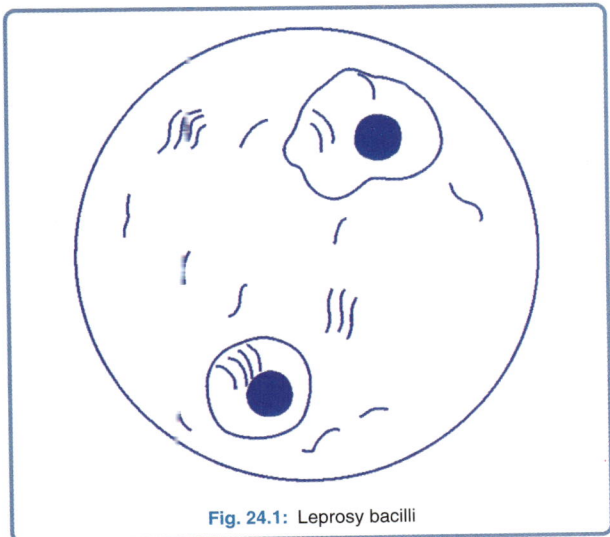

Fig. 24.1: Leprosy bacilli

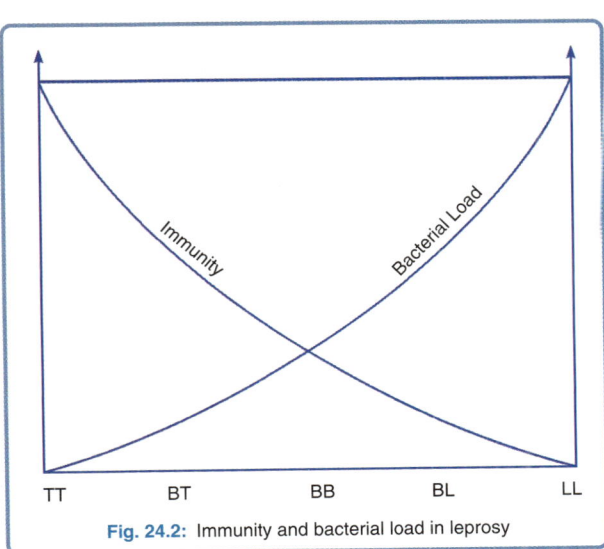

Fig. 24.2: Immunity and bacterial load in leprosy

265

Classification of Leprosy based on Clinical, Microbiologic, Pathologic and Immunologic Parameters

The commonly used Ridley-Jopling classification is based on four parameters, viz. clinical (morphology and distribution of skin lesions and nerve involvement), bacteriological (bacteriologic index on skin smears), histopathological (type of granuloma, tuberculoid or macrophage) and immunological (e.g. lepromin positivity). Trying to classify a case based only on one of these parameters may lead to errors.

Indian Classification of Leprosy

Indeterminate (I)

Tuberculoid (T)

Borderline (B)

Lepromatous (L)

Pure neuritic (P)

INDETERMINATE (I)

Clinical

One or two, poorly defined, hypopigmented, slightly erythematous, macules or patches, generally smaller than 5 cm diameter, with partial or no loss of sensation or sweating, usually over face or extremities of children are typical (Fig. 24.3).

Bacteriology

Usually negative.

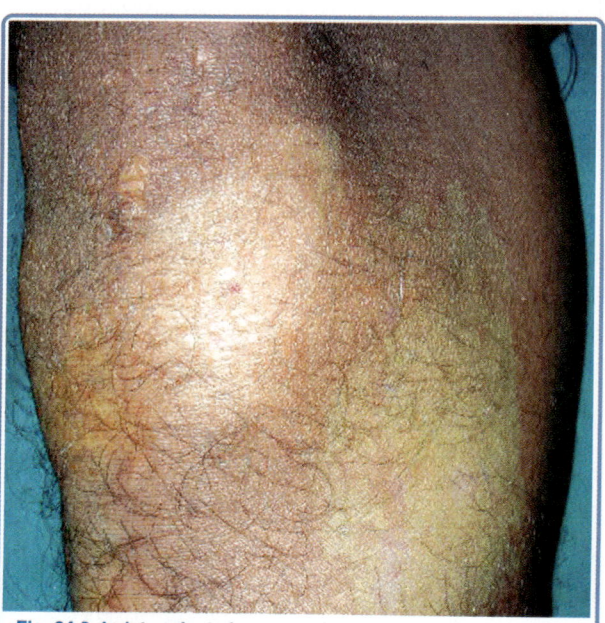

Fig. 24.3: Indeterminate leprosy—ill-defined hypopigmented patch

Histopathology

There is no granuloma; only sparse perivascular, periappendageal and peri- and intraneural infiltrate of lymphocytes.

Immunology

Lepromin negative.

TUBERCULOID (T)

Clinical

One or two, well defined, hypopigmented or erythematous atrophic patches or plaques, smaller than 10 cm in diameter (commonly 3–5 cm), with a dry surface are noted over extremities or face (Fig. 24.4). Sensations are totally lost or severely affected. Sweating is absent. A cutaneous nerve or a nerve trunk in the vicinity may be enlarged.

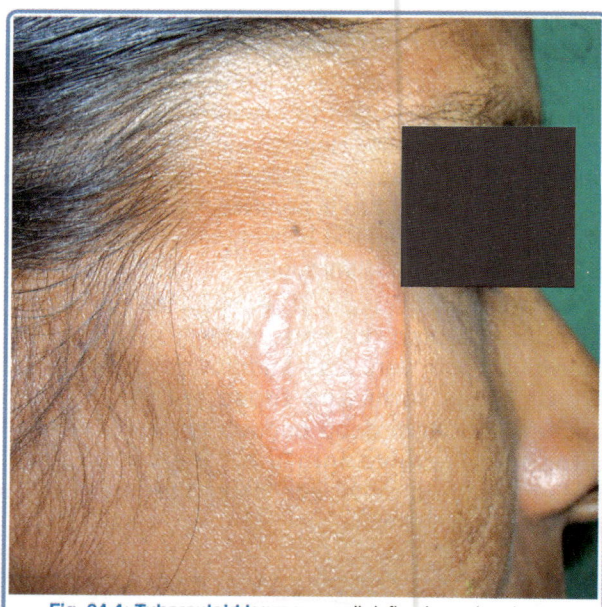

Fig. 24.4: Tuberculoid leprosy—well defined annular plaque

Bacteriology

Negative.

Histopathology

Tuberculoid granuloma consisting of epithelioid cells and lymphocytes, with prominent Langhan's giant cells, close to the epidermis; no subepidermal infiltrate free grenz zone. Granuloma is along a nerve (elongated).

Immunology

Lepromin test ++.

BORDERLINE TUBERCULOID (BT)

Clinical

One or two large (more than 10 or even 20 cm diameter) or many (up to 10 in number) smaller hypopigmented or erythematous atrophic patches or hypopigmented or erythematous atrophic patches or plaques with dry surfaces are present usually on one or two extremities (Figs 24.5–24.9). Lesions are not as well defined as in tuberculoid leprosy. Satellite lesions are smaller macules (up to 1 cm diameter) seen commonly beyond the margins of larger lesions and are a feature of BT leprosy (Fig. 24.10). Distribution of lesions is asymmetrical. Sensations and sweating over the lesions are severely affected. One or two nerve trunks in the vicinity of the lesions are commonly enlarged.

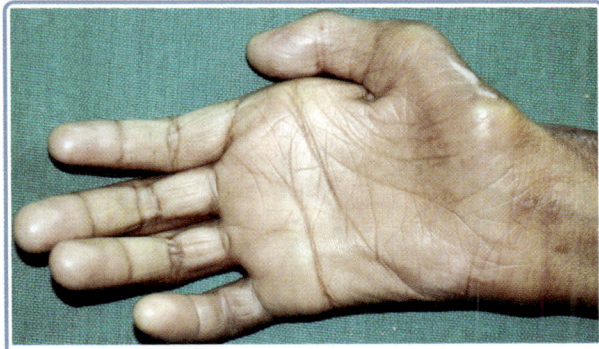

Fig. 24.7: Complete claw hand due to median and ulnar nerve affection. Note wasting of muscles, ape thumb deformity and flexion deformity of interphalangeal joints

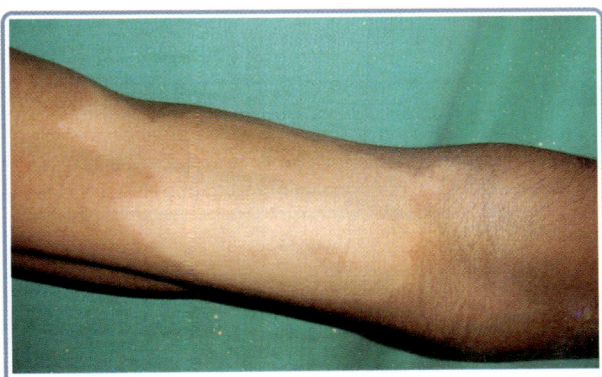

Fig. 24.5: Borderline tuberculoid leprosy—single large fairly well-defined hypopigmented, hypoaesthetic patch

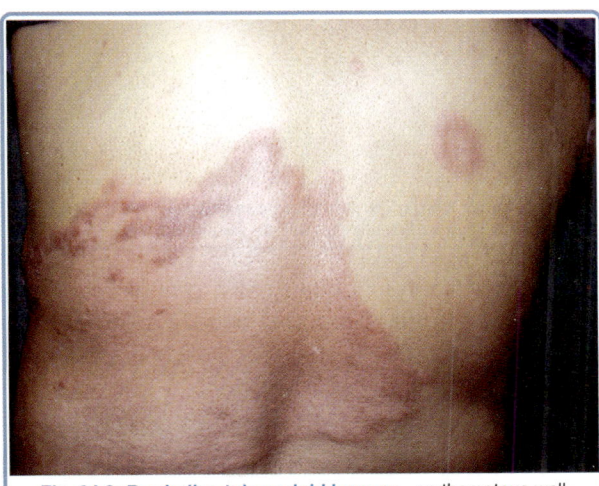

Fig. 24.8: Borderline tuberculoid leprosy—erythematous well-defined plaques with satellite lesions

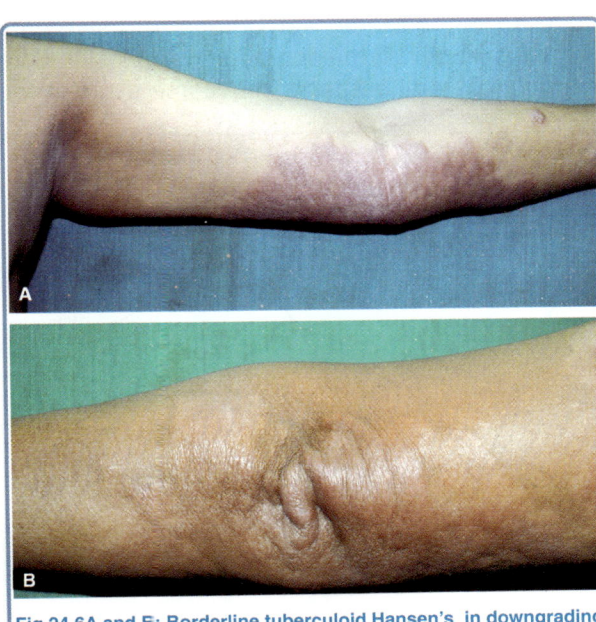

Fig 24.6A and B: Borderline tuberculoid Hansen's in downgrading reaction to borderline lepromatous disease—ill to well-defined erythematous infiltrated plaques and satellite nodules

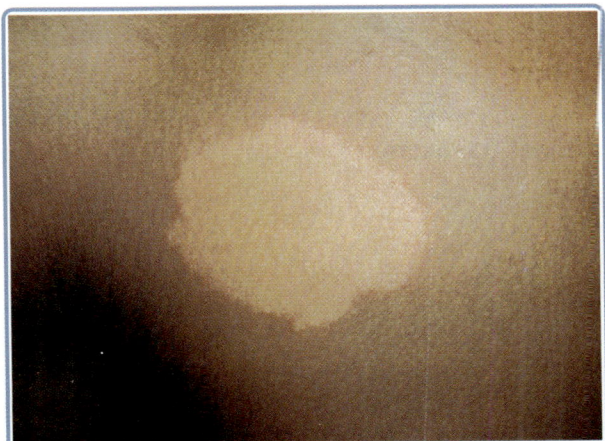

Fig. 24.9: Borderline tuberculoid leprosy—hypoanaesthetic plaque with slightly elevated sharply defined border. Note small satellite macules

Bacteriology

Usually negative; occasionally +.

Histopathology

Tuberculoid granuloma consisting of epitheloid cells and lymphocytes with absent or small and less

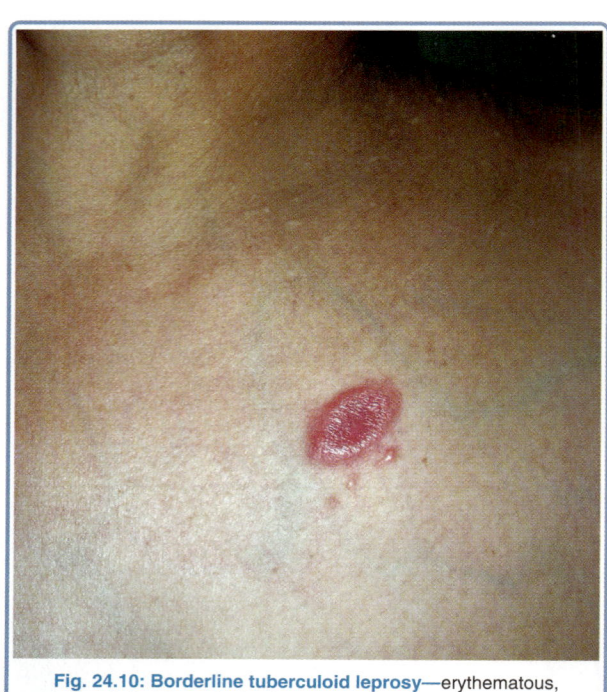

Fig. 24.10: Borderline tuberculoid leprosy—erythematous, hypoanesthetic plaque with satelite lesions

prominent Langhan's giant cells; granuloma rarely impinges on epidermis and is usually along a nerve (elongated).

Immunology

Lepromin test weak positive or negative.

MID-BORDERLINE (BORDERLINE BORDERLINE, BB)

Clinical

Compared to BT, patches and plaques increase in number but decrease in size. Rather than being

dry they tend to be more shiny or 'infiltrated', sensations and sweating are partially preserved, at least in the early phase, and lesions have a bilateral distribution involving extremities (especially proximal) and trunk.

Bacteriology

Usually 1+ or 2+, occasionally 3+.

Histopathology

Loosely arranged granuloma of histiocytes, many of which resemble epithelioid cells, along with lymphocytes and a few foreign body giant cells characterise this form. Free sub-epidermal grenz zone is present. Elongated granulomas along a nerve are still identifiable.

Immunology

Lepromin negative.

> A morphology characteristic for BB is the 'inverted saucer' like 'infiltrated' annular plaque that has a sloping periphery merging gradually with the normal skin and a punched out centre that is free of erythema or infiltration (Fig. 24.11).

BORDERLINE LEPROMATOUS (BL)

Clinical

Compared to BB, patches and plaques increase in number but decrease in size, are poorly defined, have an oily surface, sensations and sweating are partially or fully preserved and the lesions are not only bilateral but tend to become symmetrical

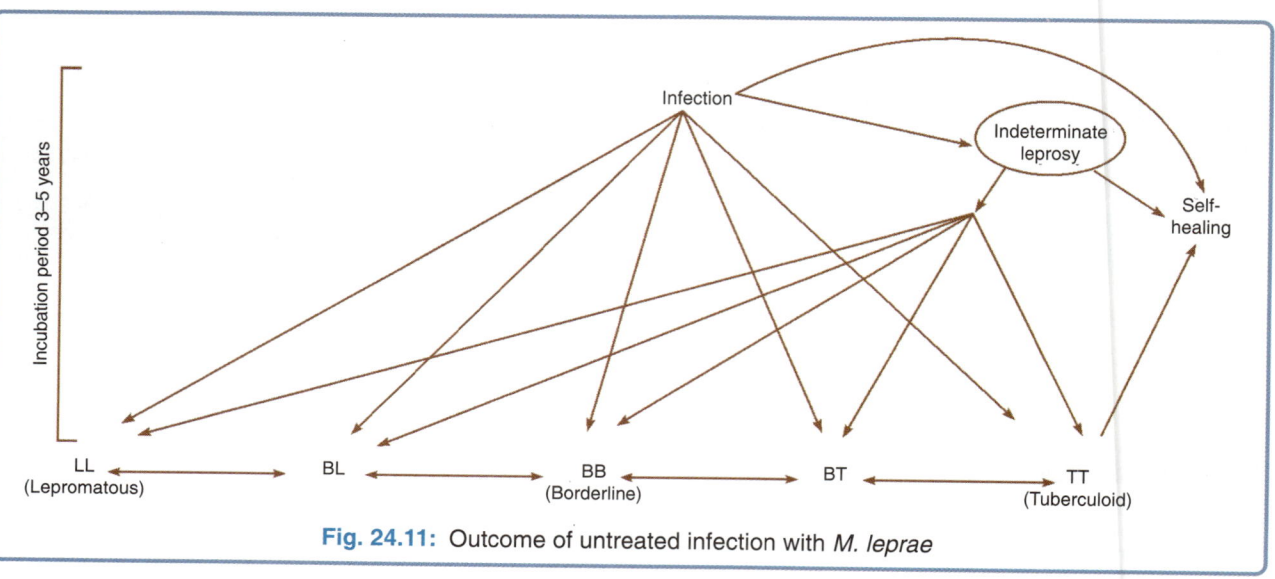

Fig. 24.11: Outcome of untreated infection with *M. leprae*

(Figs 24.12 and 24.13). Occasional erythematous infiltrated nodule may be present, usually over face (Figs 24.14–24.16). The involved skin shows little or no atrophy (observed as loss of hair follicular openings).

Bacteriology

Usually 2+ or 3+, occasionally 4+.

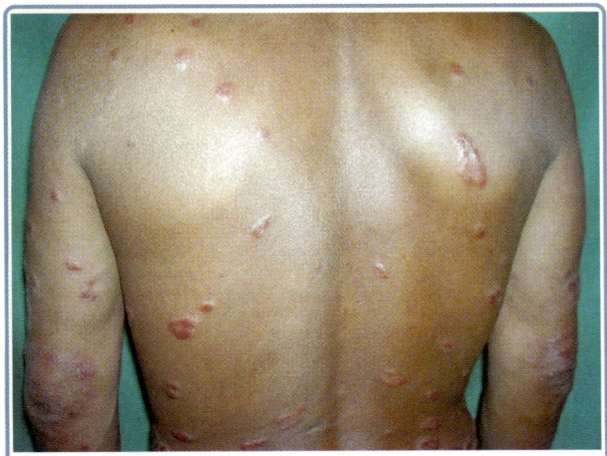

Fig. 24.12: Borderline lepromatous leprosy—erythematous nodules and plaques tending to symmetry

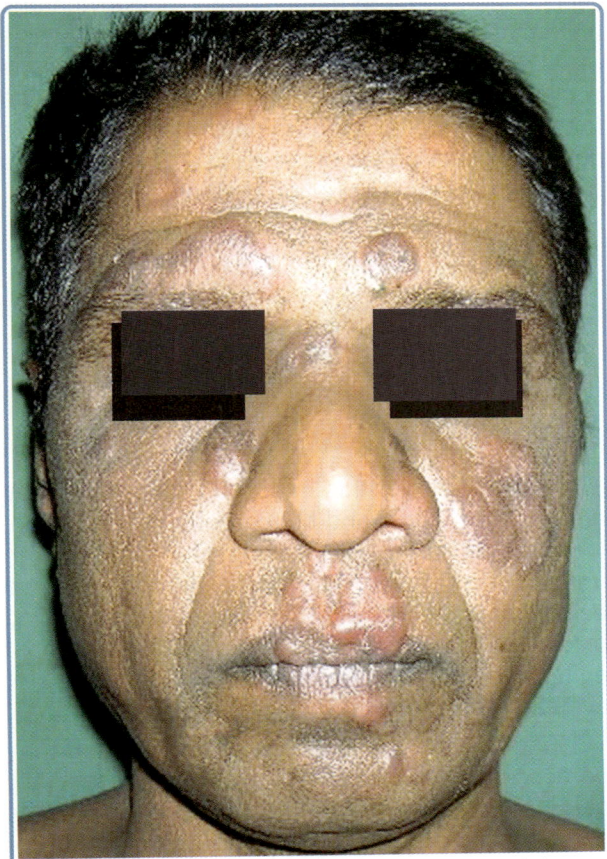

Fig. 24.13: Borderline lepromatous leprosy—nodules and plaques tending towards symmetry

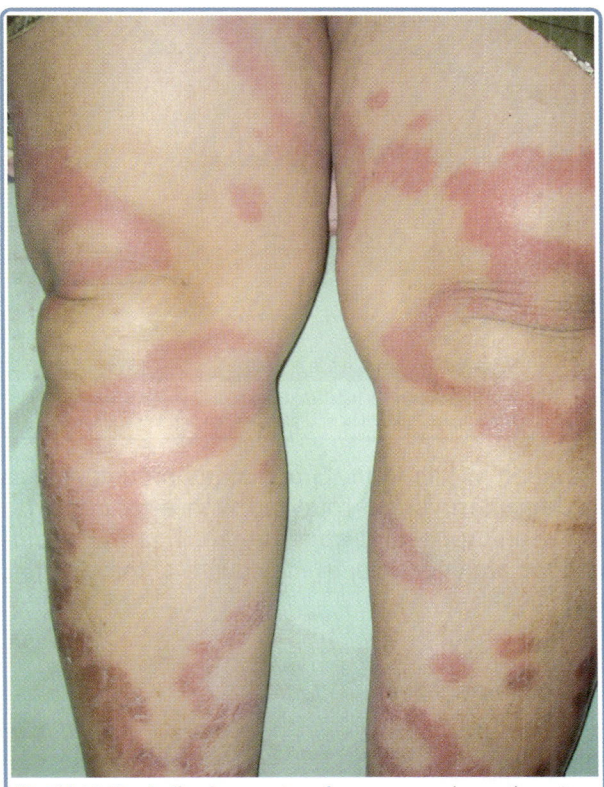

Fig. 24.14: Borderline lepromatous leprosy—annular, erythematous plaques on the legs. Note tendency to symmetry

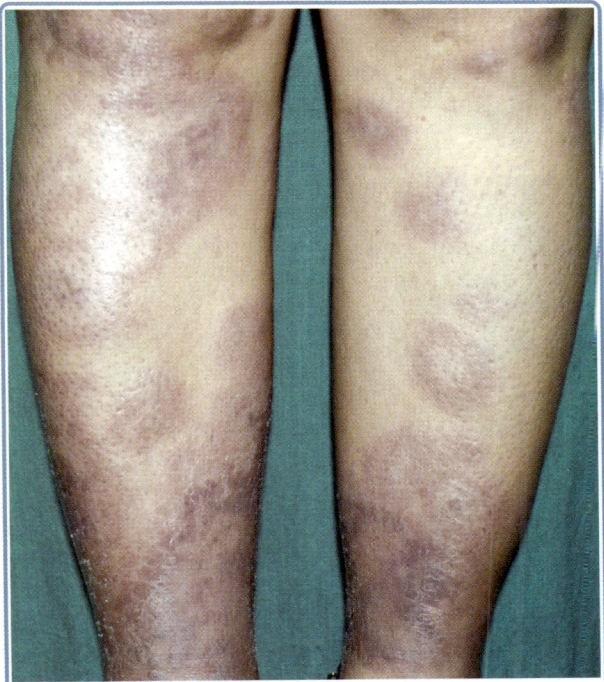

Fig. 24.15: Borderline lepromatous leprosy—erythematous plaques with ill-defined borders tending to symmetry

Histopathology

Histiocytes and lymphocytes that tend to be clustered within the poorly defined and patchy granuloma with a distinct free subepidermal zone

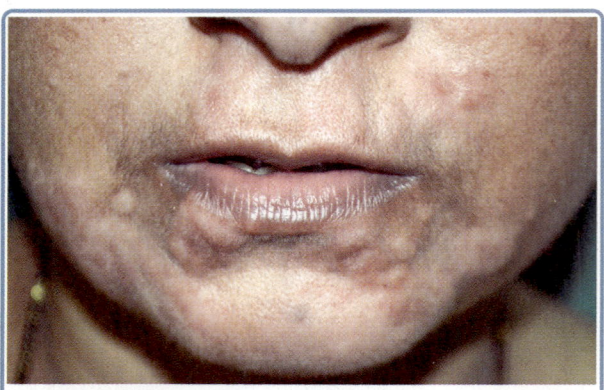

Fig. 24.16: Borderline lepromatous leprosy—erythematous infiltrated papulonodules and plaques tending to symmetry

are seen in this form. Granulomas around nerves in deep dermis are rounded with a tendency to show onion peeling appearance. Foamy macrophages are seen later in the course of the disease.

Immunology

Lepromin negative.

LEPROMATOUS LEPROSY (LL)

Clinical

Plaques are uncommon. Numerous nodules or faintly hypopigmented macules/patches characterise this type. Diffuse infiltration (erythema and oedema with a shiny appearance) of the skin of the face (Fig. 24.17) and distal extremities is

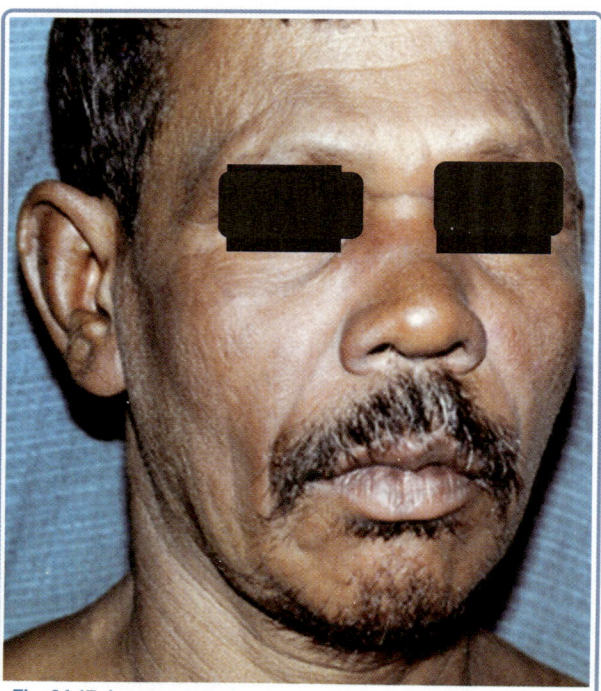

Fig. 24.17: Lepromatous leprosy—loss of eyebrow hairs along with infiltration of facial skin and ear

common. Compared to BL, lesions increase in number (innumerable), decrease in size, become ill-defined, have oily surface, sensations and sweating over the lesions are usually preserved and lesions are bilaterally symmetrical (Fig. 24.18).

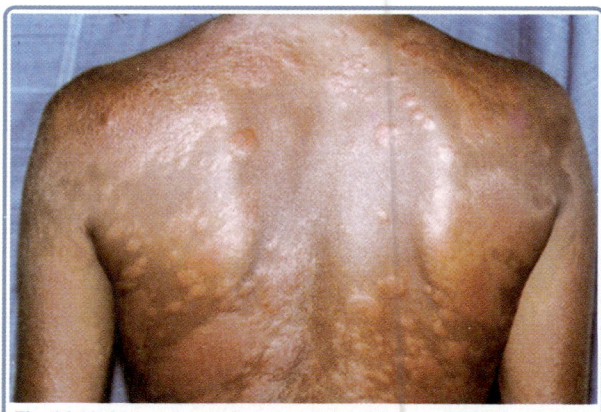

Fig. 24.18: Lepromatous leprosy—bilaterally symmetrical, infiltrated, shiny nodules and plaques

Bacteriology

Usually 3+ or 4+, occasionally 5+ or 6+.

Histopathology

Diffuse granuloma of monomorphic histiocytes and uniformly scattered lymphocytes involve the whole of dermis except the subepidermal free grenz zone. Foamy macrophages, some of which may be foamy giant cells, predominate over histiocytes during the later phase of the disease. Nerves in the deep dermis show an onion peel appearance.

Immunology

Lepromin negative.

OTHER CLINICAL FEATURES OF LEPROMATOUS LEPROSY

Early symptoms of this infectious form of leprosy are unconventional and hence likely to be missed. Nasal stuffiness, i.e. persistent rhinitis with consequent nasal discharge, which may be occasionally tinged with blood, is often neglected by the patient. Bilateral oedema of feet is most evident in the evening and is due to the loss of sympathetic tone of the vessels.

Tingling and numbness appear later and may be accompanied by thickening of facial (especially ears and forehead) skin. As the disease progresses diffuse infiltration (mild erythema and oedema) of face (Fig. 24.19), hands and feet becomes evident. Later still, nodules appear over ear rims and lobes

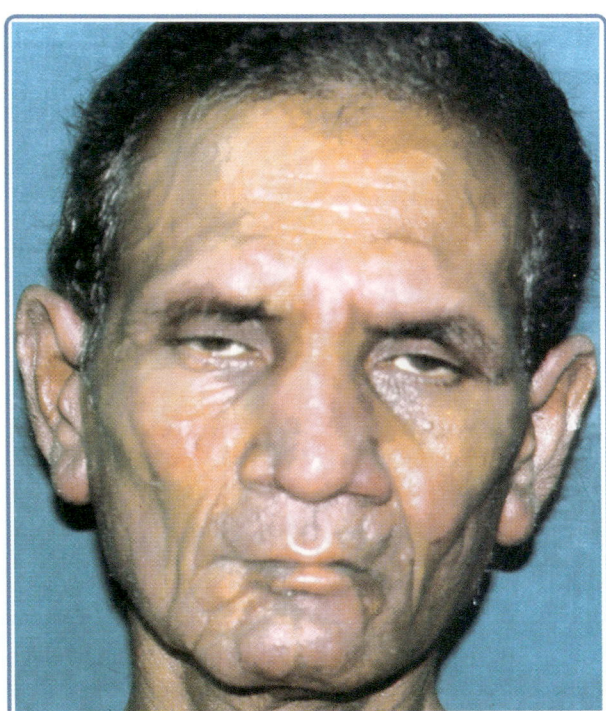

Fig. 24.19: Lepromatous leprosy—bilaterally symmetrical diffuse infiltration, nodules and plaques involving face. Note: Partial loss of lateral eyebrows and leonine facies

(Figs 24.20 and 24.21), forehead and malar region. Diffuse thickening leads to accentuation of forehead creases (leonine facies).

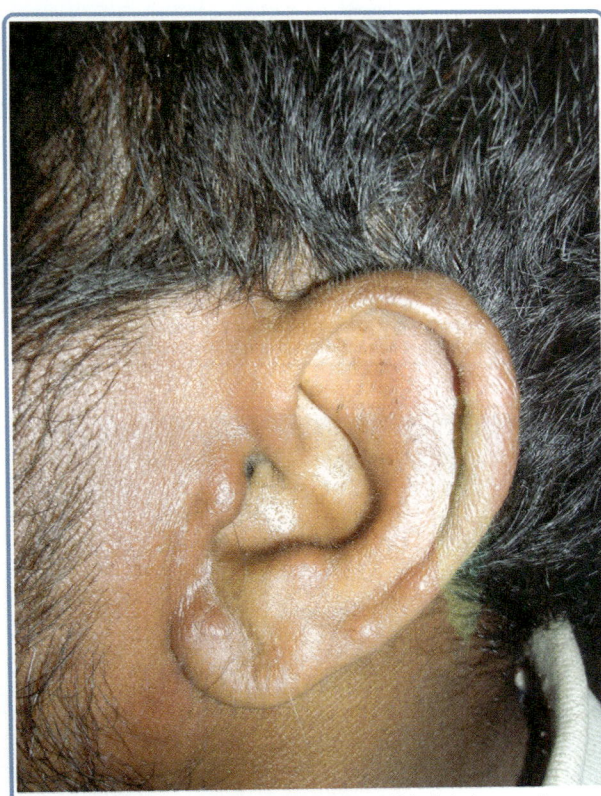

Fig. 24.20: Early infiltration of ear rim and lobule in lepromatous leprosy

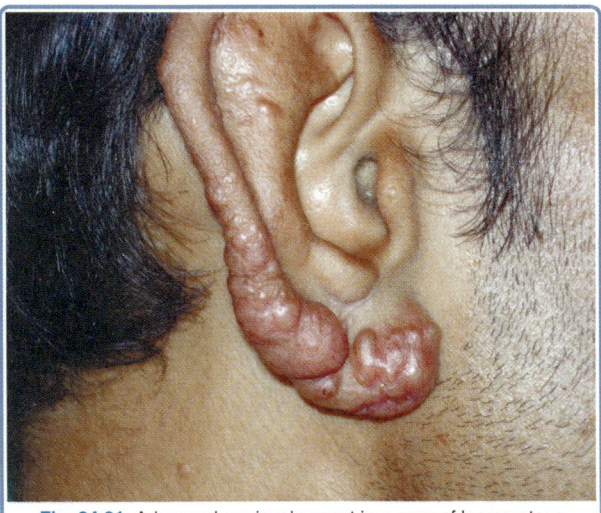

Fig. 24.21: Advanced ear involvement in a case of lepromatous leprosy

Lucio Leprosy

Lucio leprosy is a diffuse and non-nodular form of leprosy seen in the Mexican people. Diffuse facial involvement gives a beautiful look known as 'lepra bonita' or 'beautiful leprosy.'

Complications of Leprosy

These can result from four mechanisms, viz. leprous infiltration, sensory loss, autonomic nerve damage and motor damage.

Leprous Infiltration

Further progression of facial involvement in LL leads to loss of upper incisors, saddle nose (Fig. 24.22) and perforation of nasal septum or palate. Leonine facies is usually accompanied by loss of lateral half of eyebrows (Fig. 24.19). Diffuse hand or foot swelling may overlie leprous dactylitis (Fig. 24.22).

Effects of Sensory Loss

Symmetrical glove and stocking type anaesthesia occurs in LL, whereas in other types of leprosy, only particular regions are anaesthetic according to the nerves involved. Long-term effects of this sensory loss include gradual **shortening of fingers** and toes that results from repetitive subclinical trauma; **traumatic ulcers and scars** follow handling of tools, burns while cooking, smoking, etc. (Figs 24.23 and 24.24). **Trophic ulcers** over pressure bearing parts of the foot is an extremely common cause of disability in leprosy. They result from the repetitive subclinical trauma of walking, running, or jumping encountered by a dry fissured foot that lacks pain sensation. Heads of first and fifth metatarsal and

Chapter 24

Leprosy (Hansen's Disease)

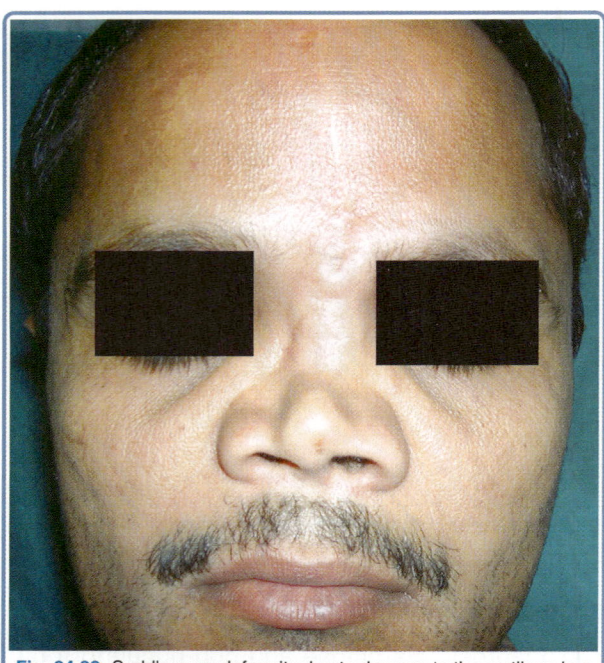

Fig. 24.22: Saddle nose deformity due to damage to the cartilage in a case of lepromatous leprosy

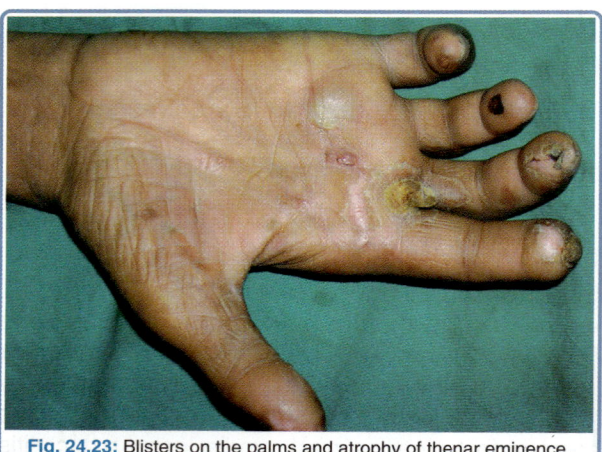

Fig. 24.23: Blisters on the palms and atrophy of thenar eminence, complete claw hand deformity and ulceration/absorption of terminal digits in leprosy

heel (Figs 24.25 and 24.26) are the commonest sites of callosities and subsequent ulceration.

Effects of Autonomic Nervous System Affection

Loss of sweating leads to **dryness** of feet, **fissuring** of soles and **ichthyosis** (dry skin with thick polyangular scales resembling fish scales) of extensor aspects of extremities. Loss of vascular tone leads to **oedema feet.**

Effects of Motor Damage

These differ according to the nerve affected. **Function of muscles** is compromised early, much

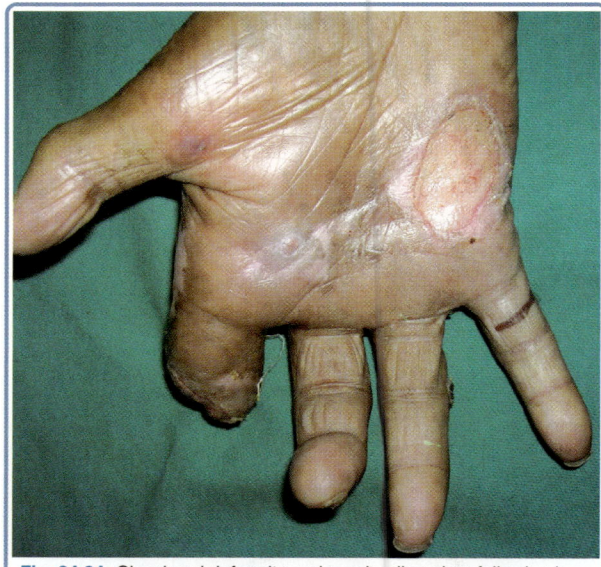

Fig. 24.24: Claw hand deformity and non-healing ulcer following burn in an anaesthetic hand. Note: Autoamputation of index finger

before **deformity** sets in. Ulnar and median nerve palsy affect hand function, whereas lateral popliteal palsy compromises walking. Paralysis of ulnar nerve at the elbow leads to **ulnar claw** (hyperextension of metacarpophalangeal (MP) joints and flexion of interphalangeal (IP) joints involving the fourth and fifth fingers and flattening of hypothenar eminence)

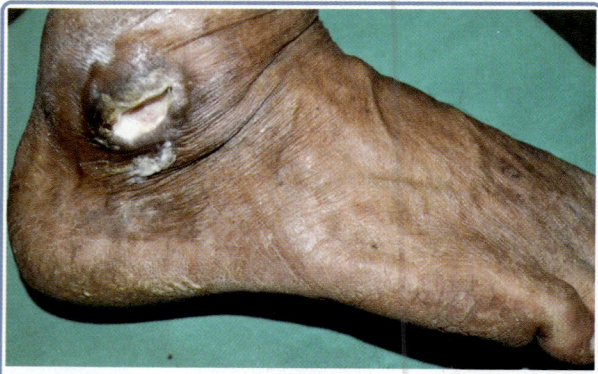

Fig. 24.25: Trophic ulcer over lateral malleolus due to cross-legged sitting posture in a patient with resolved lepromatous leprosy

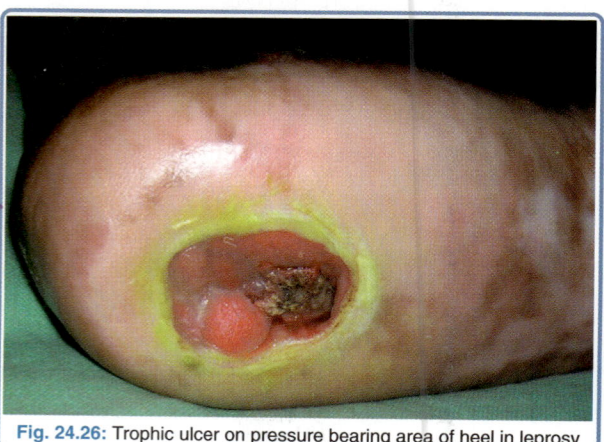

Fig. 24.26: Trophic ulcer on pressure bearing area of heel in leprosy

(Fig. 24.27). Median nerve palsy at the wrist leads to **median claw** or ape thumb deformity. Palsy of radial nerve in the arm results in **wrist drop. Foot drop** occurs due to lateral popliteal affection at the knee, whereas **hammer toes** are the result of posterior tibial palsy at the ankle. **Facial palsy** occurs due to involvement of facial nerve at its point of emergence from the skull. Other motor nerves are uncommonly involved.

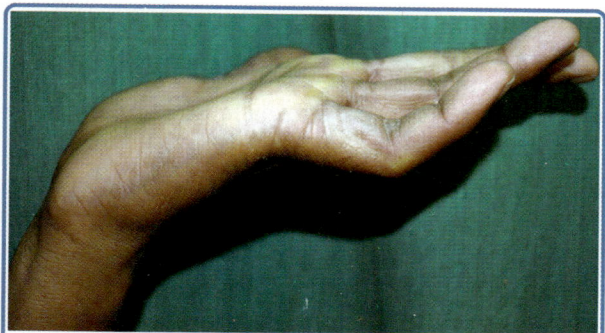

Fig. 24.27: Pure neuritic leprosy—complete claw hand demonstrating extensor deformity in metacarpophalangeal joints and flexion deformity of proximal interphalangeal joints

Diagnosis

Demonstration of *M. leprae* in the skin **is not** always possible in many cases of tuberculoid, borderline tuberculoid and indeterminate leprosy. These patients constitute the majority of leprosy cases and hence, a correlation of clinical features with findings of skin biopsy is essential to reach a diagnosis of leprosy in them.

Cardinal signs of leprosy

Ordinarily most patients with leprosy can be diagnosed as such if at least one and preferably two of the following cardinal signs are present. They include:

- Presence of acid-fast bacilli in skin lesions.
- Loss or diminished sensation over a skin lesion (patch or plaque).
- Thickened peripheral nerves, especially in leprosy endemic regions (Fig. 24.28).

Investigations in Leprosy

Skin smears

Taken by the slit and scrape method and stained with Ziehl-Neelsen technique, they provide a rapid method for diagnosis, classification and monitoring of therapy. Smears are taken from both ear lobes, forehead, chin and a skin lesion.

Bacteriological index signifies the density of bacilli in smears and is indicated as 0, 1+, 2+, 3+,

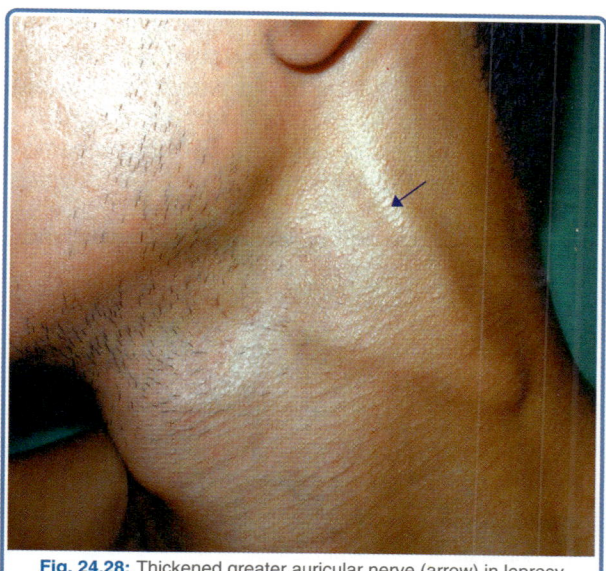

Fig. 24.28: Thickened greater auricular nerve (arrow) in leprosy

4+, 5+ and 6+. As a broad guideline, index of 0 corresponds with TT and some BT cases, 1+ to 2+ with some BT and BB cases, 2+ to 3+ with some BB and BL cases and 3+ to 6+ with LL cases. Current anti-leprosy therapy recommendations require it to be discontinued after 1 year in multi-bacillary cases irrespective of the bacteriological indices.

Morphological index (MI) indicates the proportion of live bacilli in smears. *M. leprae* may stain as solid rods, fragmented rods or granules. Solid rods are considered live bacilli. As it depends on live bacilli, MI gives a better indication of infectivity of a case. It falls rapidly to zero within 4–8 weeks of starting therapy in multi-bacillary cases.

Skin Biopsy

In tuberculoid leprosy, there is a well defined tuberculoid granuloma, consisting predominantly of epithelioid cells and lymphocytes, that impinges on the epidermis. Granuloma commonly involves and destroys cutaneous nerves.

In lepromatous leprosy, a diffuse granuloma of foamy macrophages involves the entire reticular dermis but spares the papillary dermis. Stains for acid-fast organisms reveal them to be present intracellularly within macrophages. An intermediate picture is seen in borderline varieties of leprosy. Please *see* pages 267–268 for details.

Sweat Test

This is an important clinical test that differentiates hypopigmented macules of leprosy from other macules. It compares the amount of sweating from affected site with that from a corresponding unaffected site on opposite side. Test sites are injected with 0.2 ml of 1:1000 pilocarpine nitrate, painted with iodine and powdered with starch. Starch powder turns blue in the presence of sweat. A rapid method is to use bromophenol blue impregnated paper for comparison with amount of sweat. The dye turns blue on contact with sweat.

Other Investigations

These are rarely needed.

Nerve conduction

Slowed in involved nerve trunks.

Nerve biopsy

Useful for patients in whom only nerves are affected. Only the purely sensory nerves can be biopsied.

Nasal smears

Demonstrate *M. leprae* in LL.

Histamine test

Injection of histamine fails to cause flare in leprosy macules as compared to macules due to other causes.

PGL-1 antibody in serum

Indicates that a person is exposed to leprosy bacillus but may or may not have the disease.

Lepromin Test

Lepromin test is an inradermal test in which lepromin antigen is used to assess the immunity against lepra bacilli. After injection, injection site is examined at 48th hour and after 4 weeks. Reaction can be categorised as early reaction of Fernandez (48 hours) and late reaction of Mitsuda (4 weeks). The late reaction of Mitsuda is better indicative of patient's immunity than the Fernandez reaction. Strongly positive lepromin test is seen in tuberculoid leprosy as immunity against lepra bacilli is good, whereas it is negative in lepromatous leprosy as there is no immunity against lepra bacilli. This test is not diagnostic for leprosy.

MANAGEMENT OF LEPROSY

During the last 20 years anti-leprosy therapy has undergone a sea of change. Dapsone mono-therapy is completely outmoded and has been replaced by a multidrug therapy (MDT) consisting of two or three drugs for paucibacillary and multi-bacillary leprosy respectively.

Fixed Duration MDT for Pauci-bacillary (Smear Negative) Leprosy

For the purpose of treatment, patients with less than 5 lesions are considered as paucibacillary irrespective of smear results. This includes:

- Self-administered dapsone 100 mg daily (at bedtime) and
- Supervised administration of rifampicin 600 mg (preferably before food) once a month (called a pulse) for 6 months.

Fixed Duration MDT for Multi-bacillary (5 or More Lesions) Leprosy

This includes:

- Self-administered dapsone 100 mg daily.
- Self administered clofazimine 50 mg daily (after food).
- Supervised administration of rifampicin 600 mg and clofazimine 300 mg once a month (called a pulse). Therapy is to be continued for a **fixed period** of one year in **spite of the results of skin smears**. The twelve pulses are to be completed within a maximum of 18 months.

The dosages given above are for adults. Proportionately lower dosages are used for children. It is extremely important to ensure patient compliance during the complete course. The fixed duration of therapy is advised irrespective of the changes in skin lesions or presence or absence of reactions because it has been observed over the years that patients who stop therapy after 1 year behave in exactly the same manner with respect to clinical and bacteriological features when compared to patients who continue therapy till smear negativity.

There may not be any visible change in the skin lesions in patients with macules and patches during or even at the end of therapy. Lost sensations and muscle function may or may not be regained in part or full.

Clinical implication: This has to be explained to the patient before or at least during the early part of therapy. Otherwise there is risk of patient either losing faith in the therapy or, on the contrary, continuing therapy indefinitely, without informing the doctor.

Newer Drugs in Leprosy

Single dose MDT for single lesion leprosy

A single dose of rifampicin 600 mg, ofloxacin 400 mg and minocycline 100 mg (ROM therapy) is effective for most of the patients with single lesion leprosy (tuberculoid or indeterminate).

However, due to unacceptably high relapse rate, routine use of single dose therpay is now given up. Similarly, use of ROM pulse therapy (use of rifampicin, ofloxacin and minicycline for 1 week every month) is associated with increased chance of lepra reactions and relapses and is therefore not recommended for routine use. Unfortunately, resolution of lesions is not hastened with these crash courses of antibiotics.

ADVICE TO LEPROSY PATIENTS UNDER THERAPY

- **Medical Therapy**

  - ❑ Ensure regularity.
  - ❑ Maintain records of drugs and investigations.
  - ❑ Do not discontinue unless specifically told to do so by the doctor/clinic where the therapy was begun.
  - ❑ If he/she falls ill, disclose about the therapy to the caring doctor.
  - ❑ If any exacerbation of skin lesions occurs with or without weakness of hands or feet, pain or fever, do not discontinue therapy but report immediately to the doctor.

- **Prevention of Trophic Ulcers for Insensitive Feet**

  - ❑ Use sandals that **are well** fitting, soft (without nails), have thick microcellulose rubber insoles (for equitable distribution of pressure) and with a back strap (in case of footdrop).
  - ❑ Inspect feet at night for any wounds and to attend to these immediately (complete rest, clean and dress) **even if they are not painful**.
  - ❑ Appply petroleum jelly to soles after bath and at night.
  - ❑ Do not stand in one position for long time, do not run or jump or walk long distances, if it can be avoided.

- **Prevention of Hand Injuries for Insensitive Hands**

  - ❑ Take extra care while smoking, using sharp instruments or handling tools, which require application of pressure or a tight grip.
  - ❑ Women or men who cook must use insulating grips or use utensils with insulated handles while cooking.
  - ❑ In case of injury, give complete rest and dress it.

SOCIAL ASPECTS

Social Importance of Leprosy

Additional Care for Lepromatous Leprosy Cases

- *Care of eyes (insensitive or paralytic)*

  - ❑ Wear eyeglasses preferably with side shields for protection from foreign bodies.
  - ❑ Use moistening eye drops 3–4 times a day.
  - ❑ Consciously close eyes 5 times every 5 minutes.
  - ❑ Examine eyes at night for redness and if present show a doctor.

- *Care of nose*

  - ❑ Avoid picking the nose since, due to absence of pain, ulcer/perforation may start this way.
  - ❑ Irrigate the nose with a solution of 1% each of sodium bicarbonate, sodium borate and sodium chloride to clear crusts.
  - ❑ Use lubricant paraffin jelly daily for prevention of ulcers/crusts in the nose.

A peculiarity of leprosy is the high social stigma attached to its diagnosis. Social stigma arises from deformities secondary to nerve damage in leprosy. It arose at a time when there were no medicines for leprosy and the mechanisms for development of the deformities were ill-understood. In today's world, when deformities due to leprosy can be prevented and corrected to a large extent and when effective drugs that render a patient virtually non-infectious in 24 hours are available, the social stigma is totally misplaced.

This is especially so because **the real danger of leprosy transmission is from an undiagnosed case.** Moreover, only lepromatous cases and some borderline lepromatous cases (which constitute less than 20% of all leprosy cases) are infectious cases, the rest being practically non-infectious. Besides, leprosy is much less contagious than other diseases transmitted through the droplet infection route, i.e. chickenpox. It requires prolonged contact and a weakened host immunity for the disease to occur. This is borne out by the fact that the rate of conjugal leprosy (transmission from a spouse) is less than 5%. Even when bacteriologically cured, because of residual nerve damage, leprosy can cause trophic ulcers, weakness of hands or feet and deformities. This is responsible for affecting working capacity of an individual and leads to loss of wages. Hence, it

Chapter

24

Leprosy (Hansen's Disease)

TABLE 24.1 : Summary of leprosy

	Indeterminate	TT	BT	BB	BL	LL
Number of lesions	1 or 2	Usually single	Single large or many small, up to 10 cm	Several	Numerous	Innumerable
Size	Small, usually < 5 cm	3–5 cm	>10 cm	Variable, some >10 cm	Variable, <10 cm	Small usually <5 cm
Border	Ill defined	Well defined	Well defined in parts	Ill defined	Poorly defined	Poorly defined with diffuse infiltration
Morphology						
Primary lesion	Macule, patch	Macule, patch, plaque	Patch, plaque	Patch, plaque	Patch, plaque and nodule	Macule, patch and nodule
Atrophy	+/–	++	++	+/–	+/–	+/–
Surface	–	Very dry scale	Dry	Slightly shiny	Shiny	Shiny/Oily
Distribution	Face/extremity	Face/extremity	Any one region	Limbs, trunk	Trunk, limbs	Diffuse
Symmetry	Asymmetrical	Asymmetrical	Asymmetrical	Bilateral	Bilateral, tending to symmetry	Bilateral, symmetrical
Sensation	+/–	Absent	Markedly diminished	Partially preserved	Partially or fully preserved	Usually preserved
Sweating	Normal	Absent	Absent	Decreased	Decreased	Normal or Decreased
No. of enlarged nerves	None	0 to 1	0 to 2	Many	Many	All nerve trunks
AFB in lesion	–	–	+/–	1+ to 2+	2+ or 3+	3+ or 4+ occasionally 5+ or 6+
Histopathology	Lymphocytic infiltrate	Tuberculoid granuloma	Tuberculoid granuloma	Granuloma of histiocytes and lymphocytes	Ill-defined granuloma of histiocytes and lymphocytes	Diffuse granuloma of histiocytes foamy macrophages
Grenz zone	–	–	+/–	+	+	+
AFB	–	–	+/–	+	++	+++
Infectivity in untreated state	Nil	Nil	Nil	Nil	Usually not infective	Infective
Lepromin test	–	++	+/–	–	–	–
Treatment	DDS, rifampicin	DDS, rifampicin (single dose)	DDS, rifampicin	DDS, rifampicin and clofazimine	DDS, rifampicin and clofazimine	DDS, rifampicin
Clofazimine	–	ROM for single (lesion leprosy)	–	–	–	–
Duration of therapy	6 months	6 months	6 months	1 year	1 year	1 year

is extremely important for such patients to understand the mechanism of developing these complications and ways to prevent them.

LEPRA REACTIONS

Sudden exacerbations in clinical activity of the disease process in leprosy are termed reactions. They represent hypersensitivity reactions that occur in the disease course (Figs 24.29 and 24.30). Traditionally, reactions are classified into two types (Table 24.2).

Neuritis is common to both types of reactions and manifests as pain, numbness, sensory loss, muscle weakness, deformity and tenderness in the region of affected nerve trunks.

Diagnosis of Lepra Reactions

As majority of lepra reactions occur during anti-leprosy therapy it is vital to identify the early warning signs of reactions and especially neuritis that commonly accompanies them and that is responsible for much of the disability caused.

The warning signs include pain and tenderness of skin lesions or affected limbs and crops of new painful skin lesions with fever and arthralgia. Even when actual signs of nerve damage like sensory loss or weakness appear, it is frequently possible

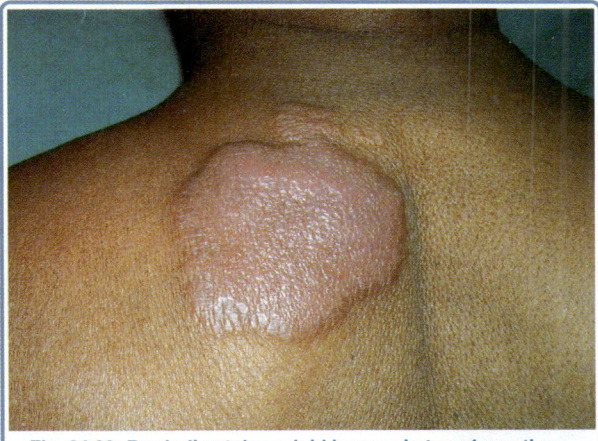

Fig. 24.29: Borderline tuberculoid leprosy in type 1 reaction—erythematous oedematous tender well-defined plaque

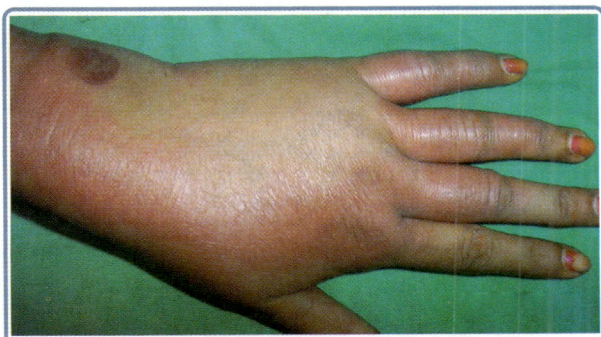

Fig. 24.30: Borderline tuberculoid leprosy in type 1 reaction—erythema, edema and dactylitis resembling cellulitis

TABLE 24.2: Lepra reactions	
Type 1	**Type 2**
Occurs in borderline leprosy.	Occurs in LL or BL leprosy.
Type IV hypersensitivity (cell-mediated immunity).	**Type III** hypersensitivity immune complex disease.
Change in protective **immunity** either for better (upgrading—from BL to BT) or for worse (downgrading—from BT to BL).	**No change** in protective immunity. Patient's leprosy type does not change.
Common **during first 6 months** of beginning therapy when immunity is boosted by anti-leprosy treatment complexes.	Common **after first 6 months** of initiating therapy when antigen released from killed bacilli forms circulating immune.
No or **mild constitutional** disturbance.	**Severe constitutional** symptoms and signs (fever, arthralgia, bodyache, prostration) common.
Existing skin lesions change (lesions show erythema, erythema, oedema hyperaesthesia, tenderness)	Existing lesions unaltered.
New lesions uncommon	**New lesions** (called erythema nodosum leprosum) occur as a rule and appear as crops of transient (last 3–10 days) red, tender, dermal or subcutaneous nodules over face and extremities (Figs 24.31–24.34).
Oedema of hands/feet uncommon.	Common.
Other systems unaffected.	Systemic affection commonly includes iritis, arthritis, periosteitis, orchitis, glomerulonephritis and lymphadenitis.
Blood analysis normal.	Raised/ESR and polymorphs.

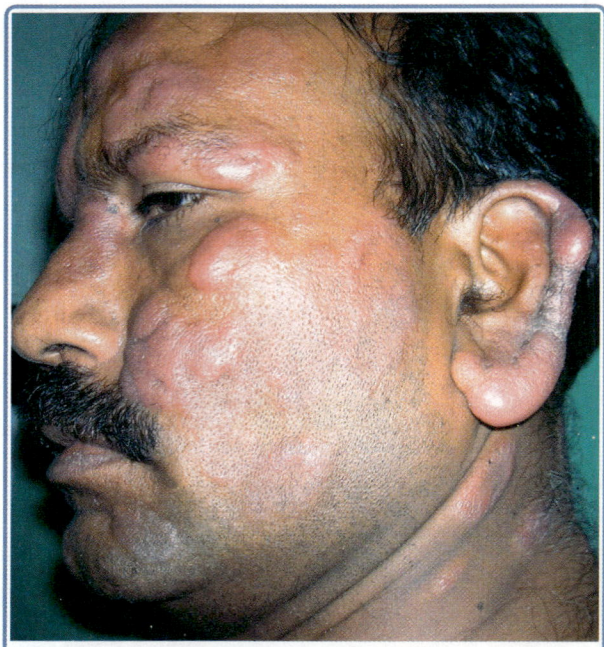

Fig. 24.31: Erythema nodosum leprosum—inflammatory nodules and plaques over face and ear

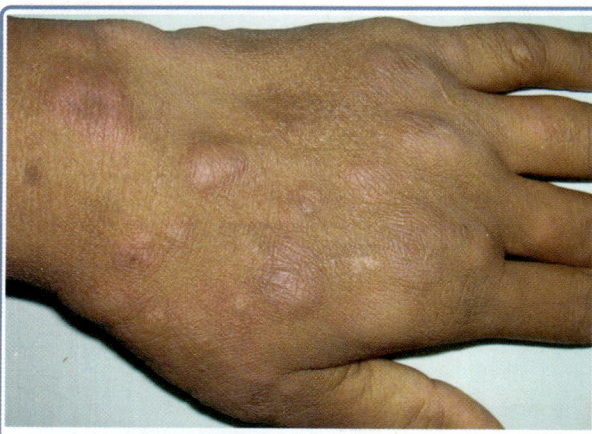

Fig. 24.32: Erythema nodosun leprosum—tender, erythematous nodules in lepromatous leprosy with type 2 lepra reaction

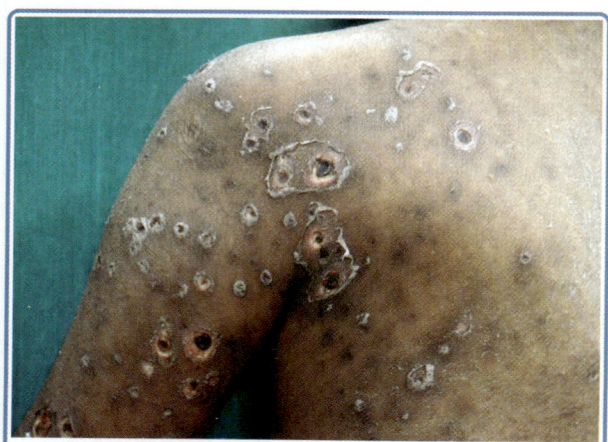

Fig. 24.33: Necrotic erythema nodosum leprosum—numerous symmetrical punched out ulcers and crusted plaques

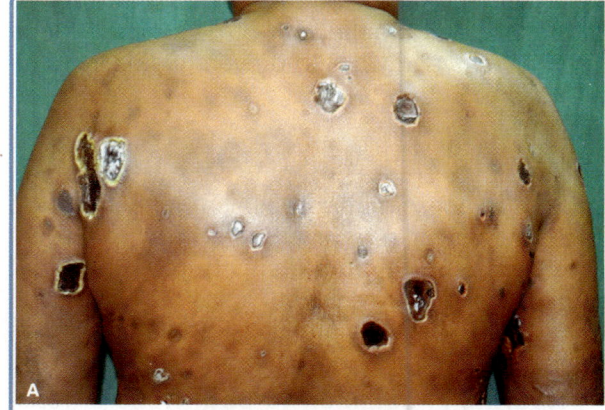

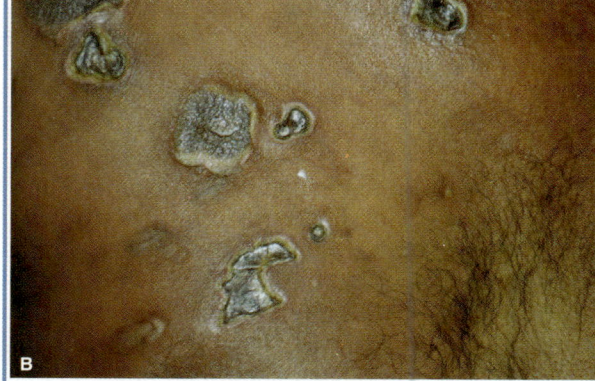

Fig. 24.34A and B: Lucio phenomenon (severe type 2 reaction in diffuse lepromatous leprosy)—widespread large and deep necrotic ulcers accompanied by severe constitutional signs and symptoms

to reverse the damage partially or completely by instituting prompt therapy.

TREATMENT OF LEPRA REACTIONS

Type 1: Downgrading type 1 reactions are usually mild and are due to lack of therapy which allows a patient to downgrade along the leprosy spectrum (e.g. from BT to BL). Therefore, they are best treated with initiating proper anti-leprosy therapy and NSAIDs. If significant neuritis is present, oral steroids may be given.

Upgrading type 1 reactions are common and severe than downgrading types and occur during the first 6 months of initiating anti-leprosy treatment. In presence of neuritis, oral prednisolone 40 mg/day, promptly instituted could make the difference between recovery and permanent palsy. As a general guideline, steroids should be slowly tapered, after the first two weeks, by 5 mg per week. In absence of neuritis, oral chloroquine phosphate 250 mg two to three times a day or ibuprofen 400 mg t.d.s. are helpful.

Type 2: Type 2 lepra reactions respond dramatically to systemic steroids. Dosage and tapering schedule of steroids is similar to type 1 reactions. However, relapses are frequent with steroid reduction. Oral NSAIDs, clofazimine (200–300 mg per day for many weeks), chloroquine, colchicine (0.5 mg t.d.s.) and zinc (220 mg OD), supplement steroid action and allow their smoother tapering. In unresponsive or relapsing reactions thalidomide 100 mg 3–4 times a day is the drug of choice. However, it is absolutely contraindicated in women of child-bearing age group due to its teratogenicity. Iritis, orchitis, glomerulonephritis need to be appropriately attended to.

> **Summary:** *Type 1 reaction:* Sudden oedema and erythema of existing lesions of leprosy with or without pain indicate type 1 reaction. Neuritis of the nerve trunk in the vicinity is common. Type 1 reaction signifies change in immune status for better (within 6 months of initiating therapy) or for worse (lack of treatment). Neuritis is an indication for systemic steroid treatment, which avoids nerve damage.
>
> *Type 2 reaction:* Reaction tends to begin 6 months after initiating therapy for leprosy and is due to immune complex deposition. Crops of symmetrical, tender, bright red nodules and plaques occur over face and extremities (erythema nodosum leprosum). Lesions are transient lasting 2–10 days but new crops appear with severe constitutional disturbance. Neuritis may lead to nerve palsies. Iritis, orchitis, periosteitis, myositis are common. High dose systemic steroids, instituted promptly and tapered gradually, avoid damage to nerves and organs.

Lucio Phenomenon

Lucio phenomenon is an uncommon and unusual reaction seen in patients with lucio leprosy. Skin lesions undergo severe necrosis and ulceration.

Prevention of Disability due to Leprosy

While deformity implies structural abnormality of a limb or face, disability includes even functional impairment like loss of sensations. Deformities in leprosy commonly result from either:

- Affection of motor nerves (e.g. ulnar/median palsy leads to ulnar/median claw, lateral popliteal palsy results in foot drop).
- Affection of sensory nerves results in loss of sensations, exposing the part to repetitive trauma and subsequent trophic ulcers. Hence, prevention of nerve damage or, at least, its early detection and prompt treatment are effective methods of preventing disability due to leprosy.

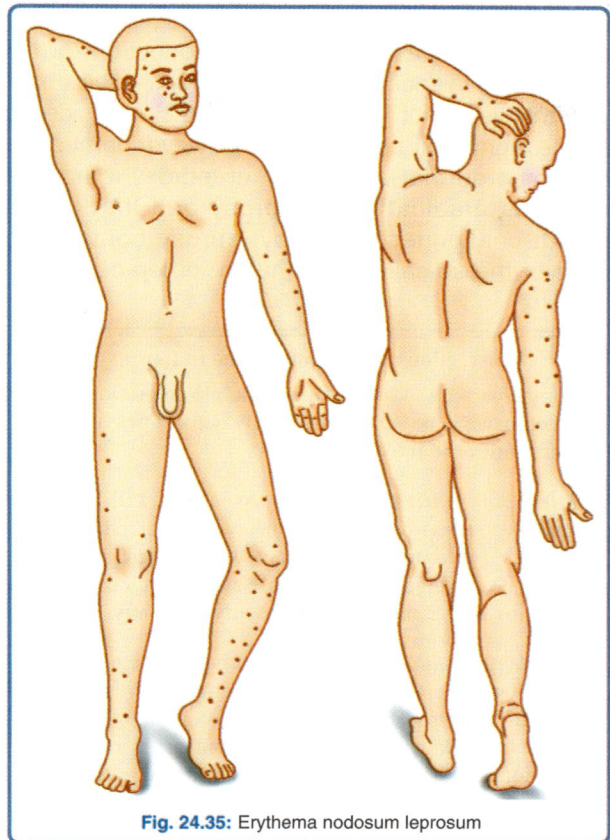

Fig. 24.35: Erythema nodosum leprosum

Steps in Disability Prevention

These include:

- **Identify patients at risk:** Patients in reactions or those who are likely to develop reactions, those with existing disability or those with enlarged nerve trunks even in absence of overt signs of neuritis.
- **Give preventive advice while** supervising and ensuring regular therapy. (Please *see* section on Advice to Leprosy Patients).
- **Be alert to early warning signs** of leprous neuritis, e.g. pain, tingling along a nerve, worsening of sensation or muscle power.
- **Treat neuritis promptly** with systemic steroids (prednisolone 40 mg/day for many weeks) while anti-leprosy therapy is continued.
- **Physical therapy during neuritis:** Rest and passive splints initially; passive exercises, active exercises and dynamic splints, later.

Elimination of Leprosy

In 1991, the 44th World Health Assembly passed a resolution to eliminate leprosy as a public health problem by the year 2000. The assembly defined "elimination" of leprosy as public health problem as reduction in the registered prevalence of leprosy

Chapter
24

Leprosy (Hansen's Disease)

patients receiving MDT to less than 1 per 10,000 population. It was proposed that reduction to this level of prevalence effectively interrupted the chain of transmission of leprosy and could be considered as the significant achievement. However, it must be remembered that elimination of leprosy is not the same as eradication of leprosy and that public health challenges posed by leprosy continue in spite of the so-called "eliminaton" of leprosy.

Correction of Deformities due to Leprosy

For the purpose of management, mobile deformities due to leprosy can be divided into early deformities, mobile deformities and fixed deformities.

Early deformities are usually associated with active neuritis and treatment is that of neuritis (i.e. prednisolone 40–80 mg/day tapered over many weeks). Rest, passive and active exercises and suitable splints are crucial in restoring power and reverting an early deformity.

Mobile deformities due to motor imbalance (e.g. a claw hand) can be corrected by a tendon transplant surgery, which redirects functional tendons so as to restore cosmetic looks and function to a hand or a foot. Short duration, mobile deformities in young persons are ideally suited for surgical correction. Transplanting extensor carpi radialis longus or brevis tendon for correcting ulnar claw and flexor superficialis tendon of ring finger for correcting thumb deformity are two of the common operations in vogue.

Importance of physiotherapy in preparation of and follow up after surgery cannot be overemphasised. Presurgical massage, wax baths improve deformity angles by softening the soft tissue contracture and improving blood supply. Pre-surgical muscle retraining prepares a patient for effective usage of the redirected muscle after surgery thereby improving the final result.

Fixed deformities can only be helped by oil massage, passive and active exercise, taking care that the insensitive limbs are not damaged. Provision of moulding hand grips for articles of day to day use reduces chances of trophic ulcers and improves function.

Due to the effective implementation of multi-drug therapy (MDT) programme during the last 20 years, estimated global burden of leprosy cases declined from 10–12 million cases in mid-1984 to 1.5 million in 1997. In 2001, WHO declared that the historic target of global leprosy elimination was achieved. In 1985, 122 countries in the world had leprosy prevalence of over 1 case per 10,000 population. By 2006, this number came down to six countries viz. Brazil, Democratic Republic of Congo, Madagascar, Mozambique, Nepal and United Republic of Tanzania.

On 30th January 2006, the Ministry of Health, Government of India formally announced that India achieved the elimination target (leprosy prevalence as on 31st December 2005 was 0.95 per 10,000).

On March 2006, 22 states and five union territories in India had achieved prevalence levels below 1 per 10,000; six states (Bihar, Chhattisgarh, Jharkhand, West Bengal, Orissa and Uttar Pradesh) and two union territories (Delhi and Dadra and Nagar Haveli) still had prevalence above 1 per 10,000.

MCQs

1. *Mycobacterium leprae* is peculiar in its:
   a. Slow duplication time
   b. Need for cooler body temperatures
   c. Ability to invade nerves
   d. All of the above

2. Immunity in this type of leprosy is the poorest:
   a. Lepromatous
   b. Borderline
   c. Tuberculoid
   d. Indeterminate

3. The bacterial load in this type of leprosy is the highest:
   a. Lepromatous
   b. Borderline
   c. Tuberculoid
   d. Indeterminate

4. The first stage in evolution of leprosy is:
   a. Intermediate
   b. Late latent
   c. Indeterminate
   d. Borderline

5. Skin lesions tend to get symmetrical in this form of leprosy:
   a. Lepromatous
   b. Borderline lepromatous
   c. Tuberculoid
   d. Borderline tuberculoid

6. Skin lesions are very well defined in this form of leprosy:
   a. Lepromatous
   b. Borderline
   c. Tuberculoid
   d. Indeterminate

7. Skin lesions are never annular in this form of leprosy:
   a. Lepromatous
   b. Borderline lepromatous
   c. Tuberculoid
   d. Borderline tuberculoid

8. Multiple nerve trunks are affected in this form of leprosy:
   a. Indeterminate
   b. Borderline lepromatous
   c. Tuberculoid
   d. Borderline tuberculoid

9. Bacteriological index in leprosy is an estimate of:
   a. Number of leprosy bacilli in the skin biopsies
   b. Number of live leprosy bacilli in skin smears
   c. Proportion of live leprosy bacilli in skin smears
   d. Number of leprosy bacilli in skin smears

10. Morphological index in leprosy is an estimate of:
    a. Number of leprosy bacilli in the skin biopsies
    b. Number of live leprosy bacilli in skin smears
    c. Proportion of live leprosy bacilli in skin smears
    d. Number of leprosy bacilli in skin smears

11. The index arrived at by counting solid staining leprosy bacilli in skin smears is:
    a. Granuloma index
    b. Bacillary index
    c. Bacteriological index
    d. Morphological index

12. The type of leprosy affecting a person is decided by:
    a. Pathogenicity of bacilli
    b. Host immunity
    c. Infecting dose
    d. Duration of disease

13. Leprosy bacilli are transmitted by:
    a. Food contamination
    b. Skin to skin contact
    c. Droplet infection
    d. Insect bite

14. Incubation period of leprosy is:
    a. 1–2 months
    b. 6–12 months
    c. 1–2 years
    d. 3–5 years

15. Elimination of leprosy refers to:
    a. Number cases of leprosy in a year
    b. Number of cases less than 1 in one lac population
    c. Number of cases less than 1 in 10,000 population
    d. Number of cases less than 1 in 1,000 population

16. Ridley-Jopling classification of leprosy is based on:
    a. Clinical features
    b. Bacteriological features
    c. Immunological features
    d. All of the above

17. Indeterminate leprosy lesion is usually a:
    a. Well defined macule
    b. Ill-defined macule
    c. Ring-shaped plaque
    d. Circular plaque

18. Lepromin test is positive in this type of leprosy:
    a. Lepromatous
    b. Borderline lepromatous
    c. Tuberculoid
    d. Indeterminate

Chapter 24

Leprosy (Hansen's Disease)

19. **Loss of sweat function is most evident over lesions of this form of leprosy:**
    a. Lepromatous
    b. Borderline lepromatous
    c. Tuberculoid
    d. Borderline tuberculoid

20. **Macrophage granuloma is seen in this form of leprosy:**
    a. Lepromatous
    b. Borderline tuberculoid
    c. Tuberculoid
    d. Indeterminate

21. **Depressed bridge of nose is seen in this form of leprosy:**
    a. Lepromatous
    b. Borderline tuberculoid
    c. Tuberculoid
    d. Indeterminate

22. **This is an early sign of lepromatous leprosy:**
    a. Nasal stuffiness
    b. Glove and stocking anaesthesia
    c. Depressed bridge of nose
    d. Asymmetrical enlargement of nerves

23. **Tuberculoid granuloma is seen on skin biopsy in this type of leprosy:**
    a. Lepromatous
    b. Borderline tuberculoid
    c. Lupus vulgaris
    d. Indeterminate

24. **Type I reactions are usually seen in this form of leprosy:**
    a. Lepromatous   b. Borderline
    c. Tuberculoid   d. Indeterminate

25. **Type II reactions are usually seen in this form of leprosy:**
    a. Lepromatous
    b. Borderline tuberculoid
    c. Tuberculoid
    d. Indeterminate

26. **Oedema feet could be a presenting sign of this form of leprosy:**
    a. Lepromatous
    b. Borderline tuberculoid
    c. Tuberculoid
    d. Indeterminate

27. **Loss of lateral eyebrows is seen in this form of leprosy:**
    a. Lepromatous
    b. Borderline tuberculoid
    c. Tuberculoid
    d. Indeterminate

28. **Nodules are seen in this form of leprosy:**
    a. Lepromatous
    b. Borderline tuberculoid
    c. Tuberculoid
    d. Indeterminate

29. **Leonine facies is a sign of:**
    a. Lupus erythematosus
    b. Lepromatous leprosy
    c. Erythema nodosum leprosum
    d. Systemic sclerosis

30. **Trophic ulcers in leprosy result from:**
    a. Loss of sensation   b. Loss of nutrition
    c. Loss of blood supply   d. Loss of power

31. **The most commonly affected nerve trunk in leprosy is:**
    a. Ulnar nerve   b. Median nerve
    c. Lateral popliteal nerve d. Sural nerve

32. **Loss of autonomic nerve function in leprosy leads to:**
    a. Ichthyosis   b. Plantar fissuring
    c. Oedema feet   d. All of the above

33. **Glove and stocking anaesthesia is seen in this type of leprosy:**
    a. Lepromatous
    b. Borderline tuberculoid
    c. Tuberculoid
    d. Indeterminate

34. **This is not a cardinal sign of leprosy:**
    a. Presence of acid-fast bacilli in skin lesions
    b. Reduced sensation over skin lesions
    c. Thickening of peripheral nerves
    d. Glove and stocking anaesthesia

35. **This nerve in the neck is commonly enlarged in leprosy:**
    a. Facial
    b. Transverse cervical
    c. Greater auricular
    d. Supraclavicular

36. **This is a sign of radial nerve palsy:**
    a. Ape thumb   b. Partial claw
    c. Wrist drop   d. Complete claw

37. **A test that is of great diagnostic value in leprosy is:**
    a. Slit skin smears   b. Skin biopsy
    c. Lepromin test   d. Sweat test

38. **A form of leprosy that does not have any skin lesions is:**
    a. Neural
    b. Borderline tuberculoid
    c. Tuberculoid
    d. Indeterminate

39. **WHO recommends therapy of borderline lepromatous leprosy with:**
    a. Dapsone
    b. Clofazimine
    c. Rifampicin
    d. All of the above

40. **Pauci-bacillary leprosy refers to those cases where:**
    a. Lot of lepra bacilli are demonstrable in the skin smears
    b. A few lepra bacilli are demonstrable in the skin smears
    c. No lepra bacilli are demonstrable in the skin smears
    d. Lepra bacilli are demonstrable in normal looking skin

41. **Multi-bacillary leprosy refers to those cases where:**
    a. Lot of lepra bacilli are demonstrable in the skin lesions
    b. A few lepra bacilli are demonstrable in the skin lesions
    c. No lepra bacilli are demonstrable in the skin lesions
    d. Any number of lepra bacilli are demonstrable in skin

42. **As per WHO recommendation for antileprosy therapy rifampicin needs to be given:**
    a. Daily
    b. On alternate days
    c. Once a week
    d. Once a month

43. **The recommended duration of theapy in pauci-bacillary leprosy is:**
    a. 6 months
    b. 1 year
    c. 2 years
    d. Till lesions heal completely

44. **The recommended duration of therapy in multi-bacillary leprosy is:**
    a. 6 months
    b. 1 year
    c. 2 years
    d. Till lesions heal completely

45. **In fixed duration therapy of leprosy treatment is administered for a fixed duration irrespective of results of:**
    a. Activity of lesions
    b. Skin smears
    c. Skin biopsy
    d. All of the above

46. **Which of the following drugs is not useful against *M. leprae*?**
    a. Cephalexin
    b. Ofloxacin
    c. Minocycline
    d. Clofazimine

47. **ROM therapy consists of all *except*:**
    a. Minocycline
    b. Ofloxacin
    c. Rifabutin
    d. Rifampicin

48. **Type I lepra reactions are commonly seen:**
    a. Before initiating antileprosy therapy
    b. Within a few days of starting antileprosy therapy
    c. Within six months of starting antileprosy therapy
    d. After completion of antileprosy therapy

49. **Type II lepra reactions are commonly seen:**
    a. Before initiating antileprosy therapy
    b. Within six months of starting antileprosy therapy
    c. After six months of starting antileprosy therapy
    d. After completion of antileprosy therapy

50. **This is not a side-effect of clofazimine:**
    a. Ichthyosis
    b. Pigmentation
    c. Gastritis
    d. Anaemia

51. **The dosage of clofazimine for leprosy reaction is:**
    a. 50 mg alternate days
    b. 50 mg daily
    c. 100 mg daily
    d. 300 mg daily

52. **Type I lepra reactions cause this serious complication:**
    a. Orchitis
    b. Nerve paralysis
    c. Arthritis
    d. Iridocyclitis

53. **Type II lepra reactions may cause:**
    a. Periosteitis
    b. Worsening of existing skin lesions
    c. Trophic ulcers
    d. Gangrene

54. **First line treatment of nerve paralysis in Type I lepra reactions is:**
    a. Oral steroids
    b. Nerve decompression
    c. Rest followed by exercise
    d. Clofazimine

55. **Type II lepra reactions respond promptly to:**
    a. Oral steroids
    b. Oral thalidomide
    c. Oral clofazimine
    d. Injectable methylene blue

56. **Skin smears are negative in which type of leprosy?**
    a. Indeterminate
    b. Neuritic
    c. Lepromatous
    d. Borderline

57. **The most common type of leprosy in India is:**
    a. BT
    b. TT
    c. LL
    d. BL

58. **Virchow's cells are seen in:**
    a. HSP
    b. TEN
    c. Congenital syphilis
    d. Leprosy

59. **Lepra cell is a:**
    a. Plasma cell
    b. Neutrophil
    c. Lymphocyte
    d. Histiocyte

60. **Satellite lesions are seen in:**
    a. Tuberculoid leprosy
    b. Lepromatous leprosy
    c. Borderline tuberculoid
    d. Histoid leprosy

61. **Inverted saucer-shaped ulcers are found in:**
    a. BT
    b. BB
    c. BL
    d. Indeterminate

62. **All are true about lepromatous leprosy** *except*:
    a. Presence of globi
    b. Subepidermal free zone
    c. Decreased cell-mediated immunity
    d. Presence of granuloma subdermally

63. **Earliest sensation to be lost in Hansen's disease:**
    a. Pain
    b. Temperature
    c. Vibration
    d. Touch

64. **All lesions are seen in leprosy** *except*:
    a. Erythematous macule
    b. Hypopigmented patch
    c. Vesicle
    d. Flat and raised patches

65. **Symmetrical multiple lesions are seen in which type of leprosy?**
    a. Borderline
    b. Neuritic
    c. Lepromatous
    d. Tuberculoid

66. **Which of the following is indication of active leprosy?**
    a. New skin lesions
    b. Nerve tenderness
    c. Erythema
    d. All

67. **Lepromin test is positive in:**
    a. Lepromatous
    b. Indeterminate
    c. Histoid
    d. Tuberculoid

68. **Drug of choice for type 2 lepra reaction:**
    a. Steroid
    b. Thalidomide
    c. Clofazimine
    d. Dapsone

69. **Thalidomide is drug of choice for:**
    a. Lepra 1 reaction
    b. Lepra 2 reaction
    c. Both
    d. Nerve abscess

70. **DOC in type 1 reaction with severe neuritis:**
    a. Thalidomide
    b. Clofazimine
    c. Dapsone
    d. Systemic corticosteroid

71. **Antileprotic drug also used in lepra reaction is:**
    a. Rifampicin
    b. Dapsone
    c. Ciprofloxacin
    d. Clofazimine

72. **Lucio reaction is seen in:**
    a. TB
    b. Leprosy
    c. Syphilis
    d. LGV

73. **Treatment of severe ulnar neuritis in borderline tuberculoid leprosy is:**
    a. MDT only
    b. MDT + steroid
    c. Wait and watch
    d. MDT + thalidomide

74. **Best method of treatment of ulnar nerve abscess in leprosy:**
    a. High dose of steroid
    b. Incision and drainage
    c. Thalidomide
    d. Low dose of corticosteroid

75. **Treatment of acute neuritis in type 1 reaction is all** *except*:
    a. MB MDT
    b. Steroid
    c. Thalidomide
    d. Incision and drainage

76. **Most effective drug against** *M. leprae* **is:**
    a. Dapsone
    b. Rifampicin
    c. Clofazimine
    d. Prothionamide

ANSWERS

1-d,	2-a,	3-a,	4-c,	5-a,	6-c,	7-a,	8-b,	9-d,	10-c,
11-d,	12-b,	13-c,	14-d,	15-c,	16-d,	17-b,	18-c,	19-c,	20-a,
21-a,	22-a,	23-b,	24-b,	25-a,	26-a,	27-a,	28-a,	29-b,	30-a,
31-a,	32-d,	33-a,	34-d,	35-c,	36-c,	37-a,	38-a,	39-d,	40-c,
41-a,	42-d,	43-a,	44-b,	45-d,	46-a,	47-c,	48-a,	49-c,	50-d,
51-d,	52-b,	53-a,	54-a,	55-b,	56-b,	57-a,	58-d,	59-d,	60-c,
61-b,	62-d,	63-b,	64-c,	65-c,	66-d,	67-d,	68-a,	69-b,	70-d,
71-d,	72-b,	73-b,	74-b,	75-c,	76-b				

SECTION 3

Sexually Transmitted Infections including HIV Infection

Sexually Transmitted Infections

Definition

Sexually transmitted infections (STIs), (sexually transmitted diseases, STDs) are a group of infections transmitted through sexual contact.

The principal STIs include:

- Syphilis
- Gonorrhoea
- Chancroid
- Donovanosis
- Lymphogranuloma venereum
- Herpes simplex
- Condyloma acuminata
- Hepatitis B
- Human immunodeficiency virus (HIV) and
- Genital infections due to:
    - Chlamydia
    - Mycoplasma
    - Candida
    - Trichomonas Vaginalis
    - Pubic louse
    - Scabies
    - Molluscum contagiosum virus

> The term venereal diseases was used previously to designate the first five diseases in the above list.

PREVENTION OF STIs (COUNSELLING FOR STI PATIENTS)

This assumed great importance in recent times with the emergence of HIV infection as presence of many STIs increases the risk of transmission and acquisition of HIV. The various measures that can be advised include:

- Abstinence from sex—impossible for most people.
- Avoid sex with sex workers, as the chance of their being a carrier for STIs, especially. HIV infection, is very high. Some years ago as many as 60% of sex workers in Mumbai were HIV positive, although this proportion has now come down due to effective control measures.
- Restrict to one sexual partner. Avoid casual sex or sex with someone whose antecedents are unknown.
- If you must, then use a good quality condom **every time**. Learn how to use a condom in a proper way. Some of the spermicidal jellies (e.g. nonoxynol 9) are also active against bacteria and viruses.
- After sex, pass urine and wash genitalia as soon as possible with plenty of water and soap.
- Prophylactic use of antibacterials like cotrimoxazole or tetracycline after an unprotected exposure is controversial. In any event, it is not useful for prevention against HIV.
- Sex education forms an essential part of prevention of STIs as it is only through such discussion that advice regarding condom usage can be disseminated to the young.
- Today, improving awareness of STIs in the community, with special reference to HIV infection, is a national priority. Prior knowledge of the far reaching medical and social consequences of HIV infection will go a long way in reducing risk taking behaviour in the young.
- **Pre-test counseling**

    This refers to talking to persons with a history of activities with high risk of acquiring HIV infection (most commonly, unsafe sex) **before collecting blood for a test** for HIV infection. A little knowledge about HIV infection with respect to its mode of transmission, unique nature, virtual incurability and long-term treatment is necessary for all persons with a history of unsafe sex, even if they have never had any other STI. They must also be told about the fact that proper use of condom can prevent transmission of HIV infection. Without such information (and consent for doing the HIV test) screening test for HIV infection should not be performed.

    Confronting a person with the possibility of a positive test result and what would be his or her reaction to such an eventuality, even before the test is done, greatly reduces the risk of an extreme reaction like suicide. It also motivates the person to alter his or her high risk behaviour, if the test turns out to be negative. A positive test result in an asymptomatic person does not mean he/she is suffering from AIDS and is likely to die in the near future. This fact needs to be emphasised to persons before enzyme-linked immunosorbent assay (ELISA) test, because there could be a time interval of up to 10 years (or even longer in many cases) between infection and development of any symptoms of HIV disease.

Counselling Persons with ELISA Report

It takes about 2–3 months from the point of infection with HIV for the antibody based ELISA test to become positive. This ELISA negative period is called the window period. All persons with a history of unsafe sex within the last 3 months should therefore be advised to repeat ELISA test 6 months after the last exposure.

Summary: Important sexually transmitted infections include HIV infection, syphilis, gonorrhoea, chancroid, donovanosis, lymphogranuloma venereum, herpes simplex, condyloma acuminata, non-gonococcal urethritis, hepatitis B, pediculosis pubis and scabies. Prevention of STIs is extremely important in the HIV era. Restricting to one sexual partner and, if this is impossible, use of condom during each and every unsafe intercourse are the two most important behavioural changes that need to be integrated into lifestyle in order to protect from HIV infection.

Vertical Transmission of STIs

This refers to transmission of infections, that are usually transmitted sexually among adults, from an infectious mother to her progeny.

Several STIs are transmitted in this fashion. Transmission may occur antepartum (transplacentally, e.g. syphilis, HIV) or intrapartum (during the passage through birth canal, e.g. gonorrhoea, herpes, chlamydia) or rarely postpartum (breast milk).

Syphilis

It is transmitted to the foetus transplacentally during the second trimester. With each subsequent pregnancy, the severity of infection reduces. Severe infection results in abortion, stillbirth or congenital syphilis presenting at birth. Milder infections result in a normal looking baby who develops features of congenital syphilis months or even years later.

Gonorrhoea

Gonococcal ophthalmia occurs in infants born to mothers who are asymptomatic carriers of gonococcal infection. Keratoconjunctivitis, corneal ulcer and blindness may follow, if it is not treated promptly.

Herpes Simplex

Herpes simplex virus II has propensity to cause disseminated herpes simplex infection in neonates born to mothers suffering from active primary genital herpes infection. Due to high morbidity and mortality associated with such neonatal infection, caesarian section is advised if the membranes have not ruptured or at least within 4 hours of rupture of membranes.

Chlamydial Infection

Pneumonia occurs in neonates born to mothers who are carriers of genital infection with chlamydia. Such maternal infection may be asymptomatic or may present as symptomatic cervicitis, urethritis or pelvic inflammatory disease.

HIV Infection

This can be transmitted ante, intra or postpartum from mothers who are HIV positive. Chances of transmission are about 35%. Severity of infection depends upon the viral load in the mother during pregnancy. Majority of the infections are intrapartum or due to transplacental transfer of HIV that occurs after 28 weeks of gestation.

Condyloma Acuminata

Intrapartum transmission is responsible for laryngeal papillomatosis in children.

Summary: Vertical transmission of STIs refers to transmission from mother to her progeny either transplacentally, intrapartum or through breast milk. Most important STIs that are transmitted are syphilis (transplacental), herpes genitalis (intrapartum) and HIV infection (all 3 ways). Vertical transmission of syphilis can cause abortion, stillbirth or congenital syphilis. That of HIV results in paediatric AIDS that is usually fatal in early childhood. Transmission of herpes genitalis induces disseminated neonatal herpes infection that has high morbidity and mortality.

SYPHILIS (LUES)

This treponemal infection is known over the years for its ability to present in many different ways. Being a potentially serious infection every doctor has to be on guard not to miss this easily treatable condition. It is caused by the spirochaete, *Treponema pallidum* (Fig. 25.1). It may be acquired as a sexually transmitted infection or may be transferred transplacentally as congenital syphilis.

ACQUIRED SYPHILIS

Acquired syphilis is a sexually transmitted infection that is systemic from the beginning. Left untreated, acquired syphilis runs course through various stages viz. incubation period (9–90 days), primary chancre (lasts for one to several weeks), episodes of mucocutaneous eruptions of secondary syphilis (individual episode lasts for one to several weeks), latent stage (may last indefinitely) and tertiary syphilis (appears 2–10 years after initial infection).

The initial two years of infection are termed as early syphilis (infectious) and include the incubation period, primary, secondary and early latent phases. After the second year of infection, the disease is termed as late syphilis (non-infectious) and this includes late latent syphilis, benign tertiary syphilis, cardiosyphilis and neurosyphilis. In the present antibiotic era, late syphilis is encountered rarely.

Summary: Acquired syphilis is sexually transmitted. After an incubation period of about 2–4 weeks, if untreated, it passes through primary, secondary stages and may later go into the tertiary stage. The first 2 years of infection are termed early syphilis (infectious) and the latter part called late syphilis (non-infectious).

PRIMARY SYPHILIS

A primary sore (hard chancre) and regional lymphadenopathy are the clinical components. Signs and symptoms regress spontaneously in 2–6 weeks even without therapy.

Patient Profile

Young adults practising unsafe sex are affected. Males are more commonlly affected. The commonest age group involved is between 25–35 years.

Morphology

A 'clean looking' rounded or oval ulcer, about 1–2 cm in diameter, with sloping or punched out edges is typical. Floor of the ulcer is formed by

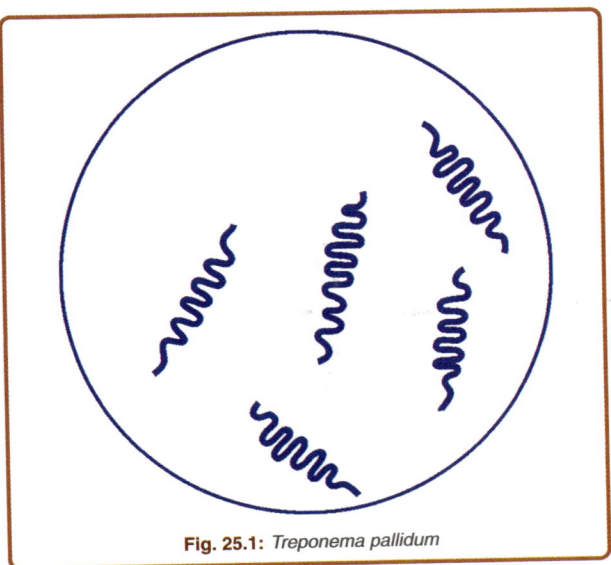

Fig. 25.1: *Treponema pallidum*

pale granulation tissue and is covered by thin serosanguinous discharge. The ulcer base is indurated and manipulation does not induce bleeding.

Distribution

Prepuce, shaft and glans of penis are common sites in males whereas labia majora and cervix are common sites in females. Affection of perianal and other extragenital sites is uncommon. Regional lymph nodes are painless, moderately enlarged, non-tender discrete and firm or rubbery in consistency.

Diagnosis

History of unsafe sex, an incubation period of 9–90 days, and presence of a single, painless ulcer with typical morphology are highly suggestive. Smear of serous discharge from the ulcer, when examined under the dark ground microscope, displays treponemes in abundance. Although, commonly positive the serum venereal disease research laboratory (VDRL) test may remain negative till the ulcer is 2 weeks old. Serum fluorescent antibody absorption (FTA-ABS) test is usually positive. It is mandatory to screen for associated HIV infection.

Therapy

It is that for early syphilis. (Please *see* therapy of syphilis).

Summary: Primary syphilis consists of a chancre and regional lymphadenopathy. The hard chancre is seen as a single, painless, rounded, indurated ulcer, with pale granulation and serosanguinous discharge in the floor and which does not bleed on manipulation. Smear for dark ground microscopy demonstrates treponemes. Serum VDRL is positive later in the course of the ulcer. Therapy is that of early syphilis.

SECONDARY SYPHILIS

Secondary syphilis usually presents as mucocutaneous lesions with or without other signs and symptoms (Figs 25.2–25.6). Occasionally, it may resent with other manifestations like fever, joint pains, lymphadenopathy or cranial nerve palsies, singly or in combination without any mucocutaneous lesions. History of and scar of genital sore are common.

Patient Profile

Same as primary syphilis.

Chapter
25

Sexually Transmitted Infections

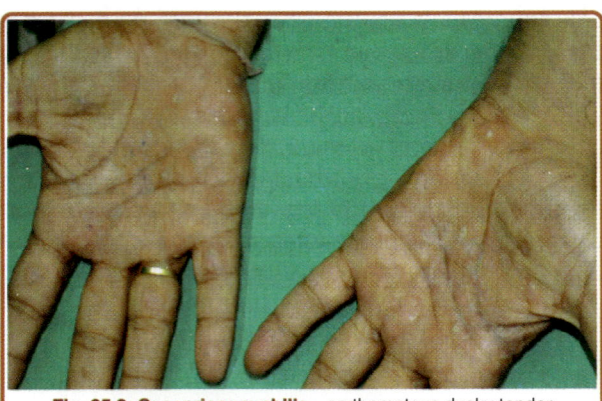

Fig. 25.2: Secondary syphilis—erythematous dusky tender maculopapules over palms

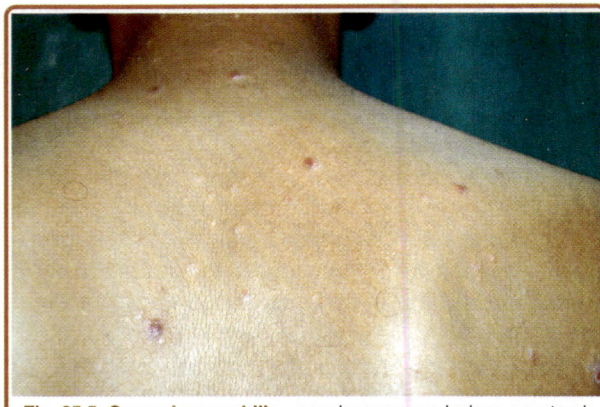

Fig. 25.5: Secondary syphilis—papulosquamous lesions over trunk in secondary syphilis

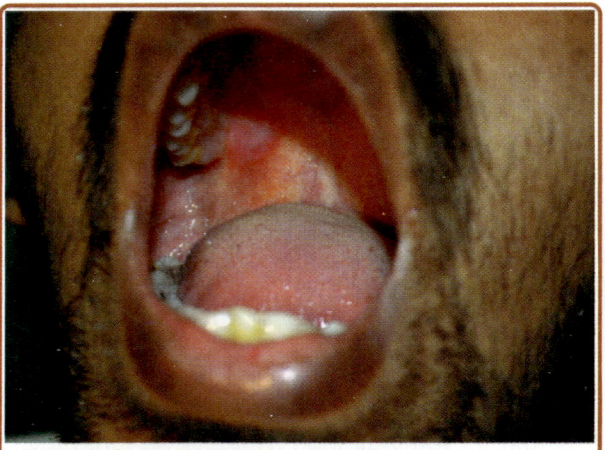

Fig. 25.3 : Secondary syphilis—erythematous mucous patch over palate with grayish centre

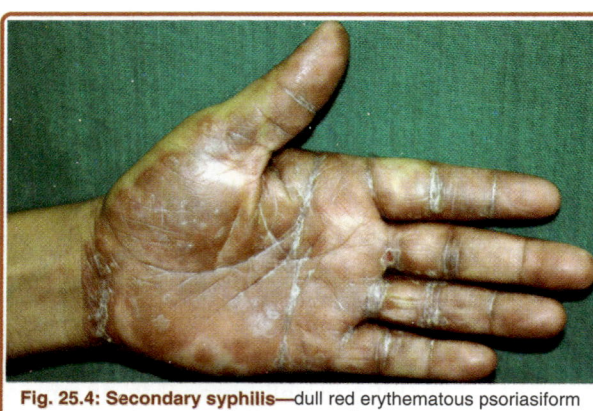

Fig. 25.4: Secondary syphilis—dull red erythematous psoriasiform plaques over palms

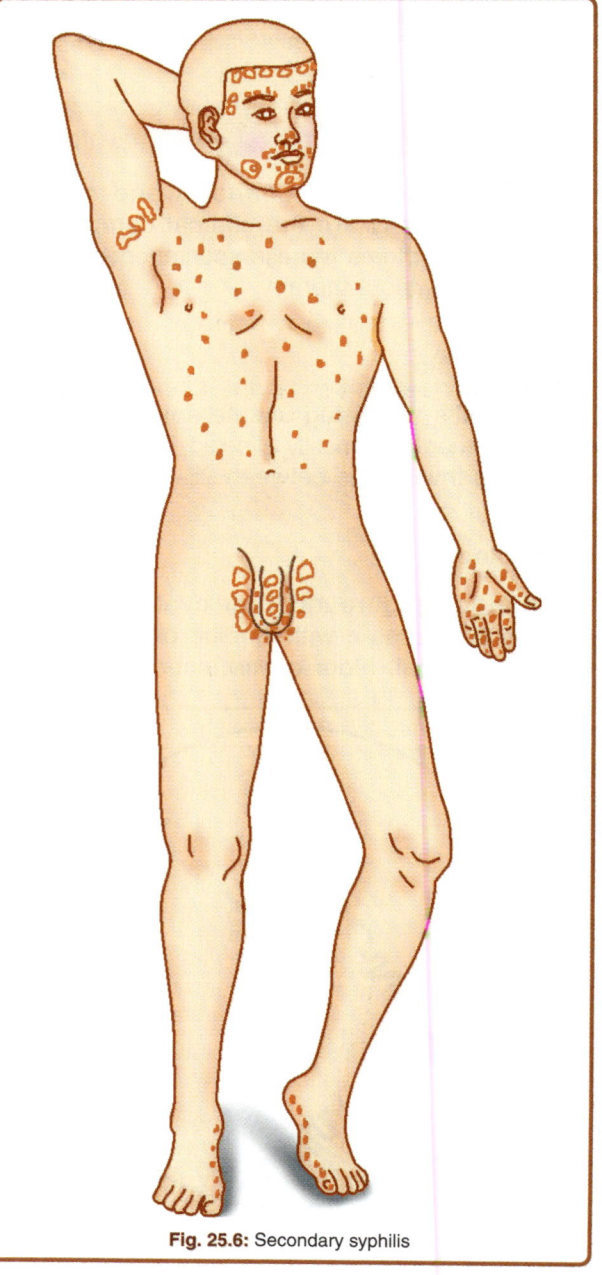

Fig. 25.6: Secondary syphilis

Morphology

Rash of secondary syphilis can be of a variety of types or combinations of them. Some of the common types are:

- **Macular** (roseolar rash)
- **Papular and papulosquamous**—dull red coloured papules with or without scales Fig. 25.7).

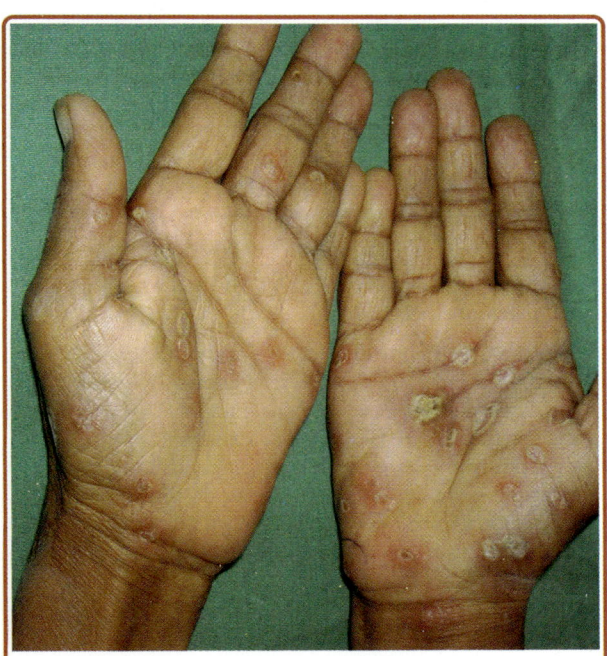

Fig. 25.7: Secondary syphilis—desquamating papules and plaques surrounded by zone of erythema

- **Pustular**—non-follicular pustules
- **Acneiform**—follicular papulopustules resembling acne
- **Annular**—ring-shaped plaques

The skin lesions show the sign of deep dermal tenderness, i.e. application of firm pressure with a small blunt object like the head of a matchstick or common pin causes pain.

Uncommon morphologic variants of secondary syphilitic rash include nodular, noduloulcerative, pustuloulcerative, rupial and corymbose.

Distribution

Nonpruritic, symmetrical rash with a tendency to affect flexor aspects of the body. Palms/Soles, flexures, mucosae, orifices and periorificial regions are preferentially affected.

Palms and Soles

Dusky red coloured, tender macules or papules on palms and soles with a tendency to become scaly or keratotic with tie are typical (Fig. 25.7).

Scalp

Skin lesions occur over scalp and tend to coalesce along the forehead scalp margin (corona veneris). Small patches of ill defined, incomplete, non-inflammatory, non-scarring alopecia result in a 'moth eaten' appearance.

Mucosae, Mucocutaneous Junctions and Body Folds

White coloured or Pale pink papules and plaques, with a broad base and moist surface at these sites are termed as condyloma lata (Fig. 25.8). Over mucosae and mucocutaneous junctions, superficial erosions with grayish surface and erythematous halo are observed. These mucous patches (also called mucous erosions) may coalesce and form irregular erosions or ulcers (serpiginous ulcer). Condyloma lata and mucous patches along with the primary chancre are the moist lesions of early syphilis.

Clinical implication: Moist lesions of syphilis are highly infectious. Hence, it is essential to examine, investigate and follow-up or treat the sexual partner of such person.

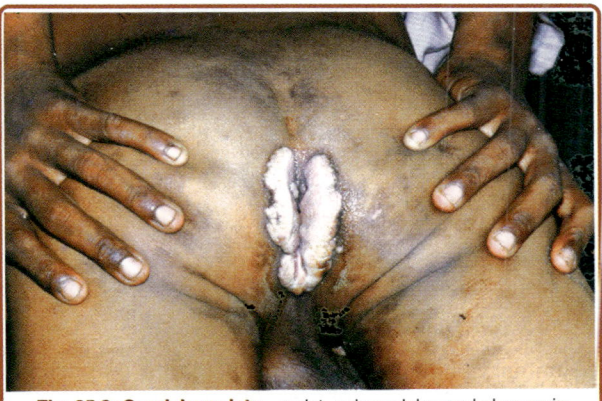

Fig. 25.8: Condyloma lata—moist, pale nodules and plaques in perianal area

SYSTEMIC MANIFESTATIONS OF SECONDARY SYPHILIS

Generalised lymphadenopathy occurs, particularly involving the epitrochlear, cervical, occipital, preauricular and postauricular, axillary and inguinal lymph nodes. Nodes are moderately enlarged, non-tender, discrete and firm (described as shotty or rubbery) in consistency.

Fever, malaise, body ache, headache, joint pains and less commonly, joint swellings are present. In rare instances, paralysis of facial muscles, extraocular muscles or deafness may occur due to involvement of cranial nerves.

EVOLUTION OF SECONDARY SYPHILIS

Secondary syphilis usually presents within the first 6 months of infection. Left untreated, skin and

Chapter
25

Sexually Transmitted Infections

mucosal lesions heal without scarring, after a variable interval of 2–6 weeks. Lesions may leave behind dyspigmentation and skin atrophy.

During the first 2 years of infection, if left untreated, rash of secondary syphilis may recur. During early infection rash tends to be widespread, symmetrical and has standard morphology. Later, lesions become fewer, asymmetric, large and unusual in morphology.

INVESTIGATIONS AND DIAGNOSIS

Confirmation of clinical diagnosis by demonstration of treponemes or a positive antibody test is necessary. If clinical findings coincide, a VDRL titre of 1:8 or more is taken as diagnostic. This is because false positive high titre VDRL results are uncommon. Please *see* following section on investigations in syphilis for more details.

When clinical findings are strongly suggestive of secondary syphilis but the VDRL is negative, repeat it in dilutions to rule out prozone phenomenon. Other possibilities in such a case are, associated HIV infection or the clinical diagnosis may be wrong.

THERAPY

Please *see* section on therapy of syphilis, later.

> **Summary:** Secondary syphilis presents with muco-cutaneous lesions, generalised, non-tender, shotty lymphadenopathy, arthralgia and fever. The lesions are non-pruritic, symmetric, widespread and dull red in colour. Deep dermal tenderness is positive over the skin lesions which may be macular, papular, papulosquamous, pustular, acneiform or annular. Condyloma lata and mucous patches are the moist infective lesions that occur over genitalia, flexures, mucocutaneous junctions and mucosae.
>
> Dark ground illumination for treponemes from the moist lesions and positive serology [VDRL test or a specific test like *Treponema pallidium* haemagglutination assay (TPHA) establish the diagnosis. Procaine penicillin (fortified) 1–2 MU IM OD for 10 days is curative. A single injection of benzathine penicillin 2.4 MU IM is also effective. Tetracycline or Erythromycin can be given (500 mg QDS for 14 days) in case of penicillin hypersensitivity. A stringent post-treatment follow up is advocated particularly in HIV positive persons.

> ### Latent Syphilis
>
> Infection with *T. pallidum* may persist without causing any signs or symptoms and may be detected during accidental screening. According to whether the condition is diagnosed during the first 2 years of infection or later, it is termed as early latent or late latent syphilis.

> **Clinical implication:** Late latent syphilis is managed like late syphilis whereas early latent syphilis is treated with a regimen for early syphilis

> #### Benign tertiary syphilis
>
> **Benign Tertiary Syphilis of Skin and Mucosae (Mucocutaneous Gumma)**
>
> In today's antibiotic era, with several of the commonly used antibiotics being effective against *T. pallidum*, tertiary syphilis is extremely uncommon. However, with the emergence of HIV infection, accelerated progression of syphilis to tertiary stage and relapses after adequate therapy are being reported. Hence, in future, tertiary syphilis may be observed. Gummatous lesions of tertiary syphilis may affect any organ in the body but are most common in the skin or mucosae.
>
> **Patient Profile**
>
> Middle aged and elderly men and women are affected. However, it may occur in younger individuals with HIV infection.
>
> **Morphology**
>
> One or a few, slowly progressive, asymptomatic, erythematous, noduloulcerative or indurated plaques that tend to heal at one end or in the centre, with formation of tissue paper scars and progress at the other end or peripherally. This pattern leads to formation of serpiginous or annular plaques. The ulcer in the centre, is punched out and deep, with pale floor covered with abundant white slough. Lesions that remain untreated for long duration cause destruction of tissues, e.g. perforation of palate.
>
> **Distribution**
>
> Although, any part of the body may be affected, head, face and nasal, oral, pharyngeal and laryngeal mucosae are frequently involved. Result may be nasal septal or palatal perforation or mutilation of the face. Ulcerative lesions may have underlying bony or soft tissue gumma.
>
> **Diagnosis**
>
> Serologic tests for syphilis and a skin biopsy can confirm the diagnosis. Treponemes are not demonstrable in the lesions or in blood.

> **Clinical implication:** Since there are no treponemes in the skin lesions, a patient of tertiary syphilis is non-infectious.

Therapy

Please *see* section on therapy of syphilis.

Summary: Benign tertiary syphilis of the skin and mucosae presents as painless, indolent, single or a few, indurated plaques or noduloulcerative lesions with annular or serpiginous outline. Spontaneous healing leads to tissue paper scarring. Face, head, nasal and oropharyngeal mucosae are frequently affected. Diagnosis can be confirmed with serologic tests and skin biopsy. Therapy is that of late syphilis.

Cardiovascular and neurosyphilis (quaternary syphilis): These are relatively uncommon. Predominant features of cardiac syphilis are aortic regurgitation, aortic aneurysm, arrhythmias and angina. Neurosyphilis can present in a variety of ways; meningovascular syphilis, tabes dorsalis and general paresis are some of the popular syndromes.

INVESTIGATIONS FOR SYPHILIS

Diagnosis of syphilis can be confirmed in the laboratory by either demonstrating the organism or antibodies against it.

Demonstration of *Treponema Pallidum*

Dark ground illumination microscopy of smears from moist genital or mucosal lesions of primary or secondary syphilis provides the quickest test for diagnosis of early syphilis. Such smears can also be made from lymph node aspirate, if mucocutaneous lesions are absent.

Silver impregnation staining of smears can also demonstrate the organism. Biopsy of mucocutaneous lesions of early syphilis can also be stained by the silver impregnation method.

DEMONSTRATION OF ANTIBODIES TO *TREPONEMA PALLIDUM*

Tests for Non-specific Antibody

Serum venereal disease research laboratory

This is the screening and monitoring test for syphilis because it is easy to perform, inexpensive, highly sensitive and can be quantitated. It becomes positive about 1–2 weeks after the appearance of primary sore and remains positive, if the disease is untreated. In treated patients, its titre (highest dilution at which test is positive) falls gradually (over months or years) depending upon the duration of the disease, finally becoming negative.

Rapid plasma reagin test

Rapid plasma reagin (RPR) test checks for the same non-specific antibody responsible for the VDRL test except that the test result is available within minutes.

Tests for Specific Antibody

These are usually performed only when clinical features and serum VDRL result do not tally (suspected false positive or false negative VDRL) or it is extremely important to confirm the VDRL test positivity, e.g. in medicolegal cases or in pregnant mothers. These tests are highly specific but, unlike VDRL, they may not become negative after successful therapy. The commonly used specific tests are TPHA and FTA-ABS test.

Treponema pallidum haemagglutination assay

This is an easy to perform test that can be quantified for monitoring patients after therapy.

Fluorescent treponemal antibody absorption test

This is a test that becomes positive, the earliest. It requires special equipment and trained staff. It is not a quantitative test.

Skin biopsy

This is useful in the diagnosis of secondary syphilis. A superficial and deep perivascular lymphoplasmocytic infiltrate with a mixture of histiocytes is observed.

Cerebrospinal fluid studies

These are necessary in cases of late syphilis and selected cases of secondary syphilis (e.g. with cranial nerve palsies) in order to demonstrate and treat CNS involvement. CSF shows raised proteins, lymphocytes and positive VDRL as well as specific tests.

Summary: Diagnosis of syphilis depends on demonstration of either the organisms (by dark ground illumination from smears of moist lesions) or the antibodies to it. VDRL test is the commonest used screening test for syphilis. However, it can give false positive results and hence sometimes its results may need to be confirmed with specific tests like TPHA and FTA-ABS test. A VDRL titre of 1:8 usually indicates infection, if the clinical findings coincide. After therapy, VDRL titre falls gradually and this is useful for monitoring the response. Skin biopsy is rarely needed for diagnosis. It shows a lymphoplasmocytic and histiocytic infiltrate. CSF studies may be done in cases of late syphilis.

Chapter 25

Sexually Transmitted Infections

THERAPY OF SYPHILIS

For the purpose of treatment, it is important to find out if the patient is:

- In the first **2 years of infection**, i.e. if it is early syphilis or late syphilis.

Clinical Implication: In patients with a history of frequent unsafe intercourses, it is difficult to be sure about this only on the basis of history. For practical purposes, patients with lesions of primary and secondary syphilis are then taken as suffering from early syphilis.

- Suffering from HIV infection.
- **Early syphilis** (includes primary, secondary and early latent syphilis):
  - In *HIV negative cases*—a single dose of benzathine penicillin 2.4 MU IM after test dose for 10 years
  - In *HIV positive cases*—benzathine penicillin is effective in cases of early HIV infection in which there is not show any signs of advanced immune deficiency. It is used in the dose of 2.4 MU IM after test dose every week for 3 weeks with careful follow-up. Procaine penicillin (fortified) 24 lac IU IM OD after test dose for 14 days, preferable with probenecid, is necessary only, if the patient has any signs of advanced immune deficiency.

- **Late syphilis** (except neurosyphilis)
  - In *HIV negative* cases—procaine penicillin G 1.2 MU IM OD for 20 days can be used. Benzathine penicillin is not advisable for its poor penetration into CSF. However, it may be used (2.4 MU IM every week for 3 consecutive weeks), if CSF examination is normal.
  - In *HIV positive* cases—crystalline penicillin G 2–4 million IU IV 4 hourly, preferably with probenecid, for 14 days is the drug of choice. If the patient can't get hospitalised, daily injections of procaine penicillin 24 lac IU IM OD for 14 days with probenecid 500 mg QDS can be substituted. Other drugs are best used only if penicillin hypersensitivity can not be overcome by desensitisation. A careful follow up after the therapy is a must.

Penicillin is the drug of choice for the treatment of syphilis. Hence, antibiotics other than penicillin can be used only in individuals with proved penicillin hypersensitivity. The antibiotics include erythromycin (for pregnant women) or tetracycline 500 mg QDS for 14 days or doxycycline 100 mg BD for 14 days.

Same drugs need to be taken for 30 days in cases of late syphilis. Cephalosporins, e.g. ceftriaxone 1 g IM OD for 10–14 days or cephalexin 500 mg qid orally for 2 weeks can also be used but may show cross-hypersensitivity to penicillin.

Jarisch-Herxheimer Reaction

This is also called therapeutic shock and is due to sudden release of treponemal antigens, from killed treponemes, as a result of institution of therapy. Fever, headache, body ache, joint pains, hypotension and vomiting may accompany exacerbation or appearance of new mucocutaneous lesions. The reaction begins within hours of penicillin injection and lasts 12–24 hours.

Follow-up After Treatment of Syphilis

All patients treated for syphilis, need an extended follow-up to ensure that there is no relapse. This is all the more important in HIV positive cases. Follow-up includes a clinical check-up and a VDRL test performed every 3 monthly for 2 years. VDRL titre falls to one-fourth of original in successfully treated individuals. The test may take several months or even years to become negative. In patients with late syphilis, it may never become negative.

Summary: Penicillin injections, after test dose, is the treatment of choice for syphilis. While a single injection of benzathine penicillin, 2.4 MU IM ATD, can be used for early syphilis in the HIV negative, it should be avoided in others. Procaine penicillin, 8 lac IU IM OD AD for HIV negative and 24 lac IU for HIV positive, for 10–14 days is the preferred therapy. For persons with late syphilis, crystalline penicillin 4 lac IU IV 4 hourly is preferred over procaine penicillin unless CSF studies rule out asymptomatic neurosyphilis. For persons with penicillin hypersensitivity, oral erythromycin or tetracycline, 500 mg QDS for 14 days can be used. After treatment, patients need to be followed-up every 3 months with a serum VDRL, to confirm a cure.

CONGENITAL SYPHILIS

Treponemes cross the placenta from an infected mother to the foetus after the trimester. Routine antenatal screening of mothers with a serum VDRL test is advised to present this dangerous possibility.

Clinical implication: Therapy of syphilis during pregnancy—prompt institution of therapy is important. Avoid drugs other than penicillin because they are either contraindicated (e.g. tetracyclines) or have poor penetration across the placenta (e.g. erythromycin). Avoid benzathine penicillin beause it does not cross placenta very well. If any of these are used, it is mandatory to treat the baby at birth.

Severity of this transplacental infection varies according to the duration of infection in the mother. Older the infection, milder the affection. Thus, this may cause abortion or stillbirth (in severest infections) or present as congenital syphilis at birth or later in infancy or childhood (in mildest infections).

Early Congenital Syphilis

During the first 2 years of life, the infection is termed as early congenital syphilis (infectious). Most common age of presentation is between 2–6 months and the complaints— low birth weight, failure to thrive, weak or hoarse cry, persistent rhinitis with or without epistaxis, generalised lymphadenopathy, hepatosplenomegaly, fever, pseudoparalysis due to metaphysitis and a mucocutaneous eruption similar to secondary syphilis in adults. Syphilitic dactylitis, choroiditis and meningoencephalitis are uncommon.

Diagnosis can be confirmed by a smear for treponemes obtained from wet mucosal lesions. A high titre of VDRL test (especially when this is compared to mother's VDRL titre) is usual. Specific test like TPHA are also positive X-ray of painful long bones (especially tibia) may show metaphysitis. Therapy comprises procaine penicillin 50000 IU per kg body weight IM OD after test dose for 10 days. Benzathine penicillin 50000 IU per kg IM single dose (half in each buttock) can also be used but is not preferred due to improper absorption and poor penetration into CSF.

Late Congenital Syphilis

This is now rare. After the first 2 years of life, the infection is called late congenital syphilis (non-infectious). Mucocutaneous lesions resemble those of late acquired syphilis. Interstitial keratitis occurs after 6 years of age and if not treated with steroids, may lead to blindness. Clutton's joints represent an arthritis with joint effusion that does not revert after antisyphilitic therapy. Persistent periosteitis leads to periosteal thickening (sabre tibia). Neurolabyrinthitis results in eight nerve deafness, vertigo and tinnitus. Interstitial keratitis, eighth nerve deafness and Hutchinson's teeth are collectively termed as Hutchinson's triad that is diagnostic of late congenital syphilis.

Diagnosis depends on clinical features, thorough obstetric history, examination and investigation of mother and father and a positive serum VDRL or TPHA. Therapy is similar to acquired late syphilis.

Stigmata of Congenital Syphilis

These are residua of the past-inflammatory processes due to congenital syphilis and hence may be seen in untreated and treated patients for the rest of their lives. Some popular stigmata include Hutchinson's teeth (peg-shaped incisors), mulberry molars, depressed bridge of nose, frontal bossing and rhagades.

Summary: Transplacental transmission of syphilis leads to, with decreasing severity of infection, either abortion, stillbirth, congenital syphilis at birth or later. Most cases are diagnosed during the first year of life (early congenital syphilis). This manifests as low birth weight, failure to thrive, rhinitis, hoarse cry, hepatosplenomegaly, skin rash resembling secondary syphilis and painful limbs due to metaphysitis. Diagnosis depends on clinical features and demonstration of treponemes and a positive serology. Treatment consists of procaine penicillin 50000 IU/kg body weight IM OD for 10 days.

URETHRITIS

Gonococcal urethritis is still the commonest cause of urethritis in India. Other organisms that may cause urethritis (non-gonococcal urethritis) include chlamydia, mycoplasma, trichomonas and candida. Uncommonly, when urethritis is not due to any specific infectious cause, it is termed as non-specific urethritis. Due to the longer length and type of cells lining the male urethra, urethritis is much more common and symptomatic in the males.

GONOCOCCAL URETHRITIS

This is the commonest cause of urethritis in India. This STI is caused by *Neisseria gonorrhoeae,* a gram negative diplococcus.

Patient Profile

Although, transmission from males to females is easier, in females the infection is commonly asymptomatic or causes mild or vague symptoms. Hence, most patients are males. The age group affected is 20–30 years.

Symptoms and Signs

A typical male patient presents with complaints of burning while micturition and purulent urethral discharge that stains the underclothing. Examination discloses profuse, purulent discharge with or without milking the urethra in addition to stains on the underclothing (Fig. 25.9). The urethral meatus is red and oedematous (meatitis). Complaints of frequency and urgency are uncommon and indicate infections of posterior urethra.

In females, the primary site of infection is the endocervical canal (endocervicitis). However, asymptomatc urethritis is present in at least 75%. Discharge is rarely complained of and burning micturition, frequency and urgency are common than in males.

Differential Diagnosis

In a patient with phimosis (inability to retract the prepuce) the discharge appears to be subprepucial

Chapter
25

Sexually Transmitted Infections

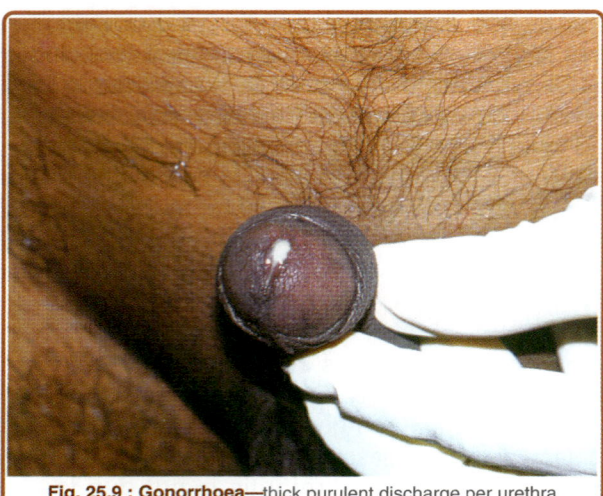

Fig. 25.9 : Gonorrhoea—thick purulent discharge per urethra

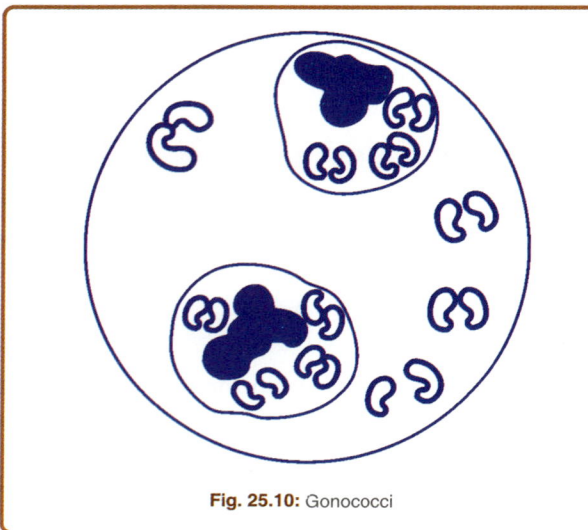

Fig. 25.10: Gonococci

as in erosive balanitis and balanoposthitis due to other causes. In such a case, after mopping all excess discharge, careful examination of the meatus through the narrowed preputial sac opening coupled with milking of urethra reveals the discharge to be urethral and not subprepucial. A smear and culture will demonstrate the gonococci.

Chlamydial urethritis can be distinguished by its longer incubation period, less profuse or scanty thin mucoid or mucopurulent discharge instead of the profuse thick purulent discharge in gonorrhoea and demonstration of chlamydia on Giemsa stained smear as against gonococci on Gram stained smear and culture.

COMPLICATIONS OF GONORRHOEA

In Men

These are observed uncommonly, in the recent times, due to the availability of effective antibiotics.

They include posterior urethritis, urethral stricture, cystitis, prostatitis, seminal vesiculitis, epididymo-orchitis and urethral fistulae (water can perineum).

In Women

Due to the relative paucity of symptoms in initial gonococcal infection in females (gonococcal cervicitis) and the reluctance of women to seek medical attention for these symptoms, complications of gonorrhoea are still commonly seen in women.

Chronic cervicitis, vulvitis, urethritis, Bartholinitis and Bartholins gland abscess, cystitis and more importantly, salpingitis, pelvic inflammatory disease, infertility and risk of ectopic pregnancy are complications of neglected gonococcal infection in females. Symptoms of gonorrhoea in females therefore include low back pain, dysuria, discomfort or pain in lower abdomen, menorrhagia, dyspareunia, and uncommonly, discharge per vaginum and fever. Per vaginal examination reveals an inflamed cervix with or without discharge from endocervical canal or cervical erosions. Bimanual examination discloses tenderness on cervical movement or of the uterus or its adnexa. Pelvic abscess may follow. The endocervical discharge reveals Gram-negative gonococci on smear and culture.

Complications in Both Sexes

Proctitis or Pharyngitis following anal or oral sex respectively and disseminated gonococcal infection can occur in both sexes. Disseminated infection may present in the septicaemic phase or, later, in the arthritic phase. Dissemination occurs more frequently in the HIV infected.

Gonococcal Conjunctivitis in Neonates (Ophthalmia Neonatorum)

It is seen in neonates born mothers with genital infection, presents as purulent conjunctivitis with profuse discharge. Keratitis may occur, if treatment with systemic or topical penicillin is not prompt. Conjunctivitis occurs uncommonly in adults and needs similar therapy.

Summary: Gonorrhoea presents most commonly as an acute uncomplicated urethritis in males. Affected young adult male complains of burning while passing urine and purulent discharge per urethra. Examination reveals thick, profuse, purulent urethral discharge. In women, it presents as gonococcal cervicitis with or without asymptomatic urethritis. Diagnosis can be confirmed with smear and culture of urethral or endocervical discharge. Complications in males include prostatitis, cystitis, epididymitis and urethral stricture/fistulae. In women, bartholinitis, salpingitis, pelvic inflammatory disease and infertility are common complications.

TREATMENT OF GONORRHOEA

Gonorrhoea, once diagnosed, is treated according to whether it affects males or females and if it is complicated or otherwise.

Uncomplicated Gonorrhoea in Males

Single dose treatments are effective and preferred. Ceftriaxone 250 mg IM with 1 g of azithromycin 2 g orally or cefixime 400 mg or ciprofloxacin 500 mg orally as a single dose are less effective. Other drugs like spectinomycin (2 g IM), kanamycin (2 g IM) have also been used, in single doses, with success. As dual infection, chlamydia is common, additional treatment for chlamydia should be given, if drugs other than azithromycin are used.

Uncomplicated Gonorrhoea in Females

Most of these are asymptomatic contacts of male patients. Treatment is same as for males. However, in view of poor facilities for monitoring response to therapy in our country and the long term repercussions of inadequate therapy, longer therapy is advisable.

Treatment of Complicated Gonorrhoea

In Males

Strains of gonococci causing disseminated gonococcal infection are usually sensitive to penicillin. Hence, crystalline penicillin 2–4 MU IV 6 hourly is the treatment of choice. Third generation cephalosporins like ceftriaxone 1 g/day or cefotaxime 1–2 g BD or spectinoycin 2 g IM every 12 hour for 7–10 days are very effective. Other complications of gonorrhoea in males, like endocarditis are uncommon but need extended duration of antibiotics for 3–4 weeks.

In Females

Mild to moderate pelvic infections and related complications respond to oral ciprofloxacin 500 mg BID for 7–10 days. Serious pelvic infections need therapy with intravenous drip of ciprofloxacin 200 mg BID to bring it under control. If the organisms are sensitive to penicillin, crystalline penicillin is effective. If mixed infection (anaerobic or chlamydia) can't be ruled out, intravenous metronidazole may be added together with oral doxycycline.

Summary: Uncomplicated gonorrhoea in men responds well to single dose ceftriaxone, cefixime or azithromycin. Other drugs like kanamycin 2 g IM spectinomycin 2 g orally also work well in a single dose. For women, although single dose therapy may be nearly as effective, multiple dose regimes are preferred because of chances of serious complications. Additional treatment for chlamydia should be provided if cephalosporins or kanamycin or spectinomycin are used to treat gonococcal infections.

DIAGNOSIS OF URETHRITIS

Urethritis can occur in both sexes. However, in females it rarely causes any symptoms. Neisseria gonorrhoeae, Chlamydia trachomatis and ureaplasma urealyticum are the principal pathogens that cause urethritis in males and urethritis and related genital infections in females.

In Males

Clinical Features

Profuse purulent discharge associated with a short incubation period (few days) clinically favours the diagnosis of gonococcal urethritis. When the discharge is scanty and mucoid or mucopurulent and is associated with a long incubation period (10–30 days) it is suggestive of either chlamydial or ureaplasmal urethritis. In this later group discharge may be so scanty that patient may not be aware of it and discharge may only be elicited on milking the urethra or manifest only as a damp urethral meatus.

Investigations

Without a good laboratory back-up, it is difficult to reliably differentiate between these types of urethritis. Confirmation of urethritis requires demonstration of more than 5 pus cells per high power field in an early morning initial (not midstream) urine sample. Smear of discharge or, when this is scanty, early morning smear from urethra demonstrates gonococci on Gram stain and chlamydia on Giemsa stain. The material thus collected can be inoculated (or put in a transport medium—Stuart's medium and sent to the laboratory) directly on to various media (Thayer Martin medium for gonococci, mouse fibroblast culture for chlamydia and a special medium for mycoplasma).

In Females

Clinical Features

Urethritis may be suspected by the symptoms of burning micturition, urgency and frequency. However, as stated earlier, they are uncommon and other symptoms of accompanying cervicitis or pelvic infection like low back pain, menorrhagia, fever, discharge per vaginum are more common. Hence, unless urethritis is caused secondary to upper urinary tract infection (which can be detected by demonstrating plenty of pus cells in mid-stream urine sample as against early morning initial urine sample in lower urinary infection) a vaginal speculum examination should be performed in all cases. Signs of cervicitis are a red, oedematous, cervix with or without purulent discharge from the endocervical canal. Palpation elicits tenderness of cervix or uterus or its adnexa.

Investigations

As in males, material for bacteriologic examination need not be collected. However, urethral smears give poor results and hence endocervical discharge is the best material collected upon speculum examination. Material is processed as in case of males.

Chapter 25

Sexually Transmitted Infections

Summary: Urethritis is symptomatic in males and frequently silent in females. Clinically, profuse purulent urethral discharge and a short incubation period favours gonorrhoea whereas its absence indicates other organisms. More than 5 pus cells/hpf in early morning urine indicates urethritis. Smear and culture of material (urethral discharge or scrapping in males and endocervical discharge in females) is required to establish the diagnosis of gonorrhoea (Gram stain. Thayer Martin medium), chlamydial (Giemsa stain, Thayer Martin medium), chlamydial (Giemsa stain, tissue culture) or mycoplasmal (Gram stain, tissue culture) infections.

NON-GONOCOCCAL URETHRITIS

Any urethritis that is not caused by gonococci is included under this title. Common causes of non-gonococcal urethritis are chlamydia trachomatis and mycoplasma (ureaplasma urealyticum). Other organisms like herpes simplex, gram-negative bacilli (*Escherichia coli*, Proteus, Klebsiella), trichomonas, candida, human papilloma virus and condyloma acuminata occasionally cause urethritis.

Chlamydial Urethritis

This is the most common cause of non-gonococcal urethritis and is important because it can cause female genital infections and all its accompanying complications (including sterility and ectopic pregnancy) similar to gonorrhoea.

Mycoplasmal Urethritis

Although, the pathogenic status of these organisms was doubted for many years, now with increasing reports of this infection in males and females (with resultant complications), it is an established condition.

Please *see* 'diagnosis of urethritis' for further details on clinical features and investigations in non-gonococcal urethritis.

Therapy

Erythromycin 500 mg QDS for 14 days or doxycycline 100 mg BD for 14 days are effective against both these common non-gonococcal pathogens. Alternatively, tetracycline 500 mg QD for 10–14 days can also be given. Azithromycin 1 g single dose. Cotrimoxazole (2 tabs BD for 10 days) is effective against chlamydia but not against mycoplasma.

Summary: Urethritis due to non-gonococcal causes is termed as non-gonococcal urethritis. Common causes are chlamydia trachomatis and mycoplasma. Unusual causes include herpes genitals, candidiasis, trichomoniasis and

secondary to upper urinary tract infection. Diagnosis is suspected when a male presents with burning micturition, but with scanty mucoid or mucopurulent discharge per urethra. Urine shows increased pus cells. Urethral smear and culture is negative for gonococci but positive for chlamydia or mycoplasma. Treatment consists of oral erythromycin or tetracycline 500 mg QDS for 14 days.

Postgonococcal Urethritis

This term is used to describe non-gonococcal urethritis that is unveiled after successful therapy of what initially looks like gonococcal urethritis. In fact, to begin with, there is a combined infection and gonorrhoea being controlled with initial therapy, urethritis due to other organisms becomes apparent after 10–14 days.

Non-specific Urethritis

When no cause, infective or otherwise, is detectable for urethritis, it is termed as non-specific. However, with improvement in facilities for diagnosis, this is being seen less frequently. Management consists of plenty of oral fluids, alkalinising the urine and avoidance of any suspected exacerbating factors.

GENITAL ULCERATIVE DISEASE (INCLUDING DIFFERENTIAL DIAGNOSIS OF GENITAL ULCERS)

Any ulcerative condition of the genitals can be included under the term genital ulcerative disease. However, by convention, it is applied to genital ulcers caused by STIs as these necessitate a different technique in patient management. Since the **presence of genital ulcerative disease greatly increases the chances of HIV transmission,** efficient management of ulcers caused by STIs has become extremely important.

Genital ulcers can broadly be classified into those due to STIs and non-STIs. **STIs** resulting in genital ulceration are **chancroid, primary syphilis, donovanosis, herpes simplex** and lymphogranuloma venereum. The first four, which are common causes of genital ulceration in India, are compared in **Table 25.1.**

Non-STIs Causes of Genital Ulcers

Scabies

Ulcers are superficial and accompany erosions, vesicles, pustules and papules over genitalia and other sites of scabies affection, e.g. web spaces, wrists and axillae. Scabies can be transmitted sexually in adults.

TABLE 25.1 : Differential diagnosis of ulcer on genitalia

	Chancroid	Donovanosis	Primary syphilis	Herpes genitalis
Causative organism	Haemophilus ducreyi	Calymmatobacterium granulomatis	Treponema pallidum	Herpes simplex virus type 2
Incubation period	2–7 days	8–80 days	9–90 days	3–6 days
Symptoms	Painful	Variable	Nil	Painful
Onset	Acute	Insidious	Insidious	Acute
Lesions preceding ulcer	Vesiculopustule	Papule	Papule	Grouped vesicles
No. of ulcers	Multiple	Single/Multiple	Single	Multiple
Size of ulcers	0.5–2 cm	2–10 cm	1–2 cm	2 mm to 3 cm
Base	Soft	Variable	Indurated	Soft
Tenderness	+	+	–	+
Bleeding	+	++	–	–
Floor of ulcer	Slough	Dark red granulation tissue	Pale granulation tissue	Slough
Slough	++	+/–	–	–/+
Depth	Deep	Deep	Variable	Superficial
Raised above the surface	+/–	++	+/–	–
Edge of ulcer	Undermined	Rolled out, variable	Variable, sometimes punched out	Sloping
Discharge	Purulent, profuse	Serosanguinous profuse	Serosanguinous, scanty	Serosanguinous, variable
Surrounding skin	Red	Variable	Normal	Variable
Progress	Fast	Slow	Slow, self-healing	Fast, self-healing
Smear	Gram's stain—gram-negative bacilli in parallel chains	Wright's stain—coccobacilli within macrophage	Dark ground illumination—T. pallidum	Wright's stain—multinucleated epithelial giant cells
Standard therapy	Cotrimoxazole, erythromycin	Streptomycin, cotrimoxazole and erythromycin	Injectable penicillin	Acyclovir

Chapter

25

Sexually Transmitted Infections

Traumatic ulcers

Ulcers have a clean floor, are angulated or linear and follow known trauma.

Ecthyma

Multiple rounded ulcers with thick heaped up purulent crusts seen usually in persons with poor hygiene.

Behcet's syndrome

Recurrent superficial or deep ulcers resembling and associated with oral aphthous ulcers, along with scars, are seen over penis, scrotum and vulva. Iritis and arthritis are associated.

Summary: The term genital ulcerative disease is used to denote genital ulcers caused by STIs as against non-STI causes like Behcet's syndrome or traumatic ulcers. Their effective management is important as they can significantly increase the risk of transmission of HIV between sex partners. STI causes of genital ulcers include chancroid, syphilitic chancre, donovanosis, herpes simplex and lymphogranuloma venereum.

CHANCROID (SOFT CHANCRE)

This is the commonest cause of genital ulceration in India though in urban areas, that position is being taken by herpes genitalis, caused by *Hemophilus ducreyi,* a gram-negative bacillus that, on smears, has a tendency to be arranged in parallel short chains resembling rail tracks. The incubation period is 2–7 days.

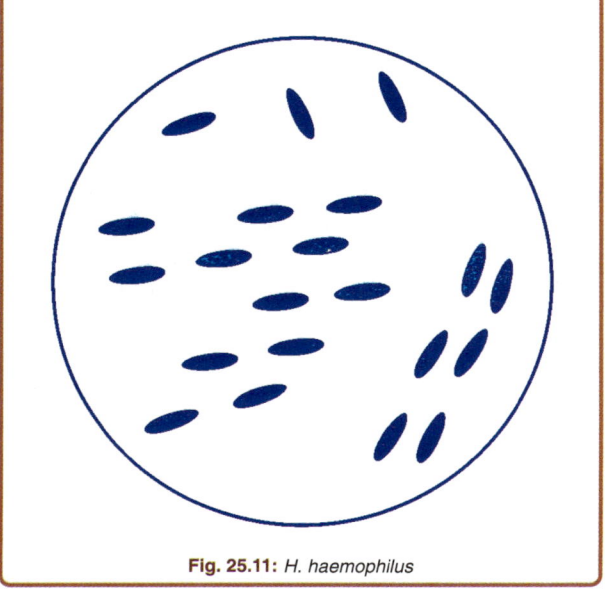

Fig. 25.11: *H. haemophilus*

Patient Profile

If affects young adult males with poor personal hygiene and practising unsafe sex. It is thought to be the disease of 'the socially unenlightened and the economically unfortunate'. It is less common in women, who probably act as carriers. Uncircumcised men are affected more commonly.

Morphology

Acute onset of multiple or single, 0.5–2 cm diameter, ulcers with ragged undermined edges and floor covered with slough and purulent discharge is characteristic (Figs 25.12 and 25.13).

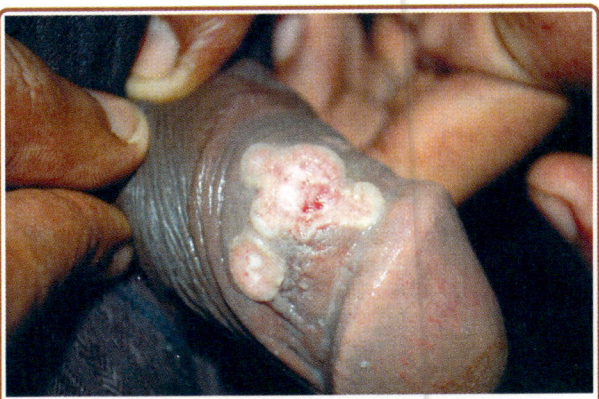

Fig. 25.12: Chancroid—multiple painful, coalescing ulcers with undermined edges and purulent discharge

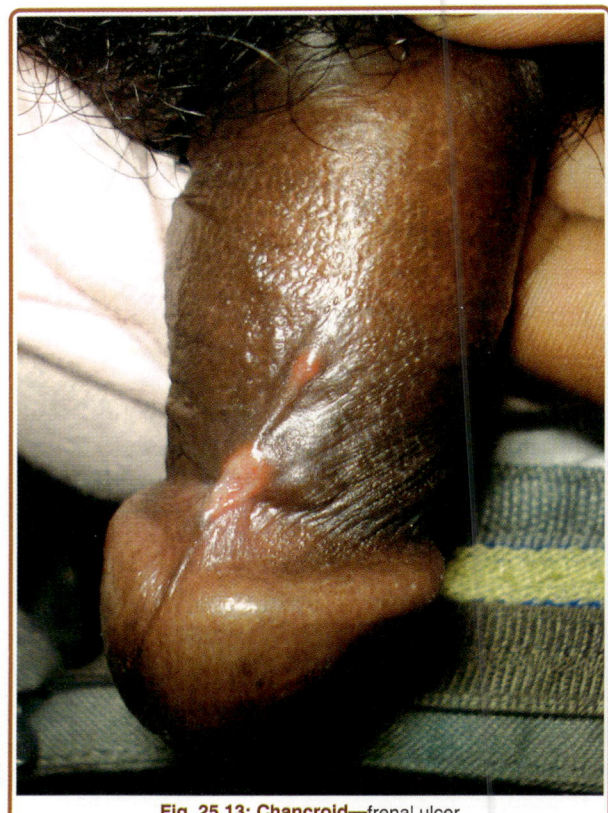

Fig. 25.13: Chancroid—frenal ulcer

Surrounding skin is red and oedematous. The ulcers are painful, tender, have a soft, non-indurated base and bleed on manipulation.

Distribution

Undersurface and less commonly, outer surface of prepuce, coronal sulcus and glans are common sites. When outer prepuce is involved, the disease spreads by contiguity (autoinoculation) to scrotum, inner thighs and lower abdomen.

Investigations

It is difficult to demonstrate the bacilli in every case by smear or culture (blood enriched agar). Routine screening for syphilis with a serum VDRL is a must. Counselling all STI patients about the risk of acquiring HIV infection and ways to avoid it, is mandatory. It is prudent to screen all STI cases with an ELISA for HIV only after such counselling and after obtaining explicit consent for HIV testing.

Complications

Complications are common in absence of therapy and they include the following:

Inguinal bubo

About 30% of cases develop tender suppurative inguinal lymphadenopathy (inguinal bubo) about a week after the initial ulcer/s (Fig. 25.10). In absence of proper therapy, the bubo enlarges and softens in the centre, the overlying skin becoming red, and then bursts in a week's time, through a single opening. The resulting sinus discharges pus and then its mouth forms a large ulcer that resembles the genital ulcer.

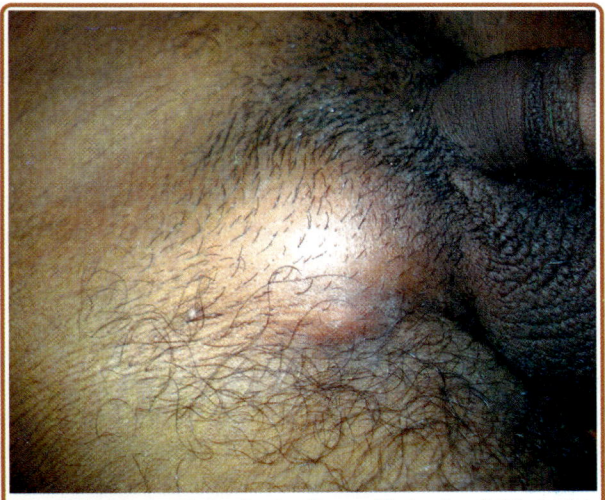

Fig. 25.14: Inguinal bubo due to chancroid—tender, slightly erythematous, unilocular and suppurative swelling of inguinal lymph nodes

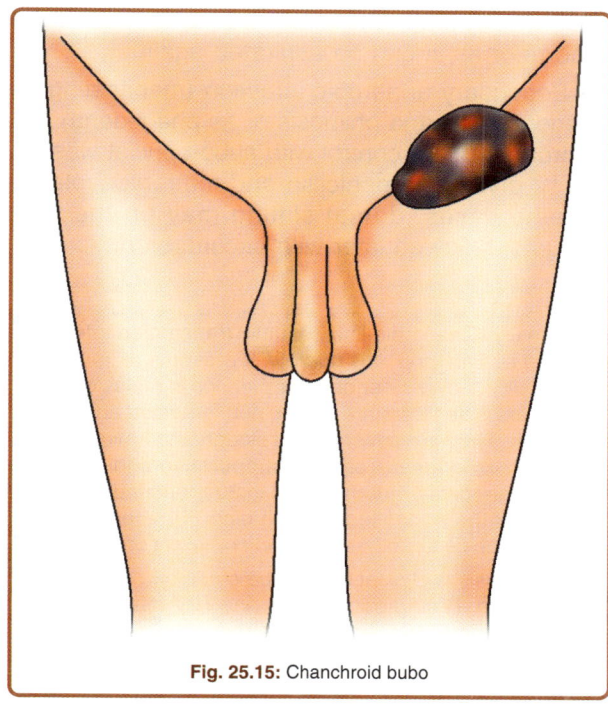

Fig. 25.15: Chanchroid bubo

Phagedena

Secodary infection with anaerobic fusospirochaetal organisms results in large, foul smelling destructive ulceration of the genitalia.

Balanoposthitis and phimosis

Diffuse erythema, erosions and purulent discharge from the undersurface of prepuce and glans penis (balanoposthitis) frequently leads to inability to retract the prepuce (phimosis).

Therapy

Ensurng good hygiene by frequent washes with a mild antiseptic solution (e.g. 1:10000 $KMnO_4$) is a must. In cases with phimosis, subprepucial washes of $KMnO_4$ can be administered with the help of an infant feeding tube.

Tetracyclines and penicillins are not recommended for treatment of chancroid. To enhance compliance, single-dose treatment with effective antibiotics are preferred. Single dose treatment with newer antibiotics like azithromycin 1 g orally or ceftriaxone 250 mg intramuscularly is effective. Erythromycin 500 mg QDS for 7 days or ciprofloxacin 500 mg BD for 3 days are also effective.

As soon as, the bubo starts softening in the centre, non-dependent aspiration of pus should be done with a wide bore needle (No. 16 or 18). Any delay in this procedure can lead to the bursting of the bubo and the resulting large ulceration of the

Chapter 25

Sexually Transmitted Infections

sinus mouth may take many weeks to heal. If the bubo reforms, it can be aspirated again.

Secondary anaerobic infection (manifesting as balanoposthitis and phimosis or as phagedena) can be brought under control with subprepucial washes and IV crystalline penicillin and metronidazole. In extreme cases, dorsal slitting may be the only recourse, followed later with circumcision.

Summary: Chancroid is a sexually transmitted infection caused by *Haemophilus ducreyi*. It presents as multiple, painful ulcers over inner or outer prepuce in males or labia in females. The ulcers are tender, non-indurated and bleed on touch. They are covered with slough and have ragged undermined edges. A tender, suppurative and inguinal lymphadenopathy (bubo) occurs in 30% and if untreated, rupture of the nodes leads to an ulcer. Phagedena and balanoposthitis are other common complications.

Diagnosis is clinical but can be confirmed with smear and culture. Ruling out syphilis and HIV infection by a VDRL and an ELISA, is a must. Frequent washes with a mild antiseptic solution for the ulcers and aspiration for the bubo are needed. Single dose treatment with ceftriaxone or azithromycin is recommended. Erythromycin or ciprofloxacin is also effective. Balanoposthitis and phagedena need crystalline penicillin and metronidazole to control the anaerobic infection.

DONOVANOSIS (GRANULOMA INGUINALE)

Calymmatobacterium granulomatis, the gram-negative coccobacillus, is responsible for this relatively uncommon STI, that is mainly restricted to the tropics. Incubation period is 3 weeks to 3 months after which a slowly progressive, relatively painless ulcer is visible.

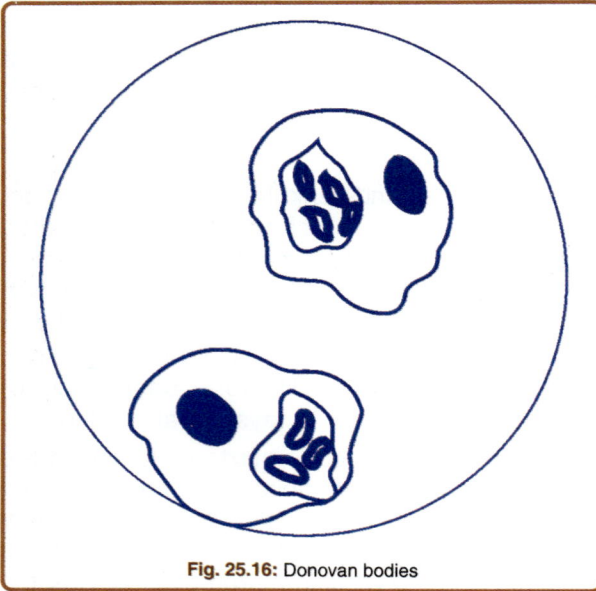

Fig. 25.16: Donovan bodies

Patient Profile

It affects young adults, practising unsafe sex. Male to female ratio is 2:1.

Morphology

The beefy red (dark red and smooth surfaced) granulation tissue forming the floor of these rounded ulcers is typical (Fig. 25.17). Pain, discharge, tenderness and induration are variable. Bleeding from the granulation tissue is usual. The floor of the ulcer is frequently elevated above the surrounding normal skin (ulcerogranulomatous lesion) and the edges is commonly rolled out.

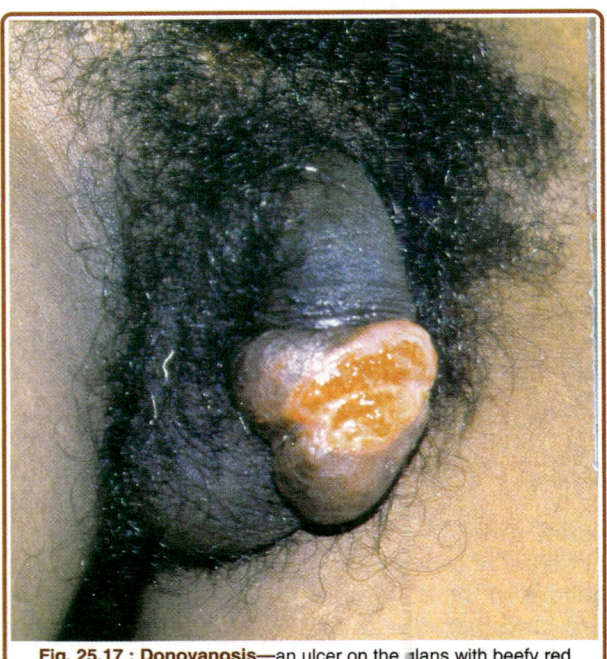

Fig. 25.17 : Donovanosis—an ulcer on the glans with beefy red granulation tissue on its floor

Distribution

Prepuce, glans and shaft of penis are common sites in males. Labia and vagina, vestibule are common sites in females. Inguinal, perianal, anal and perianal regions may be affected either in an isolated manner or by extension from other areas. Single, slow progressing lesions are common than multiple lesions, which may occur due to contiguity with the initial lesion.

Complications

Inguinal bubo does not occur. Perilymphatic spread to inguinal region leads to subcutaneous granulomata (pseudobubo) that resemble inguinal lymphadenopathy. Long standing genital lesions result in significant scarring, disfigurement of genitalia, fistulae and strictures. Lymphoedema and squamous cell carcinoma are rare, late complications.

Diagnosis

Clinical features are extremely helpful. Diagnosis can be confirmed by a Giemsa (or Wright's) stained smear of granulation tissue from ulcer that demonstrates numerous intra-cytoplasmic safety pin shaped organisms (Donovan bodies) within macrophages. Calymmatobacterium is difficult to culture (yolk sac) but is seen in Giemsa stained sections of biopsy.

Treatment

Recommended regimens include azithromycin, 1 g orally on first day, then 500 mg orally, once a day or doxycycline, 100 mg orally, twice daily for at least 2 weeks. Alternatively, erythromycin, 500 mg orally, 4 times daily or tetracycline, 500 mg orally, 4 times daily or trimethoprim 80 mg or sulphamethoxazole 400 mg, 2 tablets orally, twice daily for a minimum of 14 days. Healing occurs over a few to many weeks depending upon the size of the ulcer. Treatment should be continued until all lesions have completely epithelialised. Surgical correction is required for fistulae and strictures.

Summary: Donovanosis is a STI caused by *Calymmatobacterium granulomatis*. It induces a relatively painless ulcer with elevated beefy red granulation in the base that bleeds on touch. The edges are rolled out and a smear of the granulation reveals dumbbell shaped coccobacillary organisms within macrophages. Complications include pseudobubo, scarring, lymph stasis and carcinoma. Treatment consists of azithromycin or doxycycline for 2–4 weeks. Cotrimoxazole, tetracycline or erythromycin are also effective.

DIFFERENTIAL DIAGNOSIS OF INGUINAL LYMPHADENOPATHY

Some common STIs associated with inguinal lymphadenopathy are chancroid, primary or secondary **syphilis, lymphogranuloma venereum,** herpes simplex, HIV infection and rarely as secondary bacterial infection accompanying other STIs like condyloma acuminata, genital scabies and donovanosis.

Non-STI causes of inguinal lymphadenopathy are **tuberculous lymphadenitis, septic lymphadenitis,** filariasis, regional spread from squamous cell carcinoma or other malignancies and as a part of generalised lymphadenitis in a variety of disorders including haematologic malignancies, collagen vascular disorders, leprosy and sarcoidosis. The five common (highlighted) conditions are compared in detail in Table 25.2. The rest are described in brief.

Sexually Transmitted Infections

Herpes simplex

Within a few days of the genital lesions unilateral or bilateral, mild to moderate, tender, enlarged soft discrete nodes appear. They are more common and more noticeable during a primary attack.

HIV infection

Following a variable incubation period soft to firm, non-tender, discrete, multiregional or occasionally only inguinal lymphadenopathy appears and persists without symptoms indefinitely. HIV tests are positive, lymphopenia, thrombocytopenia may be associated and biopsy shows follicular hyperplasia.

Secondary septic lymphadenitis due to other STIs

Features of other STIs are obvious. Unilateral or Bilateral, mild to moderate, tender, enlarged soft discrete nodes that rarely progress to suppuration.

> Non-lymph node swellings that need to be differentiated from inguinal lymphadenitis are furuncles and skin abscesses in the inguinal region (including hidradenitis suppurativa), inguinal hernia, tuberculous cold abscess unrelated to lymph nodes, pseudobubo of donovanosis and mycetoma of inguinal region.

Non-sexually Transmitted Infections

Filariasis

Recurrent attacks of fever with rigors associated with epididymo-orchitis or funiculitis or oedema of a lower limb in a patient from a filariasis endemic zone is typical, Eosinophilia, raised erythrocyte sedimentation rate (ESR) and immunoglobulins are helpful. Microfilariae can only be demonstrated in smears taken during fever.

Summary: The differential diagnosis of the common causes of inguinal lymphadenopathy is presented in Table 25.1. Other than these, herpes simplex, HIV infection and scabies among the STIs and filariasis among the non-STIs also cause inguinal lymphadenopathy.

Chapter 25

Sexually Transmitted Infections

TABLE 25.2 : Differential diagnosis of inguinal lymphadenopathy

	Chancroid	Syphilis	Lymphogranuloma venereum	Tuberculosis	Septic
• Preceding genital lesion	+	+	+/−	−	−
• Interval between genital lesion and inguinal lymphadenopathy	1 week	1 week	2–4 weeks	−	−
• Pain	++	−	+	+/−	++
• Fever	−	−	+/−	+/−	+
• Evolution	Fast	Slow	Slow	Slow	Fast
• **Lymph nodes**					
□ Confluence	+	−	+	+	+
□ Consistency	Firm to soft unilocular	India rubber	Firm to soft multilocular	Firm to soft multilocular	Firm to soft unilocular
□ Colour of skin	Bright red	Normal bluish red	Bluish red	Bright red	Oval
□ Shape of bubo	Oval	−	Roughly dumb bell shaped	Variable	
□ Groove sign	−	−	+	−	−
□ Tenderness	++	−	+	+/−	++
□ Bursting	+	−	+	+/−	+
• **Sinuses**					
□ Number	Single	−	Multiple	Variable	Single
□ Discharge	Purulent	−	Serosanguinous	Serosanguinous	Purulent
□ Mouth of sinus	Ulcerated	−	Inflamed	Inflamed	Inflamed
□ Blood count	Neutrophilia	Lymphocytosis	Lymphocytosis	Lymphocytosis	Neutrophilia
□ S. VDRL	−	+	±	−	−
• **FNAC**					
□ Cells	Pus cells	−	Caseation, pus cells, epithelioid cells	Epitheloid cells, caseation	Pus cells
□ Organism	gram −ve bacilli	DGI—*T. pallidum*	Giemsa-chlamydia	AFB	Gram +ve/−ve bacteria

LYMPHOGRANULOMA VENEREUM

This uncommon STI, caused by *Chlamydia trachomatis*, is characterised by primary sore at the site of infection and the secondary syndrome due to regional lymph node affection. Most patients present with the secondary syndromes as the lymph node affection is chronic, progressive and troublesome as against the self-healing superificial sore of the primary stage (Fig. 25.18).

Patient Profile

Young or middle-aged adults, practising unsafe sex, are affected. Male to female ratio is 5:1.

Primary Stage

A small relatively asymptomatic superficial ulcer or erosion over the penis in males and labia in females, 5–10 days after infection. It heals spontaneously without scarring.

Secondary Stage

The inguinal bubo of lymphogranuloma venereum appears 2–4 weeks (occasionally few months) after the primary lesion. It involves inguinal nodes both above and below the inguinal ligament. The inguinal ligament, separating these groups of nodes, forms a horizontal groove between them (groove sign) (Figs 25.19–25.21) This sign is sometimes absent as only nodes above the ligament may be involved.

The lymph nodes are matted, moderately tender and are in different stages of evolution, i.e. some are firm, others softening in the centre while still others may be soft and about rupture. The overlying skin is erythematous with violaceous tinge. As it evolves, the bubo softens, points and finally ruptures with multiple openings. The discharge is initially purulent and later serosanguinous. Later still, clear lymph may ooze from the openings. The openings of these sinuses do not ulcerate as in the case of chancroidal bubo (please *see* Table 25.2 for differential diagnosis).

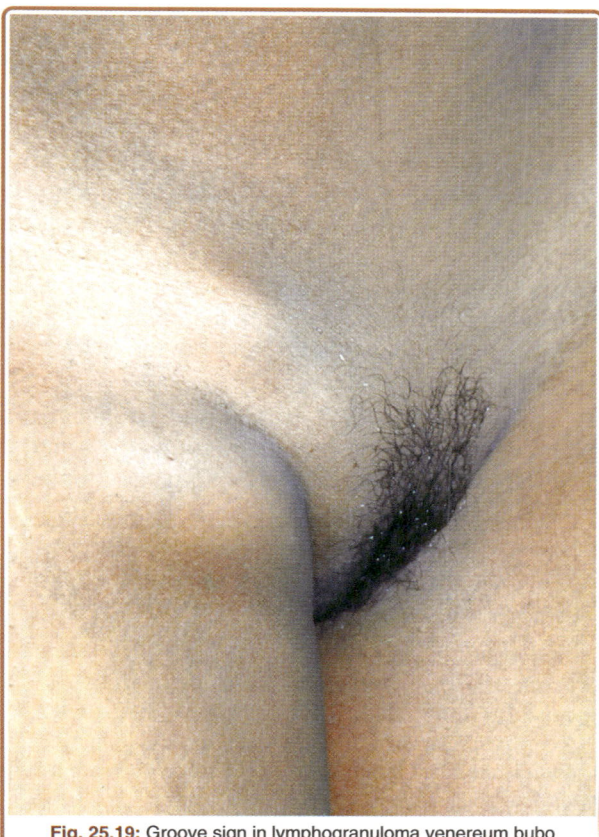
Fig. 25.19: Groove sign in lymphogranuloma venereum bubo

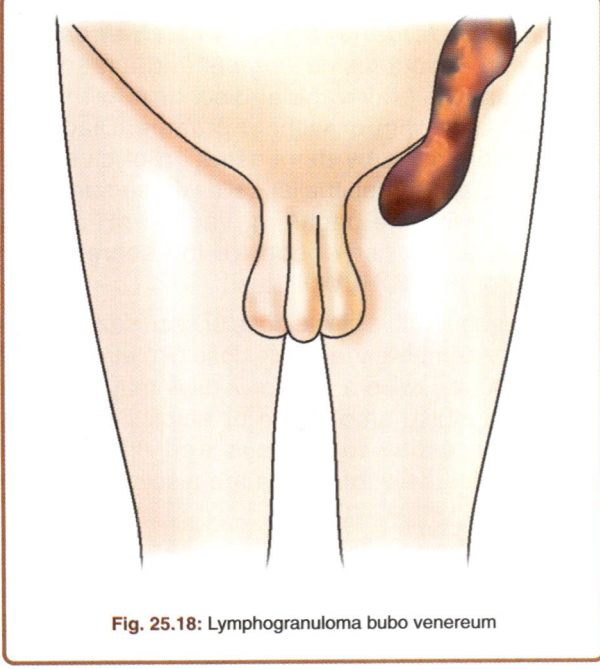
Fig. 25.18: Lymphogranuloma bubo venereum

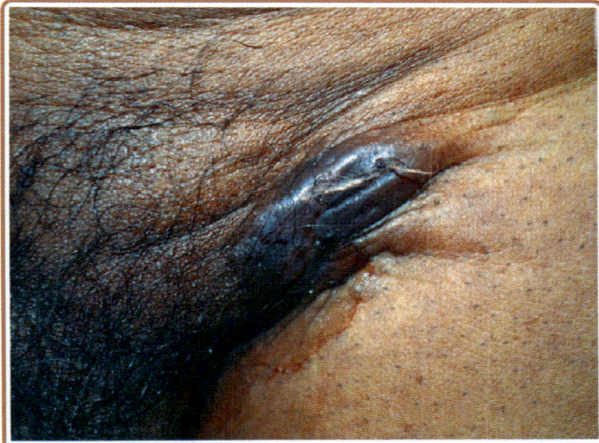
Fig. 25.20: **Donovanosis**—psuedobubo in the groins due to subcutaneous granuloma

Chapter **25**

Sexually Transmitted Infections

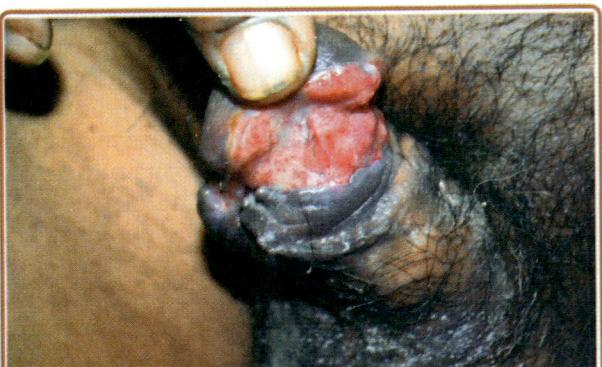

Fig. 25.21: Donovanosis—long standing large ulcer with red granulation tissue

Therapy

Doxycycline 100 mg BD or erythromycin 500 mg QDS for 2–4 weeks is the standard therapy. Pregnant women may be treated with erythromycin 500 mg QDS for the same duration. Azithromycin 1 g/week for 4 weeks is also effective. Softened points of the bubo can be aspirated with a wide bore needle. Non-steroidal anti-inflammatory drugs (NSAIDs) relieve symptoms and hasten healing of the bubo.

Large masses due to lymphoedema can be excised with plastic reconstruction of genitals. Strictures and fistulae too need surgical attention.

Systemic Manifestation of Lymphogranuloma Verereum

During the secondary phase, constitutional symptoms like fever, malaise, body ache and headache are common.

Investigations in LGV

Blood examination reveals raised ESR, lymphocytosis, raised serum globulins and a false positive VDRL. Serologic testing for chlamydia, if available, may be undertaken. Organisms from the node aspirate are difficult to demonstrate with Giemsa stain and so is tissue culture. Lymph node biopsy may be helpful for diagnosis.

Uncommon Presentations of LGV

Whenever the primary lesion is situated away form the external genitalia, it leads to a different presentation. These include:

- *Rectal syndrome*—presents as rectal stricture.
- *Anal syndrome*—presents as anal ulcer and proctitis.
- *Urethral syndrome*—presents as urethritis.

Late Complications of LGV

The chronic lymphadenitis that LGV causes results in obstruction to lymphatic drainage. Thus, the region (genitals) drained by the affected nodes shows non-pitting oedema, firm swelling, distortion of shape (ram's horn penis in males and esthiomene in females). Lymph may ooze from the skin lesions (lymphangiectasia) caused by dilation of lymphatics. Ulcers, with secondary bacterial infections, urethral, rectal and vaginal strictures and fistulae and squamous cell carcinoma are late complications.

Summary: Lymphogranuloma venereum is a sexually transmitted infection, caused by *Chlamydia trachomatis* that affects promiscuous adult males. Primary lesion is a self healing genital sore. After a few weeks, regional lymph nodes become enlarged, matted and form an inguinal bubo situated on both sides of the inguinal ligament. The bubo is multilocular, pointing and bursting through many openings. The chronicity of the secondary lymphadeno-pathic stage leads to lympoedema, distortion of genitalia (ram's horn penis and esthiomene), urethral, vaginal and rectal strictures and fistulae. Infection responds to Cotrimoxazole, tetracycline or erythromycin. Complications need surgical correction.

TRICHOMONIASIS

This is caused by a protozoan parasite, *Trichomonas vaginalis*. Typically, it affects females and males are rarely affected. Clinically, the condition presents as vulvovaginal itching with copius, foul smelling, frothy white discharge and erythema or erosions on vaginal mucosa. Males may develop urethritis and or prostatitis. Diagnosis is confirmed by demonstration of flagellate, motilea and pyriform organisms in a hanging drop preparation of the discharge.

Treatment with secnidazole 2 g single dose is effective. Alternatively, metronidazole 2 g single oral dose or 400 mg twice a day for 5 days or 200 mg thrice a day for 7 days may be used. Sexual partners of the patients should be treated for trichomoniasis. Pregnant females in first trimester can be treated with clotrimazole intravaginal pessaries.

BACTERIAL VAGINOSIS

This is a vaginal infection caused by mixed flora containing *Gardenella vaginalis (Hemophilus vaginalis)*, *Mycoplasma homnis* and anaerobes. Homogenous, gray vaginal discharge with fishy smell is seen with or without pruritus. Diagnosis can be confirmed by demonstration of clue cells (clue cells are the epithelial cells whose surface is peppered with the bacteria), vaginal pH greater than 4.5, and a fishy odoor of the secretion on addition of the KOH (Whiff test).

Treatment with a single dose of secnidazole 2 g is effective. Alternatively, a single dose of metronidazole 2 g or 400 mg twice a day for 7 days may be used. Other drugs like amoxycillin or ampicillin 500 mg 3–4 times a day for 7 days and clindamycin 300 mg twice daily for 7 days are also useful.

PELVIC INFLAMMATORY DISEASE

Pelvic inflammatory disease (PID) is a spectrum of upper genital tract infectious diseases caused by the microorganisms that ascend from the cervix and vagina. Blood borne infections or post-delivery (puerperal) or post abortion infections are to be excluded. STIs, use of intrauterine devices (IUD), vaginal douching, and presence of HIV infection increase the risk of PID. *Neisseria gonorrhoeae, Chlamydia trachomatis, Mycoplasma hominis,* and *Mycoplasma genitalium* are the common causative organisms of PID. Other organisms like *Ureaplasma urealyticum,* and anaerobes like streptococci and peptostreptococci are also responsible.

Clinical symptoms are variable ranging from asymptomatic disease to acute surgical emergencies. Symptoms like fever, chills, rigors, nausea vomiting, lower abdominal pain, abnormal vaginal bleeding or discharge are common presentations. Clinical examination may reveal tenderness and or guarding over the lower abdomen, vaginal discharge, cervicitis, palpable mass in pelvis, features of urethritis or proctitis. Complication like salpingitis or peritonitis due to rupture of tubo-ovarian abscess can occur. Investigations include staining and culture of vaginal or cervical discharge, ultrasonography of abdomen and pelvis, endometrial biopsy, cul-de-sac aspiration of peritoneal fluid and laparoscopy. Mild cases can be managed with combinations of oral doxycycline, azithromycin, fluoroquinolones, metronidazole or clindamycin to cover up for the mixed infection. Syndromic approach to patients who are not seriouisly ill consists of single-dose therapy for uncomplicated gonorrhoea (cephalosporins are recommended) plus doxycycline, 100 mg orally, twice dialy, or tetracycline, 500 mg orally, 4 times daily for 14 days plus metronidazole, 400 mg orally, twice dialy for 14 days.

However, severe cases need indoor management with parenteral antibacterials like ciprofloxacin, third generation cephalosporins, clindamycin and metronidazole. Surgical intervention may be needed in cases with rupture of pelvic abscess causing peritonitis. Recommended syndromic treatment options for PID for patients who are seriously ill and must be managed as inpatient consists of:

1. Ceftriaxone, 250 mg by intramuscular injection, once daily plus doxycycline, 100 mg orally twice daily, or tetracycline, 500 mg orally 4 times daily plus metronidazole, 400–500 mg orally or by intravenous injection, twice daily, or chloramphenicol, 500 mg orally or by intravenous injection, 4 times dialy.

2. Clindamycin, 900 mg by intravenous injection every 8 hours plus gentamicin, 1.5 mg/kg by intravenous injection every 8 hours.

3. Ciprofloxacin, 500 mg orally, twice daily, or spectinomycin 1 g by intramuscular injection, 4 times daily plus doxycycline, 100 mg orally or by intravenous injection, twice daily, or tetracycline, 500 mg orally, 4 times daily plus metronidazole, 400–500 mg orally or by intravenous injection, twice daily, or chloramphenicol, 500 mg orally or by intravenous injection, 4 times daily.

For all three regimen, therapy should be continued until at least 2 days after the patient has improved and should then be followed by either doxycycline, 100 mg orally, twice daily for 14 days, or tetracycline, 500 mg orally, 4 times daily, for 14 days.

PRACTICAL MANAGEMENT OF STIs (SYNDROMIC MANAGEMENT OF STIs)

In the HIV era, efficient management of STIs has become a national priority because:

- HIV and other STIs commonly affect the same person as their mode of transmission is similar.

- Presence of an ulcerative STI increases the chances of HIV transmission 10-fold and that of an inflammatory STI (e.g. urethritis, cervicitis, vaginitis) increases it by four fold.

- STIs when associated with HIV in the same patient are more severe and frequently unresponsive to conventional treatment.

Hence, correct and prompt treatment of STIs should be administered by the primary care physician by following a standard protocol even in the absence of facilities for establishing the correct diagnosis. Such an approach is based on identifying the correct syndrome in a patient and treating accordingly. This is called the syndromal approach to STI management.

All common STIs can be divided into the following well defined syndromes that can be identified without any facilities:

- Genital ulcer
- Urethral/cervical discharge
- Inguinal bubo
- Vaginal discharge

- **Genital ulcer: In both males and females**

If history of recurrences and vesiculation is present, the most likely diagnosis is herpes genitalis (Fig. 25.22) which is treated with oral acyclovir 400 mg 3 times daily for 5–7 days. If not vesicular, then treat with injection benzathine penicillin 2.4 MU IM after test dose (half in each buttock, preferably treat the spouse as well, if possible after a VDRL of

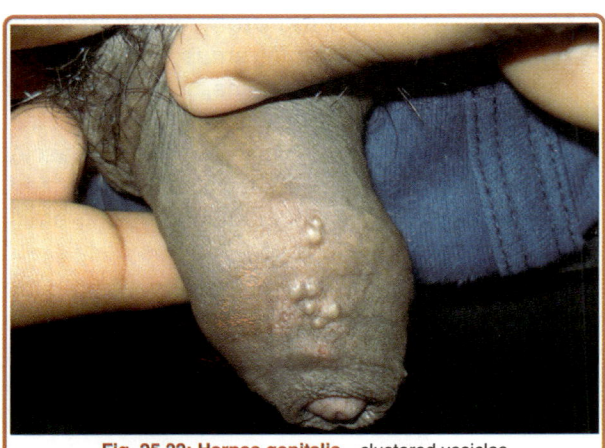

Fig. 25.22: Herpes genitalis—clustered vesicles

both azithromycin 1 g single dose. In patients allergic to penicillin, azithromycin 1 g single dose is given. In addition to doxycycline 100 mg BD for 15 days. Use erythromycin 500 mg QDS for pregnant patients.

- **Urethral discharge in males and cervical discharge in females**

  Neisseria gonorrhoeae and Chlamydia trachomatis are the major pathogens causing urethral and cervical discharge. Hence, any

syndromic management of a patient with these discharges should adequately cover these two organisms. Recommended syndromic treatment includes therapy for uncomplicated gonorrhoea plus therapy for chlamydial infection, i.e. cefixime 400 mg single dose azithromycin 1 g orally as a single dose. Patients should be advised to follow-up after 7 days, if symptoms persist.

Persistent or recurrent symptoms of urethritis may result from drug resistance, poor compliance or reinfection. In some cases, there may be infection with *Trichomonas vaginalis (T. vaginalis)*. If symptoms persist or recur after adequate treatment for gonorrhoea and chlamydia in the index patient and partner(s), the patient should be treated for *T. vaginalis* infection with secnidazole 2 g single dose. If the symptoms still persist at follow-up, the patient must be referred to an STI clinic capable of managing such cases.

- **Inguinal bubo**

  If genital ulcer is associated, treatment is similar to the genital ulcer syndrome. If fluctuant bubo is present, aspirate through non-dependent healthy skin by a wide-bore needle.

TABLE 25.3: Sexually transmitted infection syndromic approach

STI/RTI syndromic diagnosis	Name of the kit prescribed	Colour coding of the kit	Contents of the kits (Name of the drugs)
Urethral discharge (UD) Cervical discharge (CD) Ano-rectal discharge (ARD) Painful scrotal swelling (PSS) Presumptive treatment (PT)	Kit-1	Gray	1 tablet of azithromycin (1 g)/ 2 tablets of azithromycin (500 mg) and 1 tablet of cefixime (400 mg) stat
Vaginal discharge (VD)	Kit-2	Green	Tablet secnidazole 2 g and Tablet fluconazole 150 mg stat
Genital ulcer disease—non-herpetic (GUD-NH)	Kit-3	White	Injection benzathine penicillin 2.4 MU + 1 tablet azithromycin 1 g
Genital ulcer disease—non-herpetic (GUD-NH)—for patients allergic to penicillin	Kit-4	Blue	Capsule doxycycline100 mg BD for 14 days and tablet azithromycin 1 g stat
Genital ulcer disease—herpetic (GUD-H)	Kit-5	Red	Tablet acyclovir 400 mg TDS for 7 days
Lower abdominal pain (LAP/PID)	Kit-6	Yellow	Tab cefixime 400 mg stat Tab metronidazole 400 mg BD for 14 days Capsule doxycycline 100 mg BD for 14 days
Inguinal bubo (IB)	Kit-7	Black	Capsule doxycycline 100 mg BD for 21 days and 1 tablet of azithromycin 1 g stat

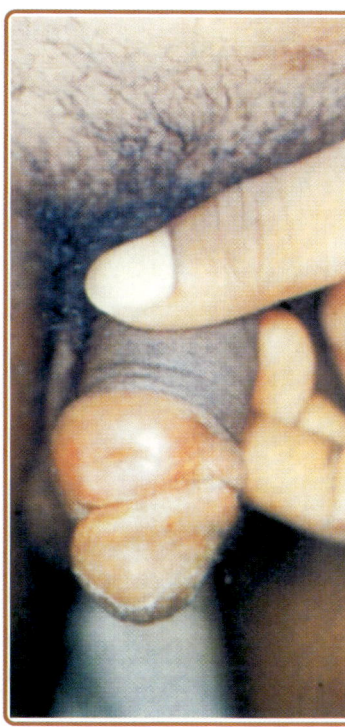

Fig. 25.23: Primary chancre—indurated, non-tender and 'clean-looking' ulcer, the floor of which has pale granulation tissue that does not bleed

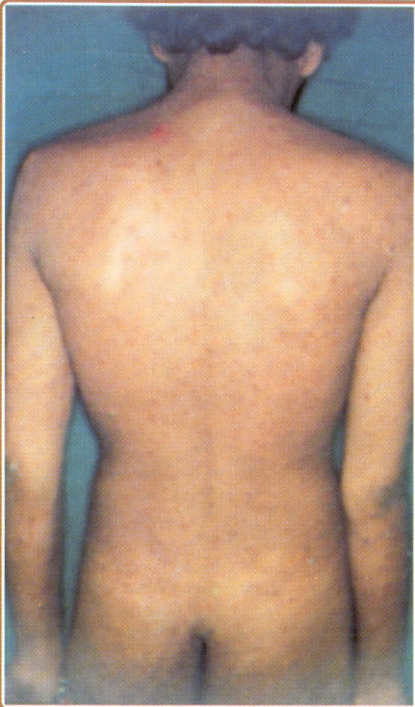

Fig. 25.24: Secondary syphilis (papular)—Generalised symmetric eruption of asymptomatic red papules, some of which are scaly. Deep dermal tenderness was positive.

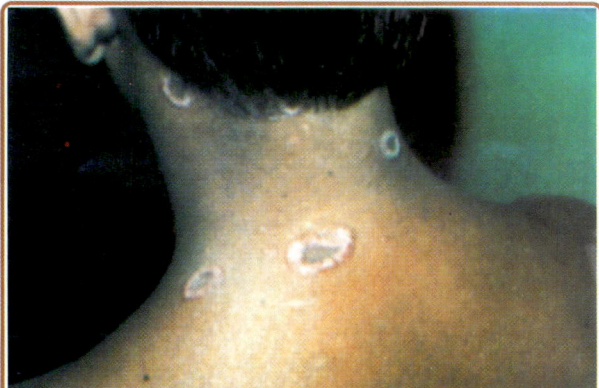

Fig. 25.25: Unusual morphological expressions of secondary syphilis—annular (ring shaped) scaly plaques

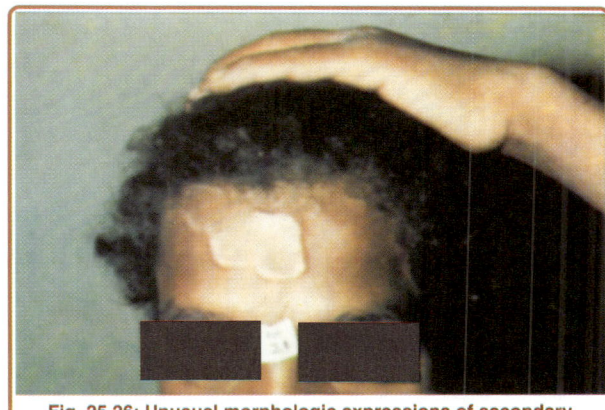

Fig. 25.26: Unusual morphologic expressions of secondary syphilis—circinate plaque on forehead

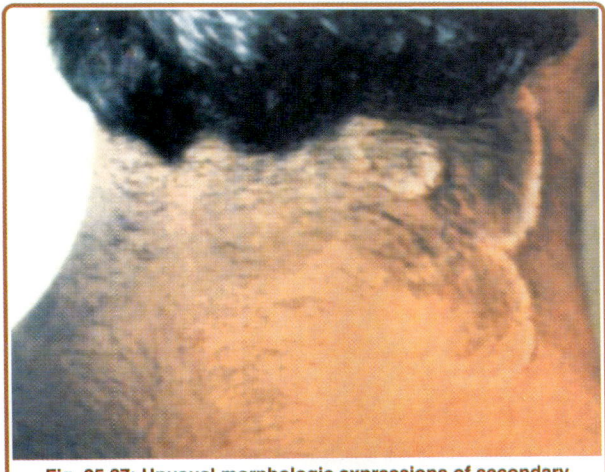

Fig. 25.27: Unusual morphologic expressions of secondary syphilis—arciform (like an arc or incomplete circle) plaque

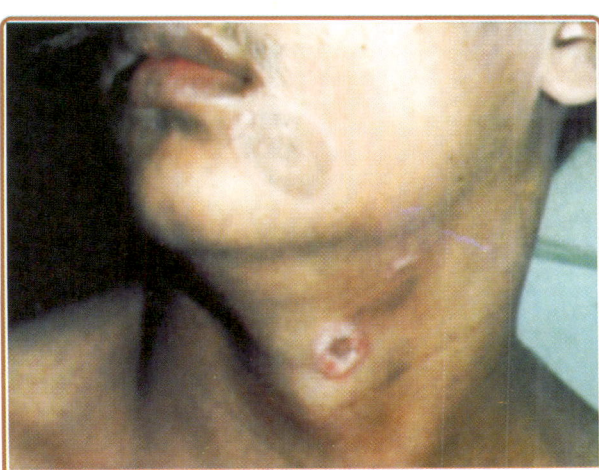

Fig. 25.28: Unusual morphologic expressions of secondary syphilis. Concentric rings (cockade) over chin

Chapter

25

Sexually Transmitted Infections

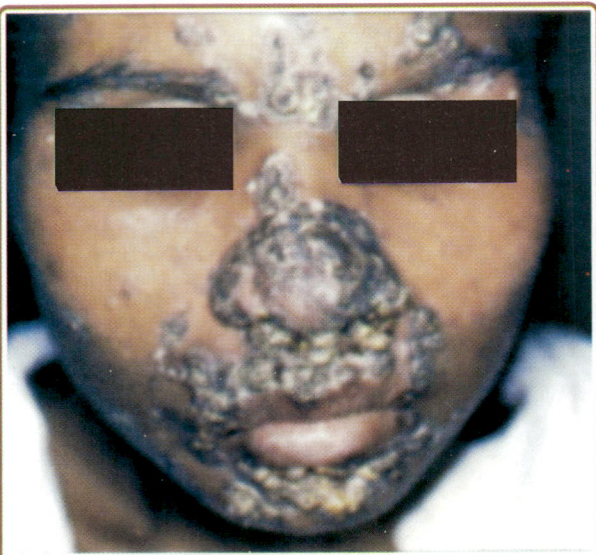

Fig. 25.29: Secondary syphilis (rupial)—Heaped up, dirty brown or yellowish scales cover red papules. Scattered molluscum contagiosum lesions suggest underlying HIV infection

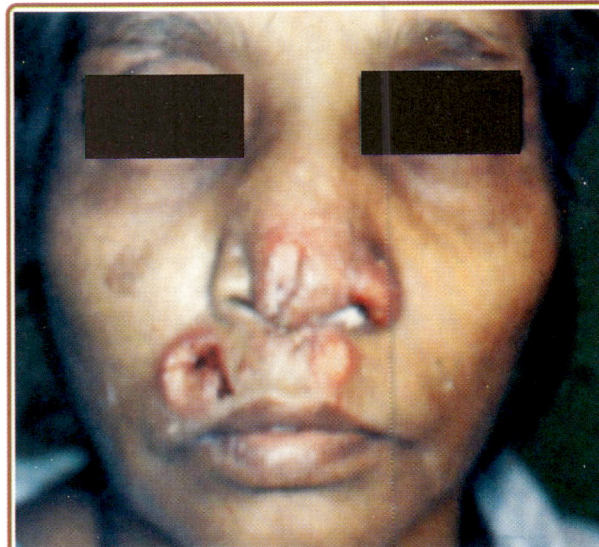

Fig. 25.30: Tertiary syphilis—a few asymptomatic ulcerated nodules over nose and lip in this middle aged lady were associated with nasal septal perforation (note collapse of tip of nose)

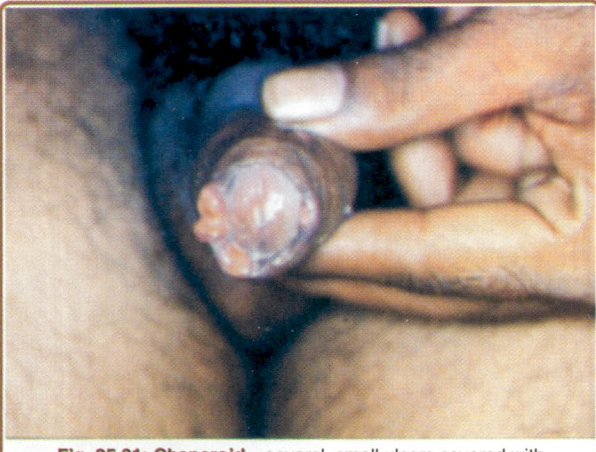

Fig. 25.31: Chancroid—several, small ulcers covered with seropurulent discharge and slough over inner prepuce. The ulcers bled on touch, were tender and non-indurated

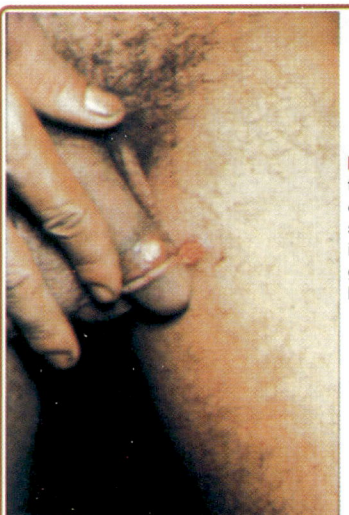

Fig. 25.32: Chancroid—this tender penile ulcer has an erythematous margin with slough and purulent discharge in the floor. Spread by contiguity, to the thigh, as seen here, is uncommon

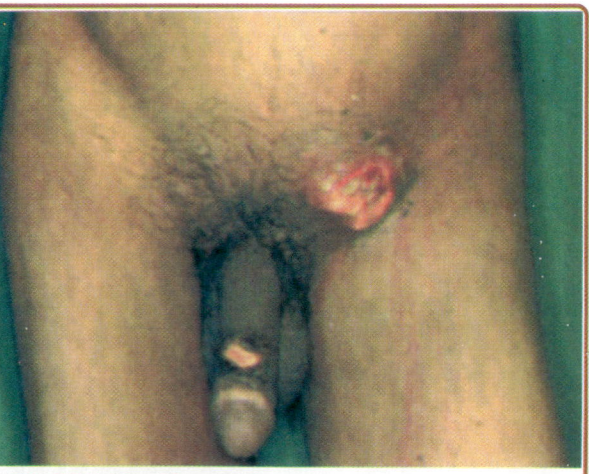

Fig. 25.33: Giant Chancroid—a penile ulcer covered with slough associated with a larger inguinal ulcer of similar morphology which followed rupture of an inguinal bubo

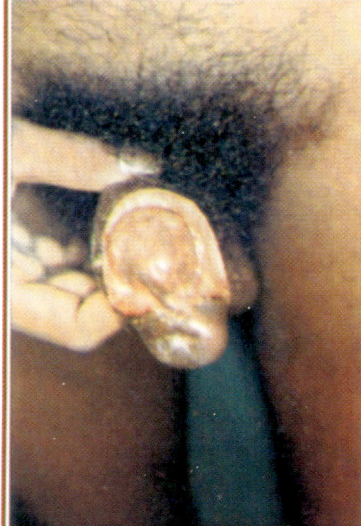

Fig. 25.34: Phagedenic chancroid—destruction of prepucial sac by this ulcer led to an abnormal opening revealing the glans penis. Such florid presentations are common in HIV disease

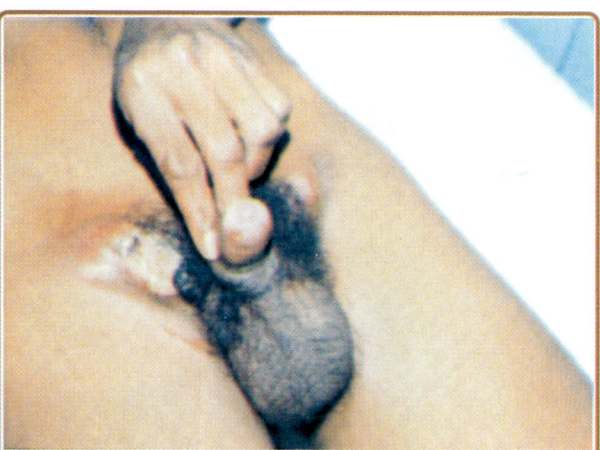

Fig. 25.35: Bilateral inguinal bubo due to chancroid in different stages of evolution—the left has burst, forming an ulcer. The right has a central softening and is about to burst

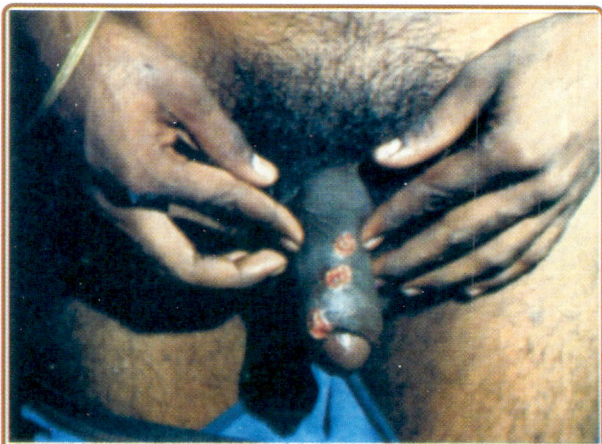

Fig. 25.36: Donovanosis (early)—three, 2–3 cm sized, ulcers—the floor of which is covered with beefy red bleeding granulation tissue

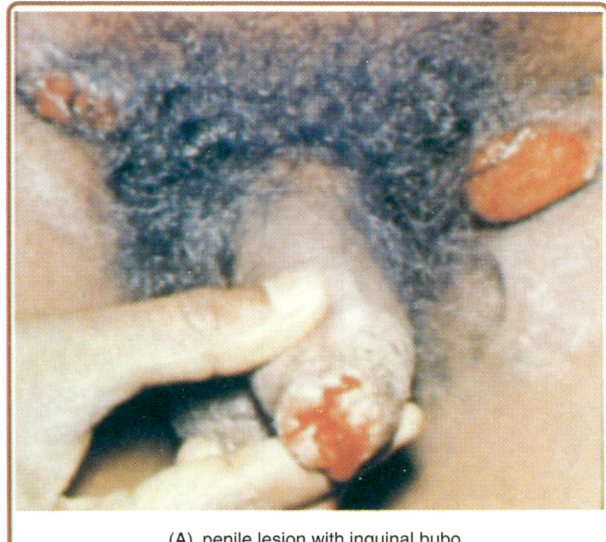

(A) penile lesion with inguinal bubo

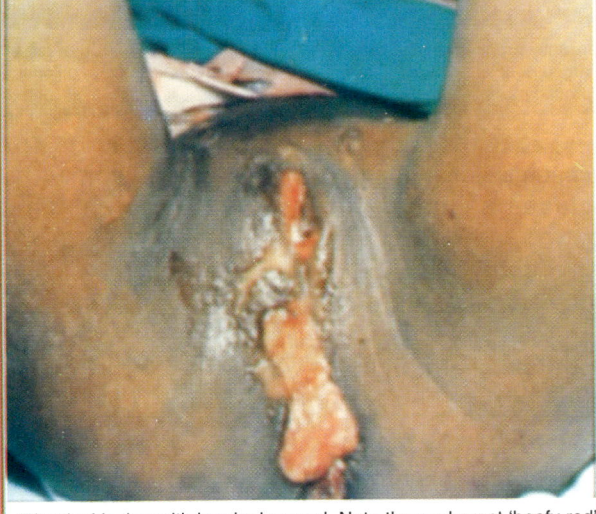

(B) vulval lesion with inguinal spread. Note the exuberant 'beefy red' granulation tissue that bleeds easily.

Fig. 25.37: Donovanosis (advanced)

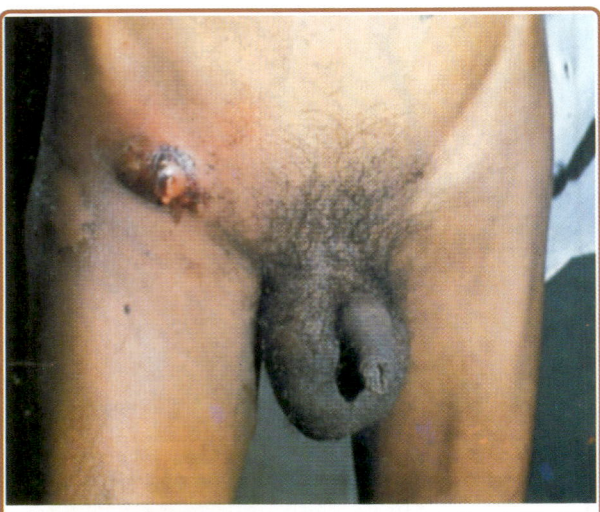

Fig. 25.38: Septic bubo—suppurative enlargement of inguinal lymph nodes without a history of genital sore or exposure to STDs. Fever and an infected leg ulcer were other clues

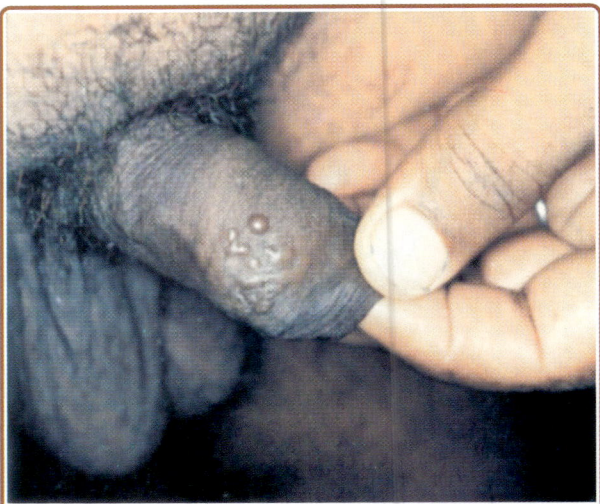

Fig. 25.39: Herpes genitalis—tiny grouped vesicles containing clear fluid over penis. Relative absence of inflammation suggests recurrent attack

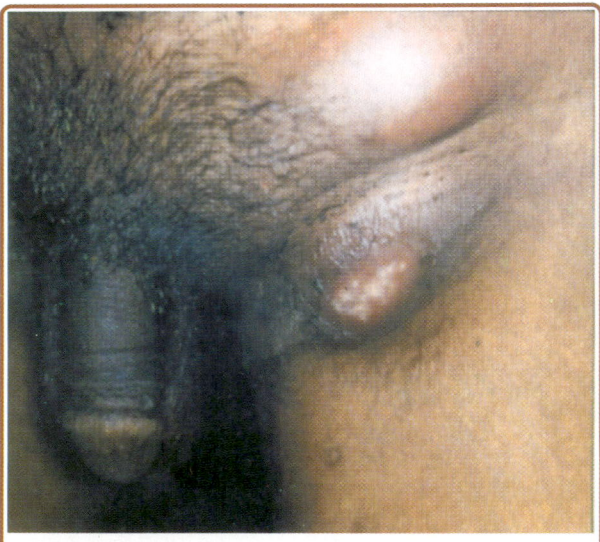

Fig. 25.40 : Lymphogranuloma venereum—groove sign is due to the inguinal ligament separating the enlarged nodes above and below it. Lower part of bubo has burst forming multiple sinuses

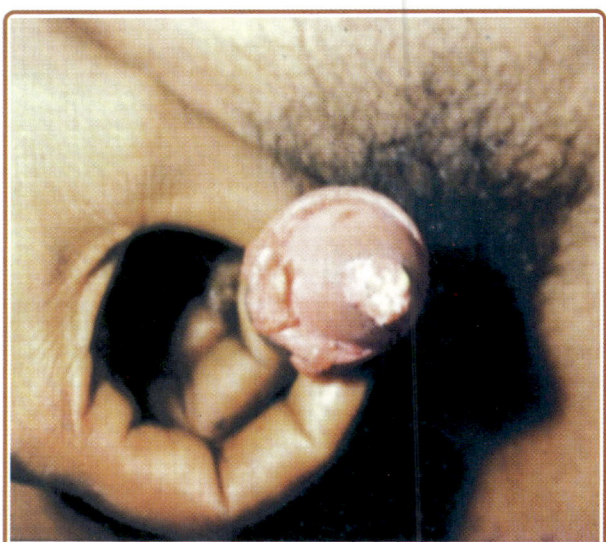

Fig. 25.41: Condyloma acuminata—several, pink, moist, conical pedunculated papulonodules and cauliflower like masses on the prepuce and glans penis

If no genital ulcer is present, recommended syndrome treatment includes azithromycin 1 g single dose plus doxycycline and 100 mg BD, orally for 21 days. Use erythromycin 500 mg QDS for pregnant women.

- **Vaginal discharge without lower abdominal pain**

  ❑ **In women not at risk for STIs:** Metronidazole orally 400 mg BD for 7 days with fluconazole 150 mg orally single dose. In pregnant women use clotrimazole metronidazole vaginal pessary once a day for 7 days.

❑ **In women at risk for STIs** (contacts of STI patients, past history of STIs or sex workers and in those with additional cervical discharge): In addition to the above treatment (oral metronidazole and fluconazole with clotrimazole pessaries) additional treatment must be given to take care of gonococcal and chlamydial genital infections and trichomonal and candidal vaginitis. Alternatively, one may use azithromycin 1 g, fluconazole 150 mg and secnidazole 1 g orally as a single dose. In pregnancy, only oral erythromycin and miconazole/clotrimazole vaginal pessary is advocated.

- **Vaginal discharge with lower abdominal pain**

  All women with vaginal discharge who have lower abdominal pain should preferably be managed by gynaecologists. However, if such services are not accessible, therapeutic trial of oral metronidazole 400 mg BD for 12 days, doxycycline 100 mg BD for 14 days and single dose of cefixime 400 mg orally is to be given.

Advice and management common to all syndromes

- This is also applicable to all asymptomatic or symptomatic contacts as well as to those with a history of unsafe sex practices.
- Counsel them about safe sex and prevention of sexually transmitted infections.
- Counsel them about HIV testing.
- Explain them about the correct method of using a condom (Please *refer* to page 359).
- Offer serum VDRL and ELISA test for HIV.
- Encourage them to get sexual partners for examination, investigations and treatment.

CHANGING EPIDEMIOLOGY OF STIs

Over the last couple of decades, gradually, the major STIs have shows several different trends. Some of these are as follows:

- There is a marked reduction in the number (prevalence and incidence) of STIs in general.
- This reduction is particularly marked in the cases of bacterial sexually transmitted infections like chancroid and gonorrhoea (which were once upon a time the commonest STIs encountered in clinical practice).
- Genital ulcerative disease due to STIs like donovanosis and lymphogranuloma venereum has become uncommon. The most common cause of genital ulceration is now herpes simplex infection (herpes genitalis).
- Viral STIs like herpes genitalis and condyloma acuminata (genital warts) are now the commonest STIs encountered in clinical practice. This is because herpes is a recurring disease (most of the cases encountered in practice are secondary attacks) while condyloma acuminata is a slowly evolving, asymptomatic disease for which it is difficult to break the chain of transmission. Moreover, an asymptomatic carrier state exists for both these infections.

The probable reasons for this change in epidemiology have been many and are as follows:

- Campaigns to increase awareness of the risks of HIV infection and AIDS due to unprotected sex with multiple partners have been succeeding.
- Compaigns to promote use of condom have succeeded in increasing their availability, acceptability and use.
- Increasing access to and upgradation of STI clinics led to early diagnosis and treatment of existing STIs.
- Promotion of syndromal management at the primary health centre level also led to early diagnosis and treatment of STIs thereby breaking the chain of transmission.

Chapter
25

Sexually Transmitted Infections

MCQs

1. The causative organism of syphilis is:
   - a. *Borrelia vincenti*
   - b. *Treponema pertenue*
   - c. *Treponema pallidum*
   - d. *Treponema carateum*

2. Syphilis becomes a systemic infection with this stage of infection:
   - a. Primary
   - b. Secondary
   - c. Early latent
   - d. Tertiary

3. The incubation period of syphilis is:
   - a. 2–3 days
   - b. 8–10 days
   - c. 11–14 days
   - d. 9–90 days

4. The genital lesion of primary syphilis is called as:
   - a. Soft chancre
   - b. Hard chancre
   - c. Chancre redux
   - d. Chancroid

5. The earliest test to become positive in primary syphilis is:
   - a. Treponema pallidum immobilisation test
   - b. Treponema pallidum haemagglutination assay (TPHA)
   - c. Fluorescent treponemal antibody absorption (FTA-ABS) test
   - d. Venereal disease research laboratory (VDRL) test

6. In which serological test for syphilis are the results available at the earliest?
   - a. TPHA test
   - b. VDRL test
   - c. FTA-ABS test
   - d. Rapid plasma reagin test

7. The type of microscopy needed for demonstration of organisms in syphilis is:
   - a. Dark ground microscopy
   - b. Polarising microscopy
   - c. Light microscopy
   - d. Electron microscopy

8. *Treponema pallidum* are identified in smears by their:
   - a. Size
   - b. Colour
   - c. Movements
   - d. Organelles

9. Non-pathogenic treponemes are distinguished from *T. pallidum* by their:
   - a. Speed of movement
   - b. Type of movement
   - c. Regularity of spirals
   - d. All of these

10. The lymph nodes in secondary syphilis are:
    - a. Firm and discrete
    - b. Hard and matted
    - c. Firm and matted
    - d. Soft and supple

11. The type of bubo seen in syphilis is:
    - a. Inflammatory
    - b. Indolent
    - c. Tropical
    - d. Pseudobubo

12. The rash of secondary syphilis is not:
    - a. Pruritic
    - b. Symmetrical
    - c. Generalised
    - d. Pustular

13. The colour of rash of secondary syphilis is:
    - a. Fiery red
    - b. Orange red
    - c. Dull red
    - d. Bright red

14. The rash of secondary syphilis:
    - a. Never recurs
    - b. Occasionally recurs
    - c. Usually recurs
    - d. Always recurs

15. The type of syphilitic lesions affecting flexures are called:
    - a. Chancre
    - b. Condyloma lata
    - c. Gumma
    - d. Mucous patches

16. The rash of secondary syphilis is commonly:
    - a. Vesicular
    - b. Pruritic
    - c. Papulosquamous
    - d. Localised

17. The rash of secondary syphilis may be all *except*:
    - a. Macular
    - b. Papular
    - c. Vesicular
    - d. Pustular

18. An interesting configuration of syphilis rash is:
    - a. Linear
    - b. Annular
    - c. Zosteriform
    - d. All of these

19. A peculiar configuration of syphilis rash seen is:
    - a. Corymbose
    - b. Clustered
    - c. Arciform
    - d. All of these

20. Most common rashes of secondary syphilis are:
    - a. Macules and papules
    - b. Papules and pustules
    - c Vesicobullous
    - d. Plaques and patches

21. **Condyloma lata occurs most commonly over:**
    a. Lips
    b. Oal cavity
    c. Axilla
    d. Perianal and genital region

22. **The sign of deep dermal tenderness is seen in:**
    a. Chickenpox
    b. Maculopapular drug eruption
    c. Secondary syphilis
    d. Darier's disease

23. **The sign of deep dermal tenderness is seen in:**
    a. Vasculitis
    b. Secondary syphilis
    c. Erythema nodosum leprosum
    d. All of the above

24. **The lymph node enlargement peculiar to secondary syphilis is:**
    a. Posterior cervical   b. Epitrochlear
    c. Inguinal   d. Femoral

25. **Mucous patches are a sign of:**
    a. Erythema multiforme
    b. Stevens Johnson syndrome
    c. Secondary syphilis
    d. Behcet's syndrome

26. **Mucous patches occur most commonly over:**
    a. Tongue   b. Lips
    c. Palate   d. Glans penis

27. **All are manifestations of mucous membrane involvement in secondary syphilis except:**
    a. Mucous patches   b. Condyloma lata
    c. Pharyngitis   d. Syphilitic chancre

28. **Gummas are seen in _____ stage of syphillis.**
    a. Primary   b. Early latent
    c. Late latent   d. Tertiary

29. **Cutaneous lesions of tertiary syphilis are all but:**
    a. Painless   b. Numerous
    c. Asymmetric   d. Slowly progressive

30. **The moth-eaten alopecia is seen in which stage of syphilis?**
    a. Secondary   b. Early latent
    c. Late latent   d. Tertiary

31. **The drug of choice for treatment of syphilis is:**
    a. Erythromycin   b. Doxycycline
    c. Penicillin   d. Ceftriaxone

32. **Preferred drug for treatment of syphilis during pregnancy is:**
    a. Erythromycin   b. Doxycycline
    c. Penicillin   d. Ceftriaxone

33. **Preferred drug for treatment of syphilis in those with penicillin hypersensitivity is:**
    a. Erythromycin   b. Doxycycline
    c. Penicillin   d. Ceftriaxone

34. **Recommended drug for treatment of syphilis in pregnant women with penicillin hypersensitivity is:**
    a. Erythromycin   b. Doxycycline
    c. Penicillin   d. Ceftriaxone

35. **Recommended dose of benzathine penicillin for treatment of early syphilis is:**
    a. 12 million units   b 24 million units
    c. 1.2 milion units   d. 2.4 million units

36. **Recommended dose of procaine penicillin for treatment of infants with congenital syphilis is:**
    a. 1000 IU per kg per dose
    b. 5000 IU per kg per dose
    c. 10000 IU per kg per dose
    d. 50000 IU per kg per dose

37. **The mode of transmission of yaws is:**
    a. Sexually transmitted
    b. Person to person contact
    c. Droplet infection
    d. Water borne

38. ***Treponema carateum* causes:**
    a. Yaws   b. Pinta
    c. Syphilis   d. Bejel

39. **The only treponematosis with clinical manifestation confined to skin is:**
    a. Yaws   b. Pinta
    c. Syphilis   d. Bejel

40. **The commonest cause of non-gonococcal urethritis is:**
    a. Mycoplasma
    b. Neisseria catarrhalis
    c. Chlamydia
    d. Trauma

Chapter 25

Sexually Transmitted Infections

41. **Recommended treatment of non-gonococcal urethritis is:**
    - a. Doxycycline
    - b. Erythromycin
    - c. Penicillin
    - d. Ceftriaxone

42. **Which of the following does not usually cause urethritis?**
    - a. *Treponema pallidum*
    - b. *Neisseria gonorrhoeae*
    - c. *Chlamydia trachomatis*
    - d. *Ureaplasma urealyticum*

43. **The genital area most commonly affected in gonococcal infection in women is:**
    - a. Vulva
    - b. Vagina
    - c. Cervix
    - d. Uterus

44. **A serious long term sequel of non-gonococcal genital infection in women is:**
    - a. Ethiomene
    - b. Mutilated genitalia
    - c. Urethral stricture
    - d. Infertility

45. **The gonococci preferentially affect organs lining:**
    - a. Stratified squamous epithelia
    - b. Transitional epithelia
    - c. Columnar epithelium
    - d. Ciliated columnar epithelium

46. **A serious systemic complication of gonococcal urethritis is:**
    - a. Orchitis
    - b. Birt Hogg Dube syndrome
    - c. Fitz Hugh Curtis syndrome
    - d. Cystitis

47. **Which of the following drugs is not recommended for treatment of uncomplicated gonococcal urethritis?**
    - a. Penicillin
    - b. Ceftriaxone
    - c. Kanamycin
    - d. Ciprofloxacin

48. **In syndromic management of urethral discharge, the recommended dose of azithromycin is:**
    - a. 250 mg
    - b. 500 mg daily for 3 days
    - c. 1 g daily for 3 days
    - d. 1 g single dose

49. **Gonorrhoea in women usually causes:**
    - a. Vulvitis
    - b. Vaginitis
    - c. Cervicitis
    - d. Endometritis

50. **The best area to take a swab for genital discharge in women is:**
    - a. Posterior vagina
    - b. Lateral vagina
    - c. Posterior fornix
    - d. Fourchette

51. **The best area to take a swab for suspected gonorrhoea in women is:**
    - a. Posterior vaginal wall
    - b. Anterior vaginal wall
    - c. Posterior fornix
    - d. Cervix

52. **Syndromic management of vaginal discharge in women at high risk for STIs includes administration of:**
    - a. Fluconazole
    - b. Azithromycin
    - c. Secnidazole
    - d. All of these

53. **Clap is a synonym of:**
    - a. Gonococcal urethritis
    - b. Syphilis
    - c. Kissing chancroid
    - d. Split pea papule of secondary syphilis

54. **Which of the following STIs is associated with lymphadenopathy?**
    - a. Donovanosis
    - b. Gonorrhoea
    - c. Herpes simplex
    - d. Condyloma acuminata

55. **A pathogenetic factor in the developmet of Kaposi's sarcoma is infection with:**
    - a. Herpes simplex type II
    - b. Herpes simplex type I
    - c. Human herpes virus 6
    - d. Human herpes virus 8

56. **Sugar fermentation reactions are used for identification of species of:**
    - a. Streptococci
    - b. Neisseria
    - c. Atypical mycobacteria
    - d. Chlamydia

57. **Condyloma acuminata is:**
    - a. A type of seborrhoeic keratosis
    - b. Genital squamous cell carcinoma
    - c. A feature of secondary syphilis
    - d. Manifestation of papilloma virus infection

58. **Condyloma acuminata usually manifests as:**
    - a. Genital ulcer
    - b. Genital discharge
    - c. Genital growths
    - d. All of these

59. **Condyloma acuminata is differentiated from condyloma lata by their:**
   a. Pale colour
   b. Pink colour
   c. Whitish colour
   d. Beefy red colour

60. **Which of the following are not infectious lesions of syphilis?**
   a. Condyloma lata
   b. Mucous patches
   c. Chancre
   d. Gumma

61. **Preferred treatment for uncomplicated widespread condyloma acuminata is:**
   a. Topical acyclovir
   b. Oral acyclovir
   c. Topical podophyllin
   d. Oral podophyllin

62. **The organism causing molluscum contagiosum is a:**
   a. Polyoma virus
   b. Papilloma virus
   c. Picorna virus
   d. Pox virus

63. **Molluscum contagiosum in the HIV infected is caused most commonly by:**
   a. MCV1
   b. MCV2
   c. MCV3
   d. MCV4

64. **The predominant causative organism of herpes genitalis is:**
   a. Herpes simplex virus type II
   b. Herpes simplex virus type I
   c. Both (a) and (b)
   d. Human herpesvirus (HHV 6)

65. **The causative organism of herpes labialis is:**
   a. Herpes simplex type 1 and 2
   b. Herpes simplex type 2 and 3
   c. Human herpes virus 1 and 2
   d. Human herpes virus 6 and 8
   e. Papilloma virus

66. **The causative organism of donovanosis is now known as:**
   a. *Corynebacterium minutissimum*
   b. *Propionibacterium acnes*
   c. *Klebsiella granulomatis*
   d. *Calymmatobacterium graulomatis*

67. **The organisms of donovanosis have microscopic appearance resembling:**
   a. Telephone handle
   b. School of fish
   c. Common pin
   d. Target

68. **The classical description of granulation tissue in donovanosis is:**
   a. Pale
   b. Beefy red
   c. Pink
   d. Yellowish

69. **Which of the following is not a complication of donovanosis?**
   a. Subcutaneous granulomata
   b. Esthiomene
   c. Inguinal bubo
   d. Squamous cell carcinoma

70. **Esthiomene is a complication of:**
   a. Herpes genitalis
   b. Syphilis
   c. Chancroid
   d. Donovanosis

71. **Common presentatiion of lymphogranuloma venereum is:**
   a. Lymphadenopathy
   b. Genital discharge
   c. Genital ulcer
   d. Genital granuloma

72. **Which of the following is not a complication of lymphogranuloma venereum?**
   a. Esthiomene
   b. Discharging sinuses
   c. Rectal stricture
   d. Paraphimosis

73. **Lymphogranuloma venereum usually causes enlargement of:**
   a. Horizontal chain of inguinal lymph nodes
   b. Vertical chain of inguinal lymph nodes
   c. Both chains of inguinal lymph nodes
   d. Pelvic lymph nodes

74. **Which clinical sign is positive in lymphogranuloma venereum?**
   a. Stricture
   b. Constriction
   c. Groove
   d. Ridge

75. **Organisms causing lymphogranuloma venereum belong to which group?**
   a. Klebsiella
   b. Chlamydia
   c. Haemophilus
   d. Neisseria

76. **Type of bubo in lymphogranuloma venereum is:**
   a. Multilocular
   b. Unilocular
   c. Painless
   d. Suppurative

77. **Most of the recent outbreaks of lymphogranuloma venereum are caused by which serovar of C. trachomatis?**
   a. L1
   b. L2
   c. L3
   d. L4

78. **Multiple painful ulcers over glans without induration is suggestive of:**
   a. Lymphogranuloma venereum (LGV)
   b. Granuloma inguinale
   c. Chancroid
   d. Secondary syphilis

Chapter
25

Sexually Transmitted Infections

79. **Beefy red foul smelling genital granuloma with a bleeding ulcer on touch is seen in:**
    - a. LGV
    - b. Chancroid
    - c. Primary syphilis
    - d. Donovanosis

80. **Most frequent cause of recurrent genital ulceration in sexually active male is:**
    - a. Herpes genitalis
    - b. Aphthous ulcers
    - c. Syphilis
    - d. Chancroid

81. **The commonest trophozoite infection by sexual intercourse is:**
    - a. Entamoeba histolytica
    - b. Trichomonas vaginalis
    - c. Treponema pallidum
    - d. Giardia intestinalis

82. **The skin lesions of secondary syphilis includes all of the following *except*:**
    - a. Macules
    - b. Vesicles and bullae
    - c. Nodule
    - d. Papulosquamous

83. **Condyloma latae are seen in:**
    - a. Congenital syphilis
    - b. Primary syphilis
    - c. Secondary syphilis
    - d. Tertiary syphilis

84. ***Treponema pallidum* causes:**
    - a. Condyloma acuminata
    - b. Condyloma lata
    - c. None
    - d. Both (a) and (b)

85. **The lesion characteristic of secondary syphilis is:**
    - a. Ulcer
    - b. Condyloma acuminata
    - c. Condyloma lata
    - d. Gumma

86. **Which stage of syphilis is most contagious?**
    - a. Primary syphilis
    - b. Secondary syphilis
    - c. Early latent syphilis
    - d. Late latent syphilis

87. **Soft sore is caused by:**
    - a. *H.ducreyi*
    - b. *Calymmatobacterium granulomatis*
    - c. *Chlamydia trachomatis*
    - d. *Treponema pallidum*

88. **Hard chancre is seen in:**
    - a. Chancroid
    - b. Syphilis
    - c. Tularaemia
    - d. All of these

89. **Chancre redux is clinical feature of:**
    - a. Early relapsing syphilis
    - b. Late syphilis
    - c. Chancroid
    - d. Recurrent herpes infection

90. **Genital warts are most commonly caused by:**
    - a. Human papillomavirus (HPV6)
    - b. HPV 16
    - c. HPV 18
    - d. HPV 33

91. **Verruca vulgaris is caused by:**
    - a. HPV
    - b. Epstein-Barr virus (EBV)
    - c. HIV
    - d. Cytomegalovirus (CMV)

92. **Type of human papilloma virus associated with Ca cervix:**
    - a. Types 6, 12, 18, 30
    - b. Types 16, 18, 31, 33
    - c. Types 6, 8, 11
    - d. Types 3, 10, 19

93. **Podophyllum resin is indicated in the treatment of:**
    - a. Psoriasis
    - b. Pemphigus
    - c. Condyloma acuminata
    - d. Condyloma lata

94. **Topical immunomodulator used for the treatment of genital warts is:**
    - a. Imiquimod
    - b. Podophyllin
    - c. Interferon
    - d. Acyclovir

Chapter 25

Sexually Transmitted Infections

ANSWERS

1-c,	2-a,	3-d,	4-b,	5-c,	6-d,	7-a,	8-c,	9-d,	10-a,
11-b,	12-a,	13-c,	14-b,	15-b,	16-c,	17-c,	18-b,	19-d,	20-a,
21-d,	22-c,	23-d,	24-b,	25-c,	26-c,	27-d,	28-d,	29-b,	30-a,
31-c,	32-c,	33-b,	34-c,	35-d,	36-d,	37-b,	38-b,	39-b,	40-c,
41-a,	42-a,	43-c,	44-d,	45-c,	46-c,	47-a,	48-d,	49-c,	50-c,
51-d,	52-d,	53-a,	54-c,	55-d,	56-b,	57-d,	58-c,	59-b,	60-d,
61-c,	62-d,	63-b,	64-a,	65-a,	66-c,	67-a,	68-b,	69-c,	70-d,
71-a,	72-d,	73-c,	74-c,	75-b,	76-a,	77-b,	78-c,	79-d,	80-a,
81-b,	82-b,	83-c,	84-b,	85-c,	86-b,	87-a,	88-b,	89-a,	90-a,
91-a,	92-b,	93-c,	94-b						

HIV Infection and AIDS

The impact of human immunodeficiency virus (HIV) infection on modern medicine as well as human life during the last 25 years stands unmatched. The HIV epidemic soon turned into a pandemic and this infection has now become endemic in many countries including India.

HUMAN IMMUNODEFICIENCY VIRUS

It was initially identified as the underlying cause for the epidemic of pneumocystis carinii pneumonia and Kaposi's sarcoma affecting homosexuals in the United States of America in the year 1984. It is a retrovirus with an affinity for CD4 receptor bearing cells in the body. Hence, it selectively infects, replicates within and destroys T4 helper/inducer lymphocytes that are the key cells in mounting an effective cellular immune response. Loss of this effector arm of immune function results in a plethora of infections and malignancies.

A retrovirus is an RNA virus that replicates in host cells through the step of reverse transcription in which DNA copies of the virus are made from RNA by the action of RNA depend DNA polymerase (reverse transcriptase). This viral DNA than incorporates into host cell nucleus and manufactures viral proteins necessary for replication.

The HIV has a central core with regulating proteins and enzymes and a surrounding envelope (Fig. 26.1). The envelope proteins (glycoprotein 41) and gp120 are important for pathogenicity and antibodies against them have diagnostic significance. The core protein antigen p24 is detectable very early in the course of the disease even when there is no other sign of the infection.

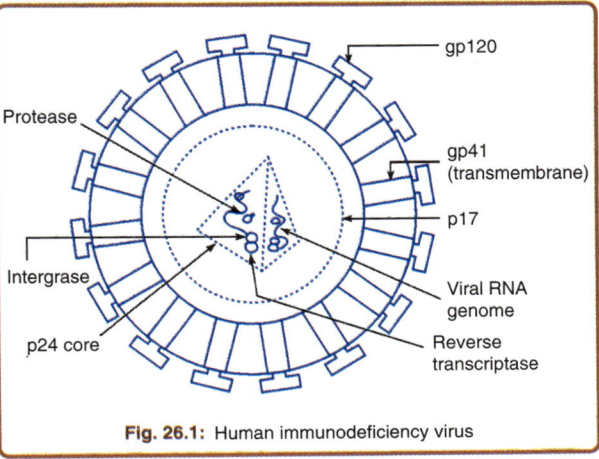

Fig. 26.1: Human immunodeficiency virus

There are two types of HIV, 1 and 2. HIV 1 (subtype c) is predominant in India accounting for about 90% of the cases. HIV 2 (subtype a), which is endemic in Africa, affects about 10% of the HIV infected in India. However, most of these cases have dual HIV 1 and 2 infection. Other subtypes of HIV 1 (a, b, e) and exclusive HIV 2 infections are uncommon.

Clinical implication: Compared to HIV 1, HIV 2 has low replication rate, so infections with HIV 2 have lower viral loads and consequently are slowly progressive, with a longer latent period, a higher life expectancy and a reduced ability of the virus being transmitted transplacentally or by breast feeding.

The HIV can be cultivated in the laboratory on a culture of T helper cells and peripheral blood monocytes (PBMC) and syncitium formation in the culture correlates with faster progression of the disease.

Summary: HIV belongs to the family of retroviruses that need the enzyme reverse transcriptase for multiplication. The virus has an envelope made of glycoproteins that are crucial to the pathogenicity of the virus. Antibodies against them are of diagnostic importance. The central core has the RNA fragment and the enzymes. A core antigen p24 is important for early diagnosis. HIV 1 subtype c is the agent causing HIV infections in India. HIV 2 is responsible for a minority of infections. HIV has affinity for the CD4 receptors and thus selectively kills the T helper lymphocytes. Loss of T cell function leads to infections and malignancies.

IMMUNOPATHOGENESIS OF HIV INFECTION

The HIV has a peculiar affinity for CD4 receptors. Hence, all CD4 receptor-bearing cells like T lymphocytes and macrophages are selectively infected and the virus uses the cellular machinery of these cells to continuously replicate within the body. gp120 is an envelope protein essential for attachment of HIV on cell surface and C-chemokine receptor type 5 (CCR5), C-X-C receptor 4 (CXCR4) act as co-receptors. Once it has completely used up the cell machinery for its own replication, the cell dies releasing hundreds of virions that are ready to infect few cells (Fig. 26.2).

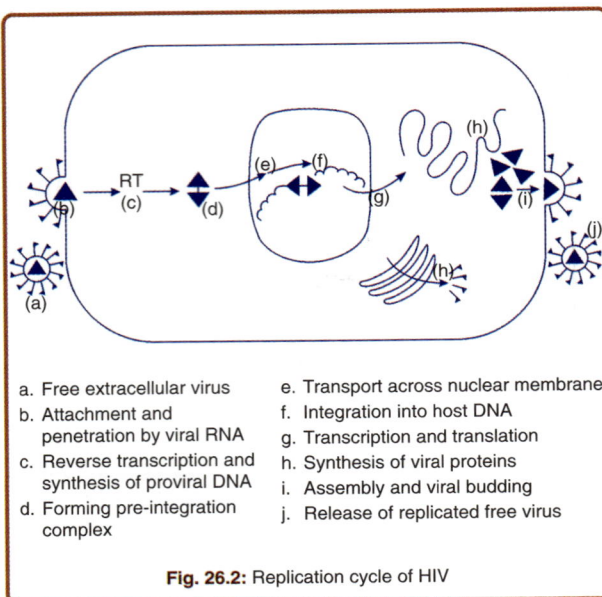

a. Free extracellular virus
b. Attachment and penetration by viral RNA
c. Reverse transcription and synthesis of proviral DNA
d. Forming pre-integration complex
e. Transport across nuclear membrane
f. Integration into host DNA
g. Transcription and translation
h. Synthesis of viral proteins
i. Assembly and viral budding
j. Release of replicated free virus

Fig. 26.2: Replication cycle of HIV

eventual downfall of the patient (Fig. 26.3). Please *see* diagrams on pages 322 and 335 for temporal correlation for clinical events in HIV disease with viraemia and CD4 count.

Summary: With its affinity for CD4 receptors, HIV selectively targets T helper cells. The dying T cells release hundreds of virions that further magnify the infection. Early in the infection, the virus is neutralised by CD8 positive cells in the blood and is therefore confined to the lymph nodes. This results in persistent generalised lymphadenopathy which lasts for a few years. Polyclonal B cell activation occurs in some patients. With disease progression, immune system gets exhausted and the virus appears in the blood. This tends to reduce CD4 cell count by destroying them. Loss of this effector arm of immunity leads to a variety of infections and malignancies.

CD4 positive T cells (T4 helper/inducer) being central to the mounting of cellular and humoral immunity against variety of infections, the result of the HIV attack is a plethora of infections with pathogenic and opportunistic organisms. Immune surveillance against malignancies also suffers leading to malgnancies.

In the early phase of HIV disease, HIV specific CD8 T cells appear in the blood following sero-conversion and their increasing number contributes to the reversal of CD4/CD8 ratio that characterises HIV infection. These virus specific CD8 T cells are responsible for preventing the appearance of the virus in the peripheral blood. During this stage the virus is more or less contained by CD4 T cells within lymphoid organs. This leads to persistent generalised lymphadenopathy that is histo-pathologically characterised by follicular hyperplasia resulting from continuous immune activation. The continuous immune stimulation throughout the disease leads to polyclonal B cell activation that is responsible for some of the disease manifestations.

As the disease progresses, continuous viral replication leads to immune exhaustion manifesting as increase in the viral load in peripheral blood and decrease in CD4. Compromised immunity leads to a variety of opportunistic infections. Such concomitant infections hasten the immune exhaustion. At this stage, lymphadenopathy resolves as follicular hyperplasia in lymph nodes gives way to fibrosis.

During this stage, the virus replicates in CD4 T cells in peripheral blood thereby killing them, leading to a reducing CD4 count. The recurrent or intractable infections and malignancies that result due to poor immune surveillance bring about the

EPIDEMIOLOGY OF HIV INFECTION

As reported in 2013, India is estimated to have around 1.16 lakhs annual new HIV infections among adults and around 14,500 new HIV infections among children. Of the 1.16 lakhs, estimated new infections among adults, the six high prevalence states account for only 31% of new infections, while the ten low prevalence states of Odisha, Jharkhand, Bihar, Uttar Pradesh, West Bengal, Gujarat, Chhattisgarh, Rajasthan, Punjab and Uttarakhand together account for 57% of new infections. The greater vulnerabilities in these states are being given higher focus in the acquired immuno-deficiency syndrome (AIDS) control programme.

The total number of people living with HIV (PLHIV) in India is estimated at 21 lakhs. Children (less than 15 years) account for 7% (1.45 lakhs) of all infections, while 86% are in the age group of 15–49 years. Of all HIV infections, 39% (8.16 lakhs) are among women. The estimated number of PLHIV in India maintains a steady declining trend from 23.2 lakhs in 2006 to 21 lakhs in 2013. The four high prevalence states of South India (Andhra Pradesh, Karnataka, Maharashtra, and Tamil Nadu) account for 53% of all HIV infected population in the country.

HIV epidemic in India is concentrated among high risk groups and heterogeneous in its distribution. The vulnerabilities that drive the epidemic are different in different parts of the country. Overall trends of HIV portray a declining epidemic at national level, though interstate variations exist. Both prevention and treatment strategies have yielded good impacts as reflected in the reduction in new infections as well as AIDS-related deaths in the country.

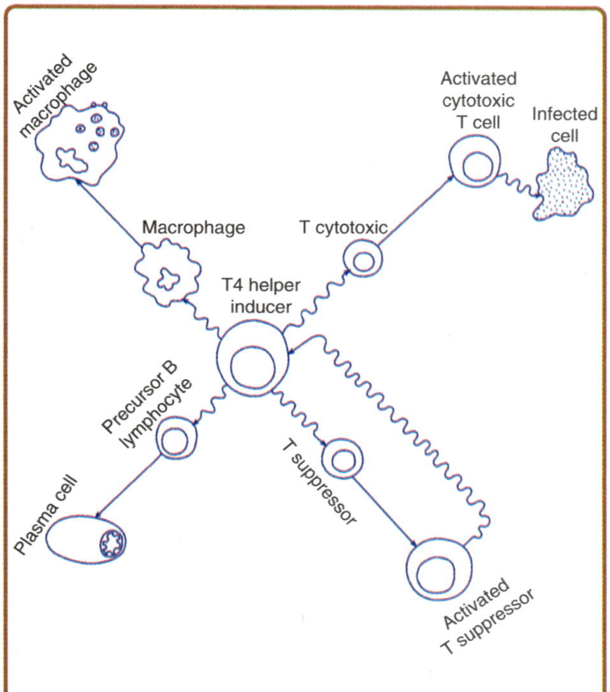

Fig. 26.3: Central role of T4 helper/inducer cell in immunity

Government of India launched the free anti-retroviral therapy (ART) programme on 1st April, 2004, starting with eight tertiary-level government hospitals in the six high-prevalence states of Andhra Pradesh, Karnataka, Maharashtra, Tamil Nadu, Manipur and Nagaland. As on March 2013, there are around 18.13 lakhs PLHIV registered at the 400 ART Centres functioning all around the country. Currently near 6.5 lakhs are on first line ART.

It is estimated that the scale up of free ART since 2004 has saved over 1.5 lakhs lives in the country till 2011 by averting deaths due to AIDS-related causes.

At the current pace of scale up of ART services, it is estimated that around 50,000–60,000 deaths annually will be averted in the next 5 years. With increasing coverage of treatment and decreasing AIDS-related mortality, a significant number of people are likely to require first and second line ART treatment in the coming years.

Transmission of HIV Infection

In India, heterosexual intercourse is responsible for transmission of 85% of cases. Intravenous drug abuse, homosexuality, and blood and blood product transfusions are responsible for a small but substantial number. In children, transmission of HIV infection from mother to her child can occur during pregnancy and labour or due to breast feeding. Children may also get infected through sexual abuse.

HIV infection can also be transmitted by donation of semen or organs. However, with screening of donors, this can be almost totally eliminated. A few cases of HIV transmission to health care workers due to needle stick injuries or contact with body fluids or tissues are known. However, as compared to hepatitis B virus, which easily spreads by this mode (seroconversion rate 30%), spread of HIV by this method, is less likely (overall seroconversion rate after exposure in the health care setting is 0.3%) and the risk to health care workers is negligible, if universal precautions are observed. (Please *see* prevention of HIV infection).

Patient Profile

Spread of HIV infection in a community shows three stages. In the first stage only persons with high-risk activity like having unsafe sex with multiple partners are involved. This phase was seen in the early 1990s in India. In the second phase, spouses (mostly housewives) or partners of individuals with high-risk activity are affected. In the third phase, the disease appears in the children born of HIV infected mothers. In India, the second and third phases have started showing their effects and hence the patient profile has changed during the last decade to include housewives and children.

Ten years back, most cases reported were males in the age group of 21–45 years. About 60% of these were unmarried. During the last decade this patient profile has shown a tilt towards affection of young married women and children. Currently about 40% of the newly detected cases are in women and children who constitute about 25% of the total cases.

Summary: About 3 million persons are estimated to be infected with the HIV in India. Although the average prevalence rate of HIV infection in the general adult population is 0.36%, in some of the states and cities it exceeds 1% of the adult population. Women and children are increasingly (25% of total and 40% of newly detected cases) infected. The major route of HIV transmission is heterosexual (85%). Perinatal transmission (5%), blood transfusions (1%), intravenous drug abuse (4%) and homosexual intercourse (5%) account for the other cases.

Chapter 26

HIV Infection and AIDS

NATURAL HISTORY OF UNTREATED HIV INFECTION

Infection with HIV does not cause any immediate symptoms or signs. A brief self-limiting flu-like illness is noted in a small proportion of the cases (others being asymptomatic) 1–3 months after the infection. This is followed by an asymptomatic phase that lasts for a variable period of 6 months to 10 years (average 4–5 years). Minor problems like herpes zoster or molluscum contagiosum may occur during this 'early stage of HIV disease'. An 'intermediate stage of HIV disease' characterised by recurrent but typical bacterial, mycobacterial, fungal and parasitic infections and infestations with fever, lymphadenopathy and weight loss follows and lasts for another 2–4 years. Serious and atypical infections like extrapulmonary or disseminated tuberculosis and unusual infections like cryptococcosis are seen during 'late stage HIV disease' which is commonly termed as AIDS and is usually fatal within 6 months to 2 years.

The duration of different stages mentioned above are applicable to untreated cases only and that too in about 75% of patients. In addition to these typical progressors, there are some who progress very rapidly (clinical latent phase lasting for just 2 years, rapid progressors, 20%) and others who progress very slowly (clinical latency of 10 years or more, long-term non-progressors, less than 5%). Infective dose, pathogenicity of the virus and the quality of supportive, prophylactic and specific therapy are some of the factors that determine the rate of progression. As more and more patients are availing the benefit of antiretroviral therapy, the above described typical progression of untreated HIV infections is fast becoming uncommon. In patients on antiretroviral

therapy, the intermediate stage of HIV disease gets prolonged as long as effective antiretroviral therapy is continued (Fig. 26.4).

Summary: Primary infection with HIV manifests within 6–12 weeks of the infection in a minority as a flu-like self healing illness. The rest go undiagnosed, being considered to be suffering from a transient viral infection, or may be asymptomatic. After a variable asymptomatic phase (average 4–5 years but can vary from 2–10 years) minor infections like herpes zoster or molluscum contagiosum may occur. Lymphadenopathy may be seen during this stage. Within 1–2 years this progresses to more internal infections that may be initially typical and later atypical. They include bacterial, mycobacterial, viral, fungal and parasitic infections and infestations with associated weight loss, fever and diarrhoea. This phase lasts 1–3 years. Serious infections (e.g. cryptococcosis, toxoplasmosis, systemic candidiasis, and cytomegalovirus) soon supervene and death results from one of these within the next 1 year. Malignancies like squamous cell carcinoma, lymphomas and Kaposi's sarcoma occur during this last stage. However, such typical progression is becoming uncommon with widespread use of antiretroviral therapy which prolongs the length of the intermediate stage till effective antiretroviral treatment is continued.

CLINICAL FEATURES AND STAGES OF HIV INFECTION

Primary Infection Illness (Seroconversion)

- About 50% of the infected develop a symptomatic primary illness. However, it is

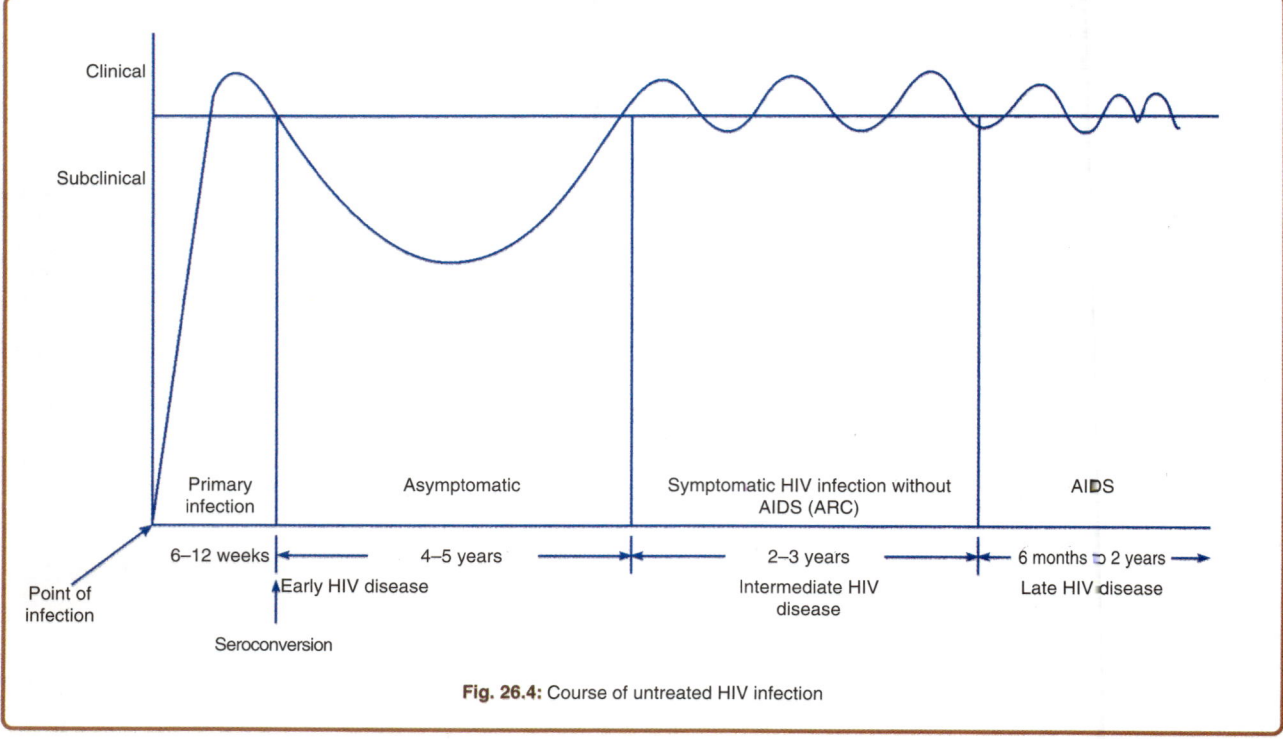

Fig. 26.4: Course of untreated HIV infection

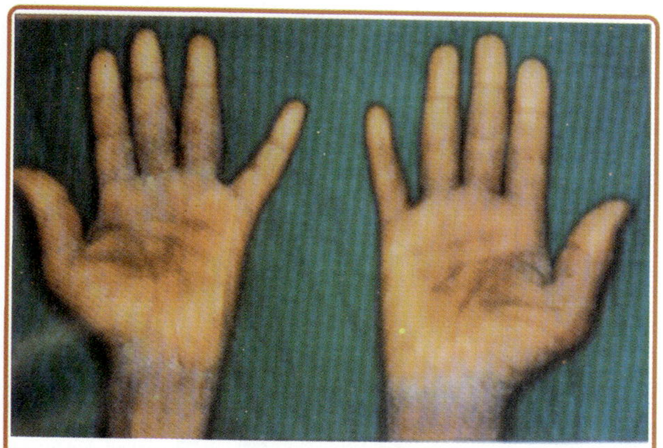

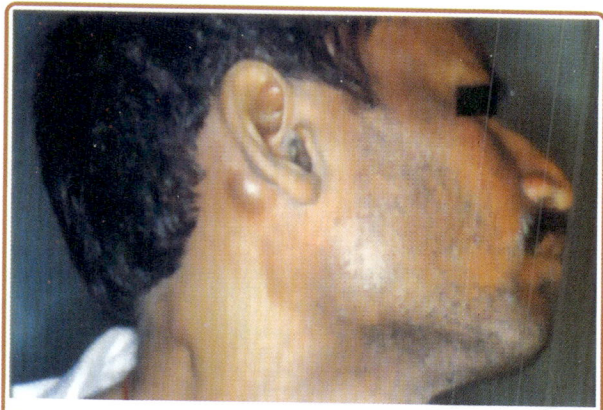

Fig. 26.5: Keratotic scabies (Norwegian scabies)—keratotic (rough surface) greyish plaques over palms in an HIV infected person. This type of scabies is highly infectious

Fig. 26.6: Seborrhoeic dermatitis with lymphadenopathy—ill defined dull red erythema and fine yellowish scales over beard area with non-tender, firm discrete, postauricular and other nodes

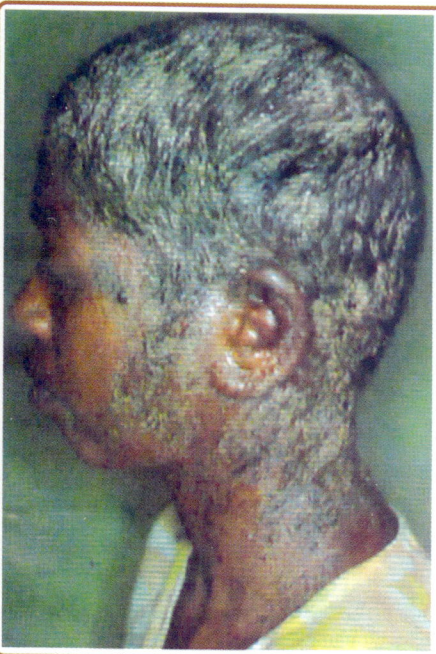

Fig. 26.7: Seborrhoeic dermatitis—Thick, yellowish greasy scales covering erythema over scalp and face severe and widespread disease like this is sometimes seen with HIV disease

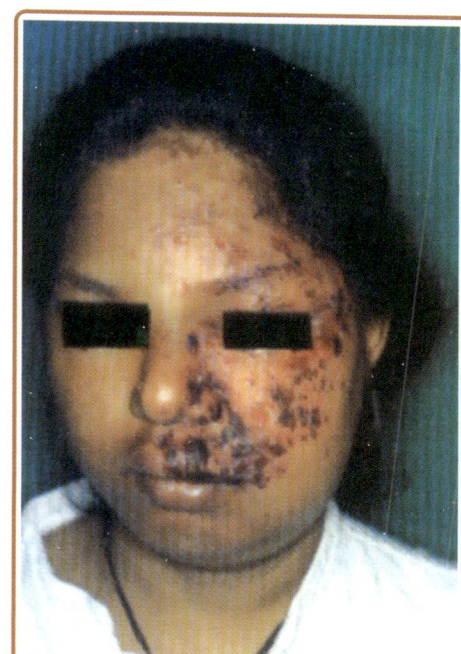

Fig. 26.8: Herpes zoster pphthalmicus—haemorrhagic vesicle sand erosions on a background of erythema and oedema in HIV disease. Ophthalmic and maxillary nerves are affected

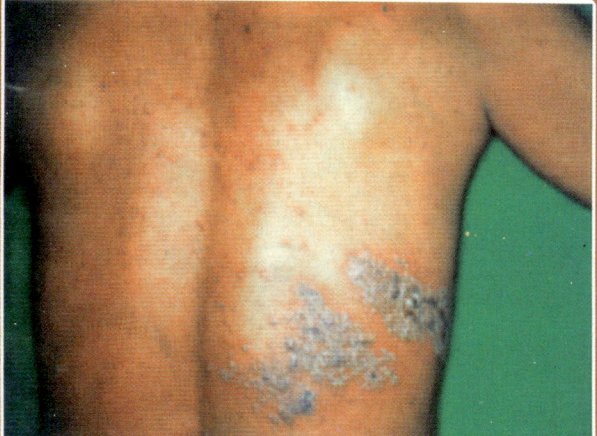

Fig. 26.9: Herpes zoster with disseminated skin lesions in HIV disease— grouped vesicles based on erythema in segmental pattern. Note numerous scattered lesions over rest of the trunk

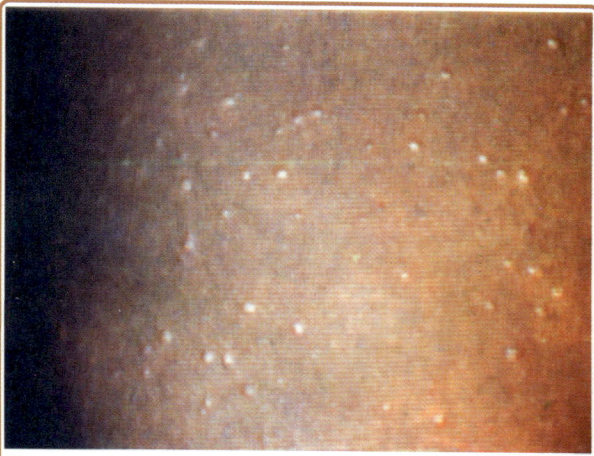

Fig. 26.10: Widespread extragenital (eruptive) molluscum contagiosa in HIV positive—tiny, yellowish or skin coloured, shiny papules, many with central umbilication, over the back

Chapter
26

HIV Infection and AIDS

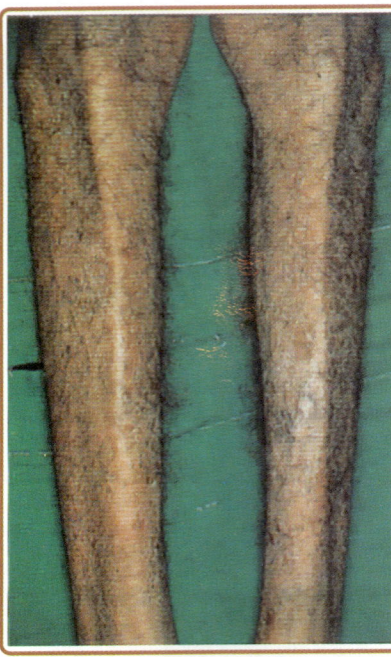

Fig. 26.11: Acquired Ichthyosis in HIV disease—dryness and small rectangular white scales over both legs in an HIV positive. Note marked wasting of legs due to advanced HIV disease

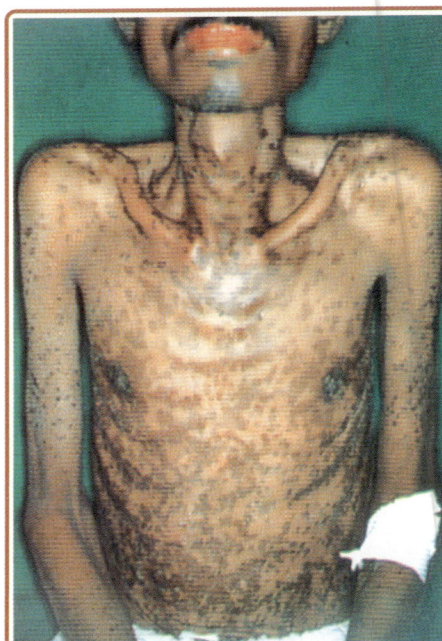

Fig. 26.12: Sulphonamide induced Stevens Johnson syndrome—Widespread reddish brown patches with bullae, lip erosions and pronounced wasting due to advanced HIV disease

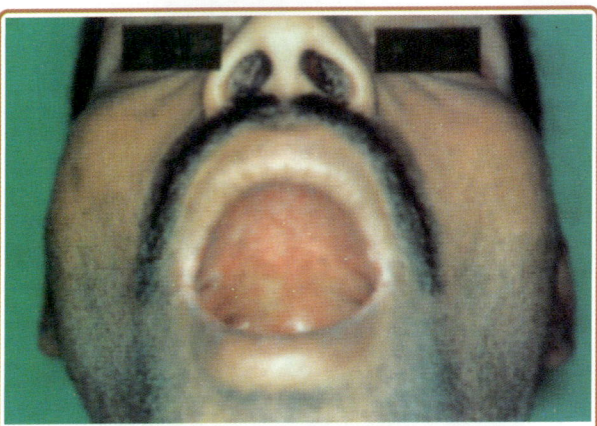

Fig. 26.13: Candidal stomatitis (oral thrush)—curdy white discharge overlying erythema and erosions on palate. Oral thrush in a healthy-looking young male suggests HIV infection

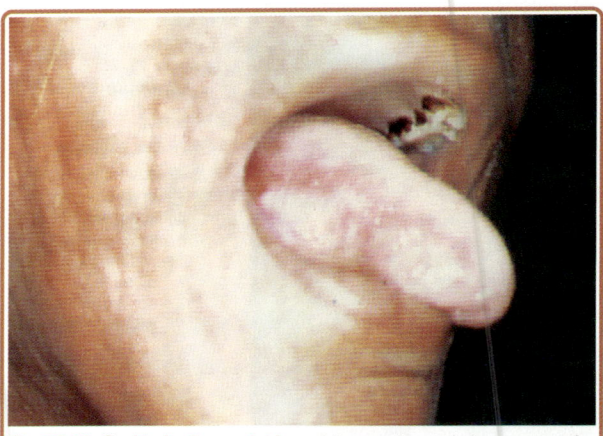

Fig. 26.14: Oral hairy leucoplakia—white papules and plaques over the side of tongue in HIV disease. The 'ribbed' appearance of lesions is typical but is not always present

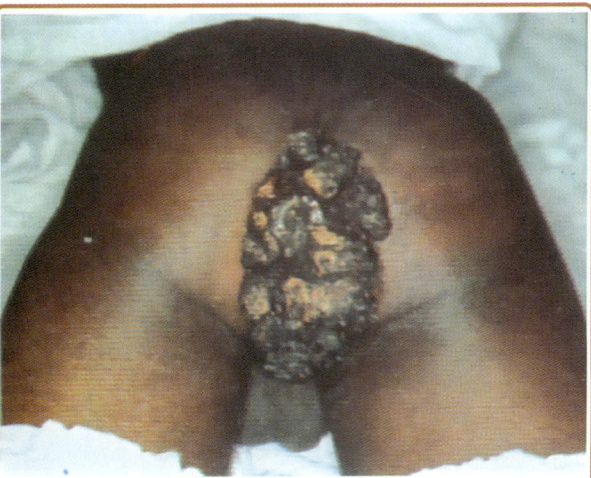

Fig. 26.15: Squamous cell carcinoma in HIV disease—Large, pedunculated, papillated, pink, exophytic tumour that bleeds on minor trauma. Biopsy differentiate from condyloma acuminata

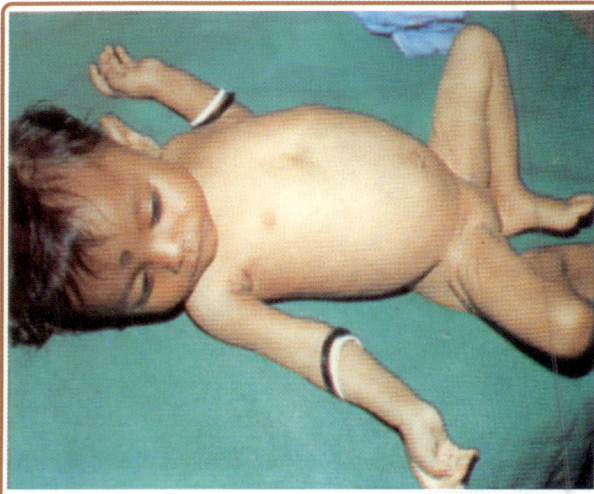

Fig. 26.16: Paediatric HIV infection—failure to thrive is a common presentation of paediatric HIV infection

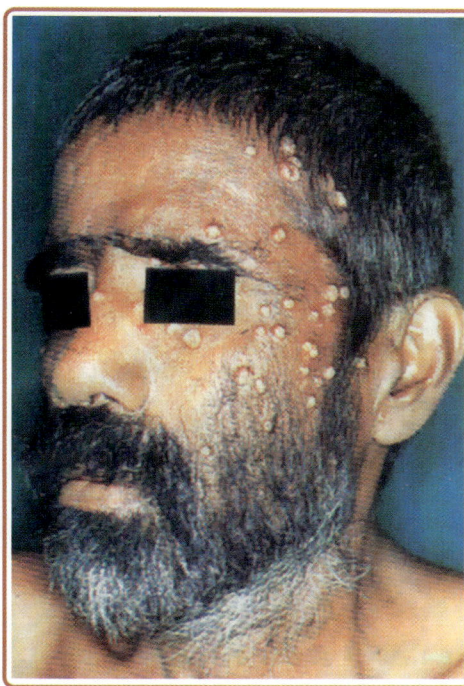

Fig. 26.17: Molluscum contagiosum—numerous, pearly while, shiny umbilicated papules over face. Extragenital location in adults suggests underlying HIV infection

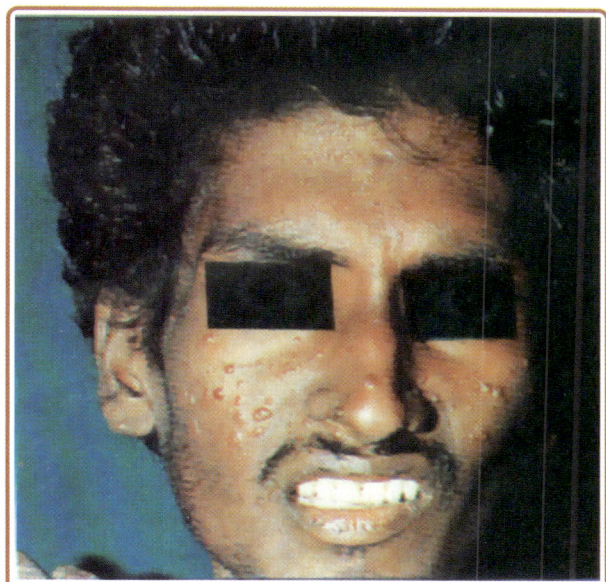

Fig. 26.18: Cryptococcosis—multiple, erythematous or skin coloured papules and nodules over face in a young adult. Some of the lesions are umbilicated or ulcerated in the centre and resemble molluscum contangiosum

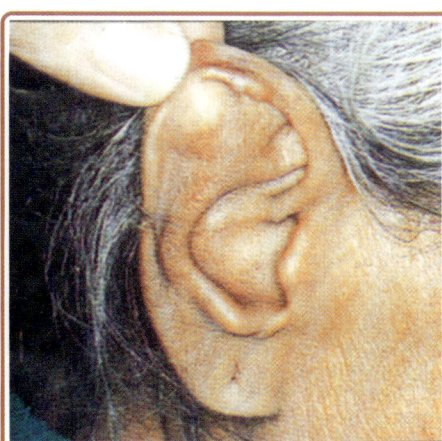

Fig. 26.19: Cryptococcosis—asymptomatic, multiple, pearly white or skin colour papules over ear rim in an elderly woman. HIV does not spare any age or sex

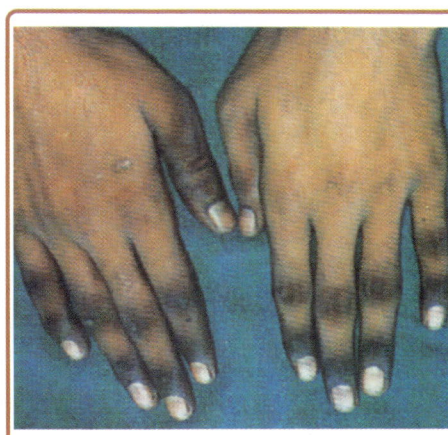

Fig. 26.20: Addisonian pigmentation—asymptomatic, symmetric, ill-defined, hyper-pigmentation over dorsa of hands. Exposed regions life face and forearms are also involved in about 50% patients with late HIV disease

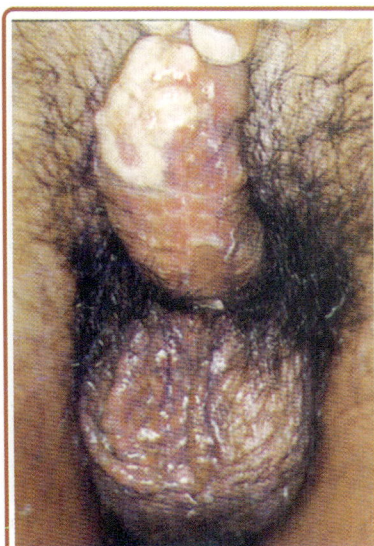

Fig. 26.21: Ulcerative herpes genitalis— ulceration with polycyclic outline affecting undersurface of penile shaft. Confluence of lesions, deeper ulceration and persistence of lesions for 1 month indicated unusual severity due to HIV infection

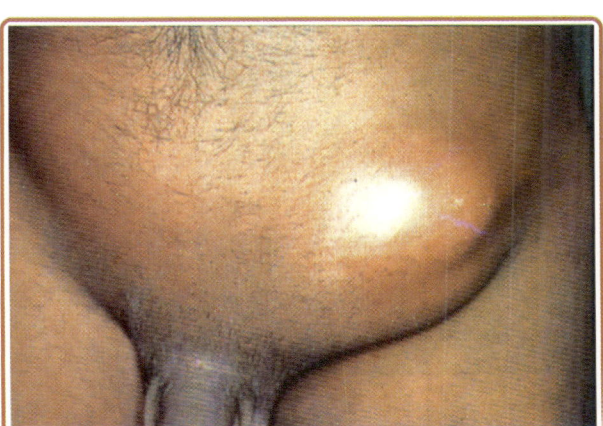

Fig. 26.22: Molluscum contagiosum—numerous, pearly white, shiny umbilicated papules over face. Extragenital location in adults suggests underlying HIV infection

Chapter 26

HIV Infection and AIDS

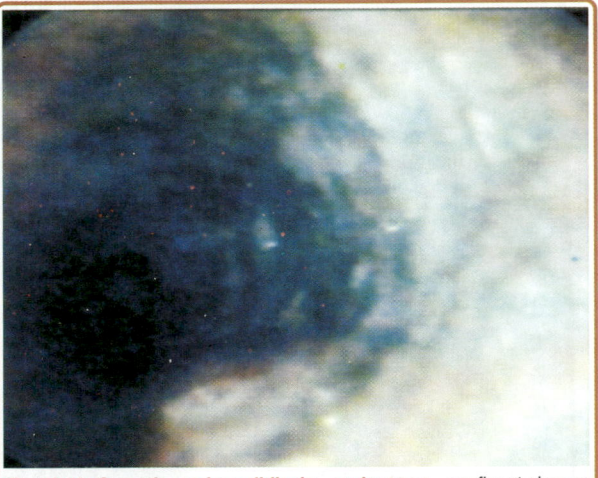

Fig. 26.23: Oesophageal candidiasis—endoscopy—confluent plaques formed by curdy white discharge due to oesophageal candidiasis in late HIV infection

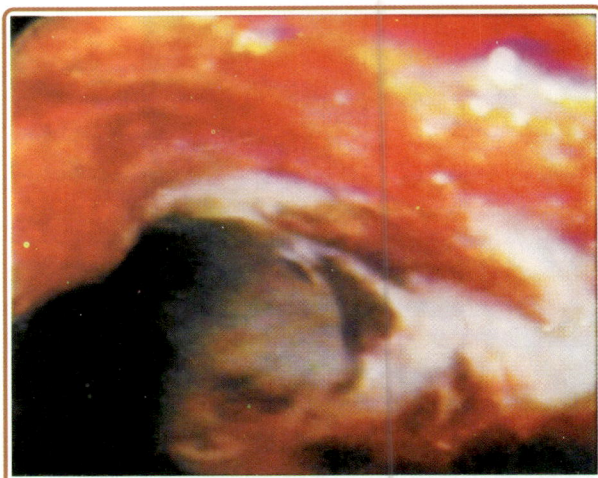

Fig. 26.24: Oesophageal herpes simplex—multiple, small vesicles and superficial erosions with erythematous flare

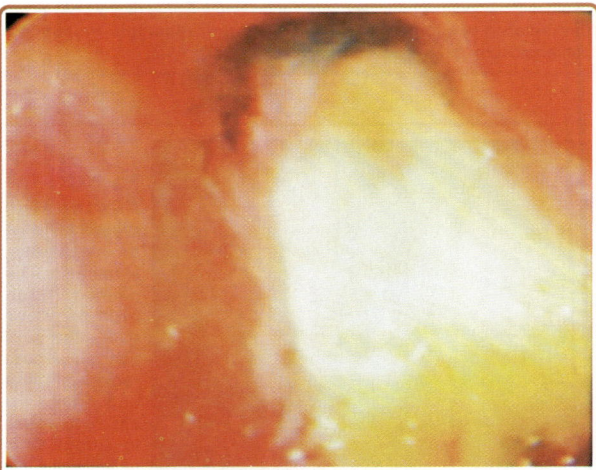

Fig. 26.25: Hypertrophic oesophageal candidiasis—endoscopy—well-defined, yellowish white plaque at lower end of oesophagus

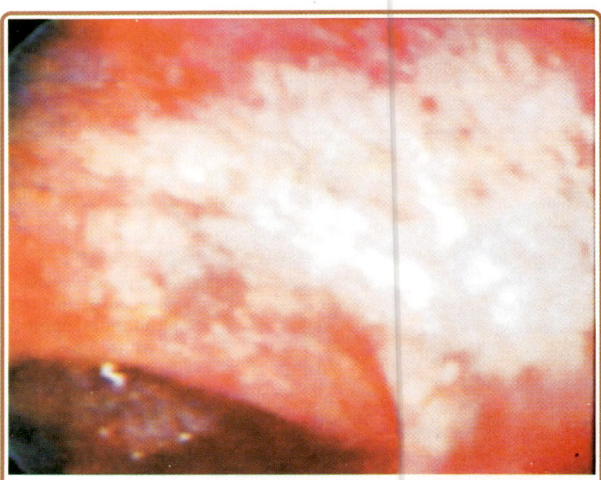

Fig. 26.26: Cytomegalovirus colitis—diffuse erythema, punctate haemorrhages and superficial erosions on colonoscopy

Chapter 26

HIV Infection and AIDS

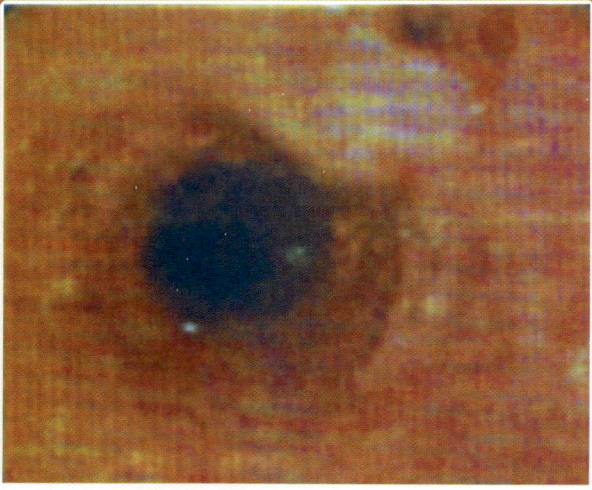

Fig. 26.27: Oesophageal tuberculosis—endoscopy reveals an abnormal opening which may be either a discharging sinus (in case of lymph node affection) or broncho-oesophageal fistula (in case of lung tuberculosis)

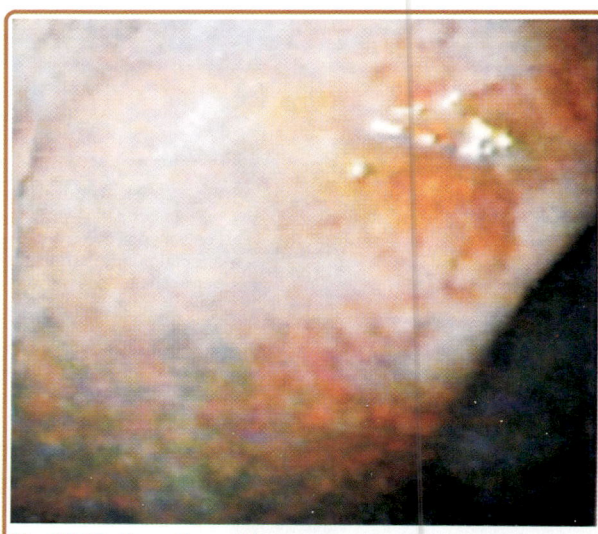

Fig. 26.28: Herpetic colitis—grouped superficial erosions with oedematous margins and surrounding erythema

rarely diagnosed, as it resembles a common respiratory viral infection like influenza.

- After a variable incubation period of 4–24 weeks (average 2 months), there may be a brief period of illness resembling influenza or infectious mononucleosis. Fever, body ache, joint pains, headache, rhinitis, pharyngitis, stomatitis and lymphadenopathy are the usual symptoms. A maculopapular erythematous or urticarial rash is sometimes present.

- This is self-limiting (lasting 1–3 weeks) and many patients do not give any history of such an episode.

- During this stage, the plasma viral load is very high as no prior immunity to the infection is present.

- Antibody tests for HIV turn positive (sero-conversion) at the end of the phase.

- Uncommonly, vomiting, diarrhoea, hepatitis, leucopenia, thrombocytopenia, aseptic meningitis and a Guillain Barre like polyneuritic illness may occur.

Summary: About 50% of infected persons develop a flu like illness 6–12 weeks after the infection. Constitutional signs and symptoms, rhinitis, pharyngitis, lymphadenopathy and maculopapular rash lasting 1–3 weeks are common. The plasma viral load is very high during this period at the end of which serum enzyme-linked immunosorbent assay (ELISA) turns positive.

Early HIV Disease (Latent HIV Infection/Asymptomatic HIV Infection)

- This phase has a highly variable duration, range being 2 years to more than 10 years, with an average (in Indian population) of 5 years.

- During this phase the patient may be totally symptom free or may have minor mucocutaneous features (e.g. folliculitis, dermatophytosis, seborrhoeic dermatitis, hairy leucoplakia or aphthae) or lymphadenopathy that when incidentally noticed or investigated reveal the underlying HIV infection.

- Other mucocutaneous manifestations that may point to underlying HIV infection include a variety of other sexually transmitted diseases like chancroid, syphilis, donovanosis, genital herpes simplex, condyloma acuminata or molluscum contagiosum. Non-sexually transmitted disease features include typical attacks of herpes zoster, seborrhoeic dermatitis and thrombocytopenic purpura.

Although, the term 'latent' is used for this stage, as it becomes evident from the above paragraph, it does cause symptoms and signs. However, these are minor and may not immediately indicate HIV infection, as the patient is in otherwise good health. In fact, the latent stage gradually merges into the symptomatic stage and the later into AIDS.

- Lymphadenopathy of HIV infection (also called persistent generalised lymphadenopathy) commonly involves many lymph node groups.

- The lymph nodes are small or moderately enlarged, painless, non-tender, firm and discrete.

- They do not suppurate and the overlying skin is normal. Biopsy reveals follicular hyperplasia.

- Other causes of lymphadenopathy in HIV infected persons include syphilis, tuberculosis, lymphogranuloma venereum and non-Hodgkin's lymphoma.

Summary: Without medical intervention, the usual duration of this phase in Indians is 4–5 years. Persistent generalised lymphadenopathy (PGL) is the only sign of this relatively asymptomatic phase. Lymph nodes are 1–3 cm sized, non-tender, firm and discrete. Recurrent minor fungal and bacteria infections [including sexually transmitted infections (STIs)] of the skin occur. Molluscum contagiosum, typical herpes zoster or unresponsive seborrhoeic dermatitis could serve as clinical markers of this phase in adults. Plasma viral load is low and CD4 count is normal.

A plethora of mucocutaneous manifestations punctuate the natural course of HIV infection in Indian patients (Table 26.1 and Figs 26.5–26.28).

Intermediate Stage HIV Disease: (AIDS Related Complex/Symptomatic HIV Infection without AIDS)

- During this period, lasting 2–4 years, patient's health is obviously affected, the gradual progression presenting as weight loss, loss of appetite, fever and typical presentations of pulmonary or extra-pulmonary tuberculosis.

- Recurrent diarrhoea, sinusitis, bronchitis and bacterial pneumonias are also common.

- Unusually severe or extensive or unresponsive sexually transmitted diseases, herpes zoster or oral candidiasis and anaemia constitute other features.

- Although, no serious opportunistic infections are demonstrable, the CD4 counts gradually fall.

Chapter **26**

HIV Infection and AIDS

TABLE 26.1: Mucocutaneous manifestations of HIV infection

SEXUALLY TRANSMITTED DISEASES Typical or Unusually florid or Non-responsive Syphilis Chancroid Donovanosis Herpes genitalis Condyloma acuminata Molluscum contagiosum **OTHER INFECTIONS** **Viral** *Herpes zoster :* Typical or unusually severe with dissemination *Warts :* Typical or Widespread Oral hairy leucoplakia (EBV) **Bacterial** Unusually extensive or florid pyoderma Bacillary angiomatosis **Mycobacterial** Scrofuloderma Orificial tuberculosis Atypical mycobacterial infections **Fungal** Candidiasis *Dermatophytosis :* Typical or Widespread Cryptococcosis Penicilliosis Histoplasmosis **Parasitic** Crusted scabies Demodicidosis **Malignancies** Sqamous cell carcinoma Lymphoma Kaposi's sarcoma	**Autoimmune Diseases** Thrombocytopenic purpura Vasculitis Lupus erythematosus Reiter's disease **Drug Eruptions** Maculopapular rash Stevens-Johnson syndrome Toxic epidermal necrolysis **Other Inflammatory Skin Disorders** Seborrhoeic dermatitis Psoriasis Papular eruption of HIV Eosinophilic folliculitis **Miscellaneous Changes** Hyperpigmentation Ichthyosis Xerosis Premature graying of hair Prurigo **Oral Cavity Lesions** Aphthous ulcers Candidiasis Oral hair leucoplakia **Herpes Labialis/Stomatitis** Typical or unusually severe with dissemination Mucous patches of syphilis Periodontitis Addisonian pigmentation Viral warts Kaposi's sarcoma Squamous cell carcinoma

Summary: If untreated, the intermediate symptomatic phase of HIV infection lasts 2–4 years. Typical systemic infections like pulmonary tuberculosis or scrofuloderma occur commonly. Others include recurrent upper and lower respiratory tract bacterial infections, unresponsive or severe STDs, severe herpes zoster or oral candidiasis, CD4 counts fall steadily and plasma viral load rises gradually during this phase. Mild to moderate constitutional symptoms and signs, i.e. fever, anorexia, weight loss and night sweats are usual.

Late Stage HIV Disease (AIDS)

- **Serious opportunistic infections** occur in this phase including:

  ❑ Disseminated or multiple attacks of pulmonary or extrapulmonary tuberculosis,

  ❑ Cryptococcosis [central nervous system (CNS, skin, lungs)]

  ❑ Candidiasis (visceral-oesophageal and disseminated)

  ❑ Toxoplasmosis (CNS, eye and lungs)

  ❑ Cytomegalovirus infection (eye, colon, oesophagus and lungs)

  ❑ Herpes simplex and zoster (encephalitis, radiculitis)

  ❑ *Pneumocystis carinii* (lungs)

❏ Atypical mycobacterial infections (lungs), diarrhoea due to unusual organisms like cryptosporidium or isospora

❏ John Cunningham (JC) polyoma virus (PML, progressive multifocal leucoencephalopathy)

● **Malignant tumours** like:

❏ Non-Hodgkin lymphoma,

❏ Cervical and anorectal carcinomas and

❏ Kaposi's sarcoma occur.

However, Kaposi's sarcoma is much less common in Indians. Infection with human herpes virus 8 (HHV 8) has been identified as a cofactor for the development of Kaposi's sarcoma. Kaposi's sarcoma in AIDS is distinctly different from Kaposi's sarcoma in immuno-competent persons. In AIDS, it presents as asymptomatic multiple, flat erythematous macules and papules of varying sizes involving the extremities, trunk, face and mucosae. Because of its slow evolution over several years, by itself, Kaposi's sarcoma is rarely fatal in AIDS cases. The patient usually falls victim to one of the opportunistic infections.

● **Direct effects of HIV infection** like:

❏ Malabsorption due to persistent diarrhoea,

❏ Wasting or 'slim disease' resulting from severe weight loss,

❏ HIV encephalopathy,

❏ Retinopathy.

Summary: Serious internal opportunistic infections like disseminated tuberculosis, cryptococcal meningitis, cerebral toxoplasmosis, cryptosporidial diarrhoea are common causes of death during late stage HIV infection in Indian patients. Herpes encephalitis, pneumocystis carinii pneumonia or cytomegalovirus infections may also occur and may lead to death. In Indian patients, malignancies like squamous cell carcinoma and lymphoma are more frequent when compared to Kaposi's sarcoma. Later, severe weight loss follows, HIV encephalopathy or peripheral neuropathy or HIV enteropathy are some late effects due to long standing HIV infection.

Diagnosis of HIV Infection and AIDS

In addition to the history of high risk activity and the clinical features mentioned above, at least three positive ELISA tests for HIV antibodies (using different kits on the same sample) are necessary to make a diagnosis of HIV infection. The three ELISA tests should be done by different kits using different methodologies (please *see* 'investigations in HIV infection').

Other tests like polymerase chain reaction (PCR) test or western blot (WB) test are more specific for HIV infection and should be used whenever available to confirm the diagnosis of HIV infection (Table 26.2). Alternatively, one may use quantitative estimation of plasma viral load or viral culture, though these are more expensive.

It must be remembered that ELISA test is high on sensitivity and slightly low on specificity. Hence, when used to check for HIV infection in non-high-risk groups like antenatal clinic attendees, it has higher likelihood of false positive results. Hence, while testing non-high-risk groups, ELISA positive results should preferably confirmed by specific tests like western blot or PCR.

Summary: Diagnosis of HIV infection is based on demonstration of circulating antibodies to HIV antigens in patient's blood by ELISA test. A positive ELISA test must be confirmed with a repeat ELISA done using a different kit based on a different method. For symptomatic patients, the sample should be reactive with 2 different kits. For asymptomatic patients, the sample should be reactive with three different kits. In case of equivocal results, confirmation can be obtained by western blot test or qualitative PCR test. Alernatively, quantitative estimation of plasma viral load or viral culture may be done, if available.

INVESTIGATIONS IN HIV INFECTION

These can be divided into those needed for diagnosis of HIV infection and those used to monitor the response to antiretroviral treatment and to rule out opportunistic infections.

Tests Used for Diagnosis of HIV Infection

HIV infection can be diagnosed by demonstrating:

1. *Antibodies against virus:* ELISA and WB tests

2. *Viral antigens:* p24 antigen assay

3. *Viral nucleic acid material:* Qualitative DNA PCR and quantitative plasma viral load

4. *Viral culture*

1. Antibodies Detection Tests

ELISA Test for HIV

Serum enzyme-linked immunosorbent assay (ELISA) is the commonest test used for screening for HIV infection. It is the most inexpensive and sensitive (99% sensitivity) test available. However, it is not absolutely specific (98% specificity) and hence, false positive results are possible and this should be kept in

Chapter
26

HIV Infection and AIDS

TABLE 26.2 : Tests for diagnosis of HIV infection						
Test	Primary illness	Early disease	Intermediate disease	Late disease	Advantages	Disadvantages
ELISA	±	+ve	+ve	+ve	Inexpensive, suited for large number of samples	False positive or negative occurs in 1%
WB	±	+	+ve	+ve	Diagnostic, if positive	False negative common in early infections, expensive
p24	++	±	±	+ve	Becomes +ve earlier than ELISA, used for diagnosis of initial infections	False negative common in intermediate and early stage
Qualitative PCR	+	+	+	+	Diagnostic most sensitive for diagnosis of initial infections	Gives no information about severity of viraemia
Viral load	+++	+	++	+++	Quantitative, used for prognosis or for monitoring therapy	Very expensive
Viral culture	+	±	±	+	Positive early, used for prognosis available False negative common	Very expensive, not easily
Spot tests (e.g. Latex aggl.)	–	+	+	+	Inexpensive, suited for small no. of samples, rapid test	High (1–5%) false positive and false negative rates

mind especially when dealing with no history of activities with high risk of acquiring HIV infection. The procedure followed for performing the test varies between laboratories and faulty procedure may result in false positive or negative results.

Children born to HIV infected mothers may show a false positive ELISA test even if they are not infected with HIV. This occurs due to passive transfer of antibodies from mother to child. Please *see* section on paediatric HIV infection for further details.

Other causes of **false positive ELISA test** include:

- ❑ Faulty laboratory techniques, including contamination or mixing of samples or heat inactivation of sera, ELISA Kit or equipment faults, etc.
- ❑ Leprosy, malaria, and other causes of polyclonal B cell activation (lupus erythematosus and other collagen vascular diseases).
- ❑ Positive antinuclear antibody test
- ❑ Lymphoreticular malignancies
- ❑ Immunoglobulin G (IgG) administration or multiple transfusion recipients or transplant recipients or multiparous women.

- ❑ HIV vaccines and infection with other retroviruses.

Now, ELISA kits are available which can differentiate between HIV 1 and HIV 2 infections. It is advisable to confirm HIV 1 and HIV 2 coinfection by additional tests like WB or PCR for HIV 1 and HIV 2.

Clinical implication: A positive ELISA result is usually reported only after double reconfirmation and this should be ideally confirmed with a WB test. If the latter test is not available or impossible due to economic constraints, confirmation of diagnosis can be obtained by repeating ELISA test on a new blood sample using a different ELISA kit and methodology.

False negative ELISA test

It may result from:

- ❑ A patient being in the window period (window period—time between HIV infection and the appearance in the blood of detectable antibodies to the virus. This time averages 4 weeks to 3 months but virtually all patients seroconvert within 6 months. A negative serologic result during the window period cannot exclude HIV infection)
- ❑ Due to laboratory errors or

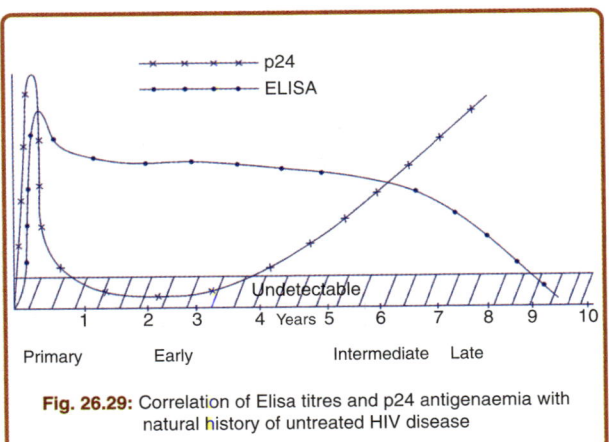
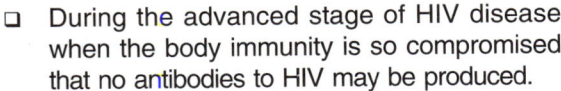

Fig. 26.29: Correlation of Elisa titres and p24 antigenaemia with natural history of untreated HIV disease

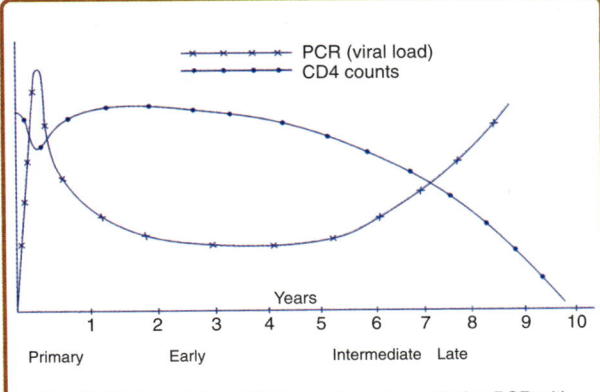

Fig. 26.30: Correlation of CD4 counts and quantitative PCR with natural history of untreated HIV infection

❑ During the advanced stage of HIV disease when the body immunity is so compromised that no antibodies to HIV may be produced.

❑ HIV 2 infection or infection by N or O subtype of HIV.

Western blot test for HIV

This highly specialised and expensive test detects antibodies to different antigens of HIV 1 and 2. Patient's serum is made to react against these different antigens blotted on a paper and the bands of the various reacting antibodies are noted. Presence of at least 2 envelope antigens and one core antigen is necessary for establishing the diagnosis of HIV infection. The test is highly specific (99.9%) but not so sensitive (95%) and hence is used only for confirming a positive ELISA test result.

Interpretation of western blot results

❑ *Positive*—reactivity to gp120/160 plus either gp41 to p24.

❑ *Negative*—no bands observed.

❑ *Indeterminate*—a few bands may be present but not fulfilling the criteria for positive test.

Clinical implication: Cases that fail to satisfy these criteria but are not totally negative are reported as indeterminate. A repeat test, after 3 months, is advised in such patients.

2. Antigen Detection Test for p24 Antigenaemia

p24 antigen assay detects presence of a major core protein, p24 and becomes positive at least 2 weeks before the ELISA test and is therefore used for:

❑ Diagnosis during the 'window period' before ELISA test is positive. However, the majority of patients in the window period are negative with this test as the test becomes positive only towards the end of the window period.

❑ In children less than 15 months of age to differentiate a false positive ELISA/WB due to maternal antibodies.

p24 antigen assay is specific but sensitivity is low (30–40%); hence, viral load is being more frequently used.

3. Detection of Nucleic Acid Material

Such tests are highly sensitive but expensive and may not be available everywhere.

❑ Qualitative PCR (proviral DNA detection).

❑ Quantitative tests for detection of the viral RNA viz. reverse transcription (RT)-PCR method and the branched chain DNA (bDNA) method. These tests detect the number of viral particles (virions) in blood and are being increasingly used to predict prognosis and monitor efficacy of antiviral therapy.

4. Viral culture and the ability of cultured virus to form syncitium in cell culture. Besides T cells, recently peripheral blood monocyte cells (PBMC) are used for HIV culture.

Summary: ELISA test for antibodies to HIV is the commonest screening test used for diagnosis of HIV infection. If repeated by two different methods, ELISA test is virtually diagnostic of HIV infection in the setting of high-risk behaviour. The ELISA test may be false negative during the window period (the first 6–12 weeks after infection).

Chapter
26

HIV Infection and AIDS

If resources are available a WB test or a qualitative PCR may be done to confirm the diagnosis especially in the absence of high-risk behaviour. p24 antigen assay is used for diagnosis of HIV infection during the window period and in the first 15 months of life in children to differentiate from false positive ELISA test due to maternal antibodies. Plasma viral load estimation is used only when antiretroviral therapy is seriously considered as it is used for monitoring response to such therapy.

TESTS TO MONITOR THE RESPONSE TO ANTIRETROVIRAL TREATMENT AND TO RULE OUT OPPORTUNISTIC INFECTION

Investigations for monitoring efficacy of therapy include plasma viral load, CD4 count and CD4/CD8 ratio. Viral load should ideally be done twice before starting therapy and then monthly for 3 months and 3 monthly thereafter. The viral load reduces rapidly to one-hundredth of the pretreatment value within the first 3 months. It should be done along with the CD4 and CD8 counts to check for parallel improvement in immunological parameters. While considering the cost of antiretroviral therapy, the hidden cost of monitoring investigations for drug efficacy as well as adverse reactions need to be taken into account. This is because, a basic monitoring investigation like plasma viral load can cost about ₹ 4,000/- every time. Hence, in resource restricted settings, CD4/CD8 counts and viral load may be done at baseline and 6 monthly thereafter.

CD4 Count

CD4 counts are useful to assess the level of immunocompromision, helps to decide when to initiate antiretroviral treatment, to monitor response to ART to decide when and which prophylaxis to start for prevention of opportunistic infections (OIs).

Normal CD4 count varies from 500–1500 cell mm³. In resource limited settings or developing countries CD4 count is widely used as an important parameter to monitor ART. CD4 count is not as reliable as viral load because besides HIV infection, several other factors affect CD4 count. CD4 count can be repeated at an interval of 3–6 months depending upon the circumstances (Table 26.7).

During an effective antiretroviral treatment CD4 count is expected to rise by 50–100 cell/mm³ per year.

CD4 Cell Counts and Risk of Opportunistic Infections

When CD4 cell counts decline, the risk of manifesting different opportunistic infections increase. Some of these OIs appear around particular CD4 count as given in the following Table 26.3.

TABLE 26.3: Correlation of CD4 cell count with opportunistic infections

CD4 cell count	Opportunistic infection
200–500	Tuberculosis, herpes zoster
50–200	Cryptococcosis, toxoplasmosis, *Pneumocystis carinii* pneumonia (PCP)
< 50	Cytomegalovirus (CMV) infection, *Mycobacterium avium* complex (MAC) infection

Hence, patients with CD4 count ≤ 250 cells/mm³ should be started on cotrimoxazole prophylaxis (480 mg BD or 960 md OD). This will protect against *Pneumocystis crainii* pneumonia (PCP) and toxoplasmosis and additionally against other bacterial infections.

If CD4 count is < 200 cells/mm³, then prophylaxis for *Mycobacterium avium* complex (MAC) infection should be started with azithromycin 1200 mg/week or clarithromycin 500 mg BD. Though, fluconazole is not the ideal drug for prophylaxis of cryptococcosis in resource restricted settings as in India, it can be used to prevent cryptococcal meningitis in endemic areas when CD4 count is < 100 cells/mm³.

Plasma Viral Load

This gives an indication of the number of viral particles in blood and is therefore important to determine disease progression, prognosis and monitoring the response to antiviral therapy. During the last few years plasma viral load has emerged as the most reliable indicator in management of HIV infection. Following an effective ART viral load should be undetectable or < 50 cells/mL at the end of 4–6 months.

The test can be done by two methods—RT-PCR and bDNA test. The test is frequently used to decide whether ART should be begun in an HIV infected person. However, the test is expensive and may not be indicated in resource restricted settings when a patient is likely to be unsuitable for antiviral therapy in the immediate future. In poor patients, it is wiser to avoid expenditure on expensive tests like viral load and save the money for therapy of opportunistic infections that may develop in future. In developing countries it is mainly used to support initiation of ART or to confirm ART failure.

Laboratory Evidence of Immunodeficiency

Absolute lymphocyte count is the simplest test that is available in any laboratory. When this dips below 1000 it is a rough indication of the declining number of CD4 receptor positive T lymphocytes (T4 or helper/inducer cells). However. since there is an increase in number of CD8 positive cells in HIV infection, CD4 count is much more reliable indicator of immunodeficiency in HIV infection. Hence, if facilities and finances are available for doing serial CD4 counts, they should be repeated 3–6 monthly to monitor immune status in HIV infection. CD4 count is above 500 during the early phase of HIV infection. It falls below 500 during the intermediate phase and below 200 during the late phase of the disease.

Other Immunologic Abnormalities

- **CD4/CD8 ratio < 1 (Normal 1.5–2):** Since CD4 cell count reduces and CD8 cell count increases with the progress of HIV infection, their ratio is more dependable indicator of the progress of HIV infection and the state of immunodeficiency than either of those counts alone.

- **Raised** serum immunoglobulins.

- **Reduced or absent delayed cutaneous hyper-sensitivity** to recall and new antigens, e.g. Mantoux test becomes negative in advanced HIV infection.

- **Raised β-2** microglobulin.

- **Infections**

  Appropriate investigations are undertaken when a patient is symptomatic.

Gastrointestinal

Stool smear to detect a variety of organisms like *Entamoeba histolytica*, Salmonella, Shigella, Giardia, Isospora or Cryptosporidium. Acid fast stain is needed to demonstrate cryptosporidia.

Central nervous system

Cerebrospinal fluid (CSF) examination for cryptococcal meningitis or CNS tuberculosis or syphilis, computed tomography (CT) scan for tuberculoma, toxoplasmosis or PML (progressive multifocal leukoencephalopathy).

Pulmonary

X-ray chest for tuberculosis and uncommonly *Pneumocystis carinii*, cytomegalovirus infections. Sputum examination for tuberculosis and *Pneumocystis carinii* pneumonia.

Lymph nodes

Serum veneral disease research laboratory (VDRL) for syphilis, fine needle aspiration cytology (FNAC) for tuberculosis and if needed lymph node biopsy.

Skin and mucosae

Smear and/or biopsy to detect various organisms like molluscum, warts, cryptococcus, aspergillus or penicillium.

- **Tumours**

  Biopsies of skin or mucosae are needed for diagnosing Kaposi's sarcoma. However, this condition is very uncommon in HIV infected Indians. Other tumours like squamous cell carcinoma and lymphomas (Hodgkin and non-Hodgkin) are comparatively more common.

- **Direct effects of HIV Infection**

  Lymph node aspiration cytology and biopsy are useful for diagnosing persistent generalised lymphadenopathy (PGL) due to HIV infection. CT scan or MRI is necessary to detect encephalopathy that occurs in late HIV infection and fundoscopy for ocular changes.

Summary: Effects of HIV infection observed by lab investigations include:

Immuno-deficiency	: Low CD4 or T-helper cell count, reversed CD4:CD8 ratio, raised immunogobulins and negative Mantoux test
Infections	: Gastrointestinal (stool organisms like Shigella/Cryptosporidia)
	Pulmonary (sputum AFB or pneumococci or CT scan—toxoplasmosis)
	Lymph node (FNAC—*M. tuberculosis*) or skin (molluscum, cryptococci)
Tumours	: Biopsy for squamous cell carcinoma or lymphoma
Direct effects of HIV infection	: HIV encephalopathy (CT scan)

MANAGEMENT OF HIV INFECTION

Counselling HIV Positive Patients

Need for counselling

Counselling forms a solid platform to build a rapport with patients, gain their confidence, educate them about their disease, allow them to make responsible decisions and to provide them with psychological support during periods of crisis. It is an indispensable part of the medical care of HIV infected persons at all stages of the infection.

Chapter 26

HIV Infection and AIDS

Who should do counselling?

Although, persons who have specialized in this job should preferably do counselling, this is not always possible. A medical or a paramedical person, who has the time, knowledge and motivation for this is also qualified for counselling. Since, during the long asymptomatic phase no active therapy is rountinely advised, a skilled counsellor forms a vital link between the patient and the caring physician. This is because an HIV positive person commonly needs guidance about social and behavioural problems that arise due to HIV infection.

Post-test counselling

- **Revealing positive report:** Revealing a positive ELISA or WB test result of the patient becomes much easier if proper pre-test counselling has been done (please *see* pre-test counselling under Chapter 25—'Prevention of STDs', page 287). Many patients who are well informed about the consequences of HIV infection may get very upset. Time should be given to them to overcome this phase of shock and grief and provide support to the person to deal with these feelings. For persons not displaying obvious reactions, ask them what they think or feel about the report. Discuss the plans for immediate future so as to uncover and deal with any possible suicidal thoughts. Issues like which relations or friends would a patient like to reveal the positive report to, are best discussed at the time of giving the report or better still during pre-test counselling.

- **Issues involving the spouse:** Post-test counselling for the HIV positive does not end with issuance of a positive report. If a person is married, revealing the test result to the spouse, counselling the spouse and getting her or him tested for HIV has to be discussed. If the spouse is HIV negative, measures that the patient needs to take to avoid transmission of the infection to the spouse should be discussed (please *see* page 355 for correct usage of condoms). The patient should be encouraged to reveal the results of HIV testing to the spouse of his or her own. In case this is not happening for some reasons, the caring physician should caution the patient about the harm that can be caused by transmission of HIV infection to an uninfected spouse. Even after this, if the seropositive person continues to conceal the serostatus from the spouse, then in the interest of the spouse, the caring physician is within his or her own rights to reveal the serostatus to the spouse (without the permission or knowledge of the patient) and advise her or him to take care for prevention of transmission.

- **How HIV is not transmitted?**

Information about how HIV infection is not transmitted by simple touching or caressing or by sharing a room or using common clothes or utensils is important as this gives confidence to the patient to move about at home and in the community.

- **Issues of parenthood:** For married persons, who desire children, issues of parenthood including chances of transmission of infection to the baby need attention. Chances of transmisson of HIV from a seropositive mother to her progeny are about 25%. The likelihood of transmission is lesser if the blood viral load is low (as measured by quantitative PCR). The chance of transmission is highest during late HIV infection and if primary infection occurs during pregnancy/post-partum. The transmission rate can however be reduced by various measures (please *see* pregnancy and HIV), page 351.

- **Patient education for early identification of complication:** All patients should be taught to identify common symptoms of complications that may indicate a need for prompt treatment. Hence, patients with early disease must be told to seek prompt attention for skin lesions those with intermediate disease for cough, fever and diarrhoea and those with late disease educated to seek prompt attention for persistent headache, neurologic symptoms or visual disturbances.

- **Ongoing process:** Counselling is an ongoing process and regular visits should be encouraged at all stages of the infection.

Summary: Counseling is an essential part of management of HIV infection. It can be undertaken by the caring physician or any other medical or paramedical person trained in the ob. It should preferably begin with pre-test counselling. Post-test counselling is done at the time of giving out the test result, positive or negative.

For those with positive report, assess their reaction to the positive test result, discuss plans for immediate future, learn about available social support, discuss about whom

Guidelines for Medical Management of HIV Infection

The principles of management of HIV infected individuals depend on the stage of infection as mentioned under diagnosis.

Early (asymptomatic) HIV disease

Principles of management include:

- Counselling about HIV infection, how it is transmitted and how it can't be transmitted, practice of safe sex, prospects regarding marriage, parenthood, etc.
- Take nutritious food prepared hygienically at home. Carefully wash fruits and vegetables before eating or cooking. Avoid contact with pets and birds or their excreta.
- Take adequate rest and relaxation as well as regular exercises.
- Do not donate blood, semen or organs.
- Treat any minor mucocutaneous infections and inflammations. Report to the caring physician whenever ill.

Intermediate HIV Disease

- All the care for early HIV disease.
- Treat common bacterial, fungal, viral or parasitic infections and infestations with appropriate drugs. Treat pulmonary tuberculosis if present:
  - If a patient can afford serial CD4 counts and subsequent antiviral therapy (cost approximately ₹ 1–2 thousand/month) then these can be undertaken. Please *see* section on Antiretroviral therapy for details on drugs and their toxicity.
  - With decreasing CD4 count the chances of opportunistic infection (OI) increase in this stage. Hence, primary prophylaxis for prevention of OIs needs to be started.
  - More recently, ART has become available free of cost at public hospitals in India. This is expected to dramatically improve the outcome of HIV infection in Indian patients.

Late HIV Disease

- All the care for early and intermediate HIV disease.
- Diagnose and treat serious opportunistic infections like:
  - Cryptococcosis (fluconazole or amphotericin B),
  - Atypical and typical tuberculosis (standard antituberculous therapy),
  - Toxoplasmosis (pyrimethamine-sulpha-diazine),
  - Cytomegalovirus (ganciclovir),
  - Pneumocystis carinii (cotrimoxazole),
  - Cryptosporidium (supportive therapy),
  - Isospora (cotrimoxazole), etc.
- In cases of probable or actual relapse of these infections, chemoprophylaxis for them is necessary. Cotrimoxazole for prophylaxis of pneumocystis, toxoplasma and isospora is advisable.

  For all the cases with HIV infection, serial CD4 counts are to be done at an interval of 6 months. This helps to monitor the level of immunity, to take timely decision regarding prophylaxis therapy for OIs and to start ART.

WHO Clinical Staging of HIV Infection (2006)

This clinical staging helps to judge the extent of immune depletion, helps to decide when to start antiretroviral treatment and indirectly helps to monitor the success of ART.

Clinical Stage 1

- Asymptomatic
- Persistent generalised lymphadenopathy
- Seroconversion illness

Clinical Stage 2

- Moderate and unexplained weight loss (<10% of presumed or measured body weight)
- Recurrent respiratory tract infections (such as sinusitis, bronchitis, otitis media and pharyngitis)
- Herpes zoster
- Recurrent oral ulcerations
- Papular pruritic eruptions
- Angular cheilitis

Chapter **26**

HIV Infection and AIDS

- Seborrhoeic dermatitis
- Fungal finger nail infections

Clinical Stage 3

- Unexplained chronic diarrhoea > 1 month duration
- Unexplained persistent fever (intermittent or constant for > 1 month) (>37.5°C)
- Several weight loss (>10% of presumed or measured body weight)
- Oral candidiasis
- Oral hairy leucoplakia
- Pulmonary tuberculosis (TB)
- Severe presumed bacterial infections (e.g. pneumonia, empyema, meningitis, bacteraemia, pyomyositis, bone or joint infection)
- Acute necrotising ulcerative stomatitis, gingivitis or periodontitis
- Unexplained anaemia (<80 g/L), and or neutropenia (<500/µL) and or thrombocytopenia (<50,00/µL) for more than one month.

Clinical Stage 4

- HIV wasting syndrome
- Pneumocystis pneumonia
- Recurrent severe or radiological bacterial penumonia.
- Chronic herpes simplex infection (orolabial, genital or anorectal of > 1 month's duration)
- Oesophageal candidiasis
- Extrapulmonary tuberculosis
- Kaposi's sarcoma
- Central nervous system toxoplasmosis
- HIV encephalopathy
- Extrapulmonary cryptococcosis including meningitis
- Disseminated non-tuberculous mycobacteria infection
- Progressive multifocal leucoencephalopathy
- Candida of trachea, bronchi or lungs
- Cryptosporidiosis
- Isosporiasis
- Visceral herpes simplex infection
- Cytomegalovirus (CMV) infection (retinitis or of an organ other than liver, spleen or lymph nodes)
- Any disseminated mycosis (e.g. histoplasmosis, coccidioidomycosis and penicilliosis)

- Recurrent non-typhoidal salmonella septicaemia
- Lymphoma (cerebral or B cell non-Hodgkin)
- Invasive cervical carcinoma
- Visceral leishmaniasis
- Symptomatic HIV nephropathy or cardio-myopathy

Management of Common Clinical Problems in HIV Infection

Tuberculosis and HIV

In India, where TB was already the most important of public health problems, arrival of HIV infection has redoubled its prevalence. This is likely to play havoc with the country's health resources and lead to a plethora of social and medical problems. Tuberculosis is one of the most common opportunistic infection in HIV infected. More than 60% of the patients living with HIV develop TB at some stage of the disease during their life. It can occur even when an HIV infected is on antiretroviral treatment.

HIV and tuberculosis have a **two-way relationship.**

- Due to its high prevalence, a large majority of Indians suffer from subclinical primary tuberculous infection some time during their early life. Because of the faltering immune response associated with HIV infection, reactivation of this primary tuberculous infection occurs in more than 50% of HIV infected at some stage of the HIV disease.

- Such reactivation of tuberculosis leads to deterioration of general health and results in faster progression of HIV disease, thereby worsening its prognosis.

Presentations of tuberculosis in HIV infected persons differ according to their immune status that roughly correlates to the stage of HIV infection they are in:

- ***Early HIV disease:*** It resembles typical pulmonary tuberculosis as either a patch of tuberculous apical pneumonitis or pleural effusion or cavitary tuberculosis usually affecting one of the apices. Cervical tuberculous lymphadenitis with or without consequent skin involvement (scrofuloderma) involving a single group of lymph nodes is also common. Hypertrophic ileocaecal tuberculosis may occur.

- **Intermediate HIV disease:** Atypical pulmonary tuberculosis involving mid or lower zone or more than one focus in the lungs is seen. Multiple groups of lymph nodes affected usually in one or two body regions with or without skin affection. Abdominal tuberculosis affecting the lymph nodes, hypertrophic affection of large intestines or peritonitis can occur. Tuberculoma of brain and tuberculous meningitis are common.

- **Late HIV disease:** Miliary or bilateral pulmonary tuberculosis and tuberculous bronchopneumonia suggest poor immunity. Multiple lymph nodes of various body regions are affected. Ulcerative involvement of large and small intestines occurs. Tuberculous abscesses affecting various body organs like liver, spleen, brain or kidneys can occur.

Prevention and Treatment

The chance of developing TB for HIV infected Indians is 10% per year.

In order to prevent this near certain occurrence of tuberculosis in the HIV infected in India, following measures are recommended.

- Do an X-ray chest of all HIV infected upon detection of HIV infection. If any episode of cough with expectoration persists beyond two weeks, sputum smear for acid-fast bacillus (AFB) should be done. Culture is the gold standard method to diagnose pulmonary TB. Newer culture methods like Bactec or mycobacteria growth in indicator tube (MGIT) are highly sensitive and results are available within 3 weeks. Presence of circulating tuberculous antigen can be looked for by the TB gold test. Check lymph nodes. If needed, do FNAC of lymph nodes. If abdominal tuberculosis is suspected, ultrasonography (USG) of abdomen is needed. If clinical suspicion of tuberculosis persists, do not give prophylaxis for TB, as this would be inadequate as therapy for tuberculosis (if that is the case) and can lead to eventual development of drug resistant tuberculosis. In such cases observe the patient for development of further signs and investigate appropriately or if there is strong clinical suspicion, antituberculosis treatment can be started after ruling out other possible differential diagnoses.

  Mantoux test (MT) is not a reliable indicator for diagnosis of TB in the HIV infected in India as most of the people would show a positive MT. In advanced HIV infection MT can be negative though the person is having active tuberculosis. Also MT can be positive due to exposure to non pathogenic environmental mycobacteria.

- **Treatment:** Start ART irrespective of CD4 count and type of tuberculosis. Start anti-tubercular treatment (ATT) first, initiate ART as early as possible between 2 weeks to 2 months when TB treatment is tolerated. Response of tuberculous infection to therapy in early HIV infection is similar to patients without underlying HIV infection. However, as a matter of abundant caution, some authorities still advise longer (9 months to a year) therapy. Therapy of tuberculosis during the intermediate and late stage HIV infection should be longer (1–1½ years) and in case of inadequate response additional drugs may be used. Antituberculosis treatment along with ART can be complicated by increased incidences of hepatotoxicity and drug interactions. Non-nucleoside reverse transcriptase ihibitors (NNRTI) like nevirapine (NVP) are contra-indiated with rifampicin as rifampicin significantly lowers the level of NVP, so it has to be replaced with efavirenz. Hence, the preferred combination to be started after patient is stabilised on anti-tuberculosis therapy is tenofovir + lamivudine + efavirenz. Protease inhibitors (PIs) have significant interactions with rifampicin. Rifabutin can be administered.

- Also the problem of drug resistant tuberculosis or multidrug resistance tuberculosis can complicate HIV-TB coinfection due to factors like low potency and more toxicities of the drugs used to treat resistant tuberculosis, long-term treatment (18–24 months) and the high cost.

- In countries with high prevalence of TB infection chances of development of drug resistant TB are high, so prophylaxis for tuberculosis with two drugs should be avoided.

Summary: With the epidemic of HIV infection, tuberculosis has bounced back in India. Suppressed immunity in HIV infection leads to reactivation of old tuberculous infection. Such reactivation accelerates the progress of HIV infection and is responsible for higher morbidity and mortality in HIV. Typical pulmonary or lymph node tuberculosis occurs in early HIV infection whereas atypical or widespread or central nervous system (CNS) tuberculosis in intermediate and late stage HIV infection. Treatment of tuberculosis in intermediate and late stages of HIV infection should be longer than usual. In symptomatic cases, investigate carefully for tuberculosis and treat adequately if the same is detected. If not, observe them without prophylaxis.

Chapter 26

HIV Infection and AIDS

Management of Diarrhoea in HIV Infection

During the early and intermediate phases of HIV disease, amoebic and bacterial infections are common and behave similar to those in the immunocompetent. During the intermediate and late stage persistent and recurrent diarrhoea due to intestinal tuberculosis or unusual organisms (Cryptosporidium, Microsporidium, Isospora, Herpes Simplex and Cytomegalovirus) occurs. During the late HIV disease, small bowel overgrowth occurs as a result of reduced gastrointestinal (GI) motility and achlorhydria. In advanced HIV disease, infection with more than one organism is common.

At least 3 stool specimens should be examined with light microscopy. AFB stain is needed for demonstrating mycobacteria, and cryptosporidia. Microsporidium can be seen by light microscope by a concentrated trichrome stain or by endomicroscopy of duodenal mucosal biopsy. Sigmoidoscopy is of great use in the diagnosis of cases where 3 stool samples have not shown any organisms. This can help diagnose herpetic and CMV colitis. Frequency of the so-called idiopathic AIDS enteropathy reduces with increasing efforts to identify GI pathogens.

Antiretrovirals like didanosine (ddI), and protease inhibitors can also induce diarrhoea, which can recover itself in a few days after continuation of therapy (Table 26.4).

Summary: The commonest cause of lymphadenopathy in HIV infection is HIV infection itself. Persistent generalised lymphadenopathy of HIV infection occurs in its early phase. The involved lymph nodes are multiregional, symmetrical, small to medium size, non-tender and firm. No specific therapy is needed. Tuberculous lymphadenopathy is seen as matted, moderate to large nodes with central softening where they may burst. FNAC or biopsy establishes diagnosis of tuberculous lymphadenitis that responds to antituberculous therapy. Secondary syphilis, lymphogranuloma venereum, atypical mycobacterial infection and non-Hodgkin lymphoma are the less common causes of lymphadenopathy in HIV infection.

Common eye problems in HIV disease include herpes simplex, herpes zoster, dry eye syndrome and corneal ulcers of bacterial or fungal origin. While herpes simplex and zoster are treated with oral acyclovir, dry eye syndrome is managed with artificial tears. Corneal ulcer needs topical/systemic antibacterial/antifungal in addition to cycloplegics. Uveitis in HIV infected could be due to syphilis or tuberculosis or it could be secondary to a corneal ulcer. Herpes zoster is uncommonly associated with retinal necrosis that occurs as two syndromes, PORN (progressive outer retinal necrosis) and ARN (acute retinal necrosis). PORN progresses rapidly to retinal detachment and blindness and responds poorly to treatment with acyclovir. ARN, if allowed to progress leads to retinal holes and detachment but responds to extended course of systemic acyclovir.

Dysphagia is a common complaint in intermediate and advanced HIV disease. It can be severe enough to cause pain (odynophagia) and is commonly associated with retrosternal pain or burning. It is important to deal with these complaints immediately because they can lead to reduced food intake and weight loss. As candidiasis is the

most common of the conditions that produce these symptoms, it is worthwhile to treat the patient empirically for candidiasis. Supportive acid suppressive therapy is needed for all patients with odynophagia and retrosternal pain. Herpetic and CMV oesophagitis can only be diagnosed with certainty by endoscopy and biopsy and herpes should be treated with acyclovir. In patients taking numerous tablets, taking ample water with the tablets can prevent drug induced oesophageal ulcers. Severe idiopathic oesophageal ulcerations may need systemic steroid therapy.

Symptomatic therapy (e.g. loperamide, diphenoxylate, atropine and kaolin), can be given as per tolerance. Oral rehydration solution and intravenous (IV) fluids (if needed) are started pending report of stool examination. Sigmoidoscopy with aspirate smear and culture or even biopsy may be needed to reach a diagnosis. If the cause is still elusive, upper GI endoscopy or colonoscopy may be done, if available, to rule out infections. If symptoms suggest bacterial dysentery treat with oral norfloxacin or IV ciprofloxacin. Oral cotrimoxazole 2 QDS for 2 weeks is useful for isospora or microsporidiosis (which also responds partially to albendazole). TB needs four drug antituberculosis therapy for up to 1 year. Prevention of diarrhoea by avoiding unhygienically prepared food is to be stressed.

Wasting in HIV Disease

Appetite is reduced due to opportunistic infections (e.g. tuberculosis) and due to depression at being struck by the disease. Oral and oesophageal candidiasis (rarely other infections) makes eating, chewing and swallowing discomforting or at times painful (odynophagia). Drugs after taste and cause nausea or vomiting. Vomiting can also be due to CNS causes (toxoplasmosis or tuberculosis) or gastrointestinal infections. Persistent GI infections lead to malabsorption. HIV enteropathy has an additive effective on malabsorption.

Studies have shown that HIV associated wasting is due to reduced intake rather than increased energy expenditure, the causes of which are outlined above. Hence, treatment of wasting should be aimed at identifying lacunae in dietary intake and finding ways to correct them. This could mean choosing foods that are easy to chew, with a taste to the liking of the patient and more than meet the energy requirement of the patient. With the above factors in mind, food schedule can be devised to suit the patient's pocket and family background.

Drugs like metformin, anabolic steroids (e.g. testosterone and its derivatives) and thalidomide are also found to be useful for HIV related wasting.

TABLE 26.4: Management of lymphadenopathy in HIV infection

Diagnosis	Clinical features	Complications and prognosis	Investigations	Treatment
Persistent generalised lymphadenopathy (PGL)	During early and intermediate disease, more than one group excluding the inguinal nodes, persistent, non-tender, small to moderate size and soft to firm nodes.	Discomfort and anxiety. Disappears with disease progression.	S. VDRL—negative FNAC—no caseation, organisms or epitheloid cells. Biopsy—follicular hyperplasia	No specific therapy needed. Therapy is for HIV infection.
Tuberculous lymphadenitis and scrofuloderma	During all stages of HIV disease, one or a few groups of LN, moderate to large size, usualy non-tender, matted nodes with central softening and eventual bursting with sinus formation. Skin overlying nodes around sinuses inflamed.	Dissemination and poor response to therapy are seen in late HIV disease.	FNAC—caseation, organisms and/or epitheloid cells biopsy— caseating tuberculois granuloma	**Four drug AKT** * 9 months, if typical * 1 year, if atypical or multiple groups of LN or late stage HIV disease.
Secondary/Tertiary syphilis	Any stage of HIV disease. Small to moderate, non-tender, firm, rubbery, discrete nodes usually multi-regional and symmetric. Overlying skin normal. Asymptomatic, symmetric and polymorphic rash with flexura and mucosal lesions.	Secondary syphilis in HIV infected can relapse even after additional recommended therapy.	S. VDRL—positive in early and intermediate stage HIV disease. May be negative in late stage HIV disease TPHA/FTA-Abs usually positive	**Early and intermediate stage:** HIV disease—injection benzathine penicillin 2.4 MU IM after test dose once a week for 3 weeks. **Late Stage** HIV disease—procaine penicillin 20 MU IM OD ATD *10 days followed by injection benzathine as above.
Lymphogranuloma venereum	Morphology of LN similar to TB. Affects inguinal nodes, usually unilateral. Preceding genital sore may be present. Lymphoedema and lymphangiectasia of genitalia.	Poor response to therapy.	FNAC—no caseation or giant cells. Chlamydia + Biopsy— suppurative granulomas. Serology—chlamydia	Capsule tetra 500 QDS * 5 days or T cotrimoxazole 2 BD * 15 days. Anti-inflammatory drugs.
Less common causes of lymphadenopathy in HIV infection				
Non-Hodgkin lymphoma	Intermediate or late stage HIV disease. Moderate or large, firm to hard nodes of uniform consistency, multi-regional and symmetric. Overlying skin normal. Extranodal disease (GI tract, liver, lungs and CNS) is common. PUO or constitutional s/s.	Extranodal disease, low CD4 count, leucopenia and pre-existing opportunistic infections indicate poor prognosis.	FNAC—no caseation/organisms/ epitheloid cells. Biopsy for exact typing X-ray chest—LN pathy CT chest/abdomen—LN pathy unexplained, rapid, marked rise in S. LDH	Low dose chemotherapy (mb CODD; methotrexate, bleomycin, cyclophosphamide, vincristine, doxorubicin, dexamethasone). Or radiotherapy.
Atypical mycobacteriosis	Clinically similar to tuberculosis.	Poor response to drugs.	Similar to tuberculosis culture—grows atypical mycobacteria	Five-drug AKT with, if needed, second line antituberculous drugs.
Kaposi's sarcoma	Rare in India. Seen during late stage HIV disease. Moderate size, firm and discrete asymptomatic nodes with normal overlying skin.	Signifies poor prognosis. However, death usually occurs due to some other cause, e.g. opportunistic infections.	Biopsy—diagnostic of Kaposi's sarcoma	Chemotherapy

S. VDRL, serum venereal disease research laboratory

Chapter 26

HIV Infection and AIDS

Hepatitis B and Hepatitis C Infection in HIV

Hepatitis B and hepatitis C are the common coinfections which can occur during transmission of HIV. Hepatitis B infected HIV positive patients has more chances of progression to chronic hepatitis, cirrhosis and hepatic carcinoma while coinfection with hepatitis C can lead to faster progression to AIDS. So, it is important to screen HIV infected patients for hepatitis B and C infection. The screening test for hepatitis B is detection of hepatitis B surface antigen (HBsAg) in blood and anti-hepatitis C virus (HCV) antibodies for hepatitis C.

Some of the drugs used for antiretroviral treatment can cause hepatotoxicity (e.g. nevirapine) and can be active against hepatitis B virus, thus complicating the management of HIV infected.

Lamivudine (3TC), emtricitabine (FTC) and tenofovir (TDF) are drugs which are active against both HIV and hepatitis B virus. These drugs are used to treat HIV and Hepatitis B coinfection, if hepatitis B infection is active [hepatitis B e antigen (HBeAg) positive and or high viral load for hepatitis B].

ANTIRETROVIRAL THERAPY

Antiretroviral therapy has significantly reduced the morbidity and mortality associated with HIV infection (Table 26.5). First line ART, once expensive and unaffordable for the HIV infected in developing countries is now available free of cost in many government ART centres. Antiretroviral agents control the viral replication resulting in decrease in viral load and increased survival of CD4 cells. Thus, increased CD4 count increases the immunity and reduces the risk of opportunistic infections. Based on their mechanism of action, current antiretroviral drugs can be divided into:

- **Reverse transcriptase inhibitors (RTIs)**

  □ *Nucleosides (NRTIs)*

    – AZT (zidovudine, azidothymidine),
    – d4T (stavudine) (no longer used),
    – ddI (didanosine),
    – ddC (zalcitabine),
    – 3 TC (lamivudine)
    – Abacavir (ABC)
    – Emtricitabine (not available in India)

  □ *Non-nucleosides (NNRTIs)*

    – Nevirapine (NVP)
    – Efavirenz (EFV)
    – Delavirdine (DLV) (not available in India)

  □ *Nucleotide*

    – Tenofovir (TDF)

- **Protease inhibitors (PI's)**

    – Saquinavir
    – Ritonavir
    – Indinavir
    – Nelfinavir
    – Lopinavir
    – Atazanavir
    – Amprenavir (not available in India)
    – Darunavir (not available in India)
    – Tipranavir (not available in India)

- **Fusion inhibitors**

    – Enfuviritide (T-20) (not available in India)

- **Integrase inhibitors**

    – Entegravir, raltegravir (not available in India)

- **CCR5 attachment inhibitors**

    – Maraviroc (not available in India)

- **Miscellaneous**

    – Hydroxyurea (currently not used)

Combination Antiretroviral Therapy (Highly Active Antiretroviral Therapy)

Whenever treating HIV infection, combination of at least 3 drugs from different classes should be used. Most commonly used first line regimen to treat ART naive cases (patients who have never received ART in the past) is a combination of 2 NRTI + 1 NNRTI. 3TC is chosen in all regimens (Table 26.6).

Various first line ART regimens used in India in order of preference are:

– TDF + 3TC + EFV
– TDF + 3TC + NVP
– AZT + 3TC + EFV
– AZT + 3TC + NVP

Efavirenz is used as an option to NVP in following situations.

1. Nevirapine toxicities like severe skin rash, hepatotoxicity, active hepatitis B or C.

2. When patient is on TB treatment containing rifampicin (rifampicin significantly decreases the level of NVP and both are known to cause hepatotoxicity).

Tenofovir + lamivudine (3TC) + EPV is used as first line ART at many centres. It is especially useful for patients:

1. with Hb < 9 g/dL
2. on concomitant ATT
3. with hepatitis B and/or C coinfection
4. pregnant women, with no exposure to single dose nevirapine in the past

Emtricitabine is considered equivalent to lamivudine in clinical efficacy. However, it is not available in India.

Triple Nucleoside Reverse Transcriptase Inhibitors

The use of triple nucleoside reverse transcriptase inhibitors (NRTI) therapy may be considered as an alternative to standard 2 NRTI + 1 NNRTI in following situations:

1. Cotreatment of tuberculosis and HIV
2. Non-nucleoside reverse transcriptase inhibitors intolerance
3. Coinfection with hepatitis B or C with hepatic dysfunction
4. Treatment of HIV-2 infection

Recommended triple NRTI combinations are 3TC + AZT + ABC and 3TC + AZT + TDF.

Advantages of Highly Active Antiretroviral Therapy

- Improves CD4 counts
- Reduces the chances of infections with common and opportunistic pathogens
- Reduces chances of development of malignancies or their progression
- Improves constitutional symptoms
- (At least temporarily) Reverses changes of HIV induced encephalopathy, diarrhoea, wasting, thrombocytopenia or myelosuppression
- It is also the only therapy available for progressive multifocal leucoencephalopathy (PML)
- Helps to reduce the chances of HIV transmission [e.g. effective prevention of mother-to-child transmission (PMTCT) helps to reduce the risk of transmission of HIV from mother to her child].

In the developing world, the main hurdle to long term therapy with antiretroviral agents, is its expense. A patient must be committed to at least a year of therapy to begin it. This because if the therapy is stopped after a few months, there is a rebound multiplication of the virus and development of resistant strains of the virus leading to faster progression of disease. However, increasingly, ART is being offered free of charge at government hospitals in

India and this is expected to dramatically improve outcomes of HIV infection in India.

Limitations of HAART

- Antiretroviral treatment does not result in a complete cure of HIV infection. None of the currently available antiretroviral drugs are proved to eradicate the HIV from blood (where virus is freely replicating and can be eliminated with relative ease) or solid tissues of the body (where virus is mostly dormant and is therefore not amenable to drugs that act on replicating virus. Endpoint of therapy is not known. Patient has to take the therapy lifelong.
- Many of the drugs are toxic and intolerance to drugs can be a major limitation.
- Compliance to medications may be difficult due to high pill burden or due to toxicities.
- Serious side effects from the drugs are not rare. They may compel one to reduce therapy to two drugs if a suitable alternative drug can not be found.

Why Antiretroviral Monotherapy is Contraindicated?

- Monotherapy or therapy with only drugs is not recommended because chances of treatment failure and development of resistant mutations are very high which can exhaust future treatment options as cross resistance can occur to the other drugs from the same class. Such drug resistant strains can spread in a community and lead to emergence of primary resistant infections, thereby complicating anti-HIV therapy further.

Treatment of HIV-2 infection

Human immunodeficiency virus-2 is naturally resistant to NNRTIs. So, these agents are not effective for HIV-2 infection. The options to treat HIV-2 or HIV-1 and -2 mixed infection are either 3 NRTIs or 2 NRTIs + PI. However, the 3 NRTI regimen is potent as compared to 2 NRTIs + PI or 2 NRTIs + 1 NNRTI.

Nucleoside reverse transcriptase inhibitors

- *Zidovudine or azidothymidine:*
  - Zidovudine or azidothymidine (AZT) is the first drug invented for the treatment of HIV infection. A nucleoside analogue, it prevents viral multiplication by inhibiting the enzyme reverse transcriptase, that is essential for viral replication.
  - It is one of the commonest components (anchor drug) of an initial triple drug HAART regimen and is currently recommended as 600 mg/day (in combination with other agents).
  - The drug crosses the placental and blood brain barrier with efficiency and is therefore important in prevention of HIV transmission to foetus and in the treatment of HIV encephalopathy.

TABLE 26.5: Antiretroviral drugs

Drug	Dose	Side effects	Comments
Nucleoside Reverse Transcriptase Inhibitors (NRTIs)			
Zidovudine (AZT)	300 mg BD or 200 mg TDS orally as part of MDT; 500 mg/day in pregnancy from 14–34 weeks up to delivery; 2 mg/kg QDS IV during delivery; 2 mg/kg QDS orally for 6 weeks for PMTCT in neonates	Intolerance, anaemia, granulocytopenia Rarely hepatitis or myositis	Anchor drug for MDT. Used as monotherapy in PMTCT, NSAIDs, cotrimoxazole, fluconazole and acyclovir increase chance of toxicity
Tenofovir (TDF)	300 mg OD	Lactic acidosis, lipoatrophy (less than d4T), renal disfunction	Good efficacy, safety profile safety in pregnancy not established.
Lamivudine (3TC)	150 mg BD orally as part of MDT; 4 mg/kg BD in children; 2 mg/kg BD in neonates	Intolerance, other toxicities are mild and uncommon	Drug with better tolerance and compliance. Non-teratogenic cotrimoxazole increases blood levels.
Didanosine (ddI)	125 mg BD orally as part of MDT; 2–3 mg/kg in children. For better absorption take on empty stomach	Intolerance, neuropathy, pancreatitis, and lactic acidosis	Poor tolerance, interferes with ddI action. Hence, never combined with it.
Abacavir	300 mg BD orally as part of MDT; 8 mg/kg BD in children; lower dose in liver disorders	Hypersensitivity reactions, lactic acidosis, fever and fatty liver	Alcohol increases abacavir levels 41%.
Non-nucleoside Reverse Transcriptase Inhibitors (NRTIs)			
Nevirapine	200 mg OD orally for 14 days; thereafter, 200 mg BD 3–4 mg/kg BD in children	Intolerance, skin rash, Stevens Johnson syndrome	Better tolerated. Can be used during pregnancy. Induces hepatic cytochrome p-450. Hence, increases metabolism of all drugs (including protease inhibitors) metabolised by p-450.
Efavirenz	600 mg OD orally	Nervous system effects, psychiatric symptoms and maculopapular rash (self-limiting)	Preferred for first-line therapy. Decreases plasma concentrations of protease inhibitors.

TABLE 26.5 : Antiretroviral drugs (*Contd...*)

Drug	Dose	Side effects	Comments
Protease Inhibitors (PI)			
Nelfinavir Amprenavir	1200 mg BD orally (or 20 mg/kg BD if body weight < 50 kg)	Abdominal pain, diarrhoea, hyper-glycaemia, nausea, paraesthesia, skin rash, and vomiting, mood disorders, fatigue, taste perversion.	Nelfinavir is active against HIV-1 and -2. High-fat meal retards absorption. Solution also available but contraindicated in childre less than 4 years and in pregnancy and hepatic and renal failure because of toxicity from propylene glycol in oral solution.
Ritonavir	600 mg BD orally as part of MDT; should be started as 300 mg BD and increased every third day by 100 mg. Children—400 mg/m² twice daily orally (max 600 mg twice/day).	Pancreatitis	At low doses (100 mg twice daily) it acts as a pharmacoenhancer of other protease inhibitors.
Saquinavir mesylate hard gelatin capsule	Recommended only in combination with ritonavir (400 mg) as 400 mg BD orally	Abdominal pain, diarrhoea, nausea, aphthae, depression, anxiety, insomnia, headache, bodyache, peripheral neuro-pathy and rash	Bioavailability of saquinavir mesylate from hard gelatin capsules is as low as 4%.
Saquinavir soft gel capsule	1,200 mg TDS orally	Same as above	Saquinavir soft gelatin capsules should be used to initiate saquinavir therapy. Saquinavir active against HIV-1 and -2.
Enfuvirtide	Adults—90 mg BD; children—2 mg/kg BD	Local injection site reactions	

NRTI: Nucleoside reverse transcriptase inhibitor • **PI:** Protease inhibitor • **NNRTI:** Non-nucleoside reverse transcriptase inhibitor • **MDT:** Multidrug therapy • **AKT:** Anti-kochs therapy • **ART:** Anti-retroviral therapy.

Note: Intolerance includes abdominal pain, diarrhoea, anorexia, nausea, vomiting. Intolerance of variable severity, is common to most of the antiretroviral drug and its severity/persistence determines, if the drug can be continued or needs to be omitted/replaced.

Chapter
26

HIV Infection and AIDS

☐ Bone marrow suppression (anaemia, granulocytopenia) may occur in the first few months of therapy. Myopathy and hepatitis are late and rare complications.

- *Stavudine (D4T):* Stavudine (D4T) is used as an alternative anchor drug in many first line HAART regimens because it is useful for patients with low blood counts or those who develop bone marrow suppression with azidothymidine. Since, it lacks synergy of action with AZT, it is not combined with this drug. It is also useful for patient previously treated with AZT and developed side effects like anaemia or bone marrow suppression. It is preferable to avoid combining this drug with ddI for fear of metabolic acidosis.

Protease inhibitors

- These act on the viral enzyme aspartyl protease.
- They are some of the most powerful anti-retroviral agents known to us.
- They should always be combined with nucleoside analogues to avoid viral resistance.
- Boosted PIs are preferred as they have higher efficacy, less chances of development of resistance and well tolerated as compared to unboosted PIs.
- Common adverse events are anorexia, nausea and vomiting.
- Class side effects of PIs include 1. hyperlipidaemia, 2. insulin resistant diabetes and 3. lipodystrophy.
- Other long term adverse effects which can be seen are pancreatitis and nephrolithiasis. Indinavir when used in higher doses can cause nephrolithiasis (loin syndrome), hence patients on indinavir should be advised to drink at least 1.5 litres of water per day.
- Protease inhibitors are contraindicated during rifampicin therapy for tuberculosis as rifampicin can decreases the concentration of PIs in blood and combination with PIs may increase the chance of rifampicin toxicity. Hence, patients who need antituberculous therapy should finish the required antituberculous course before they can be started on protease inhibitors. If a patient is already on PIs needs rifampicin then rifabutin can be used. Alternatively, such patients may be treated with combinations that exclude protease inhibitors (2NRTIs plus 1NNRTI or 3NRTIs)
  ☐ *Boosted protease inhibitors:* Combination of two PIs is used, one of which acts to increase the blood levels of the other PI and itself doesn't have any significant

antiretorviral activity because it is used in non-therapeutic concentrations. Ritonavir is used to boost other. It inhibits the enzymes in gastrointestinal tract and increases the level of other PIs.

☐ *Doubt protease inhibitors:* Two PIs (boosted or unboosted) are used and both of them have significant antiretroviral activity.

Use of certain NRTIs combinations should be avoided while treating HIV infection.

TABLE 26.6: Antiretroviral combinations which should not be used	
NRT combinations	**Reason to avoid**
AZT + d4T	Both are antagonists of each other
D4T + ddl	Overlapping toxicities
TDF + ddl	Selection of K65R mutation and high incidence of early virological failure
TDF + ABC	Selection of K65R mutation and high incidence of early virological failure
3TC + FTC	Both are equivalent to each other, so no added benefit with the combination

When to Start Antiretroviral Therapy?

As per revised guidelines on initiation of ART as on May 2017, it has been decided to treat all patients PLHIV with antiretroviral therapy regardless of CD4 count, clinical stage, age or population. Patients who are in pre-ART care should undergo fresh CD4 count, if it is more than 3 months old and baseline investigations before ART initiation as per revised criteria. Adequate counselling and preparedness needs to be ensured before ART initiation in all PLHIV, particularly for those and high CD4 count as they are likely to be asymptomatic and more likely to default.

Side-Effects of Antiretroviral Therapy

Common side-effects of ART are listed in Table 26.7.

Investigations for monitoring of drug related adverse effects to nucleoside analogues include blood counts (including platelet counts), liver function tests, renal function tests and serum amylase. For protease inhibitors, additionally, serum lipids and blood sugars need to be periodically checked. For patients who have been on ART for more than 6 months and then develop nausea, vomiting, pain in abdomen, loss of appetite, loss of weight, malaise, weakness, myalgia, hepatomegaly drug induced hepatitis, lactic acidosis and tuberculosis [as immune reconstitution inflammatory syndrome (IRIS)] must be ruled out by relevant investigations.

TABLE 26.7: Common side-effects of antiretroviral drugs

Adverse effect	Usually involved drug(s)
Anaemia	Azidothymidine (AZT)
Lactic acidosis	D4T, ddl and AZT
Peripheral neuropathy	D4T, ddl and AZT
Lipodystrophy	Protease inhibitors (PIs), D4T
Pancreatitis	D4T, ddl and PIs
Hyperpigmentation	AZT, Emtricitabine
Skin rash	Nevirapine (NVP), Efavirenz (EFV)
Hypersensitivity reactions	Abacavir (ABC)
CNS side effects	EFV

Anaemia

This is seen mostly with the use of AZT. It develops usually within the first few months after starting AZT. Hence, monitoring of haemoglobin levels is advised during AZT therapy. Besides anaemia other haematological complications like aplastic anaemia due to bone marrow suppression can also occur. In such cases correction of the anaemia with blood transfusion and replacement of AZT with other NRTIs like D4T or TDF or ABC is recommended. Erythropoietin is useful for treatment of AZT induced anaemia.

Peripheral neuropathy

Clinically, it is characterised by tingling numbness with or without burning sensation and pain in the extremities. Lower extremities are most commonly involved. Symptoms may be very severe, disturbing the sleep. On examination affected extremities may show decreased or loss of sensations. Some may have hyperaesthesia so that walking may be difficult due to pain. D4T is the commonest drug causing peripheral neuropathy. Symptomatic treatment with amitryptylline, gabapentin, cabamazepine, or lamotrigine can be effective in some cases. In severe cases or cases not responding to above drugs switch to another antiretroviral agent is recommended.

Lactic acidosis

This is one of the serious long term adverse effect of NRTI agents. D4T is the commonest drug causing lactic acidosis. AZT and ddl can also cause lactic acidosis. Females are most commonly affected, risk factors include obesity and pregnancy. Months to years of treatment with above drugs is required to develop lactic acidosis. Some patients may be asymptomatic in spite of increased serum lactate levels. Clinical presentations can be vague like nausea, vomiting, abdominal pain, myalgia, breathlessness, loss of weight and loss of appetite. If undiagnosed, in some cases, death may occur. Diagnosis is made by demonstration of increased lacate in the serum (>5 mmol/L or anion gap of 16 mmol/L). Treatment is mostly symptomatic and includes maintenance of water and electrolyte balance and correction of acidosis. Stopping of the culprit agents for a month and change of the antiretroviral therapy is required.

Lipodystrophy

It is seen following long term use of antiretroviral drugs. NNRTIs like D4T and PIs are known to cause lipodystrophy. Lipodystrophy includes lipoatrophy, i.e. loss of fat (commonly seen with D4T) and fat accumulation (seen with PIs). Fat redistribution occurs with loss of fat from buccal pads and extremities and accumulation occurs over the upper trunk (buffalo hump appearance) and abdomen (crix belly or protease paunch). Also metabolic changes like hyperlipidaemia and diabetes mellitus can occur as associated changes increasing the risk of cardiovascular diseases.

Immune reconstitution inflammatory syndrome

It is a paradoxical worsening of clinical signs and symptoms while on ART. It is considered to be due to increase in immunity following ART. In India, the agreed practical definition would be the 'occurrence and manifestations of new OI's or existing OI's within 6 weeks to 6 months after initiating ART, with an increase in the CD4 count'. The condition may be mild or severe and occasionally even fatal. Both infectious and non-infectious conditions can occur as manifestation of IRIS. IRIS can occur at any time after initiation of ART, but usually occurs within the first 2-months after ART and is more common in patients who are started on antiretroviral treatment on low CD4 counts (<50 cells/mm^3) or when ART is started while on treatment for OI. When IRIS occurs antiretroviral treatment should be continued and opportunistic infection must be treated. Mild cases can be managed symptomatically with non-steroidal anti-inflammatory drugs (NSAIDs). Systemic steroids

Chapter 26

HIV Infection and AIDS

can be used to manage severe cases. Rarely discontinuation of ART may be required in severe cases.

Resistance to Antiretrovirals

During antiretroviral therapy mutations can occur in different genes encoding for different enzymes on which antiretrovirals act (e.g. reverse transcriptase, aspartyl protease). NNRTIs (NVP, EFV) and 3 TC have low genetic barrier. They can develop resistance rapidly with a single mutation. Nucleoside analogues (D4T, AZT) develop particuar type of mutations known as thymidine analogue mutations (TAMs). Usually, multiple TAMs are required to confer resistance to thymidine anologues. PIs, particularly boosted one are relatively resistant to develop mutations and require accumulation of multiple mutations to develop significant resistance.

Resistance to antiretrovirals is tested by following methods:

- *Genotypic test*—detects mutations in viral genome
- *Phenotypic test*—compares the different concentrations of the drug required to inhibit the viral multiplication in cell cultures
- *Virtual phenotyping*—uses of both genotyping and phenotypic data.

These tests are expensive and require expertise to interpret.

ART Failure

Causes of ART failure

- Poor adherence to the ART
- Subtherapeutic levels of drugs, which can be due to drug interactions, food interactions
- Development of resistant mutations

Types of ART failure

Antiretroviral therapy failure can be sequenced in chronological order of their occurrence into (a) virological failure, (b) immunological failure and (c) clinical failure. Virological failure can be defined as failure to achieve complete viral suppression, i.e. after effective ART viral load is expected to be undetectable or <50 cells/mL at the end of 4–6 months. Immunological failure is diagnosed by monitoring CD4 counts. Clinical failure is considered when any AIDS defining illness occurs or recurs after 3–6 months of ART. Whenever, an ART regimen fails virological failure occurs first and clinical failure is the last to occur. So, monitoring viral load on ART is more useful than CD4 count monitoring for earliest detection of failure.

Antiretroviral therapy failure can be considered in the following situations (WHO criteria): Criteria 1 to 3 relate to immunological failure while the fourth refers to clinical failure.

1. Drop in CD4 count to the base line
2. After rise in CD4 count, a drop of >50% from peak CD4 value while on treatment
3. Persistently low CD4 count <100 cells/mm³
4. Occurrence or recurrence of stage 4 event while on treatment for more than 6 months (some events like oral candidiasis, TB pleural effusion, severe bacterial pneumonias should not be considered, also IRIS syndrome should be ruled out. Stage 3 events like weight loss greater than 10%, chronic diarrhoea or fever >1 month, oral hairy leucoplakia, bacterial infections, pulmonary TB are also considered as evidence of ART failure).

Second Line Antiretroviral Therapy

In India or in developing countries, PIs are reserved for use in second line regimen when first line drugs cannot be used due to their toxicities or when there is evidence of failure of ART on first line regimen. Such second line regimen includes 2 NRTIs plus PIs (either boosted or unboosted). Ideally the new drugs used should be from entirely new class to avoid the cross resistance. TDF, ABC or ddl are the NRTIs used to construct second line regimen. Though, there is high resistance to 3TC used for first line regimen, it is now a common practice to continue 3TC for second line regimen because mutations associated with 3TC.

1. It increases susceptibility to AZT, D4T and TDF
2. It delays emergence of TAMs
3. It has residual antiretroviral activity and reduces the viral fitness and AZT may prevent or delay the emergence of the K65R mutation which can ddl and ABC.

TABLE 26.8: CD4 monitoring	
CD4 count	Follow up
CD4 of any value	Every 6 months
Between 350 and 500 and not on ART	Repeat at 3 months

(1) If AZT is used in first line, NRTI of choice in second line should be TDF. If TDF was used in first line, NRTI of choice should be AZT. If both TDF or AZT can't be used, the last option is d4T.

(2) Give only boosted PI in combination. The choices are ATV/r (LPV/r only if ATV not tolerated or for HIV-2 and pregnant women with prior exposure to NVP).

Patient education, positive prevention, counselling and linkages to care and support services, including outreach services are essential to support patients started on second line therapy.

Salvage therapy or rescue therapy

Salvage therapy or rescue therapy is used when there is evidence of virological failure to 3 different classes of drugs used. Newer drugs like darunavir, tipranavir and enfuvirtide are recommended for this purpose.

Prognosis of HIV Infection

Patterns of progression of untreated HIV infection are depicted in diagram 26.4 on page no 322. While some patients progress fast, others do not progress to AIDS at all. Factors affecting the speed of progression are:

1. **Stage of HIV infection:** As is apparent from the graph of natural history of HIV infection, life expectancy depends on the stage of HIV infection. Determine the stage by history, examination and investigations (based on duration of disease, whether opportunistic infections are present and if yes, of what type, positive p24 antigen indicates recent infection, viral load is high and CD4 count low during the late stage).

2. **Viral load:** Higher the viral load poorer is the prognosis. The viral load at the beginning of infection (primary illness) is also related to the final outcome. The initial infecting dose determines the viral load during primary illness. A person who acquires HIV infection by receiving blood from a late stage HIV patient will have very high infecting dose and initial viral load and thus has poorer prognosis.

3. **Opportunistic infections:** They are a drain on the already stretched immunity in the HIV infected. Hence, most of the opportunistic infections (especially severe systemic infections like tuberculosis, malaria) worsen prognosis. Besides, GI infections lead to reduced intake as well as malabsorption resulting in wasting.

4. **Supporting therapy:** Understanding one's disease and adjusting with it with respect to life style and family routine avoids stress. A good nutritious diet, adequate sleep and rest, regular moderate exercise and clean environment (air, water and food) prevent undue stress and avoid opportunistic infections.

5. **Antiretroviral therapy:** Such therapy improves prognosis by reducing morbidity and mortality.

ART has dramatically and substantially reduced the morbidity and mortality associated with HIV infection. Now, ART is available free of cost at government ART centres. Also these centres provide prophylaxis for prevention of OIs and other laboratory facilities free of cost. This improved standard of care has brought a new hope in the life of many HIV infected. ART has improved the quality of life of HIV infected and many HIV infected are leading a normal life.

HIV AND PREGNANCY

The Interaction

Early or asymptomatic HIV infection does not seem to alter the course of pregnancy nor does it probably alter the course of HIV infection in a significant way. In late HIV infection, the chances of intrauterine growth retardation, stillbirth and infections are significantly higher. The life expectancy of children with HIV infection is lower if the mother was in the late stage of HIV infection. Due to haemodilution in pregnancy the CD4 count shows drop and comes back to normal level or increases after delivery. But the percentage CD4 count remains unaltered during pregnancy.

Transmission Risk

The possibility of transmission of HIV infection to the progeny antepartum, intrapartum or postpartum from his/her HIV positive mother makes this an extremely important subject from the point of view of society and medicine. The 2% HIV positivity rate of non-high-risk mothers from many parts of Mumbai suggests that routine antenatal HIV testing is essential. The chances of transmission of the infection from a positive mother are approximately 25–40% in the absence of interventions (antiretroviral drugs, caesarean section and avoidance of breast feeding). However, this can be reduced to less than 2% by taking certain measures. The risk of transmission roughly correlates with the viral load in blood (as measured by the quantitative PCR or bDNA technique), which is high during the primary illness and in the late stages of HIV disease. Couples must be educated about the above facts even before conception, so that they can make an informed decision about any future pregnancy.

Risk of mother to child transmission (MTCT) is higher if:

1. Viral load >1000 c/mL
2. Mother not on antiretrovirals
3. Mother in advanced stage of HIV infection

Chapter 26

HIV Infection and AIDS

4. Vaginal delivery or traumatic interventions during labour
5. Breast feeding

Mode of Transmission

The child at risk can be infected by:

Antepartum

Transplacental transmission commonly occurs after the first 28 weeks and is responsible for about 25% of MTCTs. HIV infection may progress faster as compared to other modes of MTCT.

Intrapartum

Intrapartum trauma (injury to mother or child) accouts for the majority (70%) of infections.

Postpartum

The virus is secreted in breast milk. Near about 5–10% of the infections occur this way. Breast feeding may compromise the efficacy of measures taken during antepartum and intrapartum period. Also prolonged duration of breast feeding increases the chances of MTCT.

Management of Pregnancy in HIV Infection

Before conception

Ideally, management of pregnancy in HIV infection should begin even before conception by identifying couples with infected husband and/or wife. Once identified, they must be empowered with adequate knowledge about all aspects of HIV infection particularly with respect to chances of HIV transmission to progeny and measures to prevent such transmission. Consequences of such transmission to the child must be explained. While such information will allow some couples to avoid pregnancy many others may decide to go for pregnancy.

Antepartum

If pregnancy is confirmed early, the choice for medical termination of pregnancy is still available and, after careful explanation, the decision about it should be left to the couple. After this choice of medical termination of pregnancy is no longer available, the risk of transmission can be reduced by antiretroviral prophylaxis to mother and child. (Please *see* section on parent to child transmission (PTCT) programme in India below).

During pregnancy EFV is contraindicated in first trimester of pregnancy.

Studies have shown that ART during pregnancy, labour and delivery when combined with elective caesarean section and no breast feeding reduces the risk of MTCT to less than 2%.

Intrapartum

Avoiding intrapartum trauma and opting for elective lower segment caesarean section (LSCS) delivery further minimises the intrapartum transmission risk. Elective invasive procedures like foetal blood sampling, early episiotomy, early artificial rupture of membranes and application of vacuum or forceps are all relatively contraindicated in HIV infected mothers. If found positive at the onset of labour, she should be administered the first dose of regular ART and advised for confirmation the following day. The baby should be given syrup nevirapine for minimum 6 weeks and another 6 weeks continuation, if need be.

Postpartum

Avoiding colostrum and breast milk feeding reduces the risk of postpartum transmission. However, alongwith prophylactic ART, exclusive breast feeding is recommended. After delivery, the infant should be treated with syrup nevirapine or alternatively, zidovudine 2 mg/kg QDS for 6 weeks.

PARENT TO CHILD TRANSMISSION PROGRAMME IN INDIA

The national PTCT programme now recommends single dose regimen for the HIV infected pregnant women fixed dose combination TDF + 3 TC + EFV (FDC, single dose daily, EFV > 12 weeks). This regime has the potential to reduce the risk of mother to child (MTC) to 5% or less.

Earlier, single dose NVP was being given to ANC's at the onset of labour pains and syrup Syp NVP to the baby soon after birth. This significantly reduces peripartum HIV transmission. However, it does not reduce antepartum or breast feeding risks.

In clinical practice different situations may be encountered as discussed below:

1. Woman with HIV infection not on ART presents in labour—the mother should be administered the first dose of ART (TDF + 3TC + EFV) or a single dose of NVP (200 mg) and advised for confirmation of the tests the following day. Earlier, AZT was given as 2 mg/kg bolus followed by 1 mg/kg/hr till delivery. The infant should receive either AZT or syrup NVP for

minimum 6 weeks and extended for 6 more weeks when mother has been initiated late on ART to prevent PTCT for 6 weeks.

2. If a child is attended after delivery—give syrup NVP for 12 weeks (minimum 6 weeks).

WOMEN AND HIV

Although, HIV epidemic in India initially selectively struck males practicing unsafe sex, as the epidemic evolved, women were increasingly affected. Today, nearly 40% of the newly detected HIV infections are in women and children. It is estimated that more than 1 million women in India are already infected with HIV. The HIV prevalence rate in some antenatal clinics is as high as 2%. This has made antenatal HIV testing mandatory. Following are some of the aspects of HIV infection that concern women exclusively or specially.

Pregnancy and HIV

See section on 'Pregnancy and HIV'.

Contraception

- Contraception is particularly important to HIV infected women as many of them choose not to get pregnant. While a condom is a useful barrier contraceptive it has a relatively high failure rate. However, it has additional advantage of reducing the chances of transmission of HIV infection to the sexual partner, if this is what is desired. Oral contraceptives containing ethinyl oestradiol or norethindrone have interaction with NNRTIs and PIs, so use of alternative or additional method of contraception is recommended to avoid contraceptive failure. Intrauterine contraceptive devices probably form the safest and the most reliable mode of contraception in early HIV disease.

Genital Infections

Sexually transmitted diseases (STDs) like herpes genitalis, condyloma acuminata, syphilis, gonorrhoea, non-gonococcal genital infections and other STDs are encountered relatively commonly in HIV positive women. Vaginal candidiasis is a common problem in the intermediate stage of HIV infection. Genital herpes can be severe, extensive, ulcerative or non-healing and can be extremely painful leading to retention of urine. Secondary syphilis can be unusually florid and tertiary syphilis may occur early. Other STDs may be severe or complicated and resistant to standard therapies.

Cervical Cancer

HIV infected women are at a higher risk (2 times) for developing cervical cancer. This is probably because of the higher prevalence of human papilloma virus infections (condyloma acuminata) in a setting of immunodeficiency in the HIV infected women. Some strains of human papilloma virus are known inducers of squamous cell carcinoma and are implicated in the pathogenesis of cervical cancer. Hence, regular screening of HIV infected women for cervical cancer with Papanicolaou (Pap) smear is recommended.

PAEDIATRIC HIV INFECTIONS

Paediatric HIV infections have been seen mainly in children born to HIV infected mothers.

Mode of Transmission

Mother to child transmission is by far the most significant route of transmission of HIV in infants or children. Risk is highest during labour (intrapartum) due to the trauma and interventions. Transmission can occur by following ways:

1. Intrauterine (25%)
2. Intrapartum (70%)
3. Postpartum (5%)

Without any interventions, the chances of transmission are up to 30–40%. Transplacental transfer, intranatal trauma and secretion of virus in the breast milk are responsible for infection of children born to HIV infected mothers. With ART the risk can be reduced to < 1–10%. Some of the childhood cases are due to exchange transfusions or repeated transfusions for bleeding disorders, as a result of proper HIV screening not being performed in the past years. Rarely, sexual abuse may lead to HIV transmission.

Chapter 26

HIV Infection and AIDS

Diagnosis of Infection

Requirements for diagnosis of HIV infection in children older than 18 months remain the same as those for adults. However, the diagnosis of HIV infection in children younger than 18 months is complicated by the fact that maternal antibodies against HIV are transferred across the placenta and are detectable up to an age of 15 months. Hence, positive antibody detection tests like ELISA or WB tests in these younger children do not indicate HIV infection. For the diagnosis of HIV infection in children younger than 18 months any one of the tests for viral antigens or viral particles in blood is necessray. These include qualitative

PCR or viral load. However, as a substantial proportion of infections occur at birth or soon thereafter many of these tests may be negative at birth or during the first few months of life. Hence, it is recommended to do first DNA PCR at age of 6 weeks and another at 3 month. p24 antigen assay can also be used but it is less sensitive.

Immunization

In India, the risk to life is much more from the chances of development of infectious diseases than from a theoretical possibility of progressive infections due to live vaccines. Hence, since the immune system is not affected early in life in most HIV infected children, all children born to HIV infected mothers should be immunised with the routine immunisation schedule. Giving Bacillus Calmette-Guérin vaccine (BCG) early in life, as usual, is important.

Before starting immunisation assess clinical status of child with five vaccines.

Vaccines for polio (oral polio vaccine, OPV), measles-mumps-rubella (MMR) are to be given. Generally, if the HIV infected child is asymptomatic or midly symptomatic, vaccinations should be given. Withhold vaccine (live vaccines) for HIV-infected children who are symptomatic and severely immunocompromised. Inactivated polio vaccine (IPV) is now registered in India, and will be available soon.

Natural History

The general health remains unaffected during the first 6 months. The decision about breast feeding needs to be individualised. Prognosis depends on the viral load in the mother during pregnancy, labour and lactation. If the pregnant mother was in the late stage of HIV infection, life expectancy is commonly < 2 years. Such cases account for less than 25% of childhood HIV infections and develop symptoms during the first year of life. On the contrary, if the mother was in the asymptomatic phase during pregnancy, life expectancy can be much higher, up to 10 years (or even longer). However, about two-thirds of the paediatric infections progress at an intermediate pace in India with an average life expectancy of 5 years.

HIV infection in newborn differs that from adults in following manner:

1. Different modes of transmission
2. High rate of mortality (most of the mortalities occur in 1-year of life especially in first 6 months, if infection occurs in uterus)
3. Faster progression to AIDS as compared to adults

Primary Illness in Children

This is similar to that in adults. It is seen in less than 20% of children infected at birth within the first 6 weeks of life.

Early Paediatric HIV Disease

The common modes of presentation are:

- Failure to thrive
- Repeated upper and lower respiratory tract infections, otitis media, pneumonias and TB
- Tuberculosis is less prevalent in children as compared to adults with HIV, but still affects about 20% of cases
- Chronic or Recurrent diarrhoea
- Hepatosplenomegaly and lymphadenopathy
- Mucocutaneous manifestations are unresponsive or relapsing candidiasis, molluscum contagiosum, warts, herpes simplex and zoster, recurrent infections with pyogenic bacteria, dermatophytosis and scabies.
- Lymphocytic interstitial pneumonitis is uncommon in India.

Late Paediatric HIV Disease

This may be characterised by:

- Actual weight loss may occur. Severe wasting is common
- Serious and unusual infections, e.g. disseminated TB, CMV infection
- Chronic parotid swelling with Sjogren like symptoms is peculiar to children with HIV
- HIV encephalopathy is more common in children than in adults
- Lymphomas and cardiomyopathy are other serious manifestations.

When to Start Antiretroviral Therapy in Paediatric Population

All HIV exposed babies are given 6 weeks of nevirapine prophylaxis immediately after birth, so as to prevent PTCT. They are initiated on cotrimoxazole prophylaxis at 6 weeks of age and tested for HIV DNA PCR at 6 weeks. If PCR is positive, then a repeat DNA PCR is done. If 2 DNA PCR are positive, the HIV exposed baby is initiated on lifelong ART irrespective of CD4 count. Final confirmation of the HIV status in the baby should be done at 18 months of age by doing all 3 rapid tests, even if the first antibody test comes negative.

Even for a child freshly diagnosed with HIV, it is recommended to initiate ART as soon as possible.

Staging of HIV Disease using Clinical Criteria

Stage 1
- Asymptomatic
- Persistent generalised lymphadenopathy

Stage 2
- Hepatosplenomegaly
- Papular pruritic eruptions
- Seborrhoeic dermatitis
- Extensive wart virus infection
- Extensive moluscum contagiosum
- Fungal nail infections
- Recurrent oral ulceration (two or more episodes in 6 months)
- Angular cheilitis
- Linear gingival erythema
- Parotid enlargement
- Herpes zoster
- Recurrent or chronic upper respiratory tract infections (URTIs) (otitis media, otorrhoea, sinusitis, two or more episodes in any 6 months period)

Stage 3
- Unexplained moderate malnutrition that does not respond to standard therapy
- Unexplained persistent diarrhoea (>14 days)
- Unexplained persistent fever (intermittent or constant, for longer than 1 month)
- Oral candidiasis (outside neonatal period)
- Oral hairy leucoplakia
- Acute necrotising ulcerative gingivitis/periodontitis
- Pulmonary TB
- Severe recurrent presumed bacterial pneumonia
- Unexplained anaemia (<8 g/dL), and or neutropenia (<500/mm) and or thrombocytopenia (<50,000/mm) for more than 1 month
- HIV-related cardiomyopathy
- HIV-related nephropathy

Stage 4
- Unexplained severe wasting or severe malnutrition not adequately responding to standard therapy
- Pneumocystis pneumonia

- Recurrent severe presumed bacterial infections (e.g. empyema, pyomyositis, bone or joint infection, meningitis, but excluding pneumonia)
- Chronic herpes simplex infection (orolabial or cutaneous of more than 1 month duration)
- Disseminated or Extrapulmonary TB
- Kaposi's sarcoma
- Oesophageal candidiasis
- Central nervous system toxoplasmosis (outside the neonatal period)
- HIV encephalopathy

Management of Paediatric HIV Infections

Principles of management of HIV infection in children are similar to those in adults. Intercurrent infections with common or opportunistic organisms should be managed with appropriate anti-infective agents. Antiretroviral drugs currently approved for use in children include zidovudine, ddI, 3TC, nevirapine, nelfinavir, d4T, saquinavir, lopinavir, ABC, and FTC. Although, their dosages differ principles of therapy remain similar.

For infants and children younger than 3 years, the NRTI backbone for ART regimen should be ABC + 3TC or AZT + 3TC and LPV/r based regimen should be used. When viral load monitoring is available, substitution of LPV/r with an NNRTI can be considered after virological suppression is sustained.

For children with HIV 3 years and older (up to 10 years and <35 kg) 2 NRTI's (ABC/AZT/TDF + 3TC) along with efavirenz is the preferred NNRTI. NVP is an alternative.

Efavirenz is not recommended for use in children <3 years and or weight less than 10 kg. Tenofovir is not recommended for use in children.

Chapter 26

HIV Infection and AIDS

Homosexuality and AIDS

When the AIDS epidemic broke out in the United States of America in the year 1981, and even a few years later, AIDS was believed to affect only the homosexual population. This was thought to be due to the fact that many homosexuals in the United States of America had sex with multiple partners and the rectal mucosa is much more amenable for penetration with HIV than the vaginal mucosa. However, as the epidemic progressed, it became clear that HIV could also spread through the intravenous route and by heterosexual intercourse. By this time, the epidemic had spread to distant parts of the world and turned into a pandemic. Today, the dominant mode of HIV transmission is by heterosexual intercourse. This has therefore made it very difficult to control and hence the infection has become endemic in many parts of the world including India.

The prevalence of homosexuality in India is popularly believed to be very low (less than 5%). However, as disclosing one's sexuality is still considered a taboo in India, these figures are only predictions. Some workers feel the prevalence could be higher and this could partly be responsible for the higher incidence of HIV infection in men.

HIV Infection and Other STDs

The Association

HIV infection is transmitted as an STD in more than 85% of cases. Being associated with practicing unsafe sex, HIV infection and other STDs like chancroid, syphilis, donovanosis, herpes genitalis, molluscum contagiosum tend to occur together in the same patient.

Effect of STDs on HIV Infection

Co-existence of ulcerative STDs (e.g. syphilis or chancroid or donovanosis) causes 10-fold increase in the chances of transmission of HIV to sexual contacts. Therefore, control of HIV infection is almost directly dependent on the control of STDs in a community. Even non-ulcerative STDs (e.g. urethritis) increase the chance of HIV transmission by four times.

Effect of HIV on STDs

Presence of underlying HIV infection modifies clinical features and management of STDs. In general, STDs tend to be unusually severe in terms of morphology, extend and complications. They also respond poorly to standard therapies and may relapse after adequate treatment. Extended courses and high doses of antibiotics are frequently necessary to bring these STDs under control.

Syphilis

The mucocutaneous lesions of primary and secondry syphilis may be unusually florid (Figs 25.2–25.7 page 290). Pustular, nodular and ulcerative lesions can occur in secondary syphilis. The disease needs more stringent monitoring because of the higher chances of relapse. Accelerated progression to tertiary syphilis or neurosyphilis is known (Fig. 25.30, page 310).

Chancroid

Large ulcers with phagedena, bilateral buboes are common. Response to commonly used antibiotics may be poor.

Donovanosis

Large, complicated and unresponsive lesions are common. Squamous cell carcinoma may occur.

Gonorrhoea

Poor response to complicated infections is expected. Disseminated gonococcal infections (gonococcaemia) do occur.

Herpes Genitalis

Coalescence of adjacent lesions lead to large areas of ulceration which may take long time to heal. Oral acyclovir is indicated in such patients. If CNS involvement is suspected, IV acyclovir may be used.

Molluscum Contagiosum

Disseminated extragenital lesions in adults are a pointer to underlying HIV infection.

Condyloma Acuminata

Florid and unresponsive lesions are common. Neoplastic change to squamous cell carcinoma may occur.

Summary: Paediatric AIDS is becoming increasingly frequent. Most cases are due to transmission from mother. Intrapartum trauma is the most frequent (70%) mode of transmission. Transplacental and breast milk transmission are less frequent. Positive Elisa or WB tests do not indicate HIV infection in a child less than 18 months. Tests for HIV antigens like p24 antigenaemia or qualitative PCR for HIV are needed to diagnose HIV infection in infants. The standard immunisation schedule is recommended also to HIV infected children.

Health is unaffected in the first 6 months of life. However, life expectancy is only about 5 years as minor, recurrent upper and lower respiratory tract infections begin in the first year in some and by the 3-year in most. Failure to thrive, diarrhoea and lymphadenopathy are other common indicators. Cutaneous viral, fungal, bacterial and parasitic infections are common. Hepatosplenomegaly, lymphoid interstitial pneumonia, sicca syndrome, HIV encephalopathy, cardiomyopathy and lymphomas are all more common in children than in adults. Principles of management are similar to those in adults. Antiretroviral drugs that can be administered in children include azidothymidine, ddI, 3TC, nelfinavir and nevirapine.

PREVENTION OF AIDS/HIV INFECTION

Prevention of HIV infection is doubly important because of the seriousness of this infection and the ease with which it can be prevented.

A multi-pronged approach to prevention of HIV infection can be outlined as follows:

- *Health promotion:* Sex education and promotion of safe sex practices. The general population belonging to the sexually active age group is the most important and the largest vulnerable group. Efforts to educate this group should be mainly directed at promoting safe sex practices (please *refer* to 'Prevention of STDs', *see* Chapter 25, page 287). *See* diagram on page 355 for method of using a condom.

- **Specific protection**
  - ❑ **General population**

    Use of condoms: For correct usage of condoms (Fig. 26.31) (please refer to 'Prevention of STDs', Chapter 25).

    HIV Vaccines: *See* page 332.

  - ❑ **Health workers**

    Education about caring and nursing HIV infected persons—although risk of transmission of HIV to health care workers is small, this group is theoretically exposed to such transmission. It is probably impractical to know HIV sero-status of each patient. According to a view-point, it does help in taking extra precaution in a particular case. On the other hand, such routine screening is unable to detect patients in the window period and a negative test in such a case may produce a false sense of security, thereby actually increasing the chances of transmission to health care workers. Hence, rather than performing routine preprocedure HIV screening, it is important to treat every patient as potentially HIV positive.

    Following are the guidelines for examining/treating patients in an outpatient department (OPD):

    - Use gloves when contact with wet body surfaces (mucosae, open wounds or wet skin lesions) is likely.
    - Use gloves and goggles during endoscopy. Video-endoscopy is preferred.
    - Fluid and tissue specimens should be put in a bottle with a stopper and be carried by gloved hands.
    - Whenever possible use disposable instruments.
    - Reusable instruments should be washed by gloved hands with soap and water and then put in 2% glutaraldehyde for 20 minutes or autoclaved. Needles need to be destroyed by a needle cutter and then disposed off in a thick plastic container with tight cap. Alternatively, they can be sterilised in a plastic tray containing 1% sodium hypochlorite before being disposed off in plastic container. Needles should never be recapped as this increases the chance of needle stick injury. Surgical blades should be disposed in a way similar to needles.
    - Large equipment and furniture or floor stained with tissue fluid can be disinfected by wiping with sodium hypochlorite 1% (prepared fresh by 1:10 dilution of common household bleach).

    Following are the guidelines for operation theaters (OTs):

    - Minimum necessary staff and equipment should be present in OT during such surgery.

- The operating table should be covered with a disposable plastic sheet.
- Staff with a wound or abrasion or skin disease should stay out.
- Staff should wear sterile disposable plastic gowns, double gloves, goggles and overshoes.
- Cutting electrocautery preferred over scalpel. Clips preferred over suturing with needles. This reduces the chances of accidental cutting or penetrating trauma.
- Sharp instruments should never be handed down from one person to another. They should always be carried onto a tray. Disposal of needles and blades is done as in guidelines for OPD.
- Reusable instruments should be double autoclaved.
- Resuscitation by ventilator is preferred to mouth-to-mouth resuscitation.

- ***Protection in the workplace:***
  - ❑ No body fluids/moist surfaces/tissues should be handled with bare hands.
  - ❑ It is important to protect surgical and nursing staff during procedures (use gowns, caps, masks, gloves and goggles, the latter if there is a risk of blood splashing or spurting).
  - ❑ Besides, whenever infective material is being sent to the laboratory or for disposal it must be packed properly.
  - ❑ Infected material to be disposed, must be sterilised by using sodium hypochlorite solution before disposal.

- ***Early detection—screening of high risk groups:*** Blanket screening of all high risk individuals is not advised. However, they must be counselled about transmission and prevention of HIV infection and offered an option to undergo testing for HIV infection. The risk groups include commercial sex workers, STD cases, adults with multiple sex partners, spouses of HIV positive persons, IV drug addicts and children born of HIV positive mothers. Screening of pregnant mothers is now a routine practice.

- ***Disability limitation:*** This is achieved through counselling of HIV positive persons, prompt therapy of complications and if possible, by administration of antiretroviral drugs.

- ***Rehabilitation:*** This is the most important exercise that needs to be undertaken earnestly by the concerned physician, medical social worker (MSW) and the patient's relatives and friends.

Chapter **26**

HIV Infection and AIDS

HIV VACCINES

Vaccines stimulate the body's immune system to provide protection against infection or disease. Vaccines against HIV are being developed, and they are in various stages of clinical trial but at present none have proven effective. An effective vaccine agianst HIV infection is still a distant dream since the virus changes its genomic structure with each replication, thereby preventing emergence of protective immunity.

HIV infection broke out as an epidemic in parts of the United States in the late 70s and spread rapidly all around the globe to result in a pandemic within the next 10 years. The only approach to arresting HIV pandemic is probably preventing it through health education and if feasible, a vaccine. Following the success in culturing the HIV virus, many approaches towards vaccine development have been tried.

Envelope based Vaccines

The envelope proteins of the virus are essential for attachment of the virus to the vulnerable cells. Hence, vaccine directed against these proteins will prevent entry of virus particles into vulnerable cells thereby preventing the infection in the first place. Vaccines against both the glycoprotein (gp) molecules of envelope gp120 and gp160 have been tried. Some of these vaccines produce antibodies against these proteins whereas other make these molecules dysfunctional by covering them or altering them. The recent results of the trials has found these vaccines to be ineffective against HIV.

Viral Peptides

These comprise synthetically manufactured viral proteins. Their injection produces antibodies as well as memory cells that can identify these viral proteins as foreign and destroy them at the next contact.

Vector Controlled Vaccines

These are HIV viral proteins that are combined with another benign virus, so that they are able to reach the immune cells of the body, e.g. V520 vaccine, a weakened adenovirus that serves as a carrier for three subtype B HIV genes.

DNA Vaccines

These are genetically engineered vaccines that comprise more than one HIV proteins and hence can probably produce better immunity.

Whole HIV Vaccines

These comprise irradiated whole HIV and hence are supposed to be the most immunogenic as they have all the viral proteins.

Utility of Vaccines

Until now, only one (ALVAC vCP 1521 canary pox vector/AIDSVAX prime-boost vaccine) of the vaccines have reached phase III trials in humans for immunoprophylaxis. Even if they do, we will still need several years before utility of any vaccine is decided. Only evidence of utility of these vaccines comes from animal studies in which a gp120 based vaccine was found to have protective value for some simian immunodeficiency viruses.

The principal problems with vaccine development today is that each region of the world has its own strian of the virus. There is up to 40% variation in the genetic material between these strains. Hence, vaccine against one may not be useful against another. To complicate the problem further, the virus keeps on mutating rapidly so this variation in the genetic material keeps increasing. Because of those reasons, vaccines against HIV are not likely to be available for general use in the near future.

A more practical use of these several candidate vaccines is for immunotherapy in following situations:

- During pregnancy in an HIV infected woman to reduce viraemia and thereby reduce chances of transmission of HIV to foetus.

- For post-exposure prophylaxis, e.g. in a newborn child of an HIV infected mother or after a risky blood transfusion.

> **Summary of HIV Vaccines:** A cure has not yet been found for HIV infection. In such a scenario, an effective vaccine would have been an ideal way to arrest the march of HIV infection. Approaches to vaccine development have included targeting the viral envelope and making it dysfunctional or producing antibodies to it. Use of viral peptides or viral particles to stimulate immunity against the virus has also been tried. Combining these viral proteins with other benign viruses (vector controlled vaccines) can improve their performance. Composite DNA vaccines comprise several viral proteins and hence are stronger immune stimulators.

Chapter
26

HIV Infection and AIDS

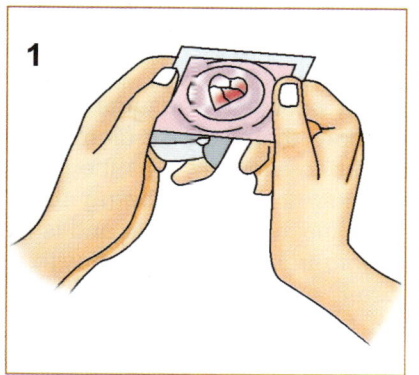

To reduce chances of tear while using, buy lubricated latex condoms. Check expiry date.

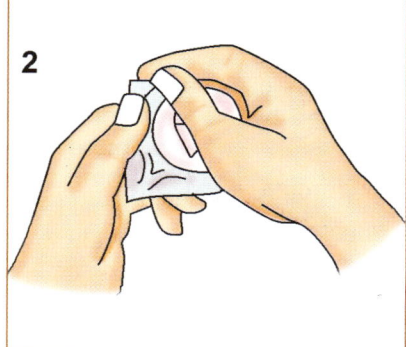

Open carefully to avoid tearing. Put condom over erect penis but before any genital contact.

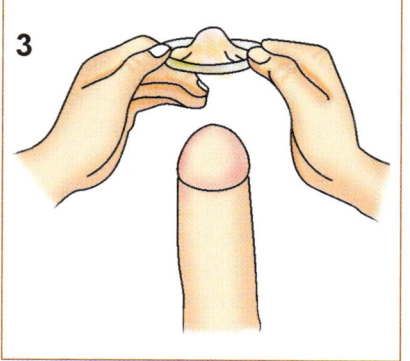

Use water based lubricant, *e.g.* KY jelly (not oil based or vaseline). Spermicidal jelly containing nonoxynol-9 (Today) is better.

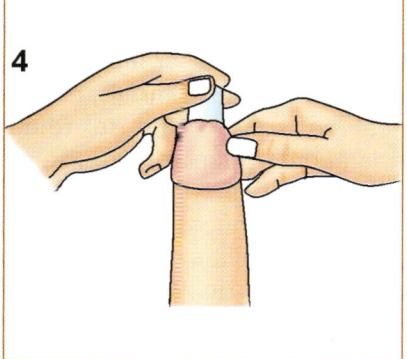

Pinch air from tip before unrolling, otherwise condom may burst during use.

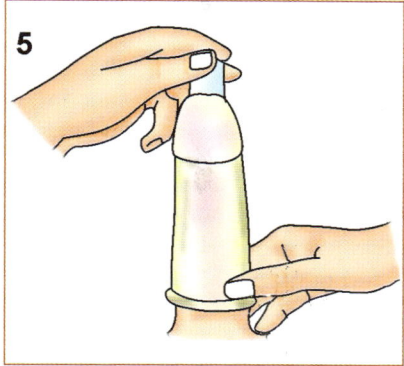

Unroll condom fully with the other hand up to the base of the erect penis.

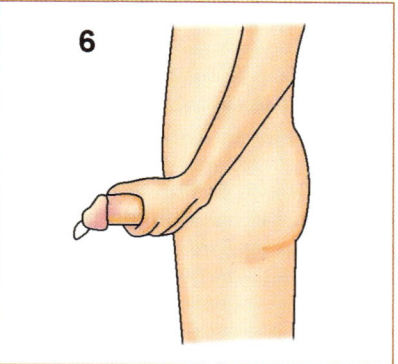

After ejaculation, remove condom by holding firmly at the base and pulling out the penis while it is still hard, taking care not to spill the semen.

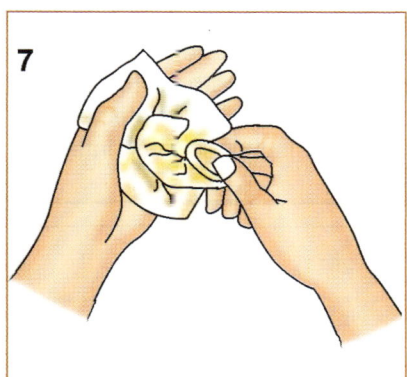

Tie a knot to prevent spillage of semen. Throw away in garbage. Use a condom only once.

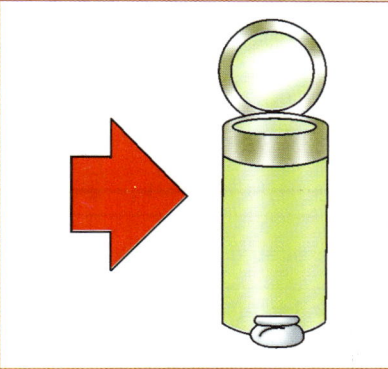

Dispose carefully in a bin.

Do not throw in toilet.

Fig. 26.31: Method of use of condom

The main hurdle to vaccine development has been the ability of HIV to mutate rapidly and form newer viral strains with a different genetic make-up. This makes vaccines against earlier strains ineffective. Till now none of the vaccines have reached final stage of clinical evaluation although some are expected to reach that stage in the next few years. A more practical use of the vaccines is in immunotherapy of an HIV infected mother to reduce the risk of transmission to her foetus or for immunotherapy of a newborn of an HIV infected mother.

POST-EXPOSURE PROPHYLAXIS

Post-exposure prophylaxis (PEP) refers to measures taken to reduce the chance of infection with HIV after a person has been exposed potentially to infective fluids or tissues. Such exposure is becoming increasingly common in the health care settings and all health care workers have to know about the risks involved in such exposure, how to

Chapter
26

HIV Infection and AIDS

avoid such exposure and if accidentally exposed, how to immediately react to the situation.

While such measures do not guarantee prevention of HIV infection, they reduce chances of establishment of HIV infection as evidenced by seroconversion.

The chance of HIV transmission for percutaneous expsoures is estimated to be 0.3% and that for mucous membranes is 0.09%.

Recognised risky exposure to HIV infections may occur in a variety of ways.

Some of the common circumstances are:

- Exposure to HIV infected fluids in a health care setting.
- An unprotected sexual encounter with an infected person,
- Baby born to an infected mother.

Uncommon circumstances include inadvertent transfusion of HIV infected blood or blood products, exposure to HIV infected fluids in a public place or sexual abuse of a child by an HIV infected person.

Factors that govern the chances to seroconversion (infection with HIV) are:

- What was the fluid? Semen and blood can be highly infective. Other fluids including vomitus, saliva, urine or foeces are relativley less infective as the number of HIV particles in these fluids is low.
- Was it a penetrating wound? Or a surface exposure? A surface exposure is much less likely to lead to infection because the virus needs a breach in continuity of the recipient's skin or mucosa.

- Was the recipient's contact area large? A large contact area (more than 12 inch diameter) is more likely to lead to infection. Was the contact over skin or mucosa? Skin, being tough, provides a better mechanical barrier and is less likely to given into trauma associated with the contact. Mucosa is more likely to be traumatised during contact.

- Did sufficient infected fluid enter the body? An injury by a hollow hypodermic needle filled with infected blood is more likely to be infective than that with a suturing needle covered with infected blood just because the amount of blood (about 0.1 mL) in the first instance is much more than the second. Similarly, because of anatomical reasons, male to female transmission is about 10 times more likely as all of the highly infective semen remains in contact with the vaginal mucosa as opposed to transient contact of penile skin with infected vaginal secretions in the female to male transmission.

- Was the infective patient in late stage of HIV infection? An HIV positive individual is most infective during the late HIV infection stage (AIDS when the immunity is at its lowest and the viral load highest) and during the window period before seroconversion. However, the latter possibility usually goes undetected. Early asymptomatic HIV infection is least infective.

TABLE 26.9: Post-exposure prophylaxis for HIV (WHO 2014)	
Number of antiretroviral drugs	An HIV post-exposure prophylaxis regimen with two antiretroviral drugs is effective, but three drugs are preferred.
Preferred antiretroviral regimen for adults and adolescents	TDF + 3TC (or FTC) is recommended as the preferred backbone regimen for HIV post-exposure prophylaxis among adults and adolescents LPV/r or ATV/r is recommended as the preferred third drug for HIV post-exposure prophylaxis among adults and adolescents, where available RAL, DRV/r or EFV can be considered as alternative options.
Preferred antiretroviral regimen for children < 10 years old	AZT + 3TC is recommended as the preferred backbone regimen for HIV post-exposure prophylaxis among children 10 years and younger ABC + 3TC or TDF + 3TC (or FTC) can be considered as alternative regimens LPV/r is recommended as the preferred third drug for HIV post-exposure prophylaxis for children 10 years and younger.
Prescribing frequency	A 28-day prescription of antiretroviral drugs should be provided for HIV post-exposure prophylaxis after initial risk assessment.
Adherence support	Enhanced adherence counselling is suggested for all individuals initiating HIV post-exposure prophylaxis.

For accidental exposure in a health care setting:

- Wash the contact area thoroughly with soap and water. If there is no penetrating injury or a raw wound, adequate washing is usually enough to prevent transmission of HIV infection.

- If there is a cut or a penetrating injury, after thorough washing with soap and water, apply proximal pressure or tourniquet and allow the wound to bleed for a few minutes.

For an Unprotected Sexual Exposure

- Washing of genitals with soap and water is of limited benefits.

- After discussing the factors affecting the chances of transmission, a decision about whether post-exposure prophylaxis is to be given is taken with active participation of the exposed person.

- The efficacy of PEP after risky sexual exposures has not been well documented. Two-drug or three-drug therapy as mentioned above may be given. The treatment needs to be started within 2 hours of exposure for substantial benefit.

Prophylaxis should be started as soon as possible preferably within 2 hours after exposure.

- If one decides to give antiretroviral drugs for post-exposure prophylaxis, they must be started as soon as possible preferably within 2 hours of exposure.

- After counselling and consent, collect blood for HIV testing as soon as possible. This is important medicolegally to prove that the person was not previously infected with HIV. If the involved person refuses testing, any future claim for compensation may be jeopardiased. Tests to diagnose HIV infection are to be done at base line, i.e. immediately after exposure, at 4 weeks, 3 months and 6 months interval to rule out HIV seroconversion.

For accidental transfusion of contaminated blood or blood products: As this type of exposure carries very high risk of infection, three-drug therapy should be started as soon as possible.

Chapter
26

HIV Infection and AIDS

MCQs

1. **The type of HIV predominance in india is:**
   a. HIV 1 subtype a
   b. HIV 1 subtype b
   c. HIV 1 subtype c
   d. HIV 2

2. **True about HIV is all *except*:**
   a. HIV has affinity for CD4 T-cell receptors
   b. It needs the enzyme reverse transcriptase
   c. Reverse transcriptase is a DNA dependent RNA polymerase
   d. The glycoprotein envelope is important for pathogenicity of the virus

3. **These cells are responsible for early neutralisation of HIV virus in the blood:**
   a. CD8 T-cell
   b. CD4 T-cell
   c. Natural killer (NK) cell
   d. Memory cells

4. **Most common mode of transmission of HIV in India is:**
   a. Heterosexual
   b. Homosexual
   c. Mother to child
   d. Injection drug abuse

5. **Malignancies like systemic lupus erythematosus (SLE), Kaposi's occur in which stage of HIV?**
   a. Stage 1
   b. Stage 2
   c. Stage 3
   d. Stage 4

6. **Which of the following is used for early diagnosis of HIV?**
   a. Latex agglutination
   b. Qualitative DNA PCR
   c. ELISA for HIV-1/2 antibodies
   d. CD4 count

7. **Unresponsive seborrhoeic dermatitis is seen in:**
   a. Stage 1 HIV disease
   b. Stage 2 HIV disease
   c. Stage 3 HIV disease
   d. Stage 4 HIV disease

8. **Most common opportunistic infection in HIV is:**
   a. Candida
   b. Herpes simplex
   c. Tuberculosis
   d. Cryptosporidium diarrhoea

9. **The chance of developing TB in HIV infected individual is:**
   a. 10%
   b. 15%
   c. 20%
   d. 30%

10. **Most common cause of lymphadenopathy in HIV is:**
    a. Secondary syphilis
    b. Non-Hodgkin's lymphoma
    c. Persistent generalised lymphadenopathy (PGL)
    d. Tuberculosis

11. **Which of the following can be used for HIV related wasting?**
    a. Chlorpromazine
    b. Thalidomide
    c. Vitamin B complex
    d. Lactobacilli

12. **All of the following are skin manifestation of HIV *except*:**
    a. Seborrhoeic dermatitis
    b. Vasculitis
    c. Eosinophilic folliculitis
    d. Pyogenic granuloma

13. **True about ELISA is:**
    a. Highly sensitive
    b. Highly specific
    c. Less sensitive
    d. None of these

14. **Causes of false positive ELISA are all *except*:**
    a. Leprosy
    b. Faulty lab techniques
    c. Lupus erythematosus
    d. Tuberculosis

Chapter 26

HIV Infection and AIDS

15. Select the false statement:
a. Quantitative viral RNA predicts prognosis
b. Western blot is highly specific but less sensitive
c. p24 antigen assay is used for monitoring disease
d. ELISA is negative in window period

16. On retroviral therapy, the CD4 count is expected to increase by:
a. 50–100 cells/mm³/year
b. 100–150 cells/mm³/year
c. 200–250 cells/mm³/year
d. 500 cells/mm³/year

17. Drug of choice of prophylaxis of mycobacterium avium complex (MAC) infection is:
a. Isoniazid
b. Rifampicin
c. Azithromycin
d. Dapsone

18. Normal CD4 count is (cells/cubic mm):
a. 1200–1500
b. 1000–1500
c. 500–1500
d. 900–1500

19. Mantoux test becomes negative in:
a. Post-measles
b. Sarcoidosis
c. Advanced HIV disease
d. All of these

20. AIDS per se can lead to:
a. Hepatitis
b. Encephalopathy with retinopathy
c. Squamous cell carcinoma (SCC)
d. None of the above

21. Drugs active against both hepatitis B and HIV are:
a. Lamivudine
b. Emtricitabine
c. Tenofovir
d. All of these

22. Nucleoside reverse transcriptase inhibitors (NRTIs) are all except:
a. Abacavir
b. Delavirdine
c. Didanosine
d. Emtricitabine

23. Alternative anchor drug in first line HAART is:
a. Ritonavir
b. Enfuvirtide
c. Stavudine
d. Nevirapine

24. Lactic acidosis caused by all except:
a. Stavudine
b. Didasone
c. Both of the above
d. None of these

25. Hypersensitivity reactions are caused by:
a. Abacavir
b. Stavudine
c. Zidovudine
d. None of these

26. Which drug is used as a pharmacoenhancer of other protease inhibitor?
a. Darunavir
b. Nevirapine
c. Ritonavir
d. Saquinavir

27. Which drugs are ineffective against HIV-2?
a. NRTI
b. NNRTI
c. Integrase inhibitor
d. Protease inhibitor

28. All are protease inhibitor except:
a. Ritonavir
b. Indinavir
c. Ropinavir
d. Tenofovir

29. Lipodystrophy is secondary to ART. All are true except:
a. Moon facies
b. Buffalo hump
c. Protease paunch
d. Diabetes mellitus (DM)

30. Resistance to antiretrovirals is tested by which of the following methods?
a. Genotyping test
b. Phenotyping test
c. Virtual phenotyping
d. All of these

31. For salvage therapy or rescue therapy which is virological failure to three different classes of drugs following drugs can be used, except:
a. Darunavir
b. Tipranavir
c. Enfuvirtide
d. Abacavir

32. The chances of transmission of HIV from mother to child in the absence of intervention is:
a. 10–20%
b. 10–25%
c. 25–40%
d. 40–50%

33. ART prophylaxis regimen used for MTCT consists of:
a. AZT alone
b. Nevirapine alone
c. AZT+3TC
d. All of these

34. Prevention of parent-to-child transmission (PPTCT) was started by National AIDS Control Organisation (NACO) in the year:
a. 1980
b. 1989
c. 2000
d. 2002

Chapter
26

HIV Infection and AIDS

35. **Which of the following is the most reliable mode of contraception in early HIV?**
    a. Oral contraceptive (OC) pills
    b. IUD
    c. Barrier
    d. Injection depomedroxyprogesterone acetate (DMPA)

36. **Transmission of HIV from mother to child is maximum in:**
    a. Intrauterine
    b. Intrapartum
    c. Postpartum
    d. Breast feeding

37. **Following tests can be used in child less than 18 months are all *except*:**
    a. Qualitative PCR
    b. p24 antigen assay
    c. Viral load
    d. ELISA

38. **Chance of HIV transmission by percutaneous is:**
    a. 0.03%
    b. 0.003%
    c. 0.3%
    d. 0.09%

Chapter
26

HIV Infection and AIDS

─────── *ANSWERS* ───────

1-c,	2-c,	3-a,	4-a,	5-d,	6-b,	7-b,	8-b,	9-a,	10-d,
11-b,	12-d,	13-a,	14-d,	15-c,	16-a,	17-c,	18-c,	19-d,	20-b,
21-d,	22-b,	23-c,	24-d,	25-a,	26-c,	27-b,	28-d,	29-a,	30-d,
31-d,	32-c,	33-d,	34-d,	35-b,	36-b,	37-d,	38-c		

SECTION 4

Dermatotherapeutics

Topical Therapy in Dermatology

Topical therapy of skin diseases brings with it the advantage reaching the site of action directly with minimum risk of systemic side-effects. However, for maximum efficacy, a topical agent needs to be dispensed in an optimised vehicle that helps in penetration of the skin barrier. Apart from the vehicle, efficacy of topical agents is influenced by:

1. Whether the skin barrier is intact or not—conditions associated with skin erosions or abrasions allow higher penetration of drug due to loss of barrier function.

2. What is the site of application—flexures and genitals allow higher penetration due to the occlusive effects of the site.

3. What is the concentration of the drug used—higher the concentration, more the effect.

4. What is the amount of the drug—certain minimum amount needs to be applied, excess does not necessarily lead to more efficacy. An application that leaves a layer of 0.1 mm thickness is considered optimum for most topicals. Ordinarily a palm sized area of the skin can be covered with one fingertip unit of cream (i.e. cream taken out of a 5 mm nozzle from tip of finger to the distal finger crease which is approximately 0.5 g).

5. What is the frequency of application—most topical agents act best when applied twice a day, higher frequency being unnecessray and lower frequency may lead to less than optimal efficacy. However, there are exceptions to this rule.

All the topical agents are mixtures of two or more of the basic phases of topical agents. These phases, liquids and oils (Table 27.1).

Side-effects of Topical Agents

Topical agents may cause side-effects at the site of application. These include burning, stinging, pruritus, irritant dermatitis and contact allergic dermatitis. They may also get absorbed into the bloodstream and cause systemic effects. This is more likely to happen in newborns and infants than adults because of their higher body surface:weight ratio.

COMMONLY USED TOPICAL AGENTS

CLEANSERS, SOAPS AND SHAMPOOS

These topical agents are used almost universally by all for the routine care of skin and hair. Soaps serve to rid the skin of oil, sweat, dust and other particles on surface through their surfactant action. Soaps are sodium or potassium salts of fatty acids and in addition to cleansing the skin they also change the skin pH (thereby reducing its resistance to bacteria) and damage the stratum corneum (which is responsible for the barrier function). To minimise these adverse effects of soaps, various approaches are used. They include:

- Low alkalinity soaps
- Neutral soaps
- Superfatted soap
- Moisturising soaps
- Syndet (synthetic detergent) soaps

All of these are useful while cleansing diseased (eczema, psoriasis) or sensitive skin.

Non-soap cleansers (e.g. cetyl alcohol and stearyl alcohol) are synthetic chemicals that have cleansing properties and may be used to cleanse the skin with or without rinsing with water. They are less damaging to the skin as compared to soaps and are preferred for cleansing of eczematous skin.

Shampoos remove dirt, grime and oil from the hair but have to be formulated to minimise damage to hair as frequent shampooing with strong shampoos may lead to hair breakage. This is achieved by adding conditioners to shampoos (conditioning shampoos or shampoo with conditioner) or by using a wash-off conditioner or leave-on conditioner after the use of a shampoo.

MOISTURISERS AND EMOLLIENTS

These are products that aim to increase water content of skin through various mechanisms. They include liquid paraffin, white soft paraffin, yellow soft paraffin, lanolin, urea, lactic acid, natural moisturising factors, squalene, cholesterol, fatty acids and ceramides.

Clinical implications: Natural moisturising factors are a group of water soluble substances (e.g. aminobutyric acid) in stratum corneum that have water binding properties. They are added to some moisturising formulations to stimulate physiologic state. However, since these substances are water soluble, repeated wetting of the skin leads to them being washed away from the stratum corneum. Hence, repeated wetting cf

TABLE 27.1: Classification of topical agents			
Type	**Sub-type**	**Preparation**	**Comments**
Liquids	Solutions	Wet dressings and soaks/baths	Used in acute inflammatory conditions, erosions and ulcers Cools and dries through evaporation Causes vasoconstriction Cleanses exudates, crusts and debris Soothing, anti-pruritic and anti-inflammatory
	Pure aqueous solution	Lotions	Suitable for hairy areas Cools and dry the affected area Leaves an uniform film of powder on evaporation
	Alcohlic or hydro-alcholic solutions	Tincture, paints	Cools and dries Paints, after applying by brush and evaporate
	Oily solutions	Oils	Suitable for treating dry dermatoses Sticky
	Emulsions	Oil in water (O/W) Water in oil (W/O)	Suitable for use in any area of glabrous skin O/W emulsions can be washed with water, but not W/O emulsions Used as lubricants Retain heat and impede water loss
Semisolids	Water-free	Ointments	Suitable for dry skin conditions More messy and occlusive Better to avoid in oozy, infected area
	Water-containing (monophasic)	Hydrogels	Suitable for glabrous as well as hairy areas
	Water-contaiing (Biphasic)	Creams (O/W or vanishing cream and W/O or oily cream)	Vanishing cream is water washable, cosmetically more acceptable and widely used Oily creams are water immiscible, difficult to wash off Emollient and lubricant Less occlusive than ointments
Solid	Powder	—	Suitable for use in body folds Promotes drying by increasing surface area

Chapter 27

the skin, evetually leads to more drying and people with dry skin should be advised not to make it wet repeatedly.

The lower stratum corneum (with thickness of less than that of a paper) is responsible for the barrier function of the skin. It achieves this by filling up the intercellular spaces of anucleate corneocytes (which act like bricks) with lipids (which act as the mortar) released from Odland bodies, intracellular organelles in the spinous and granular layer. These lipids are a mixture of ceramides, cholesterol and free fatty acids in a fixed proportion. Defects in keratinisation of epidermis (e.g. ichthyosis) or in the metabolism of these fats lead to skin dryness and resultant compromise in barrier function. Moisturisers should aim to restore barrier function to an extent and retain the body and skin moisture.

The most commonly used moisturisers among the above are white soft paraffin and liquid paraffin which are preferred for their stability, patient acceptability, efficacy and affordability. White soft paraffin and liquid paraffin act by providing an occlusive barrier to the skin, thereby preventing transepidermal water loss. Hence, for best effect, they should be applied immediately after bath on slightly hydrated skin.

Urea in lower concentrations (up to 10%) and glycerin are used popularly as hydrating agents in many of the formulations for dry skin. Squalene containing formulations of paraffins have been recently advocated for their longer lasting action.

Topical Therapy in Dermatology

Moisturising containing ceramides, cholesterol and fatty acids have been recently introduced and the claimed to stimulate the normal lipid envelope in the stratum corneum These are claimed to be beneficial in patients with atopic dermatitis but are currently expensive for regular use.

Due to their occlusive effect on the hair follicles, the paraffin moisturisers make the skin prone to folliculitis and funrunculosis. Moisturisers containing urea may cause irritation of skin while those containing lanolin may cause contact allergic.

SUNSCREENS

Sunscreen protect the skin from harmful effects of the sun, especially the ultraviolet B (UVB) (290–320 nm) and ultraviolet A (UVA) spectrum (320–400 nm). Melanin in the epidermis serves to cut off UVA, UVB and visible spectrum or radiation with excellent efficacy. However, protection with sunscreen is required when patients have abnormal sensitivity to sunlight (*see* chapter on photosensitive dermatoses) or would prefer to avoid the normal tanning or burning effects of sunlight.

Sunscreens may be chemical sunscreens that bind the skin and absorb ultraviolet light by chemical reactions without damaging the skin. These include para-aminobenzoic acid (PABA) or its esters, cinnamates, salicylates benzophenones, avobenzone, etc. Alternatively, they may be physical sunscreens that scatter or reflect UV radiation by the physical action of their granules. They include zinc oxide and titanium dioxide. These are usually micronised to make the formulations non-visible and thus cosmetically acceptable.

Most of the sunscreen formulations in the market today have a mixture of physical and chemical suncreens to achieve optimum efficacy (by blocking both UVA and UVB light) and patient acceptability. The ability of a sunscreen to block ultraviolet light is expressed as the sun protection factor. This is calculated as a ratio of ultraviolet light needed to produce minimal erythema with sunscreen to that needed without sunscreen. For a good sunscreen, this ratio should be at least 15 for normal skin and at least 30 for photosensitive skin.

Chemical sunscreens require some time to start action as chemical binding with stratum corneum is needed for their action to begin. Hence, most sunscreens (except pure physical sunscreens) should be applied about 30 minutes before going out in sun. Moreover, efficacy of most of the sunscreens lasts only for 2–3 hours requiring reapplication of the product every 2–3 hours or after excessive sweating or swimming. Side-effects from sunscreen are uncommon but may occur in persons with sensitive skin. Itching, burning, contact allergic dermatitis and more frequently exacerbation or initiation of acne lesions are side-effects seen with sunscreens.

TOPICAL STEROIDS

Improvements in actions of topical steroids have led to advances in dermatologic therapy in the last decade. Corticosteroids used topically have anti-inflammatory, immunosuppressant and anti-proliferative properties. Some of the common indications of topical steroids include eczemas of various types (e.g. lichen simplex chronicus, atopic dermatitis, seborrhoeic dermatitis, contact dermatitis, nummular eczema and pompholyx), localised psoriasis, lichen planus, vitiligo, alopecia areata, discoid lupus erythematosus and localised sclero-derma.

Depending on the efficacy of their action, topical steroids have been grouped into various classes. Class 1 steroid being most potent and the class 7 steroids being least potent (Table 2). Steroid ointments are more potent than creams or lotions and are preferred over creams or lotions in dry scaly skin lesions like lichen simplex chronicus, atopic dermatitis and psoriasis. While choosing a topical steroid for use, potency is the most important consideration and it should be decided based on the indication (or severity of a condition) and the site of application or whether it is a child.

High potency steroids and fluorinated steroids are, by and large, to be avoided in children and over face and flexures in adults for fear of causing skin atrophy. Apart from irreversible skin atrophy which may occur when potent topical steroids are used for more than a couple of weeks, other side-effects like hypopigmentation, striae, purpura, telangiectasia, perioral dermatitis (when used over face especially by ladies) and tinea incognito or scabies incognito (if used inadevertently over dermatophyte or scabies lesions). Rarely, when used over large areas, especially in children, systemic absorption of steroids may lead to iatrogenic Cushing's syndrome (Table 27.2).

CALCINEURIN INHIBITORS

Tacrolimus and pimecrolimus are calcineurin inhibitors that modulate the immune response by suppressing the activation of T lymphocytes. They provide a non-steroidal alternative for the treatment of eczemas, especially atopic dermatitis. They are available in ointment and cream forms respectively and are helpful in the treatment of mild to moderate atopic dermatitis. Currently, their use in dermatology is limited by their high cost. Used over extensive

Chapter 27

Topical Therapy in Dermatology

areas, especially in children, they may get absorbed systemically. For this reason, only tacrolimus 0.03% ointment is approved for use in children.

TABLE 27.2: Classification of topical steroids based on potency

Class 1	**(Super potent)** Clobetasol propionate ointment and cream 0.5% Betamethasone dipropionate ointment 0.05% Halobetasol propionate ointment and cream 0.05%
Class 2	**(Highly potent)** Mometasone furoate ointment 0.1%
Class 3	**(Potent)** Betamethasone dipropionate cream 0.05% Fluticasone propionate ointment 0.05%
Class 4	**(Moderately potent)** Fluocinolone acetonide ointment 0.025% Fluticasone propionate cream 0.05% Mometasone fluroate cream 0.1%
Class 5	**(Moderately potent)** Betamethasone valerate cream 0.1% Hydrocortisone butyrate cream 0.1%
Class 6	**(Mildly potent)** Desonide cream 0.05% Fluocinolone acetonide solution 0.05%
Class 7	**(Least potent)** Dexamethasone cream 0.1% Hydrocortisone 1%

TOPICAL ANTIBACTERIALS

Most of the skin infections (primary bacterial infections) are caused by gram-positive cocci while only some of them (usually secondary bacterial infections) are due to gram-negative or mixed flora. Topical antibiotics useful for infections caused by gram-positive organisms include 1% mupirocin and 1% fusidic acid. They are both available in cream and ointment form; ointments are preferred for deeper infections due to their high penetration. Mupirocin is effective against a wide variety of organisms including staphylococci [and especially methicillin resistant *Staphylococcus aureus* (MRSA)], streptococci and gram-negative bacteria.

Aminoglycosides like neomycin, framycetin and gentamycin are effective against both gram-positive and gram-negative bacteria including *Staphylococcus aureus* and beta haemolytic streptococci. Sometimes polymyxin B, effective against gram-negative bacilli including pseudomonas, and bacitracin, effective against gram-positive cocci, are combined with neomycin to improve its efficacy.

As a general rule, antibiotics that are in common use orally or parenterally (e.g. penicillins and cephalosporins) are not used topically for fear of promoting cross resistance and allergic rashes. Side-effects of topical antibacterials include stinging, burning (mupirocin), contact allergic dermatitis (neomycin, framycetin and gentamycin) and rarely systemic absorption, if used over large areas (gentamycin and neomycin). Widespread use of an antibacterial promotes development of antibiotic resistance and increases chances of contact allergic dermatitis. Hence, these effects are now increasingly seen with the newer antibiotics like mupirocin and fusidic acid.

TOPICAL ANTIFUNGALS

A range of antifungal creams are available for topical treatment of fungal infections. Table 27.3 provides a brief summary of them.

Antifungal agents are available as creams or lotions or powders. While creams are used in most instances, gels and lotions are preferred in hairy areas. Powders are used to reduce friction in flexural areas and to keep them dry. Some of them like ketoconazole, zinc pyrithionate (ZpTO) and cyclopirox have been successfully formulated in shampoos while amorolfine and cyclosporine are also available as nail lacquer.

TOPICAL ANTIVIRALS

Topical acyclovir ointment (1%) has limited utility in clinical practice as it does not substantially reduce healing times nor does it prevent recurrences of herpes infection. Since oral acyclovir or its analogues are highly effective in herpes infections addition of topical acyclovir ointment is unnecessary. Topical cidofovir is highly effective against molluscum contagiosum and herpes infections but is not available in India.

Other topical agents used in treatment of viral infections act against viruses by boosting immunity (imiquimod) or by causing necrosis of infected cells (podophyllin).

Imiquimod

Imiquimod is useful for condyloma acuminata affecting mucocutaneous junctions but is not

TABLE 27.3: Topical antifungal agents		
Group	**Drug**	**Active against**
1. Traditional	Whitfield's ointment (half strength), i.e. salicylic 3% and benzoic 6%	Dermatophytes
	Gentian violet—sulphur (sodium thiosulphite and selenium sulphide)	Candida Malassezia
2. Imidazoles	Clotrimazole, miconazole, ketoconazole, sertaconazole, etc.	Dermatophytes, malassezia and candida
3. Allylamines	Terbinafine, butenafine, and amorolfine	Mainly dermatophytes, also acts against candida and malassezia
4. Polyenes	Nystatin, amphotericin	Candida
5. Cyclopirox	Cyclopirox	Dermatophytes and malassezia

advocated for direct application over mucosae. It boosts local cell-mediated immunity against human papilloma virus by inducing interferon gamma. It is used as 5% cream available in sachets that is rubbed into the lesions thrice a week. Used in this regime, it is also useful to the treatment of molluscum contagiosum and small premalignant and malignant lesions like solar keratoses, Bowen's disease, and tiny basal cell carcinomas.

Podophyllin

Podophyllin is a cytotoxic resin extracted from the plant *Podophyllum emodi*. The active component podophyllotoxin stops cell multiplication in metaphase inducing cell necrosis. It is available as a 20% suspension in tincture benzoin which is to be painted weekly on the surface of lesions and kept on for 2–4 hours. It is the drug of choice for the treatment of condyloma acuminata (genital warts). The drug is an irritant if it spreads to surrounding normal skin or is kept for longer periods. The drug is teratogenic and is absolutely contraindicated in pregnant and lactating women.

AGENTS AGAINST ECTOPARASITES

Agents used for the treatment of scabies and pediculosis are discussed in detail in Chapter 4. Although, 5% permethrin cream is the treatment of choice in scabies, benzyl benzoate (25% emulsions), gamma benzene hexachloride (1% lotion), crotamiton (10% cream or lotion) are also useful.

Permethrin (1% cream rinse), gamma benzene hexachloride (1% lotion) and malathion (0.5% lotion) are all effective in pediculosis.

Anti-Acne Agents

Pathogenesis of acne involves blockage of follicular openings with keratin plus leading to micro-comedone formation, excess activity of sebaceous glands and subsequent overgrowth of *Propionibacterium acnes* and resultant inflammatory processes. For more details of this refer to the chapter on acne.

Anti-acne agents aim to affect one or more arms in the pathogenesis mentioned above and include topical retinoids (described in the subsequent paragraphs), topical benzoyl peroxide and topical antibacterials.

Benzoyl peroxide

This is commonly used in the topical treatment of acne. It has both antibacterial and comedolytic actions and *P. acnes* shows little tendency to development of resistance to its antibacterial effect. Hence, unlike topical antibiotics, it is used frequently for long term maintenance treatment of acne vulgaris. It is available as once daily application of 25% and 5% gel formulation and should be used with caution due to its possible irritant effects on face. Mild burning lasting for a couple of minutes is common in the initial days of treatment. However, some patients develop burning or/and itching lasting for longer periods and then may not tolerate continued use of the drug.

TOPICAL ANTIBIOTICS FOR ACNE

Erythromycin

This macrolide antibiotic is in common use for inflammatory acne vulgaris. It is used as twice daily application of 2–3% gel or solution in the treatment of papulopustular or pustular acne. It is fairly effective against *P. acnes*, though with widespread use, increasing prevalence of resistant strains has been seen. Local allergic or irritant reactions are uncommon.

Clindamycin

Clindamycin is an antibiotic of the lincosamides group that is related to the macrolides. It is used as twice daily application of 1% gel formulation in the treatment of inflammatory acne vulgaris (erythematous papules and pustules). It is highly effective against *P. acnes*, though some resistant strains of *P. acnes* are being reported. Apart from uncommon allergic or irritant reactions, if used over extensive area, clindamycin may get absorbed and rarely induce pseudomembranous colitis.

TOPICAL RETINOIDS

Retinoids are synthetic analogues of vitamin A that have multifarious effects on the skin. They act on cellular differentiation and proliferation (useful in treatment and prevention of malignancies) and stabilise keratinisation of epidermis (useful in genetic disorders of keratinisation like ichthyosis) and follicular infundibula (useful in acne vulgaris). They also affect the immune system and are therefore useful for the treatment of many inflammatory dermatoses including psoriasis.

Topical retinoids have evolved over the last two decades with increasing specificity in their site of action, thus reduction in their side-effects. They can be classified into first generation—tretinoin, second generation—isotretinoin and third generation—adapalene, tazarotene and bexarotene. Indications for topical retinoids include acne vulgaris, prevention and treatment of changes of photoaging, localised stable psoriasis, ichthyoses and keratoderma, cutaneous T-cell lymphoma (bexarotene). They have also been found to be of some value in melasma and keloids. Topical retinoids should be avoided during pregnancy due to their potential for teratogenicity. Side-effects of topical retinoids are skin irritation that gives rise to burning, itching, erythema, photosensitivity and dryness of treated skin (retinoid dermatitis).

Topical tretinoin (0.025–0.05% cream), adapalene (0.1% gel) and tazarotene (0.05% gel) are all effective in acne vulgaris but adapalene is the least irritant of them. Topical tazarotene 0.1% cream is effective in treatment of localised stable plaque type psoriasis but carries with it the risk of irritation and exacerbation of psoriasis. Tazarotene cream 0.1% is also effective in keratinisation disorders like ichthyosis, keratoderma and Darier's disease as well as topical treatment of solar keratoses.

ANTIPSORIATIC AGENTS

Coal Tar

Coal tar is effective in psoriasis as a component of the traditional Goeckerman regimen or as a stand-alone therapy. It is believed to act by its anti-inflammatory and cytostatic effects in psoriasis and eczemas like seborrhoeic dermatitis. They may be used as a paste (psoriasis and chronic eczemas) or as lotion in psoriasis or as a shampoo in seborrhoeic dermatitis and psoriasis. It is contraindicated in unstable, pustular and erythrodermic psoriasis for fear of causing irritation and exacerbation of psoriasis lesions.

Dithranol (Anthralin, Goa Powder)

Anthralin is a plant derived compound that is formulated as an ointment or paste. It is effective in psoriasis by its anti-inflammatory action and effect on cell proliferation. Its main side-effects are irritation of surrounding skin leading to worsening of psoriasis and dark brown pigmentation of healing skin in psoriasis. Because of the fear of irritation and worsening of psoriasis, it is used in short contact therapy. Patients with unstable psoriasis should not apply anthralin. While treating stable plaques of psoriasis, the surrounding normal skin should be protected with white soft paraffin and then anthralin ointment or paste should be applied carefully to the affected areas. It should be kept on for 15–30 minutes and then washed off. Improvement is seen after a few weeks and is accompanied by dark brown pigmentation which may persist for months. Anthralin is sometimes used for its irritant effects in alopecia areata with variable result.

Vitamin D3 Analogues

Calcium metabolism is affected in the pathogenesis of psoriasis. This allows for beneficial effects of this group of agents in the treatment of mild to moderate stable plaque type psoriasis. Calcipotriol is the commonly used compound from this group, though calcitriol also has comparable action. Its main side-effect is again irritation and worsening of psoriasis. Its potential for systemic absorption and inducing hypercalcaemia should always be kept in mind while using the drug over larger surface areas. Maximum permissible quantity of calcipotriol that can be applied by a patient in a week's time is 100 g.

HYPOPIGMENTING AGENTS

All hypopigmenting agents are useful for treating epidermal pigmentation disorders like melasma, freckles or post-inflammatory hyperpigmentation. Dermal melanoses may be helped by lasers. Hydroquinone is the most commonly used agent but may cause side-effects on prolonged use. It is used as a 2–4% cream along or in combination with sunscreen. Sunscreens reduce the tanning influence of sunlight and thus help in lightening the lesions. On prolonged use, hydroquinone causes paradoxical hyperpigmentation due to 'pseudo-ochronosis' resulting from systemic absorption of hydroquinone.

Other hypopigmenting formulations include Kligman's formula for treating melasma contains hydroquinone 2%, tretinoin 0.1% and hydro-cortisone 1%. Other agents like azelaic acid 20% cream or kojic acid 1–2% cream or liquorice or arbutin are also commonly incorporated in lightening creams.

PIGMENTING AGENTS

Most of these compounds exaggerate the phototoxic effects of sunlight and are used in the treatment of vitiligo. They include psoralens (trimethyl psoralen and 8-methoxy psoralen), khellin, pseudocatalase and beta fibroblast growth factor. They are discussed in more detail in the section on vitiligo. Dihydroxyacetone is an artificial tanning agent that is used sometimes to camouflage hypo or depigmented patches. It gives a temporary reddish brown colour to the affected skin.

MISCELLANEOUS AGENTS

Astringents

These are added to aqueous solutions used for soaks, baths and open wet compresses that are used in weeping eczemas by bringing about precipitation of proteins. Potassium permanganate (1:10000–1:25000) aluminium sub-acetate and silver nitrate are frequently used as astringents. Refer to Table 27.1 for the action of these soaks and compresses.

Calamine

Calamine is zinc carbonate with some iron impurities which give it the skin-like pink colour making cosmetically acceptable. It is usually formulated as a lotion (aqueous suspension) with addition of zinc oxide and glycerin. Bentonite is added as a suspending agent and the lotion should be shaken well before application. Calamine lotion has excellent soothing and anti-inflammatory properties and is useful for giving immediate symptomatic relief in acute dermatoses like sunburn and miliaria or weeping dermatoses like acute eczema. For additional relief 1% camphor or menthol may be added to the formulation. In the treatment of acne, several agents active in acne are commonly added and these include sulphur,

phenol and resorcinol in a proportion of 1–2%. In case calamine lotion is required to be used in dry skin conditions, it may be formulated as oily calamine lotion or calamine ointment that does not cause drying.

AGENT FOR HAIR GROWTH

Minoxidil

Minoxidil increases the blood supply to the follicles by its vasodilatory action and also directly stimulates growth of hair follicles. It is available as 2%, 5% and 10% solutions that are to be applied twice daily to the affected parts. It is indicated for androgenetic alopecia in males (5%) and females, (2% solution) and alopecia areata (2% in women and 5% in men). Effects of minoxidil application on scalp hair are noticeable after the third month of use. The vellus hair in androgenetic alopecia and alopecia areata tend to gain in thickness and length with minoxidil. The number of hair falling also reduces during the first 3 months. However, cosmetically significant hair regrowth can only be seen after 9 months to a year. In androgenic alopecia, the treatment needs to be continued till hair regrowth is desired by the patient. In alopecia areata substantial regrowth occurs in 6–9 months. Side-effects include dryness of hair, scalp burning, irritation and itching, and hirsutism (especially if 5% lotion is used in ladies) and hypertrichosis.

Diphencyprone and Other Contact Sensitisers

Contact sensitisers are compounds that, when applied to the skin, induce delayed type hyper-sensitivity response in the skin causing contact allergic dermatitis. They include, diphencyprone, squaric acid dibutyl ester (SADBE) and dinitro-chlorobenzene (DNCB). Once allergy develops, a controlled mild dermatitis is maintained thereafter by adjusting the concentration of the applied sensitiser.

These compounds are used for the treatment of alopecia areata if it does not respond to initial therapy with topical or intralesional steroids and minoxidil. Side-effects include allergic rashes, irritant dermatitis, contact leucoderma and hyper-pigmentation. DNCB should not be used in women of childbearing age and children, as it is mutagenic in Ame's test. Sensitisers need to be applied once a week to the affected site and a mild erythema is maintained at the site during therapy by adjusting the concentration of the solution used. Contact sensitisers have also been used for the treatment of recalcitrant warts.

Chapter **27**

Topical Therapy in Dermatology

MCQs

1. Topical application to be effective, _____ mm thick application is recommended.
   - a. 0.05
   - b. 0.1
   - c. 0.2
   - d. 1

2. One finger tip unit (FTU) consists of how much quantity of cream?
   - a. 1 g
   - b. 0.25 g
   - c. 2 g
   - d. 0.5 g

3. One FTU covers how much area of the body?
   - a. One palm size
   - b. Half palm size
   - c. Entire face
   - d. Full hand

4. Which of the following is true?
   - a. High alkalinity soaps cause less damage to the skin
   - b. Patients with dry skin should repeatedly wet the skin
   - c. Odland bodies are responsible for the barrier function of the skin
   - d. Phenylene diamine is a natural moisturising factor

5. Which of the following is a physical sunscreen?
   - a. Para-amino benzoic acid
   - b. Zinc oxide
   - c. Avobenzone
   - d. Salicylates

6. The sun protection factor for photosensitive skin should be minimum:
   - a. 30
   - b. 20
   - c. 15
   - d. 50

7. Clobetasol propionate is available in what concentration?
   - a. 0.1%
   - b. 0.05%
   - c. 0.5%
   - d. 1%

8. The most potent formulation of a given topical agent is:
   - a. Ointment
   - b. Cream
   - c. Lotion
   - d. Paste

9. The topical antibiotic preferred for pseudomonas infection is:
   - a. Bacitracin
   - b. Polymixin B
   - c. Neomycin
   - d. Gentamycin

10. Which of the following formulations is preferred in hairy areas?
    - a. Gels
    - b. Cream
    - c. Ointment
    - d. Paste

11. Topicals used for cutaneous viral infections include all except:
    - a. Cidofovir
    - b. Acyclovir
    - c. Imiquimod
    - d. Podophyllin

12. Imiquimod is available as:
    - a. 1% cream
    - b. 5% ointment
    - c. 5% cream
    - d. 2% ointment

13. Which of the following has a comedolytic action?
    - a. Erythromycin
    - b. Benzoyl peroxide
    - c. Clindamycin
    - d. Coal tar

14. Which of the following anti-acne agent is potentially teratogenic?
    - a. Tretinoin
    - b. Benzoyl peroxide
    - c. Clindamycin
    - d. Nadifloxacin

15. Topical retinoids are used in all of the following except:
    - a. Acne
    - b. Psoriasis
    - c. Darier's disease
    - d. Pityriasis rosea

16. Maximum weekly permissible dose of calcipotriol is:
    - a. 200 g
    - b. 300 g
    - c. 100 g
    - d. 150 g

17. A skin lightening agent commonly used for treatment of melasma is:
    - a. Hydroquinone
    - b. Chloroquine
    - c. Hydroxychloroquine
    - d. Monobenzyl ether of hydroquinone

18. Kligman's formula for treatment of melasma consists of:
    - a. Hydroquinone, tretinoin and hydrocortisone
    - b. Hydroquinone, tretinoin and mometa-sone
    - c. Hydroquinone, adapalene and dexametha-sone
    - d. Hydroquinone, adapalene and hydrocortisone

19. Artificial tanning agent that may be used in vitiligo is:
    - a. Monobenzone
    - b. Benzophenone
    - c. Dihydroxyacetone
    - d. Acetylbenzone

20. **Which of the following is responsible for the pink colour of calamine lotion?**
    a. Zinc carbonate
    b. Zinc oxide
    c. Iron impurities
    d. Sulphur

21. **Adjustment of the concentration of contact sensitisers is by assessment of:**
    a. Maintenance of mild erythema
    b. Vellous hair regrowth
    c. Increase by 0.5% every application
    d. All of the above

22. **Gentian violet is:**
    a. Weak antibacterial
    b. Antifungal
    c. Staining agent
    d. All of these

23. **Goa powder is:**
    a. Podophyllin
    b. Tazarotene
    c. Dithranol
    d. Coal tar

24. **Podophyllin is derived from which plant?**
    a. *Podophyllum emodi*
    b. *Podophyllum rosacea*
    c. *Podophyllum indica*
    d. *Podophyllum manea*

25. **Calamine lotion chemically is:**
    a. Zinc oxide
    b. Zinc carbonate
    c. Iron oxide
    d. Magnesium sulphate

Chapter 27

Topical Therapy in Dermatology

--- ANSWERS ---

1-b,	2-d,	3-a,	4-c,	5-b,	6-a,	7-c,	8-a,	9-b,	10-a,
11-b,	12-c,	13-b,	14-a,	15-d,	16-c,	17-a,	18-a,	19-c,	20-c,
21-a,	22-d,	23-c,	24-a,	25-b					

Systemic Therapies in Dermatology

Although, it is extremely advantageous to treat skin disorders with topical therapy, there are situations when systemic therpay is preferred either because it is effective (leprosy or tuberculosis of skin) or it is more convenient (extensive dermatitis or infections). Apart from anti-infective agents, most of the drugs used in dermatology are either anti-allergic or anti-inflammatory (including steroids) or immuno-suppressants. Others may have direct effects on keratinisation (retinoids) or are antiandrogens (used for hair loss or acne).

SYSTEMIC ANTIBACTERIAL AGENTS

β-Lactam Antibacterial Agents

These antibacterial agents have a β-lactam ring in their molecular structure and inhibit bacterial cell wall synthesis and activate bacterial autolytic enzymes. β-lactam antibiotics include penicillins, cephalo-sporins, carbapenems and mobactams. Penicillins can be natural or semi-synthetic. Semi-synthetic penicillins have ability to act against a wide range of organisms which includes gram positive, gram-negative and β-lactamase producing bacteria. β-lactamase (penicillinase) is an enzyme which can cleave the β-lactam ring, thus preventing the action of penicillins. β-lactamase inhibitors are always used in combination with semi-synthetic penicillins and they include clavulanic acid (with amoxycillin), tazobactam (with piperacillin) and sulbactam (with ampicillin). Cloxacillin, dicloxacillin, flucloxacillin, methicillin, nafcillin and oxacillin are β-lactamase resistant penicillins.

In dermatology, semi-synthetic penicillins are commonly used to treat bacterial skin infections like impetigo, ecthyma, folliculitis, furunculosis, cellulitis, and erysipelas. Injectable penicillins like benzathine penicillin, procaine penicillin and crystalline penicillins are widely used to treat syphilis. Penicillins are also useful for treatment of infections like anthrax, disseminated gonococcal infections and erysipeloid.

Doses

Ampicillin—250–500 mg QID, amoxycillin—250–500 mg TID, cloxacillin—250–500 mg QID

Some strains of *Staphylococcus aureus* are resistant to even these β-lactamase resistant penicillins and are called methicillin resistant *Staphylococcus aureus* (MRSA). MRSA are resistant to many other antibiotics as well and are responsible for many serious nosocomial infections. Vancomycin and linezolid are the drugs of choice in MRSA infections.

Common adverse effects of penicillins include skin rashes (urticaria, maculopapular rash and erythema multiforme) and, rarely anaphylaxis, which occurs only with injectable penicillins. To prevent anaphylaxis, a test dose should always be done before each course of penicillin injections. Diarrhoea can occur with the use of amino-penicillins like amoxycillin and ampicillin. Probiotic supplements may prevent or reduce the severity of diarrhoea. Infectious mononucleosis like illness can occur due to ampicillin. Infections with opportunistic pathogens like candida occur with all broad spectrum antibiotics including semi-synthetic penicillins.

Penicillins can cross react with each other and with cephalosporins (5–10% of cases). Hence, in patients with severe manifestations (anaphylactic reactions or severe IgE-mediated reaction or type IV delayed hypersensitivity reactions) of sensitivity to penicillins use of other group of penicillins and cephalosporins should be avoided.

Summery: Penicillin, ampicillin, amoxycillin, amoxycillin-clavulanate combination are the β-lactam agents used to treat infections caused by gram-positive organisms like folliculitis, furunculosis, carbuncle, etc. The drug of choice for MRSA is linezolid and vancomycin. Penicillin sensitivity test is mandatory before giving injectable penicillins for risk of anaphylaxis. The use of vancomycin is restricted to MRSA and pseudomembranous enterocolitis. It can also be used in penicillin allergic patients.

The antibacterial spectrum of macrolides is narrow. The mainly act on gram-positive and few gram-negative organisms with high level of resistance. They are used as first line for treatment of mycoplasma infections and chancroid, otherwise mainly as an alternative to penicillin.

Aminoglycosides are used mainly for gram-negative organisms, especially pseudomonas. They share common side effects of ototoxicity, nephrotoxicity and neuro-muscular blockade in varying proportions depending on the type of drug.

Trimethoprim-sulphamethoxazole (TMP-SMX) are available in fixed dose combination in a ratio of 1:4. They have a wider spectrum of action for gram-positive and gram-negative organisms and can be used for a longer duration for infections like actinomycetoma foot and prophylaxis in immunocompromised patients.

Cephalosporins

First generation cephalosporins (cefadroxil 250–500 mg BID or cephalexin 250–500 mg QID) are active against staphylococci and non-enterococcal streptococci. Second generation cephalosporins (cefixime and cefaclor) and third generation (cefotaxime and ceftriaxone) are less active against gram-positive but more active against gram-negative organisms. Dermatological indications of cephalosporins are the same as those for penicillins, i.e. treatment of skin and soft tissue infections. Single dose of injection ceftriaxone is useful to treat uncomplicated gonorrhoea. Ceftriaxone can be used to treat syphilis in patients who are sensitive to penicillins. Side effects include gastrointestinal disturbances and skin rashes.

Vancomycin

It is a glycopeptide antibiotic which acts by inhibiting bacterial cell wall synthesis. It is used to treat skin and soft tissue infections due to MRSA and methicillin-resistant coagulase-negative staphylococci in a dose of 500 mg QDS intravenously. Rapid infusion can lead to red main syndrome and shock due to release of histamine.

Macrolides

They act by binding to 50S subunit of ribosome and inhibits RNA dependent protein synthesis. Macrolides can be used as substitutes in patients allergic to penicillins. Erythromycin is mostly effective against gram-positive organisms and anaerobes. Azithromycin and clarithromycin have similar spectrum of activity as erythromycin with advantage of effectiveness against several gram-negative bacteria, atypical mycobacteria. Macrolides are also effective to treat infections caused by chlamydia, mycoplasma and ureaplasma.

Macrolides are used to treat skin and soft tissue infections. Erythromycin and azithromycin are found to be effective for acne and rosacea. They can also be used to treat sexually transmitted diseases like syphilis, chancroid, gonorrhoea, nongonococcal or post-gonococcal urethritis and donovanosis, lymphogranuloma venereum. Erythromycin is effective for bacillary angiomatosis in HIV infection. Azithromycin and clarithromycin are used to treat atypical mycobacterial infections.

Gastrointestinal upset is common with erythromycin than azithromycin or clarithromycin. Other adverse effects of erythromycin include cholestatic jaundice especially with its estolate salt. Unlike erythromycin and clarithromycin, azithromycin does not inhibit hepatic cytochrome P450 enzyme, so it can be used concomitantly with other drugs without any drug interactions.

Doses

Tablet erythromycin—250–500 mg QID × 5 days

Tablet azithroycin—500 mg TID × 3 days

Fluoroquinolones

This group of antibiotics act by inhibiting DNA gyrase activity of bacteria. They have wide range of activity against gram-negative and variable activity against gram-positive organisms. They are also highly effective against *Mycobacterium tuberculosis*, atypical mycobacteria and *Mycobacterium leprae*. Ofloxacin has been used for treatment of leprosy. In dermatology fluoroquinolones are useful to treat infections caused by gram-negative organisms, e.g. abscesses, ulcers, wound infections and anthrax. For sexually transmitted diseases like gonorrhoea single dose of ciprofloxacin or ofloxacin is effective.

Fluoroquinolones are contraindicated in pregnancy and in children as they can damage the cartilage. Most common adverse effects observed with the fluoroquinolones is gastrointestinal upset. Nalidixic acid, norfloxacin and ciprofloxacin can give rise to fixed drug eruption. Photosensitive eruption can occur with the use of lomefloxacin, ciprofloxacin, norfloxacin and ofloxacin. Long term use of ciprofloxacin can be complicated by pseudomembraneous colitis.

Doses

Tablet ciprofloxacin—250–500 mg BD for 5–7 days for soft tissue infections

Gonorrhoea—ciprofloxacin single dose 500 mg

Chancroid—ciprofloxacin 500 mg BD × 3 days

Leprosy—ofloxacin 400 mg/day [as a part of rifampicin, ofloxacin and minocycline (ROM) therapy]

Gonorrhoea—ofloxacin 400 mg single dose

Tetracyclines

These are the broad spectrum, bacteriostatic antibiotic which include tetracycline, doxycycline and minocycline. They act by inhibiting protein synthesis by binding to 30S unit of bacterial ribosomes. Tetracyclines are contraindicated in pregnancy and children less than 12 years of age. Tetracyclines are widely used for treatment of acne, rosacea, perioral and periorbital dermatitis. Infections like lymphogranuloma venereum, donovanosis, syphilis, and

Chapter 28

Systemic Therapies in Dermatology

non-gonococcal urethritis can be treated with tetracyclines. Tetracycline is the drug of choice for treatment of syphilis, if the patient has hypersensitivity to penicillin. Minocycline is used for treatment of inflammatory lesions of acne vulgaris, atypical mycobacterial infections and leprosy. Besides their antimicrobial property they possess anti-inflammatory property which is useful for treatment of some autoimmune diseases like bullous pemphigoid.

Doses

Tetracycline—	Acne	: 250–500 mg TID or QID
	Rosacea	: 250–500 mg TID or QID
	Syphilis	: 500 mg QID × 14 days for early syphilis, 28 days for late syphilis
Doxycycline—	Acne	: 100 mg BD or OD
	Rosacea	: 100 mg BD or OD
	Syphilis	: 100 mg BD × 14 days for early syphilis, 28 days for late syphilis
Minocycline—	Leprosy	: 100 mg/day
	Acne	: 50–100 mg/day

Gastrointestinal disturbances are common adverse effects with tetracyclines. Discolouration fo teeth and delayed bone growth can occur in children. Other adverse effects include phototoxicity, candidiasis, and pseudotumour cerebri. Minocycline causes blue-black discolouration of nails, skin and scars.

Trimethoprim and sulphamethoxazole

Combination of these two drugs has synergistic action in blocking the synthesis of paraminobenzoic acid (PABA). They are active against a wide range of organisms but resistance is common. This combination is drug of choice for nocardial infections including nocardial mycetoma. It is also useful for the treatment of sexually transmitted infections like donovanosis and lymphogranuloma venereum. Skin reactions (fixed drug eruption, erythema multiforme, Stevens Johnson syndrome and toxic epidermal necrolysis) are common, particularly in the HIV seropositive.

Rifampicin

It acts by inhibiting protein synthesis by binding to 30S units of bacterial ribosome. It is used in combination with other drugs to treat mycobacterium

tuberculosis infection, leprosy and atypical mycobacterial infection. Used in the dose of 10 mg/kg/day, in tuberculosis it is an important component of the multi-drug therapy. Although it is also effective against pyogenic bacteria like staphylococci the drug should be reserved for its use in tuberculosis and leprosy. In leprosy it is used as once a month pulse dose of 600 mg and such a dose kills 99.9% of dividing bacilli. However, it is unable to act on dormant bacilli (persisters) in leprosy which persist in the body even after successful therapy of leprosy.

Common side effects of rifampicin include reddish discolouration to urine, skin and skin rashes (maculopapular rash, purpura, erythema multiforme and Stevens Johnson syndrome) and, with intermittent therapy, flu-like symptoms. Hepatotoxicity and thrombocytopenia are uncommon. Rifampicin is a potent inducer of cytochrome, so when used with other drugs possibility of drug interactions should be considered and doses need to be adjusted accordingly. Please refer section on antiretroviral therapy for interactions.

Antibacterials for acne

Antibacterial agents are advised for inflammatory moderate to severe grade acne. They act by inhibiting growth of *Propionibacterium acnes*. They additionally have anti-inflammatory properties. Systemic antibacterials can be used along with topical anti-acne preparations.

Tetracycline (250–500 mg TID or QDS) or doxycycline (100 mg OD or BD) is the antibiotic of choice. However, for patients who are not responding adequately, minocycline provides an effective alternative. It should be started in the dose of 50 mg/day and then depending upon response, the dose may be increased up to 100 mg BD. Macrolides like erythromycin (250 mg QID) are also effective. More recently, azithromycin 500 mg/day for 3 days to be repeated every 10–15 days has offered a patient friendly alternatively with improved compliance.

Long term use of systemic antibiotics can lead to gram-negative folliculitis, characterised by sudden appearance of papules and pustules on face in a patient who was earlier repsonding to the treatment. Gram-negative folliculitis responds well to treatment with oral ampicillin.

Metronidazole

This is active against gram-negative anaerobes. Dermatological uses include treatment of anaerobic infections as in deep abscesses and wounds, phagedenic ulcers, noma and tropical ulcer. It is also useful to treat sexually transmitted infections like trichomoniasis, bacterial vaginosis in females and erosive balanitis and phagedena in males. The dose varies between 200–400 mg BD. In higher doses, metronidazole is effective for cutaneous amoebiasis. Metallic taste and nausea are the common side effects. Cutaneous adverse effects include fixed drug eruption and lichenoid eruptions. Disulfiram like (antabuse) reaction can occur if metronidazole is taken with alcohol. Tinidazole and secnidazole have the same spectrum but have advantage of a single dose with similar efficacy.

ANTIVIRALS

Acyclovir and its newer analogues are useful for treatment of infections caused by herpes viruses which include herpes simplex, herpes zoster and chickenpox. Newer analogues like valaciclovir and famcyclovir have the advantage of better bioavailability and less dosing frequency as compared to acyclovir. Adverse reactions are uncommon and include gastrointestinal disturbances, headache and rarely renal tubular damage due to crystal deposition.

Systemic complications due to herpes virus infection may be treated with intravenous acyclovir 5–10 mg/kg 8 hourly for 5–7 days.

Chronic suppressive therapy for herpes simplex or herpes genitalis is indicated when repeated attacks of recurrent herpes simplex affect quality of life of a person. It is administered for prolonged periods like 6 months to 2 years. However, such therapy may not reduce the frequency or severity or recurrent herpes simplex attacks after stoppage of the therapy. The dosages used are acyclovir—400 mg twice a day, valacyclovir—250 mg twice a day or famciclovir—250 mg twice a day (Table 28.1).

ANTIPARASITIC AGENTS

Ivermectin

This is an antiparasitic agent, which acts by inhibition of glutamate related chloride ion channels leading to neuromuscular paralysis of the parasite and death. It is effective for treatment of scabies and pediculosis. The dose used is 200 µg/kg of body weight as a single dose, which may be repeated after 10 days to improve efficacy.

SYSTEMIC ANTIFUNGAL AGENTS

Griseofulvin

Griseofulvin is a fungistatic agent that acts by inhibiting fungal microtubules formation. It is effective against dermatophytic infections affecting the skin, nails, scalp and hair but ineffective against other fungi and moulds. Fatty food increases its oral absorption. Common side effects include gastrointestinal disturbances, phototoxicity, hepatotoxicity and precipitation of porphyrias. It is contraindicated in hepatic failure and in patients with porphyria. Since griseofulvin is fungistatic, it needs to be used for extended periods in dermatophytic infections. It is available in micronised form and is given as tablets 250 mg twice a day (10 mg/kg/day in children) for 3–4 weeks for tinea cruris/corporis/faciei, 6 weeks for tinea manuum and capitis, 8 weeks for tinea pedis, 6 months to 1 year for fingernails and 1–2 years for toe nails (*see* Table 7.4, page 77).

Azoles

This group of antifungals act by inhibiting 14-α demethylase leading to decrease in ergosterol synthesis (essential for fungal cell was synthesis). It includes two groups of agents:

1. Imidazoles, e.g. ketoconazole
2. Triazoles, e.g. fluconazole and itraconazole

TABLE 28.1: Antiviral dosages

	Herpes simplex or genitalis	Chickenpox	Herpes zoster
Acyclovir	200 mg 5 times/day or 400 mg TID × 10 days for primary episode and for 5 days for recurrent episodes	800 mg 5 times/ day × 7 days	800 mg 5 times/ day × 7 days
Valcyclovir	1 g BD for 7–10 days for primary episode and 500 mg BD × 5 days for recurrent episodes	1 g TID × 7 days	1 g TID × 7 days
Famciclovir	250 mg 8 hourly × 7–10 days for primary episode and 125 mg BD × 5 days for recurrent episodes	250 mg TID × 7 days	2560 mg TID × 7 days

Ketoconazole

It is an imidazole derivative active against candida, dermatophyte and deep fungal infections, but due to higher incidences of adverse effects and drug interactions, it is not used as commonly as it was before. Adverse effects include gastrointestinal upset, hepatotoxicity, decreased libido and gynaecomastia. Ketoconazole is used in the dose of 200 mg once or twice a day.

Fluconazole

It is particularly active against yeasts like candida and cryptococcus, but is also effective for dermatophyte infection. It is recommended for treatment of oral, oro-oesophageal, vaginal candidiasis and cryptococcosis (orally for maintenance treatment after amphotericin B). However, it is not the drug of choice for dermatophyte infections and as far as possible use for dermatophyte infections should be avoided due to higher relapse rates and to prevent development of resistance. Adverse effects are uncommon and include nausea, vomiting, headache and elevation of hepatic transaminases. Dose differs according to indication; higher doses and longer durations are used in the immunosuppressed.

Oral candidiasis—100 mg/day × 7–10 days

Oesophageal candidiasis—100 mg/day × 14 days

Vaginal candidiasis—150 mg single dose

Pityriasis versicolor—400 mg single dose

Onychomycosis—150 mg once weekly × 3–6 months for fingernails and 9–12 months for toe-nails

Tinea cruris/corporis—150 mg once weekly × 2–4 weeks

Tinea pedis/manuum—150 mg once weekly × 2–6 weeks

Tinea capitis—6 mg/kg/day × 2–3 weeks

Itraconazole

This is a triazole with broad antifungal spectrum and is recommended for the treatment of superficial and deep fungal infections. It is highly effective against all dermatophytes including onychomycosis caused by all types of fungi and deep fungal infections like histoplasmosis, aspergillosis and blastomycosis. Although, it can be used for candida infections, fluconazole is preferred for this indication due to its high efficacy. Itraconazole is also effective in sub-cutaneous deep fungal infections like subcutaneous zygomycosis, phaeohyphomycosis and eumycotic mycetoma. Gastrointestinal upset and elevation of hepatic transaminases may occur, though the latter is less common and less serious than ketoconazole (Table 28.2).

Terbinafine

This is an allylamine antifungal which acts by inhibiting fungal squalene epoxidase leading to accumulation of squalene metabolites (toxic to fungi) and blocks ergosterol synthesis. Terbinafine is recommended for dermatophytosis and is

TABLE 28.2: Antifungal regimens		
	Continuous therapy	**Pulse therapy**
Itraconazole:		
Tinea cruris/corporis	100 mg/day × 2 weeks	200 mg/day × 1 week
Tinea pedis/manuum	200 mg/day × 2 weeks	200 mg twice/day × 1 week
Tinea capitis	5 mg/kg/day 2–4 weeks	5 mg/kg/day 1–3 pulses (each pulse consists of medication for 1 week each month with, 1 week on and 3 weeks off between successive pulses)
Onychomycosis	200 mg/day, 6 weeks for fingernails and 12 weeks for toe nails	200 mg twice/day × 1 week of every month × 3 months
Terbinafine:		
Tinea cruris/corporis	250 mg/day 2–4 weeks	—
Tinea pedis/manuum	250 mg/day 2–6 weeks	—
Tinea capitis	5 mg/kg/day 2–4 weeks	—
Onychomycosis	250 mg/day 6 weeks for fingernails and 12 weeks for toenalis	250 mg twice a day for 1 week a month for 3–4 months

effective in onychomycosis except that caused by non-dermatophyte moulds. It is less effective for infections caused by candida, malassezia and non-dermatophyte moulds and is not effective for deep fungal infections. It is contraindicated in hepatic disease and renal impairment. Common adverse effects include headache, nausea, vomiting, skin rash and elevation of hepatic transaminases.

> **Summary for antifungals:** The use of griseofulvin is restricted to the treatment of dermatophytoses. It is the drug of choice for tinea capitis in children. Oral ketoconazole is rarely used nowadays due to its side effects. The azoles as well as terbinafine can be used for dermatophytoses. Clinical failures to terbinafine have shown a sharp rise in the recent years. Higher dose and longer duration of treatment with terbinafine and terbinafine combined with itraconazole are used to combat clinical failures and resistant cases. Candidiasis and pityriasis versicolor respond well to fluconazole and itraconazole. Griseofulvin is ineffective for candida and pityriasis versicolor. Itraconzole is drug of choice for fungal infections of unknown cause and subcutaneous mycoses.

ANTIALLERGIC AGENTS

These are H1 receptor blocking agents that have been in use since several decades and provide not only symptomatic relief from pruritus, but also control the severity of allergic rashes. Their classification and other details are discussed in the chapter on urticaria for which they are commonly used. They are also useful for treatment of eczemas, and may be used in adjunctive treatment of scabies, lichen planus and other pruritic disorders.

H2 Blockers

Ranitidine is a histamine receptor blocker, that is a useful adjunct for the treatment of urticaria. It is used as 150 mg twice daily and is always combined with H1 blockers.

Doxepin

This antidepressant has strong H1 and H2 receptor blocking effets and is therefore used in the treatment of chronic urticaria.

CORTICOSTEROIDS

Corticosteroids are useful for treating variety of dermatologic conditions.

Absolute Indications

In these conditions systemic steroids need to be given in relatively larger doses (1–2 mg/kg/day of prednisolone) even in presence of relative contra-indications like hypertension or diabetes mellitus. They include autoimmune vesiculobullous diseases like pemphigus or bullous pemphigoid and collagen vascular disease like systemic lupus erythematosus and dermatomyositis, erythroderma with systemic complications and severe type 1 and type 2 (ENL, erythema nodosum leprosum) lepra reactions.

Optional Indications

These conditions frequently need systemic steroids in small doses (0.5–1 mg/kg/day of prednisolone) for rapid control and symptomatic relief. However, if relative contraindications are present, steroids may be avoided and the condition managed with topical steroids or antihistaminics or immuno-suppressants, as appropriate. These conditions include severe eczematous rashes including contact dermatitis, widespread atopic dermatitis, nummular dermatitis and autosensitisation eczema. Some autoimmune diseases like widespread lichen planus, unstable vitiligo, linear IgA dermatosis, dermatitis herpetiformis and systemic sclerosis may benefit from small doses of systemic cortico-steroids.

Long term steroid therapy can lead to weight gain, hypertension, diabetes, gastritis, precipitation of peptic ulcer, osteoporosis, myopathy, cataract, glaucoma and decreased immunity leading to reactivation of latent tuberculosis or other infections. Cutaneous adverse effects include redistribution of body fat (moon face, buffalo hump, central obesity), striae, thin and fragile skin, telangiectasia, ecchymosis and hypertrichosis.

High dose corticosteroid intravenous pulse therapy—high doses of corticosteroids (1 g of methylprednisolone or 100 mg of dexamethasone) are given intravenously over a period of 2–3 hours, on three consecutive days per month. It can be combined with immunosuppressives like cyclophosphamide given as 500 mg IV on 1 day per month. Such therapy is highly effective in controlling disease activity and is used particularly for pemphigus vulgaris, systemic lupus erythematosus, dermatomyositis, pyoderma gangrenosum and rarely for severe bullous pemphigoid. On long term use, most of the side effects of steroids are seen with this therapy. Additionally, electrolyte imbalance, cardiac arrhythmias and haemorrhagic cystitis (due to cyclophosphamide) may occur.

ANTI-INFLAMMATORY AGENTS

Antimalarials

Chloroquine and hydroxychloroquine are used in dermatology as systemic sunscreens. They minimise damaging effects of sunlight in patients with photosensitive disorders. They are effective in treatment of cutaneous lesions of lupus erythematosus, polymorphous light eruption and porphyria cutanea tarda. As an anti-inflammatory agent, it is used in type 1 lepra reaction.

Common side effects include gastrointestinal upset, hyperpigmentation of skin, lichenoid drug eruption, and urticaria. Ocular toxicity may occur as reversible keratopathy or reversible or irreversible retinopathy on long term use. An early symptom of retinopathy is halos around lighted objects. Baseline ophthalmic examination and periodic perimetry assessment at intervals of 6 months to 1 year are recommended during long term therapy for lupus erythematosus. In photosensitive disorders including lupus erythematosus, it is used in the dose of 250–500 mg/day, while in prophyria a much lower dose of 125 mg twice a week is used. The use of chloroquine is gradually declining with increasing availability of hydroxychloroquine (200 mg OD or BD) which has much less ocular toxicity. However, regular eye checkups are needed even with hydroxychloroquine.

Dapsone

This bacteriostatic agent is a sulphone which acts by inhibiting folic acid metabolism. Hence, it should not be combined with methotrexate. Besides its well known antimicrobial properties *against Mycobacterium leprae*, it possesses anti-inflammatory action, especially in neutrophilic dermatoses.

It is the drug of choice for leprosy (100 mg/day for all patients) and the autoimmune vesicobullous diseases dermatitis herpetiformis and linear IgA dermatosis. However, albeit with lesser efficacy, it is also used in the treatment of other autoimmune bullous disorders like pemphigus and bullous pumphigoid, lichen planus and nocardial mycetoma. Common side effects include haemolytic anaemia, agranulocytosis, methaemoglobinaemia, skin rashes and dapsone hypersensitivity syndrome. Dapsone caused dose related haemolysis with average reduction in haemoglobin of 1 g%. However, persons with glucose-6-phosphate dehydrogenase (G6PD) deficiency may develop severe haemolysis. Hence, screening for G6PD activity is necessary before initiating dapsone for any disorder.

Clofazimine

This is used as one of the drugs for multi-drug therapy for leprosy (50 mg/day). In higher doses (200–300 mg/day) it is used for its anti-inflammatory activity for type 2 and even type 1 lepra reactions. It is also used for treatment of atypical mycobacterial infections and vitiligo. Mahogany red-brown discolouration of skin and mucosae is the most common side effect and it is reversible (over several months) once the treatment is stopped. Xerosis and ichthyosis can occur due to clofazimine. Enteropathy and acute abdominal pain are rare complications.

Thalidomide

This is approved for treatment of ENL in the dose of 200–300 mg per day. It is highly effective in steroid dependant type 2 lepra reaction, where it allows tapering of steroids. Other dermatological uses are severe aphthous ulcerations and Behcet's disease. It is absolutely contraindicated in pregnancy due to its well known teratogenic effects. Sedation is the commonest side effect; others include paraesthesiae and pain due to peripheral neuropathy, oedema feet, constipation, xerostomatitis and xerosis of skin.

Doses: 100 mg BD or TID.

IMMUNOSUPPRESSANTS

Several immunosuppressive agents are used for treatment of autoimmune diseases. They may be used along or in combination with systemic steroids. When combined with steroids, they are used as steroid sparing agents. Their use allows smoother taper of steroid doses and reduces side effects of steroids by reducing steroid requirement.

Methotrexate

This drug is cytotoxic as well as immunosuppressant. It is a competitive and irreversible antagonist of dihydrofolate reductase required for metabolism of folic acid in DNA synthesis. It is commonly used to treat extensive psoriasis and other autoimmune diseases. It can also be used for treatment of collagen vascular disorders. Gastrointestinal intolerance, especially nausea is common. Blood counts must be checked for evidence of bone marrow suppression. Long term use must be monitored for development of hepatic fibrosis and cirrhosis. Regular monitoring of complete blood count and liver functions is recommended during methotrexate therapy. In dermatology, the drug is used in a once weekly regimen of 5–15 mg per week. Acute toxicity can occur due to accidental overdose, if the patient takes it daily. Antidote for methotrexate is folinic acid, which is available as injections or tablets and must be administered within 6 hours.

Cyclophosphamide

This is an alkylating, immunosuppressive agent. It can be used as a steroid sparing agent in auto-immune diseases. Along with corticosteroids, it is used for the treatment of pemphigus vulgaris, sclero-derma, or dermatomyositis in a dose of 50–100 mg/day. Bone marrow suppression and haemorrhagic cystitis are serious side effects and should be monitored regularly. Mesna (sodium 2-mercaptoethane-sulphonate) is used to reduce bladder toxicity when high doses of cyclophosphamide are given. Cutaneous side effects include hair loss and hyper-pigmentation of nails. The drug is contraindicated in pregnancy or lactation or even in women who wish to conceive in future.

Azathioprine

This immunosuppressive agent is useful for the treatment of collagen vascular diseases (scleroderma, dermatomyositis and systemic lupus erythemato-sus) and autoimmune vesiculobullous diseases like pemphigus vulgaris or bullous pemphigoid. The drug is used in a dose of 50–100 mg/day. Bone marrow suppression and hepatotoxicity can occur and should be monitored by regular laboratory investigations. It is contraindicated in pregnancy and lactation, but can be used in children and in women who wish to conceive in future.

Cyclosporin

This is an extremely effective immunosuppressant for T cell mediated autoimmune diseases. It is used for the treatment of severe psoriasis and atopic dermatitis in a dose of 3–5 mg/kg/day in order to achieve rapid control. However, it is not as regularly used because of its cost and fear of renal toxicity. Common side effects of cyclosporin include hypertension, nephrotoxicity (seen as raised serum creatinine), hyperkalaemia, hyperlipidaemia and hyperuricaemia. Regular monitoring of blood pressure and serum creatinine is essential.

Psoralen and Ultraviolet A Therapy

For psoralen and ultraviolet A (UVA) therapy please refer the section on vitiligo.

MISCELLANEOUS SYSTEMIC THERAPIES

Oral Retinoids

Retinoids are the semi-synthetic derivatives of vitamin A. Systemic retinoids in common use include isotretinoin and acitretin. Isotretinoin normalises follicular keratinisation and inhibits sebaceous gland activity and is used (20–40 mg/day) for the treatment of severe acne vulgaris, acne conglobata, hidradenitis suppurativa, and several keratinisation disorders of the skin like ichthyoses and keratoderma. Acitretin has anti-inflammatory and keratostatic properties and is used for the treatment of psoriasis and other disorders of keratinisation.

All retinoids are teratogenic and are therefore contraindicated in pregnancy, lactation and due to their teratogenic properties. They should be prescribed with caution in women of childbearing age only when patients agree to use two methods of contraception and with full understanding that the drug remains in the body much after stoppage of intake (2 months for isotretinoin and 2–3 years for acitretin). Exacerbaton of lesions of acne may occur during first few weeks after initiation of therapy. Common side effects are dryness of lips and skin with photosensitivity and hyperlipidaemia. Sometimes, elevation of serum transaminases may occur. On long term use in children with keratinisation disorders like ichthyosis, diffuse idiopathic skeletal hyperosteosis (DISH) affecting the vertebral column can occur.

Biologicals

Biologicals are molecules from human or animal sources modified for acting on or blocking of a specific pathomechanism. In dermatology, they are used to treat psoriasis, especially when it is associated with psoriatic arthritis. Infliximab (intravenous infusion), etanercept, secukinumab and adalimumab are used in psoriasis while vituximab is used for pemphigus.

Finasteride

Finasteride is the only oral drug currently approved for the treatment of androgenetic alopecia. It acts by inhibition of 5 reductase which converts testosterone to its active form viz. dihydrotestosterone (DHT) in the hair follicle. This prevents the miniaturising effects of testosterone on the hair follicle allowing them to grow as intermediate or terminal follicles. Recommended dose is 1 mg/day. Side effects are uncommon and include elevated transaminases and reversible loss of libido and rarely erectile dysfunction. It is contraindicated in pregnancy for fear of feminising a male foetus.

They act on tumor necrosis factor-α (TNFα) which is one of the important mediators of inflammation in psoriasis. Because they target the efferent arm of immunity, they compromise body's ability to fight infections like tuberculosis.

Chapter 28

Systemic Therapies in Dermatology

MCQs

1. **All of the following are β-lactamase resistant penicillins *except*:**
   a. Cloxacillin
   b. Methicillin
   c. Nafcillin
   d. Amoxycillin

2. **Drug of choice for MRSA is:**
   a. Linezolid
   b. Cephalexin
   c. Gentamycin
   d. Cotrimoxazole

3. **The important adverse effect(s) of penicillin is/are:**
   a. Nausea, vomiting
   b. Headache
   c. Type 1 hypersensitivity
   d. Vertigo

4. **Red coloured urine is a side effect of:**
   a. Ampicillin
   b. Linezolid
   c. Methicillin
   d. Rifampicin

5. **Which of the following is a bactericidal?**
   a. Erythromycin
   b. Doxycycline
   c. Clofazimine
   d. Ofloxacin

6. **Which of the following groups of antibacterials is safe for penicillin allergic patients?**
   a. Fluoroquinolones
   b. Azithromycin
   c. Macrolides
   d. Cephalosporins

7. **The drug interactions due to effects on cytochrome P450 are least with:**
   a. Erythromycin
   b. Azithromycin
   c. Clarithromycin
   d. Rifampicin

8. **Which of the following is contraindicated in pregnancy?**
   a. Erythromycin
   b. Ampicillin
   c. Amoxycillin plus clavulanic acid
   d. Clindamycin

9. **Drug of choice for syphilis in penicillin allergic patient is:**
   a. Doxycycline
   b. Ciprofloxacin
   c. Erythromycin
   d. Cephalosporin

10. **All are indications of tetracycline treatment *except*:**
    a. Syphilis
    b. Rosacea
    c. Bullous pemphigoid
    d. Pemphigus vulgaris

11. **Pseudotumour cerebri is caused by:**
    a. Tetracyclines
    b. Fluoroquinolones
    c. Penicillins
    d. Macrolides

12. **True about rifampicin is:**
    a. It is a potent hepatic enzyme inducer
    b. It inhibits formation of cell wall
    c. It has no drug interaction
    d. It is a potent hepatic enzyme inhibitor

13. **Rifampicin is:**
    a. Nephrotoxic
    b. Hepatotoxic
    c. Ototoxic
    d. Oculotoxic

14. **Dose of rifampicin in cutaneous tuberculosis is:**
    a. 5 mg/kg/day
    b. 10 mg/kg/day
    c. 15 mg/kg/day
    d. 20 mg/kg/day

15. **Most common side effect of oral metronidazole is:**
    a. Metallic taste
    b. Fixed drug eruption
    c. Maculopapular drug rash
    d. All of the above

16. **Mechanism of action of Ivermectin in scabies is as a:**
    a. Spasmodic agent
    b. Neuroparalytic agent
    c. Cytotoxic agent
    d. All of the above

17. **Which of the following is not an azole?**
    a. Terbinafine
    b. Itraconazole
    c. Fluconazole
    d. Ketoconazole

18. **The antidepressant used for its antipruritic effect is:**
    a. Fluoxetine
    b. Doxepin
    c. Sertraline
    d. Fluoxamine

ANSWERS

1-d,	2-a,	3-c,	4-d,	5-d,	6-c,	7-b,	8-c,	9-a,	10-d,
11-a,	12-a,	13-b,	14-b,	15-a,	16-b,	17-a,	18-b		

Procedures in Dermatology

In this era of cosmetic dermatology, an increasing number of therapeutic interventions are being practised for treatment of cosmetically important skin ailments or 'blemishes'. Moreover, some of the procedures 'enhance' the appearance of normal skin rather than aiming to treat any disease or remove any marks. In fact, there is burgeoning demand for such procedures from patients who are ready to spend a fortune to 'improve' their looks.

These interventions include electrotherapy, cryotherapy, chemical peels, lasers, dermabrasion and microdermabrasion. Besides these procedures, several dermatosurgical techniques (or minor operative procedures) are now being routinely performed by dermatologists for improvement in acne scars and for treatment of vitiligo. Of late, there is an increasing trend for injecting the skin with fillers (chemicals that physically add fullness to the skin) and botulinum toxin (which temporarily paralyses muscles of facial expression to make dynamic wrinkles disappear), so as to make the face look younger.

CHEMICAL PEELS

Chemical peeling entails application of alpha or beta hydroxy acids on to the skin in order to induce controlled exfoliation. The acids cause damage to the superficial layers of the epidermis and sometimes even the papillary dermis (deep peels) with subsequent rejuvenation within a few days. The final result is partial or complete removal of superficial epidermal lesions (e.g. solar lentigo) and reduction of wrinkles as well as improved texture of skin.

Types of Chemical Peels

1. Superficial

These exfoliate part or whole of epidermis, i.e. maximum up to dermoepidermal junction. Choice and strength of peeling agents and duration of contact determine the actual depth reached by any peeling procedure. Glycolic acid is an alpha hydroxy acid that is commonly used for superficial peels in pigmentation disorders while salicyclic acid is a beta hydroxy acid that is commonly used for treatment of microcomedones and pigmentation in acne.

2. Medium depth

These peels reach up to the papillary dermis and are helpful for treatment of pigmentation disorders and superficial scars. Trichloroacetic acid in a concentration of 30–70% is used to treat superficial scars and pigmented lesions. However, when used for pigmentation disorders, paradoxical hyperpigmentation may be seen with trichloroacetic acid especially if strict sunlight avoidance can't be practised.

3. Deep peels

These peels are rarely used nowadays, as they penetrate to the upper or midreticular dermis and may cause scarring if the depth reached is more than desired. Controlling their depth requires lot of expertise and hence fear of scarring prevent their common use.

Indications for Chemical Peels

1. **Facial rejuvenation:** For wrinkles, textural alteration, 'dull' skin, dyschromia, i.e. variable pigmentation of face due to ageing or excess sunlight exposure, elastosis due to excess sunlight exposure.
2. **Dyschromias:** For melasma, post-inflammatory hyperpigmentation, periorbital pigmentation, pigmentary demarcation lines, solar lentigo, freckles and lentigines.
3. **Acne and acne scars:** Chemical peels cause exfoliation of small comedonal plus thereby helping acne. They also improve post-inflammatory hyperpigmentation following acne lesions and, to an extent, superficial acne scars.

Side-effects of Chemical Peels

Medium depth and deep peels may cause scarring, if the depth is beyond the desired limit. Superficial peels, which are used more commonly in practise, cause irritation, burning and erythema on application in a proportion of patients. Hence, immediately after application, ice-packs are used to relief of these emergent symptoms. Photosensitivity, irritant dermatitis, and pigmentation may sometimes occur in the next few days. Strict sun-protection with a high sun protection factors (SPF) sunscreen is needed following chemical peels.

Limitations of Chemical Peels

Only superficial chemical peels are safe for general use. The medium depth and deep peels can result in scarring, if inappropriately used. Besides, strict photo protection is needed with chemical peels lest pigmentation and photosensitivity may occur.

CRYOSURGERY

Cryosurgery refers to controlled freezing to cause local cellular destruction. Hence, cryotherapy is one of the ablative modes of treatment of small neoplasms and hyperplasias. Cryogens used for cryotherapy include liquid nitrogen, nitrous oxide or carbon dioxide. Liquid N_2 is an efficient cryogen, since its temperature is extremely low ($-196°C$). However, it must be used with care, otherwise burns due to accidental freezing of normal tissue or burns to the operator may result.

Cryogen may be delivered to the skin by

1. **Spray technique:** A flask with a spray release trigger on top sprays the cryogen on skin.
2. **Probe technique:** Flow through a metal probe which touches and freezes target tissue.

Indications of Cryosurgery

Benign lesions: Viral warts, molluscum contagiosum, epidermal nevi, seborrhoeic keratoses, strawberry haemangioma, keloids and lentigines.

Malignant lesions: Bowen's disease, actinic keratosis, keratoacanthoma, leucoplakia, small basal and squamous cell carcinoma.

Procedure of Cryosurgery

A cryogen when applied for sufficient time bring down the temperature of the target tissue suddenly leading to formation of ice crystals within cells leading to cell rupture and cell death. The frozen tissue is then allowed to thaw and then frozen again for maximum effect. During the procedure of cryosurgery anaesthesia may be required depending on the site being treated and sensitivity of a person. Following cryosurgery, the area becomes erythematous within a few hours and a blister forms in 24–72 hours. The blister heals with exfoliation of the roof with which the treated portion of the target tissues is shed within a week.

Complications of Cryosurgery

Immediate: Pain, oedema and blister formation are commonly seen in 24–72 hours. Sometimes, if excess depth is reached, it may lead to tissue necrosis, ulceration and scarring. Infection and haemorrhage are rare with cryotherapy.

Delayed: Depigmentation and scarring are the most undesirable of the long term side-effects of cryotherapy. It may cause hyperpigmentation or hypopigmentation, milia formation and hypertrophic scarring.

ELECTROSURGERY

Electrosurgery refers to cutting or destruction of tissue using electrical energy. Electrosurgery has been in use for a long time being a rapid, cost-effective treatment for many benign and malignant neoplasms as well as hyperplasias like viral warts. The term electro-fulguration is used when the current jump to target tissue and chars it superficially while the term electro-dessication is used when the electrode touches the target tissue and gradually desiccates and burns it to deeper levels. The regular skin cautery is a unipolar machine that delivers a high voltage current through the target tissue to achieve these aims.

Electro-coagulation refers to use of electric current to stop haemorrhage while electro-section refers to making incisions with an electrocautery machine. Both these functions required very high frequency and this is one with surgical cautery or a radiofrequency machine. A radiofrequency cautery is a type of electrosurgery machine that has very high frequency (2–4 mega hertz), which allows all the functions of a skin cautery as well as a surgical cautery and does this without causing significant collateral damage to surrounding tissue. In addition, it also allows for radiofrequency resurfacing.

Indications of Electrosurgery

Electrocautery: Benign lesions like viral warts, molluscum contagiosum, epidermal nevi, seborrhoeic keratosis, other benign keratoses and arsenical keratoses can be easily treated with the skin cautery machine.

Surgical cautery/radiofrequency: Malignant or potentially malignant lesions like Bowen's disease, actinic keratosis, keratoacanthoma, leucoplakia, small basal and squamous cell carcinoma may be treated with the radiofrequency machine. It can also be used as a tool in other surgeries for stopping haemorrhage or cutting or dissecting tissues.

Radiofrequency machine: Radio surgical resurfacing and face lift may be done with this machine as also electrolysis for hair removal.

Complications of Electrosurgery

Complications include haemorrhage, secondary bacterial infection, scarring and keloid formation.

INTENSE PULSE LIGHT

Lasers are an expensive technology for treatment of various cosmetic problems of skin. Since one laser does not suffice to treat all types of skin blemishes, it becomes even more expensive. Hence, intense pulse light (IPL) evolved as a cost effective alternative for lasers in the treatment of skin diseases. IP uses high intensity xenon arc light that resembles sunlight in its spectrum. It delivers this light at high intensity and depends on selecting the spectrum by using a filter to select the rays needed to affect a particular type of skin lesions. Since, it can deliver all frequencies, it can be used for treatment of all types of skin lesions. However, its efficacy is usually lower than that of a laser delivering that frequency.

Intense pulse light can be used for hair reduction, skin rejuvenation, as well as treatment of vascular nevi and epidermal pigmented lesions. Complications of IPL therapy include burns, erythema, symptoms of pruritus and burning, photosensitivity and hyperpigmentation.

LASERS

Laser Properties

'Laser' is an acronym derived from light amplification by stimulated emission of radiation. Lasers are monochromatic (single wavelength) sources of high intensity light which is coherent (waves are in same phase) and collimated (traveling parallel to each other).

Use of lasers in dermatology was pioneered by Anderson who proposed the principle of selective photothermolysis. Selective photothermolysis refers to the fact that each coloured target in human body is amenable to selective ablation by a specific wavelength of light depending on its light absorption properties.

Being collimated, allows laser light to be accurately focussed into small spots that can target small lesions without damaging surrounding tissue, which happens with electrosurgery or cryosurgery. Being coherent, makes laser light to target the tissue with very high energy and being monochromatic, allows laser light to target only a specific cell or pigment which has particular optical properties. Laser light is produced within a cavity that contains a lasing medium and has mirrors at both ends to increase the power of the beam. The lasing medium may be a gas (e.g. carbon dioxide), liquid (e.g. dye) or solid (e.g. neodymium: yttrium-aluminium-garnet (Nd:YAG), erbium YAG or alexandrite). Each medium produces a specific wavelength of light, which may be in the visible spectrum or infrared spectrum or rarely in the ultraviolet spectrum (excimer laser).

Laser Targets and Parameters

Some of the common laser targets (chromophores) in dermatology are melanin (for hair reduction, for epidermal and dermal melanoses and pigmented birth marks), haemoglobin (for cherry angiomas, port wine stain and telangiectasia), or water (for ablation of small benign and malignant neoplasms).

The efficacy of a laser is dependent on the amount of energy (fluence) in a specific wavelength that it is able to deliver at the desired depth where the target is located. Hence, if the target is located deep in the skin, e.g. hair follicle, longer wavelengths delivering lower energy are preferred (long pulse Nd:YAG laser for hair reduction).

Moreover, efficacy of a laser is also dependent on its ability to selectively destroy the target cells and not to harm the surrounding tissue at the same time. Laser light delivered in short pulses reduces the amount of heat produced, thereby reducing thermal injury to surrounding tissues that could result in scarring. Hence, pulse mode lasers have an advantage over continuous mode lasers. This is how Q-switched Nd:YAG 1064 laser avoids damage to melanin containing cells in the epidermis and affects only dermal melanin.

Laser efficacy is therefore dependant on how differently it affects the target and the surrounding tissues. Pulse duration of a good laser is kept at less than or equal to the thermal relaxation of time of the target tissue. Thermal relaxation time of any target tissue is defined as the time needed for it to cool down by 50% by transfer of heat to surrounding tissues. Hence, pulse duration is an important parameter that determines efficacy of a laser as it controls the differential of damage to target and surrounding tissues.

Indications of Lasers in Dermatology

- **Ultraviolet light**
  - ❏ Excimer laser for vitiligo and psoriasis.

- **Visible light**
  - ❏ Q-switched Nd:YAG 532 for epidermal pigmentation

- ❑ Alexandrite for hair reduction, pigmented and vascular lesions and photorejuvenation
- ❑ Diode laser for hair reduction

- *Infrared*
  - ❑ Q-switched Nd:YAG 1064 for tattoos and dermal pigmented lesions like nevus of Ota
  - ❑ Long pulse Nd:YAG for hair reduction
  - ❑ Erbium YAG laser for skin resurfacing, acne scars and facial rejuvenation, carbon dioxide laser for ablation of benign and malignant neoplasms, skin resurfacing and acne scars.

Side-effects of Lasers in Dermatology

Immediate complications include pain, erythema and oedema that may be followed by bruising, blistering or crusting. These complications are reduced in good lasers by using various skin cooling methods (use of ice packs, cooling air jets or cooling laser tips) that prevent heating and damage to the epidermis and the surrounding tissues. A long term pigmentary changes may follow damage to the epidermis and this may occur over several weeks. Scarring due to extensive damage is rare but may be seen with ablative lasers like carbon dioxide laser.

DERMATOSURGERY

Several minor operations are done by dermatologist for residual skin problems left behind after medical therapy. Principally, they include surgery for residual patches of vitiligo and acne scars. Less commonly performed procedures include surgical biopsies and excisions of small lesions and to a limited extent, dermabrasion and hair transplantation.

ACNE SURGERY

Scars over face, following acne or other dermatoses, affect social interaction and self belief. They require more attention than scars over other sites. According to the type, size and number of scars, choice of method for surgery differs. Microdermabrasion brings improvement in skin pigmentation and texture while superficial scars and pigmentation improve with superficial chemical peels. Deep post-acne scars may be treated with dermabrasion or resurfacing with laser or cryotherapy. Isolated deep scars can be improved with subcision, punch microsurgery or fillers.

Hypertrophic or Keloidal scars can be treated with intralesional steroids, cryotherpay and compressive dressings.

DERMABRASION

Dermabrasion refers to controlled surgical abrasion of the skin reaching up to the level of the papillary dermis. Result is improvement in skin texture and clearing of epidermal pigmentation and superficial scars reaching up to papillary dermis. Primarily, dermabrasion is used for medium depth and deep acne scars especially when they are many in number and are spread out all over the face. Localised area of scarring may be treated with spot dermabrasion. However, it may be also used for superficial epidermal skin lesions like freckles, lentigines, melasma, seborrhoeic keratoses, and actinic keratoses. Some of the papillary derma lesions like syringoma, epiderma nevi or lichen amyloidosus need to be dermabraded carefully as risk of scarring due to deeper dermabrasion is higher. Some of the deeper papulonodular lesions like trichoepithelioma or adenoma sebaceum have been treated with dermabrasion with variable results. The procedure may be done under local or general anaesthesia. Contraindications include active acne lesions, bleeding disorders, keloids at other sites, past history of herpes labialis. Following full face dermabrasion, a patient needs to remain indoors at least for a week. Strict photoprotection is needed for at least 1 month. Immediate complications include bleeding, erythema, oedema, bacterial infection and precipitation of severe attack of herpes labialis. Late complications include photosensitivity, pigmentation, scarring and rarely hypertrophic or keloidal scarring.

VITILIGO SURGERY

Vitiligo is an acquired autoimmune disease resulting patchy depigmentation due to melanocyte loss. Patients with circumscribed stable vitiligo are usually good candidates for vitiligo surgery. Patients with larger area of involvement or unstable disease need to be treated medically before they become stable and are left with residual small patches. Various surgical approaches to the treatment of vitiligo include:

1. **Therapeutic tattooing:** Introduction of various types of pigments into the lesions for permanent camouflage, e.g. tattooing. However, this frequently leaves the patient dissatisfied because of poor colour match, irregular pigmentation and loss of pigment with time.

2. **Excision:** Small depigmented patches may be simply excised with primary closure.

3. **Skin grafting:** Taking skin from a normally pigmented area and grafting it onto depigmented patches give lasting results in stable vitiligo due to the principle of donor dominance. One may simply use Thiersch grafts, ultra-thin grafts, or the more easy to perform, punch grafts. Please refer to the section on vitiligo for more details.

4. Traumatising the depigmented patch with dermabrasion itself leads to stimulation of pigmentation from hair follicles and the margins in a fair proportion of patients. Similar function may be served by laser resurfacing or chemical peels.

5. **Melanocyte transfer:** In suction blister grafting, the blister roof carrying melanocytes is transplanted onto the dermabraded depigmented skin. While the graft falls off, melanocytes from it survive, repopulate and repigment the vitiliginous skin. In melanocyte culture grafting, patient's melanocytes from normal skin are separated cultured and then applied onto dermabraded depigmented skin. This procedure requires good laboratory back-up but gives good results.

SKIN AUGMENTATION (FILLERS)

Augmentation of facial skin is usually done for cosmetic purposes, but may be occasionally done for facial reconstruction following injury or surgery. Injectable materials used for such skin augmentation are called as fillers. An ideal filler should not evoke allergic or foreign body reactions and should have long lasting or preferably permanent action.

Fillers are used to improve or obliterate frown lines (glabellar lines), crow's feet (periorbital lines), deep smile lines (nasolabial furrows), smile lines (nasolabial lines), cheek depressions, thin lips (with lip augmentation), smokers' lines (perioral lines), marionette lines (oral commissures), worry lines (forehead lines), witch's chin (with chin augmentation), acne-scars and facial scars.

Fillers that have evolved gradually over the years include silicone, bovine collagen, hyaluronic acid, fibre and polyacrylamide. Autologous fat is used for treatment of lipoatrophy, which may follow panniculitis or may be metabolic. The rate of complications varies with each material and the expertise of the injector. Complications include allergic reactions, infections and overcorrection or undercorrection.

BOTULINUM TOXIN

Botulinum toxin is a wonder drug, which can combat some cutaneous signs of aging. Some of the facial wrinkles are caused due to overuse of some of the muscles of facial expression. Botulinum causes paralysis of the injected muscle by preventing the release of acetylcholine from motor nerve terminals leading to withering of muscle fibres. The muscle strengthens again as the nerves regenerate. Botulinum toxin also reduces sweating by blocking the sympathetic nerve fibres that control sweat glands.

Indications for botulinum toxin include wrinkles and frown lines as well as hyperhidrosis of palms, soles and axillae. The effect of botulinum toxin starts wearing off within a few weeks, but re-treatment is not usually needed for 3–6 months or even longer. However, it can be repeated as required. Contraindications are pregnancy, lactation and patients with degenerative or auto-immune diseases of skeletal muscle.

Complications of botulinum injection are local pain, oedema, or ecchymoses at the injection in eyelid muscles, undercorrection or overcorrection leading to excessive flattening of face or asymmetric results.

SKIN BIOPSY

Skin biopsy is the most commonly used and reliable diagnostic procedure in dermatology. There are many methods of doing a skin biopsy viz. punch biopsy, shave biopsy, surgical excisional biopsy and surgical incisional biopsy. A punch biopsy adequately samples the whole of the skin needed for diagnosis of inflammatory skin diseases. Hence, punch biopsy is the commonest method of doing a skin biopsy in India. It involves using a cylindrical sharp instrument called the skin biopsy punch. Punches are available in various sizes, the most commonly used being 3 mm, 4 mm and 5 mm.

Indications of Skin Biopsy

Punch biopsy is indicated for establishing diagnosis of an inflammatory or neoplastic lesions. Skin infections like leprosy, tuberculosis, leishmaniasis, mycetoma or other deep fungal infections or sometimes even warts need to be confirmed by a biopsy. Common examples of inflammatory diseases that need confirmation by biopsy include lichen planus, psoriasis, eczemas, vesicobullous disorders like pemphigus or pemphigoid or collagen vascular diseases like lupus erythematosus or scleroderma. Neoplasms like basal cell carcinoma, squamous cell carcinoma and melanoma must be confirmed by biopsy before further surgery. Skin biopsy is contraindicated in the presence of infection or bleeding disorder.

Procedure of Skin Biopsy

A biopsy should be ordinarily taken from a fully evolved, non-excoriated lesion away from joints and bony prominences. After local anaesthesia, the skin around the lesion to be biopsied is stretched with the thumb and forefinger perpendicular to relaxed skin tension lines. The punch is then driven into the skin vertically up to the subcutaneous fat. On removal of the punch, the central cylinder of tissue pops out above the surface of the rest of the skin. This cylinder of tissue is then gently lifted, snipped at the base and deposited into a prelabelled formation container. The biopsy wound heals in 5–7 days and leaves behind an oval scar smaller than the size of the punch used. If a suture is taken the scar will be even smaller. Complications are uncommon but include bleeding, infection and scarring.

MCQs

1. **The following are side-effects of cryotherapy except:**
   a. Hypopigmentation
   b. Scarring
   c. Milia
   d. Neoplasia

2. **The most common post-treatment side-effect of cryotherapy is:**
   a. Pigmentary changes
   b. Milia
   c. Scarring
   d. Infection

3. **Cryotherapy works on the principles of:**
   a. Ablation by freezing
   b. Release of reactive oxygen species
   c. Exfoliation of the skin
   d. Metaphase arrest

4. **The agents used in chemical peels are:**
   a. Acids
   b. Bases
   c. Salts
   d. Ketones

5. **For actinic keratosis which peels should be used?**
   a. Superficial
   b. Medium
   c. Deep
   d. Any of these

6. **Superficial peels penetrate up to the:**
   a. Epidermis/Dermoepidermal junction
   b. Mid-papillary dermis
   c. Upper reticular dermis
   d. Deep reticular dermis

7. **Deep peels penetrate up to the:**
   a. Papillary dermis
   b. Upper reticular dermis
   c. Mid-reticular dermis
   d. Deep reticular dermis

8. **Alpha hydroxy acids exert their epidermal effect on:**
   a. Stratum corneum and granulosum junction
   b. Granular layer and spinous layer
   c. Mid-spinous layer
   d. Dermoepidermal junction

9. **Select the true statement:**
   a. The use of alpha hydroxy acid has been shown to reverse the signs of photoaging
   b. Photosensitivity is not a contraindication for peels
   c. Sunscreens should be avoided before and after the procedure
   d. Persistent erythema after peels is a good sign

10. **Which of the following is not an indication for superficial peels?**
    a. Melasma
    b. Ephelides
    c. Post-inflammatory hyperpigmentation
    d. Actinic keratosis

11. **Is this true that 'multiple superficial peels will produce the same result as one deeper chemical peel'?**
    a. True
    b. False
    c. Depends on the chemical used
    d. Depends on the time of contact

12. **Complications of intense pulse light therapy include:**
    a. Burns
    b. Erythema
    c. Photosensitivity
    d. All of these

13. **Full form of LASER is:**
    a. Light amplification by sustained emission of radiation
    b. Light assimilation by sustained emission of radiation
    c. Light amplification by stimulated emission of radiation
    d. Light amplification by sustained eruption of rays

14. **Excimer laser produces light in the:**
    a. Microwave
    b. Visible light
    c. Ultraviolet
    d. Infrared

15. **The lasing medium is usually:**
    a. Gas
    b. Liquid
    c. Solid
    d. All of these

16. **Melanin is a chromophore for:**
    a. Acne
    b. Port wine stain
    c. Hair reduction
    d. Bowen's disease

17. **Surrounding tissue is protected because of which property of lasers?**
    a. Fluence
    b. Short wavelength
    c. Long wavelength
    d. Pulse mode

18. **Pulse duration should be:**
    a. More than thermal relaxation time of surrounding tissue
    b. More than thermal relaxation time of target tissue
    c. Less than or equal to thermal relaxation time of target tissue
    d. Less than or equal to thermal relaxation time of surrounding tissue

Chapter 29

Procedures in Dermatology

19. **Which of the following is not a mode of therapy in a patient with keloid?**
    a. Intralesional steroids   b. Cryotherapy
    c. Silicone dressings   d. Subscision

20. **All are indication of dermabrasion *except*:**
    a. Lichen amyloidosis   b. Freckles
    c. Nodulocystic acne   d. Epidermal nevi

21. **Which is true for the surgical methods for vitiligo?**
    a. Tattooing   b. Skin grafting
    c. Excision   d. All of these

22. **Autologous fat transplant is done for:**
    a. Anetoderma
    b. Lipoatrophy
    c. Smoker's cheeks
    d. Lip augmentation

23. **Which of the following is used as a filler?**
    a. Silicone
    b. Wax
    c. Paraffin
    d. Botulinum toxin

ANSWERS

1-d,	2-a,	3-a,	4-a,	5-b,	6-a,	7-c,	8-a,	9-a,	10-d,
11-b,	12-d,	13-c,	14-c,	15-d,	16-c,	17-d,	18-c	19-d,	20-c,
21-d,	22-b,	23-a							